D0072274

The Mammary Gland

Development, Regulation, and Function

The Mammary Gland

Development, Regulation, and Function

Edited by

Margaret C. Neville

University of Colorado School of Medicine
Denver, Colorado

and

Charles W. Daniel

University of California, Santa Cruz
Santa Cruz, California

PLENUM PRESS • NEW YORK AND LONDON

Library of Congress Cataloging in Publication Data

The Mammary gland.

Includes bibliographies and index.
1. Mammary glands. I. Neville, Margaret C., Date- . II. Daniel, Charles W. [DNLM: 1. Breast—growth & development. 2. Breast-physiology. 3. Breast Neoplasms. 4. Lactation—physiology. WP 800M265]
QP188.M3M36 1987 612′.664 87-18606
ISBN 0-306-42641-2

A Division of Plenum Publishing Corporation
233 Spring Street, New York, N.Y. 10013

Printed in the United States of America

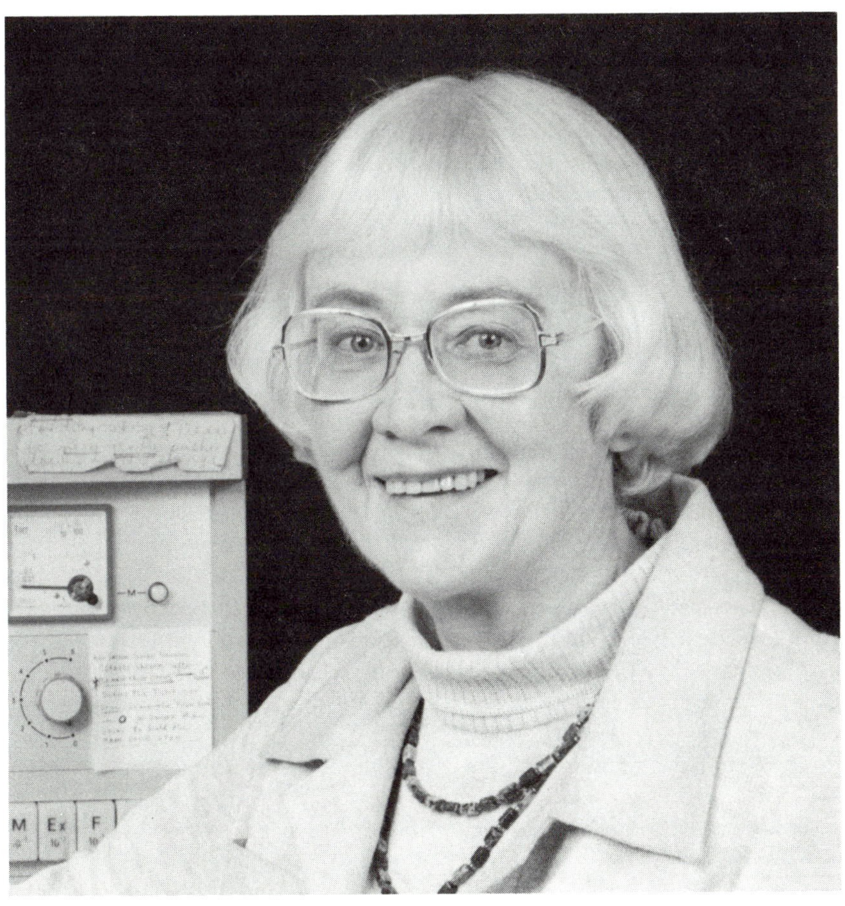

DOROTHY RIGGS PITELKA

Dorothy Riggs Pitelka was born of missionary parents in Marsovan, Turkey, but left as a small child and grew up in Colorado, where she attended the University of Colorado at Boulder, receiving a Bachelor of Arts degree, cum laude, in 1941. She entered graduate school at Berkeley the same year. In 1943 she was married to a fellow graduate student, Frank Pitelka, and in 1948 she received a doctoral degree in protozoology. During her graduate school and postdoctoral years she gave birth to three children. After a short postdoctoral stint in France in 1957–1958, Dr. Pitelka returned to the Department of Zoology, where she remained until her retirement in 1985, moving from Associate Research Zoologist to Adjunct Professor of Zoology in 1971. Although she never received a tenure-track appointment, the list of her accomplishments includes not only a superb record of research in both protozoology and mammary gland biology, but also a distinguished teaching history. She served as mentor to a long succession of graduate students and postdoctoral fellows. She was president of the Society of Protozoologists in 1967–1968, chaired the Gordon Research Conference on Mammary Gland Biology in 1977, and in 1981 served as chairman of the program committee for the Annual Meeting of the Tissue Culture Association. During the course of a distinguished career she published over 100 papers on such diverse topics as the fine structure of the buccal apparatus in paramecium (1963), the appearance of viruslike particles in mouse mammary gland (1964), cell contacts in the mammary gland (1975 and after), cell–cell and cell–stroma interactions in metastases (1983), and interactions between mammary epithelial cells (1985).

A colleague writes, "Pitelka's micrographs are the quality standard by which pictures produced by the current generation of mammary gland biologists are judged. Dorothy's ability to interpret ultrastructure and integrate this information with that derived from biochemical studies established her as a leading authority. From secretory pathways to cell–cell interaction to transcellular transport to culture of epithelial cells, her research has served as the basis for much of the current work in mammary gland biology."

A former student writes, "Dorothy unselfishly shared her time, energy, and knowledge. Her patient guidance, understanding, and enthusiasm were instrumental in enabling her students to successfully take their place in the scientific community. She was truly an inspiration for her standard of excellence in scientific research."

The authors and editors of this book share these attitudes about Dorothy Pitelka as a scientist, teacher, leader, and friend. This book is dedicated to her in recognition of her outstanding contributions to all our research.

Contributors

Mina J. Bissell • Laboratory of Cell Biology, Division of Biology and Medicine, Lawrence Berkeley Laboratory, University of California, Berkeley, California 94720

Robert D. Bremel • Department of Dairy Science, College of Agricultural and Life Sciences, University of Wisconsin, Madison, Wisconsin 53706

Robert Callahan • Laboratory of Tumor Immunology and Biology, National Cancer Institute, National Institutes of Health, Bethesda, Maryland 20892

Charles W. Daniel • Department of Biology, Thimann Laboratories, University of California, Santa Cruz, California 95064

Thomas C. Dembinski • Department of Physiology, Faculty of Medicine, University of Manitoba, Winnipeg, Manitoba R3E OW3, Canada

Anne Faulkner • Hannah Research Institute, Ayr KA6 5HL, Scotland

H. Glenn Hall • Laboratory of Cell Biology, Division of Biology and Medicine, Lawrence Berkeley Laboratory, University of California, Berkeley, California 94720

D. Grahame Hardie • M.R.C. Protein Phosphorylation Group, Department of Biochemistry, University of Dundee, Dundee DD1 4HN, Scotland

Sandra Z. Haslam • Department of Anatomy, Michigan State University, East Lansing, Michigan 48824

Jean-Pierre Kraehenbuhl • Swiss Institute for Experimental Cancer Research, Lausanne University, Lausanne, Switzerland

E. Birgitte Lane • Imperial Cancer Research Fund, Lincoln's Inn Fields, London WC2A 3PX, United Kingdom

Robert F. Loizzi • Research Resources Center and the Department of Physiology and Biophysics, University of Illinois at Chicago, Chicago, Illinois 60680

I. H. Mather • Department of Animal Sciences, University of Maryland, College Park, Maryland 20742

Michael R. Munday • Department of Pharmaceutical Chemistry, The School of Pharmacy, University of London, London WC1N 1AS, United Kingdom.

Malcolm Peaker • Hannah Research Institute, Ayr KA6 5HL, Scotland

Jeffrey M. Rosen • Department of Cell Biology, Baylor College of Medicine, Houston, Texas 77030

Irma H. Russo • Department of Pathology, Michigan Cancer Foundation, Detroit, Michigan 48201

Jose Russo • Department of Pathology, Michigan Cancer Foundation, Detroit, Michigan 48201

Teruyo Sakakura • Laboratory of Cell Biology, RIKEN, Tsukuba Life Science Center, The Institute of Physical and Chemical Research, Yatabe, Tsukuba, Ibaraki 305, Japan

Linda A. Schuler • Department of Comparative Biosciences, School of Veterinary Medicine, University of Wisconsin, Madison, Wisconsin 53706

Robert P. C. Shiu • Department of Physiology, Faculty of Medicine, University of Manitoba, Winnipeg, Manitoba R3E OW3, Canada

Gary B. Silberstein • Department of Biology, Thimann Laboratories, University of California, Santa Cruz, California 95064

Roberto Solari • Department of Immunobiology, Glaxo Group Research Limited, Greenford, Middlesex UB6 OHE, United Kingdom

Joyce Taylor-Papadimitriou • Imperial Cancer Research Fund, Lincoln's Inn Fields, London WC2A 3PX, United Kingdom

Frank Talamantes • Department of Biology, Thimann Laboratories, University of California, Santa Cruz, California 95064

Gudmundur Thordarson • Department of Biology, Thimann Laboratories, University of California, Santa Cruz, California 95064

Barbara Kay Vonderhaar • Laboratory of Tumor Immunology and Biology, National Cancer Institute, National Institutes of Health, Bethesda, Maryland 20892

Preface

Scientific interest in milk and the organ that produces this complex fluid goes back at least 400 years. An early and widely held theory suggested that milk originated in the uterus. Thus, Leonardo da Vinci* clearly depicted a system of ducts connecting the uterus and mammary glands in a graphic drawing of the human reproductive organs. This idea was finally dispelled in the 19th century, partly as a result of the detailed anatomical descriptions of the breasts and their blood supply by the English surgeon Sir Astley Cooper.† However, no sooner had the gross anatomical relation of the mammary gland been settled than application of the light microscope to sections of the lactating mammary gland produced a new set of misconceptions about the cellular mechanisms of milk secretion: The unique mechanism by which milk fat is secreted suggested to the early histologists that milk actually consisted of the tips of the mammary cells, which broke off into the lumen of the gland.

This misconception was dispelled and a firm basis was established for the understanding of milk secretion with the use of the electron microscope and the elucidation of the detailed biochemical pathways of milk secretion in the 1960s and 1970s. This work has provided the basis for a new generation of studies of mammary gland development and cell biology and regulation of mammary growth and function as described in this volume. With the exception of the dairy scientists who demonstrated sustained interest in mammary function throughout the first half of this century, most workers have used the mammary gland from time to time to ask questions related to fundamental problems in biology rather than viewing it as an organ with a basic set of properties and functions of its

*C.D. O'Malley and J.B.d.C.M. Saunders, *Leonardo da Vinci on the Human Body,* Henry Schuman, New York, 1952, p. 461.

†Astley Cooper, *The Anatomy and Diseases of the Breast,* Lea and Blanchard, Philadelphia, 1845.

own. While this has led to a certain fragmentation of our knowledge of mammary function, it has also produced major advances in the field. Thus, developmental biologists have found the developing gland of great interest because much of mammary development takes place in the adult, where the organ can often be studied more easily than in the fetus. Molecular biologists have found the lactating mammary gland to be a rich source of messenger RNA for the major class of milk proteins, the caseins, providing a foundation for more recent studies, using recombinant DNA technologies, of the molecular biology of milk secretion. Much of the recent work on mammary gland biology has been carried out by cancer biologists, partly because of the prevalence of human breast cancer, but also because certain strains of mice carry a virus (MMTV) passed through the milk that causes hormonally induced mammary malignancies. This virus is beginning to prove a powerful tool for eludication of the regulation of normal mammary cell proliferation. Finally, the regulation of mammary gland development and milk secretion requires both the correct hormonal milieu and an appropriate extracellular matrix, making this organ an excellent experimental object for studies of the molecular basis of hormone action and cell–matrix interactions. The purpose of this volume is to report advances in these areas of mammary gland biology in a series of authoritative and comprehensive review chapters by leaders in the field.

Although not a few volumes on lactation as well as breast cancer have appeared in recent years, this is the first attempt to bring the current work on the developmental, cellular, and molecular biology of the mammary gland together in one volume. The length of the volume reflects the number of topics that are currently moving forward at a rapid rate and also suggests that this volume is overdue.

This book was conceived by the Committee on Mammary Gland Biology and Lactation, which also served as an editorial board. This committee, currently chaired by Stephanie Atkinson, McMaster University, has as its goal the promotion of excellence in research and communication among scientists in the field of mammary gland biology and lactation. Other committee members, all of whom played salutary roles in the editing of this volume, include Mina J. Bissell, Lawrence Berkeley Laboratory; Robert Collier, Monsanto Corporation; William B. Heird, Columbia University; Margaret C. Neville, University of Colorado; Floyd Schanbacher, Ohio Agricultural Research and Development Center; Robert P.C. Shiu, University of Manitoba; and Barbara Kay Vonderhaar, National Cancer Institute. We thank Dorothy Scally for her unstinting secretarial service and George Tarver for his elegant rendering of many of the drawings in diverse chapters. Finally, we thank all the authors, who met deadlines amazingly well, graciously accepted the criticisms and comments of the editorial board, and provided intellectually satisfying fare for the editors and readers of this volume.

Margaret C. Neville
Charles W. Daniel

Denver and Santa Cruz

Contents

I. Developmental Biology of the Mammary Gland

1. Postnatal Development of the Rodent Mammary Gland

Charles W. Daniel and Gary B. Silberstein

2. Mammary Embryogenesis

Teruyo Sakakura

I

Developmental Biology of the Mammary Gland

1

Postnatal Development of the Rodent Mammary Gland

Charles W. Daniel and Gary B. Silberstein

1. Introduction

The mammary cycle of lobuloalveolar differentiation, lactation, and involution has been a subject of fascination to generations of biologists. Historically, much of the published mammary research has been focused on questions surrounding secretory activity, with particular emphasis on hormonal regulation during pregnancy and lactation. Another area of research interest, with perhaps an equally imposing literature, has been the problem of mammary cancer.

The mammary gland is also a fruitful subject for the developmental biologist. In the fetus, the primordial gland provides a useful model for investigations of epithelial–mesenchymal interactions and their modification by hormones (reviewed in Chapter 2 of this volume). Unlike most organs, which have completed morphogenesis by the time of birth and whose subsequent development is mainly enlargement or replication of preexisting structures, the mammary gland undergoes most of its morphogenesis in the subadult and adult animal. At these stages, unlike the fetus, it is accessible to direct in vivo study and analysis.

To the developmental biologist, this period of mammary ductal growth and branching morphogenesis provides a striking example of the orchestration of systemic and local regulatory processes. While mammary growth clearly depends on circulating hormones for stimulation

---

Charles W. Daniel and Gary B. Silberstein • Department of Biology, Thimann Laboratories, University of California, Santa Cruz, California 95064.

and for synchronization with reproductive events, it is generally accepted that other levels of control and regulation must be involved. These include interactions between epithelium and stroma, possibly involving tissue-specific growth (or inhibitory) factors, and certainly including regulatory interactions with components of the extracellular matrix.

From birth through reproductive maturity, the mammary gland develops to fill the constantly expanding mammary fat pad with a ductal network of characteristic pattern. Although this phase of development is covered in a number of useful reviews (Nandi, 1958, 1959; Munford, 1964; Topper and Freeman, 1980; Tucker, 1981; Knight and Peaker, 1982), the brief treatment given to the period of branching morphogenesis in the juvenile indicates that, historically, interest in mammary gland biology has been centered on fetal development, lobuloalveolar differentiation, or milk production during lactation. In recent years, however, there has been a surge of interest in mammary ductal morphogenesis as indicated by publications and by prominence in society meetings. This appears due to awareness of certain experimentally useful characteristics of the gland at this stage of development:

1. The mammary gland is accessible. It is one of the few organs that develops late in life, permitting developmental studies to be carried out in subadult animals and avoiding many of the notorious technical difficulties of working with fetal materials.
2. The juvenile mammary gland provides a model for developmental studies of duct formation, regulation of pattern formation, and cell lineage studies. For endocrinologists, it provides an interesting site of interaction between systemic hormones and tissue-level regulation.
3. Epithelium–stroma interactions may be studied in a unique system in which large quantities of epithelium-free stromal tissue are readily available in young animals. The invasion of stroma by advancing epithelial end buds provides one of the few examples of inductive tissue interactions outside the embryo.
4. Branching morphogenesis of the mammary gland is relevant to cancer biology. The growth of the end bud through adipose stroma provides a useful model for tissue invasion; while ductal elongation must be seen as rapid and aggressive even when compared with highly malignant tissues, its growth is tightly regulated by tissue-level homeostatic factors. Even more directly, in the rat the mammary end bud is the target tissue for certain carcinogens.

The present chapter considers the growth of rudimentary mammary ducts in the postnatal and subadult animal as they develop into the mammary tree upon which, during pregnancy, secretory structures may develop. We emphasize those aspects of mammary structure and function that may be found useful by researchers interested in basic questions of morphogenesis, tissue regulation, and functional differentiation.

2. Development of the Ductal Tree

2.1. The Neonate

In newborn female mice, the mammary parenchyma consists of branching cords of epithelial cells connected to the nipple by a single primary duct. The incipient mammary ducts are partially canalized and display up to third- or fourth-order branching. Sekhri et al. (1967) have described ducts at this stage as consisting of two to three layers of epithelial cells at the thickest point, near the nipple, and containing numerous small lumina that gradually fuse to form fully canalized mammary ducts. The ductal ends terminate in small end buds containing numerous mitotic figures.

During the first 3 weeks of life, the mammary ducts elongate and ramify slowly in females, displaying isometric growth that keeps pace with but does not exceed that of the animal (reviewed by Knight and Peaker, 1982). With elimination of maternal hormones, the terminal end buds present at birth become reduced in size or disappear, accounting for the sluggish growth rate. Growth occurring during this period appears to be ovary dependent and is abolished in response to castration, even though sexual maturation in the mouse and rat is not reached until week 4–6 of age (Rugh, 1968).

It is interesting to note that the rudimentary ductules at term are fully committed to differentiate into mammary tissue. When cultured with appropriate hormones, neonatal mouse mammary cells display functional differentiation by the formation of casein. Using even younger tissue, Ceriani (1970) demonstrated casein synthesis in 16-day fetal rat mammary cells when cultured in the presence of insulin, glucocorticoid, and prolactin. In some species, including human, secretion (witch's milk) is present in mammary glands of the newborn, a result of stimulation by maternal hormones.

Evidence supporting precocious functional differentiation, however, does not imply that the mammary anlagen is fully determined to undergo mammary specific morphogenesis. It has been known for a number of years that fetal mammary tissue responds to heterotypic salivary mesenchyme in vitro by the formation of a salivary-like pattern of branching, with adenomere formation sometimes observed (Kratochwil,

1969). Sakakura et al. (1976) placed similar heterotypic tissue recombinants in the kidney capsule of recipient mice and confirmed the ability of salivary mesenchyme to specify the growth pattern of fetal mammary epithelium. In lactating hosts, however, the salivary-like mammary epithelium developed lactose synthetase and produced milk-like secretion products. It thus appears that the secretory function of mammary epithelium is determined by the time of birth, indeed well before, but the epithelial tissue remains pleuropotent with respect to mesenchyme-directed morphogenesis. This conclusion might be taken to support the concept of a mammary stem cell lineage, here represented by a mesenchyme-responsive subpopulation of epithelial cells. Evidence for a stem cell compartment in mammary tissue will be reviewed later.

Differentiation of the mammary stroma around the time of birth is a striking feature of the mouse mammary gland. In the fetus, a condensed mesenchymal mass has been identified (Sakakura et al., 1982) which differentiates late in gestation. By term, a white adipose tissue, the mammary fat pad, is developed (Sekhri et al., 1967). As will be discussed, this white fat represents the obligatory substrate for subsequent mammary morphogenesis, interacting with the epithelium to specify developmental pattern; the boundaries of this fat pad will later demarcate the ultimate limits of glandular enlargement.

2.2. The Juvenile: End Buds and Ducts

Beginning at about 3–4 weeks of age in the mouse and slightly later in the rat, end buds reappear at the ductal tips and growth increases both in rate and degree of branching (Nandi, 1959). Growth becomes increasingly allometric, with the area occupied by mammary gland in the rat increasing 1.13 and 3.92 times faster than body surface area between 10 and 20 and 23 and 40 days of age, respectively (Sinha and Tucker, 1966). End bud formation and allometric growth appear before puberty (Cowie, 1949) but are nevertheless dependent on ovarian hormones since ovariectomy causes regression of end buds and cessation of growth within a few days.

The terminal end bud drives ductal morphogenesis in the gland by producing a supply of differentiated ductal and myoepithelial cells for elongation of the subtending ducts. In addition to providing for linear growth, end buds are the regulatory control points that determine branching, turning, and pattern formation (Fig. 1). The behavior of end buds is influenced by (1) systemic hormones that supply stimulation for growth and (2) local, tissue-level regulatory signals that influence the direction of growth and ultimately cause end bud regression. These

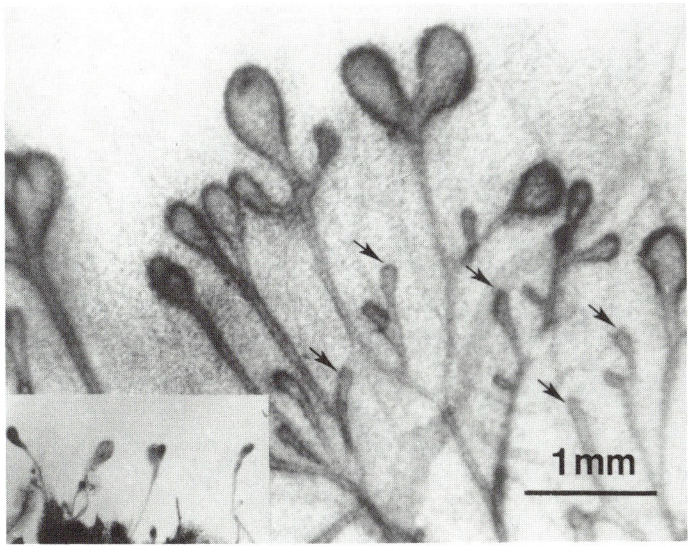

Figure 1. Expanding ductal network of 5-week-old female mouse mammary gland seen in stained whole mount. Conspicuous terminal end buds penetrate the white adipose tissue of the mammary fat pad. Branches with insufficient stroma available for elongation terminate as ductal extensions without end buds (arrows). *Insert:* Exposed end buds, freed from fat pad stroma by HCl, acetone, and collagenase treatments. From Williams and Daniel (1983).

signals cause growth to stop when the limits of the available fat pad are reached (Faulkin and DeOme, 1960). It may be noted that while much information is available on the subject of systemic hormones, nothing is known about the nature of local regulatory factors.

Although all reports of mammary development have recognized the importance of end buds as growth points, only in recent years have detailed studies of their structure and functional activities appeared (Williams and Daniel, 1983). Terminal end buds are easily visualized in situ, ranging in size from 0.1 to 0.5 mm in diameter (Fig. 2). A large end bud consists of four to six layers of cuboidal epithelium. The luminal surface is lined with cells that are continuous with, and give rise to, luminal cells in the subtending mature ducts. These are characterized by microvilli on the luminal face and junctional complexes laterally.

On the basal surface of the end bud, the outermost cell layer differs considerably from deeper regions of epithelium. These *cap cells* appear just beneath the basal lamina and are often separated from deeper cell layers by small clefts (Williams and Daniel, 1983). Cap cells are distinguished from other mammary cell types by the absence of differenti-

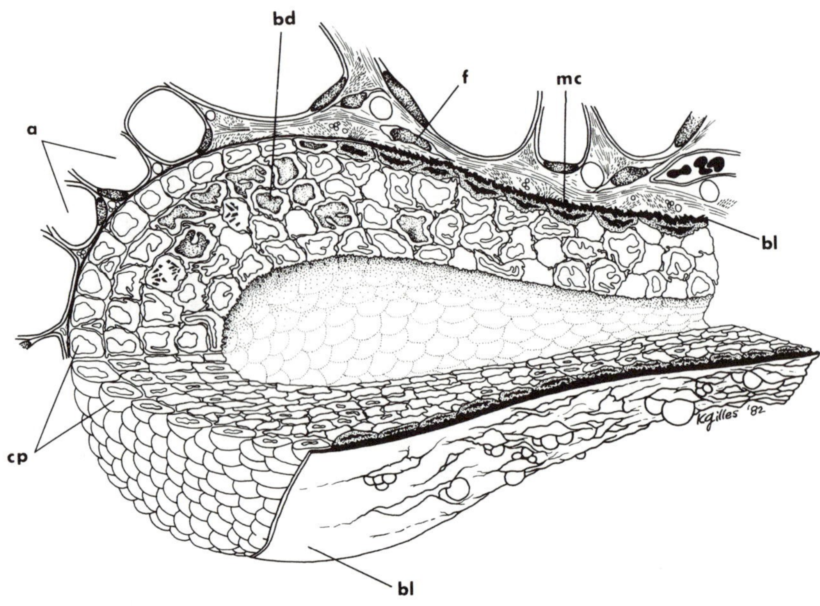

Figure 2. Composite drawing made from light and electron microscope analyses. Adipocytes (a) abut against cap cells at the tip (left). Fibrous components and fibrocytes (f) comprise the connective tissue tunic around the neck region. The basal lamina (bl) is represented as a cutaway to expose the underlying cap cells (cp). Cap cells are cuboidal but become progressively flattened toward the midregion of the end bud, then differentiate into and are continuous with myoepithelial cells (mc) in the neck region. The basal lamina overlying myoepithelial cells in the midregion is 14 times thicker than that at the tip. Mitosis is seen in the cap and body cells (bd). From Williams and Daniel (1983).

ated features. They lack cytoplasmic polarity and do not contain highly organized cytoskeletal elements. They are only loosely in contact with neighbors and no formed junctions have been seen connecting them with each other or with deeper lying cells. This lack of cell adherence can be demonstrated in vitro by dissolving the basal lamina of living end buds with hyaluronidase, after which the cap cells can be seen to dislodge and float away from the underlying, more adherent epithelium (C. W. Daniel, unpublished data).

As the basally located cap cells are followed laterally toward the neck region, they are seen to accumulate myofilaments and to develop cell processes, membrane junctions, and electron-opaque cytoplasm characteristic of myoepithelial cells. Thus, cap cells appear to represent a stem cell population for myoepithelium. Williams and Daniel (1983) also reported that although most cap cells maintained their basal location, some infiltrate the body cells of the end bud, perhaps to contribute to the population of ductal cells. This suggests that cap cells may represent a pleuropotent stem cell population, capable of differentiating into both mammary ductal and mammary myoepithelial cell types.

The structure of mammary ducts has been well described (Sekhri et al., 1967). All mammary ducts consist of two main cell types, an inner region of mammary ductal cells of varying thickness and an outer monolayer of myoepithelial cells with their closely applied basement membrane. Primary and secondary ducts may be composed of several layers of ductal epithelial cells, becoming fewer with higher orders of branching. Most terminal ducts are composed of a single layer of ductal cells. The luminal cells are fringed with short, blunt microvilli and their lateral edges display well-developed junctional complexes. Interdigitation of lateral membranes is frequently observed.

In the Sprague–Dawley virgin rat, ductal epithelial cells have been classified as light, dark, or intermediate on the basis of their cytomorphology (Russo et al., 1976a), and similar observations have been made in the mouse (J. M. Williams and C. W. Daniel, unpublished data). It is not known whether these represent stable morphotypes or if they might reflect transient changes. Cell cycle analysis in vivo (Eberhard et al., 1982) indicates differences in such parameters as transit time, labeling index, and growth fraction. In normal ducts, the dark cells predominate, but in ducts transformed following administration of carcinogens, higher proportions of intermediate cells were observed (Russo et al., 1976b), suggesting that these may represent the target cell for carcinogen action.

The outermost layer of mammary ducts consists of a monolayer of myoepithelial cells arranged with their cell processes extending laterally. Both morphological (Williams and Daniel, 1983) and immunohistochemical methods (Warburton et al., 1982) indicate that in the ducts myoepithelial cells are aligned and form a continuous sheath round the mammary ductal cells. In alveoli, the myoepithelial cells are basket-shaped and in spaces between their cell processes, mammary alveolar cells are in direct contact with the basal lamina. The functional significance of myoepithelium in secretory mammary tissue is clear, but in the virgin animal this highly organized contractile tissue has no obvious function and its significance is uncertain. It has been suggested that these ductal myoepithelial cells are capable of dedifferentiation into cap cells during the formation of lateral branches or alveoli. Williams and Daniel (1983) used scanning electron microscopy to study myoepithelium on the surface of collagenase-isolated ducts and observed that, at junctions where new lateral buds and cap cell layers were forming, individual cells displayed surface features of both myoepithelium and cap cells, suggesting transitional forms. The use of antibodies against surface antigens of specific mammary cell types could contribute to our knowledge of this important subject.

2.2.1. Basal Lamina

The basal lamina of the mammary tree is synthesized by cap cells in the end buds and by myoepithelial cells in ducts (Silberstein and Daniel, 1982a; Williams and Daniel, 1983). At the end bud tip, the lamina is about 100 nm in thickness and resembles that described by Gordon and Bernfield (1980) in mammary epithelium from midpregnant animals and in other epithelia undergoing branching morphogenesis (Cohn et al., 1977). It can be considered as an *expansion lamina,* in which its components, especially hyaluronate, are rapidly incorporated as the end bud adds new surface area to accommodate the proliferating epithelial cell mass (Silberstein and Daniel, 1982a).

It is noteworthy that in the mouse neither electron nor light microscopy has detected discontinuities in the lamina through which epithelial–stromal cell contacts might take place, and in this the end bud resembles cap-stage tooth development in mice, where inductive interactions occur across an unbroken basal lamina (Slavkin et al., 1983). In the rat, on the other hand, Dulbecco et al. (1982) have suggested that during proestrus and estrus the basal lamina becomes indistinct and there may be some intermixing of epithelial and stromal cells.

The basal lamina at the end bud tip is rich in hyaluronic acid (Silberstein and Daniel, 1982a) which may serve to reduce adhesions as the end bud invades the mammary fat pad. This suggestion is supported by the observation that the tip separates easily from surrounding stroma during microdissection, in contrast to the neck region which is bound to the stroma by extensive collagenous adhesions (Williams and Daniel, 1983). The penetration of stroma by the invading end bud represents a forceful process, demonstrated by distortion of adipocytes ahead of the advancing end buds and by indentations in the end bud basal lamina itself, resulting from the pressure of apposed adipocytes (Fig. 3). There are no reports that hydrolytic enzymes are involved in this process of tissue penetration, although the question apparently has not been investigated.

Along the end bud flanks and in the constricted neck region, the basal lamina is extraordinarily hypertrophied, becoming 13–20 times thicker than the typical 100-nm lamina found in other regions of the gland (Williams and Daniel, 1983). The excess lamina material appears

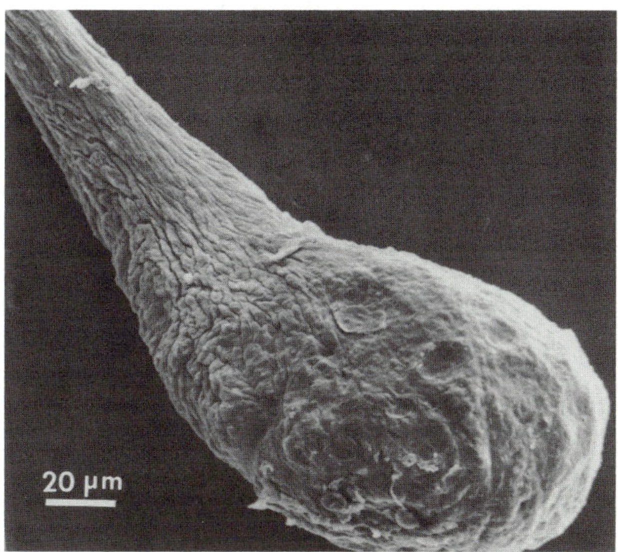

Figure 3. An end bud and part of its subtending duct isolated by HCl, acetone, and collagenase to illustrate features of differentiating myoepithelium. A smooth basal lamina covers the tip. Deep contours in the neck region are associated with extensive folding of the lamina which overlies differentiating myoepithelium. Along the duct, cell processes from myoepithelial cells become longitudinally arranged. From Williams and Daniel (1983).

to be formed from folds (Fig. 4) rather than from multilayering, which has been described in mammary tumors (Pitekla et al., 1980), in regressing mammary gland following weaning (Pitelka and Hamamoto, 1977), and in certain embryonic tissues (Meyer et al., 1981). The hypertrophied lamina in the end bud is also much thicker than that reported in other tissue. This unusual feature cannot be accounted for solely by passive folding resulting from reduction in surface area in the constricted portion of the end bud. Instead, rapid incorporation of $^{35}SO_4$ in this region demonstrates high levels of glycosaminoglycan synthesis, indicating the formation of new lamina material (Silberstein and Daniel, 1982a). The significance of this unusual specialization is unknown, but it is interesting to conjecture that the presence of this greatly thickened, anionic layer might alter the availability of ions or charged molecules, thereby influencing the activities of underlying cap cells which in this region are differentiating into myoepithelium.

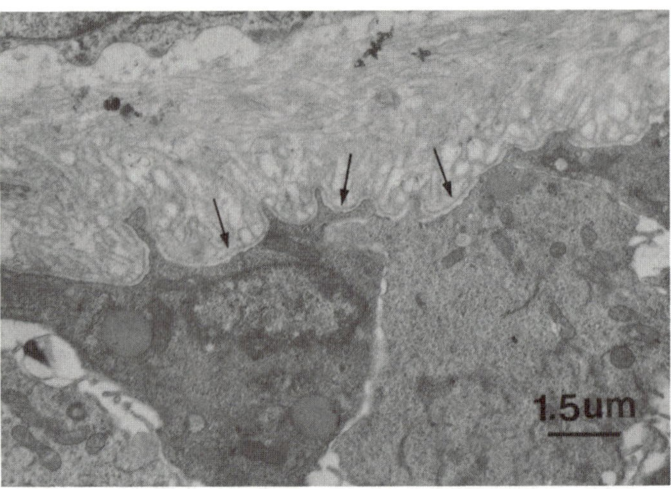

Figure 4. Basal lamina in the neck region of a large end bud is extensively folded, forming a layer more than 1 μm thick in some instances. From Williams and Daniel (1983).

2.2.2. Cell Replication

An overview of the distribution of DNA synthesis in the adolescent mammary gland can be obtained by whole-gland autoradiography of glands permitted to incorporate ^{14}C-thymidine (Fig. 5). It is apparent that most DNA synthetic activity is associated with the terminal end buds, while the subtending ducts are relatively quiescent. This pattern of peripheral growth continues in the virgin until the gland reaches its limits of travel in the mammary fat pad, when end buds regress and the ducts remain mitotically inactive until pregnancy occurs.

More detailed studies have been carried out in the rat gland. Russo and Russo (1980) infused rats for 5 days with ^{3}H-thymidine and measured the labeling index autographically, determining the growth fraction in various structures and relating them to cell cycle data obtained using the wave of labeled mitosis method (Table I). In the virgin rat gland, the terminal end buds displayed the largest growth fraction and the shortest doubling time, resulting in a calculated population doubling time of about 21 h. This very rapid doubling time, which must be regarded as somewhat uncertain because of several assumptions involved in the calculations, indicates a cellular basis for the extremely rapid growth observed in these structures.

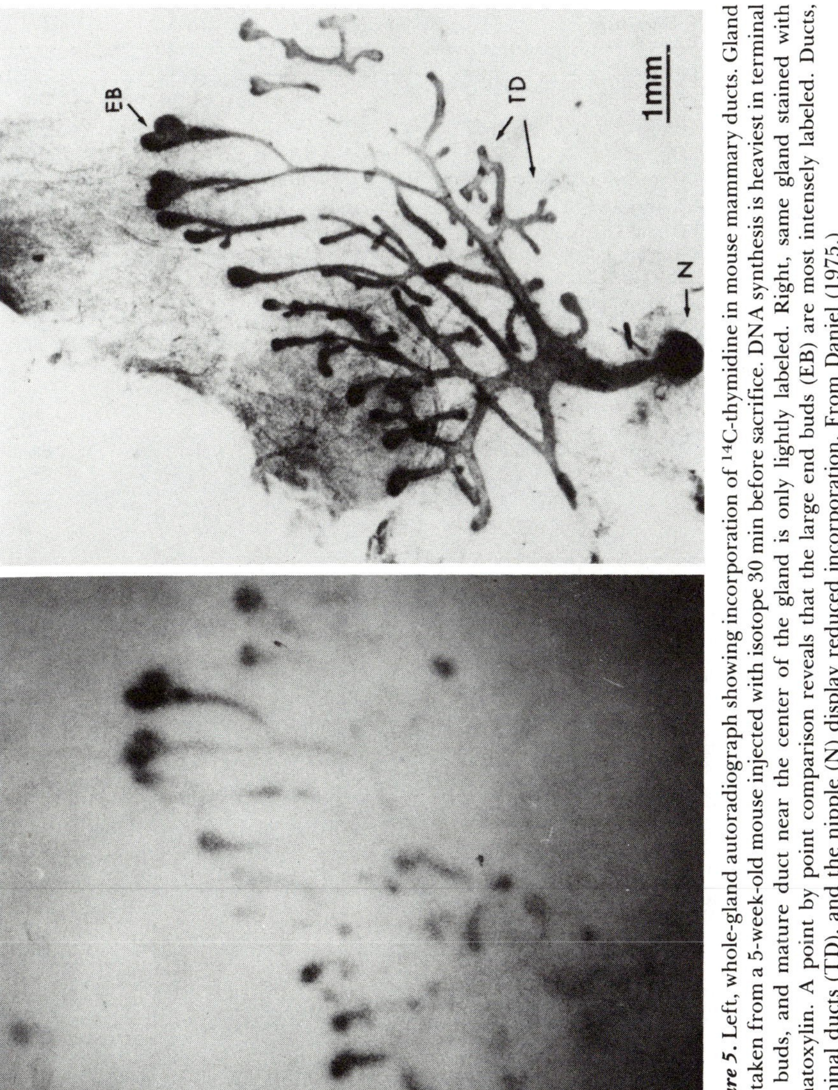

Figure 5. Left, whole-gland autoradiograph showing incorporation of ^{14}C-thymidine in mouse mammary ducts. Gland was taken from a 5-week-old mouse injected with isotope 30 min before sacrifice. DNA synthesis is heaviest in terminal end buds, and mature duct near the center of the gland is only lightly labeled. Right, same gland stained with hematoxylin. A point by point comparison reveals that the large end buds (EB) are most intensely labeled. Ducts, terminal ducts (TD), and the nipple (N) display reduced incorporation. From Daniel (1975.)

Table I. Length of T_c in the Various Structures Present in the Mammary Gland of Young Virgin, Old Virgin, and Parous Rats Corrected and Uncorrected for GF[a]

Rats	Structure	T_S[b]	GF_5[c]	T_c[d]	DNA LI[e]	T_p[f]
Young virgin	TEB[g]	7.20	0.55	11.65	0.34	21.18
	TD[h]	7.47	0.39	20.81	0.14	53.36
	AB[i]	8.67	0.13	28.18	0.04	216.75
Old virgin	TD_R	7.60	0.19	18.75	0.077	98.70
	TD and ducts	7.60	0.054	20.57	0.020	380.00
	AB and alveoli	8.20	0.030	30.75	0.008	1,025.00
Parous	TD and ducts	7.40	0.0097	23.92	0.003	2,466.66
	AB and alveoli	10.13	0.0049	49.63	0.001	10,130.00

[a] From Russo and Russo (1980).
[b] T_S, time in S phase obtained from the curve of labeled mitoses.
[c] Growth fraction: Total number of labeled cells/100 cells after 5 days of continuous infusion of [^{3}H]dThd.
[d] Cell cycle time: Calculated by counting the number of labeled cells after 1-h pulse of [^{3}H]dThd and expressed as labeled cells/100 cells.
[e] T_c Labeling Index.
[f] T_p Uncorrected T_c, or potential doubling time. See Russo and Russo (1980) for method of calculation.
[g] Terminal end buds.
[h] Terminal ducts.
[i] Alveolar buds.

Russo and Russo (1980) also studied various parts of the cell cycle and reported that the variations in cycle transit times between terminal end buds, ducts, and alveolar buds are due almost entirely to variations in G_1, with S phase requiring 7–8 h in all cases and other phases of the cell cycle showing only small variations. Bresciani (1965) also used the wave of labeled mitosis technique to measure S-phase duration in the mouse mammary gland. Although his results in the terminal end buds agree with data from the rat, with an average S-phase duration of 8.8 h, mouse ductal cells showed a longer period of DNA synthesis, averaging 12.2 h. Bresciani (1965) also reported effects of ovarian steroid hormones on the length of the S phase, indicating that in the mouse mammary gland, in contrast to most other tissues and perhaps other species, "DNA synthesis is not an unadjustable process of the proliferative cycle."

2.2.3. *Stem Cells and Other Cell Types*

Several observations suggest the presence of a subpopulation of stem cells within the mammary gland. The cycle of mammary development—pregnancy, lactation, and involution—involves massive cell replication, differentiation, and death that can be repeated many times during the life of a reproductively active female. The presence of undifferentiated cells spaced along the mammary ducts that could respond to appropriate hormonal stimulation presents an attractive model.

The presence of pleuropotent cells within the mammary ductal tree can also be inferred from transplantation experiments. A number of workers (DeOme et al., 1959; Hoshino, 1964; Daniel et al., 1968) have reported the ability of mammary transplants taken from any region of the ductal tree to regenerate normal gland following transplantation into gland-free mammary fat pads. These transplants are capable of normal growth and can differentiate into milk-producing tissue in pregnant or lactating hosts. It is important to note that regenerated glands form normal end buds with well-defined cap cell layers; it is uncertain whether these second-generation cap cells arise from dedifferentiation of myoepithelium or ductal cells, or alternatively, if they might represent a residual population of undifferentiated stem cells in the mammary ducts that are not detected by presently available techniques.

Attempts to identify mammary stem cells have been carried out both in animals and in culture. In vivo, the identification of cap cells as progenitors of ductal myoepithelium (Williams and Daniel, 1983) has been discussed earlier. In the rat, Dulbecco et al. (1982) reached similar conclusions based on studies of end buds and ducts during phases of the estrus cycle. Using thymidine autoradiography to measure DNA synthetic activity in different cell types during the phases of the estrus cycle, they suggested that cells located at the tips of the terminal end buds form the lineage of the inner ductal cells and perhaps of the myoepithelium as well. These lineages were characterized further by the use of immunological markers (Dulbecco et al., 1983). The identification of stem cells is an important matter not only because of theoretical interest, but because in rats the end buds are targets for the action of carcinogens (Russo et al., 1979), and it is likely that properties of stem cells are relevant to the behavior of mammary cancers. The conclusive identification of a stem cell subpopulation in the mammary gland awaits cloning a putative stem cell and demonstrating that its descendants are capable of regenerating a complete gland when introduced into a gland-free mammary fat pad.

Attempts to identify mammary stem cells in clonal culture have been reviewed (Rudland et al., 1980b). One of the first and most interesting cell lines, Rama 25, was derived from a DMBA-induced rat mammary tumor (Bennett et al., 1978), which has been repeatedly cloned and has given rise to a number of sublines. Rama 25, whose basic morphology is *cuboidal,* gives rise to two other cell types described as *elongate* and *droplet.* Droplet cells, which form domes in culture and synthesize small amounts of casein in response to mammogenic hormones, are identified as alveolar-like cells. Elongate cells (Rama 29) are tentatively identified as myoepithelial-like on the basis of morphology, type IV collagen production, and possible basal lamina production, although in other respects they resemble stromal-derived fibroblasts. The rate at which Rama 25 cells differentiate into droplet cells is increased by mammogenic hormones and dimethyl sulfoxide (Warburton et al., 1983).

These experiments are somewhat difficult to relate to the normal gland because the cell lines originate from tumors. Transplantation of Rama 25 cells into nude mice gives rise to tumors that may contain regions of both spindle-shaped cells and epithelial cells, again suggesting the ability of these cells to differentiate (Rudland et al., 1980a). Attempts to carry out similar experiments using normal tissue have given rise to cell lines that are morphologically similar to Rama 25 and that give rise to the two other cell types in culture (Rudland et al., 1980b). But it is not known if these cells regenerate normal gland when introduced into gland-free mammary fat pads. Indeed, the only cell line thus far able to regenerate normal gland in vivo is the COMMA-1D line (Danielson et al., 1984), which was originated from glands of midpregnant mice.

3. Growth Regulation

3.1. Systemic Growth Regulators

Our knowledge of systemic hormone effects on ductal mammogenesis comes primarily from classical endocrine ablation/replacement studies (Lyons, 1958; Lyons et al., 1958; Nandi, 1958) using the mouse and rat. A recent review of hormonal regulation of mammary development (Topper and Freeman, 1980) shows that the fundamental conclusions reached in these studies remain unchallenged. In these experiments, triply operated animals (ovariectomized, hypophysectomised, adrenalectomized), with completely regressed ductal systems, were treated for up to 30 days with steroid and peptide hormones, alone or in combination, and effects on growth were investigated.

In the mouse, Nandi reported the strongest ductal stimulation with a combination of estrogen and growth hormone, while growth hormone alone produced very mild stimulation and estrogen none at all. Deoxycorticosterone acetate (DCA), in combination with estrogen and growth hormone, stimulated very slight lobuloalveolar development. Because in intact animals the most vigorous ductal growth occurs between weeks 4 and 7 postpartum, it was unfortunate that these experiments were performed on 12-week-old animals, by which time ductal epithelia have already filled available fatty stroma. This prevents a critical evaluation of the results with respect to ductal elongation since growth is self-regulated and end buds regress on reaching the edge of the fat pad even if hormonal requirements for growth are met.

Lyons' (1958) studies were conducted on less mature glands. Systemic treatment of triply operated animals with estrogen and growth hormone stimulated vigorous end bud growth in zones where ducts faced empty stroma. An attenuated response in the duct-filled midgland appeared identical to Nandi's result in the mouse. Lyons also placed pellets containing growth hormone next to glands on one side of an estrogen-primed, triply operated animal: growth hormone strongly stimulated end bud growth while the untreated, contralateral gland was only mildly affected. In similar experiments, estrogen alone was never found to be mammogenic in the triply operated animals.

3.2. Estrogen

A direct mitogenic role for estrogen on mammary epithelium has been called into question by several in vitro studies in which estradiol added to the medium failed to stimulate proliferation of primary (Yang et al., 1980a,c; Imagawa et al., 1982) or whole-gland cultures (DuBois and Elias, 1984). In contrast, recent reports indicate that in mixed cultures of mammary epithelial and stromal cells, epithelial proliferation may be enhanced by estradiol (McGrath, 1983; Haslam and Levely, 1985; Haslam, 1986).

Plastic implants capable of delivering undenatured, bioactive molecules in situ have allowed us to investigate possible direct effects of the classical ductal mammogens (Silberstein and Daniel, 1982b). Estradiol (17-β), implanted in the glands of ovariectomized animals, stimulated local end bud proliferation (Fig. 6). Contralateral glands were unaffected and the response was specific in that 17-α estradiol was not stimulatory except at concentrations approximately 1000 × greater than that created with the 17-β isomer (C.W. Daniel, G.B. Silberstein, and P. Strickland, unpublished data).

We conclude from these experiments that estrogen may act directly as a ductal mammogen. However, because these experiments were not performed in hypophysectomized animals, it may be that some estrogen stimulated the release of pituitary factors such as growth hormone. If so, estradiol would then be acting to sensitize the gland locally and thus could still be said to have direct (nonsystemic) action on the gland. While

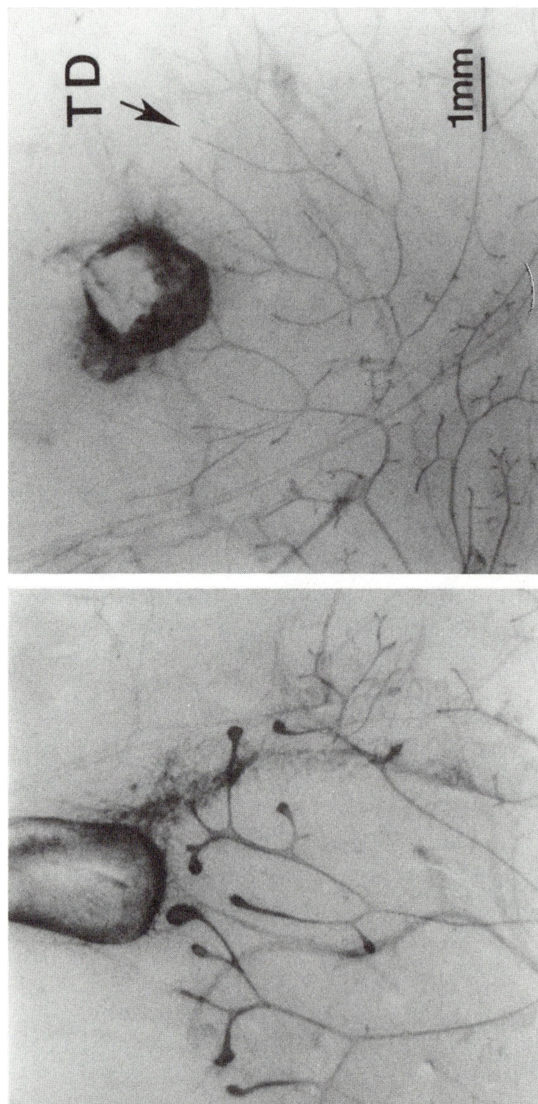

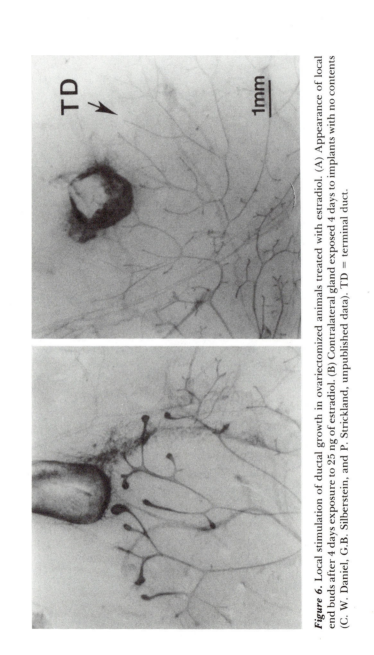

Figure 6. Local stimulation of ductal growth in ovariectomized animals treated with estradiol. (A) Appearance of local end buds after 4 days exposure to 25 ng of estradiol. (B) Contralateral gland exposed 4 days to implants with no contents (C. W. Daniel, G.B. Silberstein, and P. Strickland, unpublished data). TD = terminal duct.

still a subject for speculation, estrogen may also be acting solely as a local agent promoting local synthesis of unidentified ductal mitogens.

3.3. Growth Hormone and Prolactin

Lyons' demonstration that growth hormone implants stimulated local end bud formation was done in estrogen-primed animals; thus, stimulation could have been due to local or systemic interactions between the two hormones. Both growth hormone and prolactin can stimulate mammary epithelial proliferation in vitro (Yang et al., 1980a; Richards et al., 1983; DuBois and Elias, 1984) suggesting that these hormones could act independently of estrogen at the level of the growing gland.

Using unprimed, ovariectomized animals, we have demonstrated that bovine and mouse growth hormone placed in slow-release implants stimulated local end bud formation (G.B. Silberstein and C.W. Daniel, in preparation). Contralateral and ipsalateral glands were unaffected, indicating that growth hormone did not act systemically. Ovine prolactin and mouse prolactin were similar to growth hormone in both dose relation and the ability to stimulate local end bud growth. Insulin, important in in vitro maintenance and growth of the gland (DuBois and Elias, 1984), did not stimulate local growth (G.B. Silberstein and C.W. Daniel, unpublished data).

3.4. Epidermal Growth Factor

The inability of the classical ductal mammogens to stimulate morphogenesis or even normal levels of DNA synthesis in end buds in vitro indicates that other factors act in conjunction with the systemic hormones to achieve normal growth. Using serum supplemented medium and collagen gel cultures, Yang et al. (1980b) demonstrated that epidermal growth factor (EGF), as well as agents that raised intracellular cyclic AMP (cAMP) levels, strongly stimulated mammary epithelial proliferation. Investigating the growth of normal mouse mammary epithelium in the same culture system but with a serum-free medium, Nandi et al. (1984) reported that a combination of insulin, EGF, transferrin, bovine serum albumin, and cholera toxin stimulated cellular proliferation up to 10-fold within 10 days. Deletion experiments demonstrated that EGF and insulin were absolute requirements for growth. Later experiments (Imagawa et al., 1985) have shown that EGF at low concentrations (1 ng/ml) can synergize with prolactin and progesterone to stimulate growth.

Using slow-release implants, we have investigated the effects of implanted EGF on ductal growth in the regressed glands of ovariectomized, virgin C57/black mice. EGF stimulated local end bud growth in a dose-dependent manner (Fig. 7) with peak end bud stimulation occurring at 4 days after implantation and 3 days after the peak EGF release (not shown; S. Coleman, unpublished observations).

Autoradiographic analysis of EGF receptor activity in the hormonally intact, 5-week-old animal showed heavy concentrations of receptors in the stroma immediately adjacent to the end bud's flank, with less dense labeling in stroma surrounding the cap region. Few, if any, receptors were seen in the lumenal epithelium. Quantitative analysis of receptor levels in a mammary fibroblast cell line and the COMMA-1D mammary epithelial cell line (Danielson et al., 1984) revealed roughly 100-fold fewer receptors in the epithelial cells than in fibroblasts, supporting our observations with the intact gland. The EGF effect was specific insofar as other peptide growth promotors—insulin, platelet-derived growth factor, transforming growth factor beta, and transferrin—had no effect when implanted.

The question of which cellular compartment is sensitive to EGF—epithelium or stroma or both—requires further study. The presence of numerous stromal receptors for EGF suggests that the stroma may be the site of primary action. However, it is well established that stimulation of EGF receptors causes receptor down-regulation, so that the absence of epithelial receptors in the parenchyma may actually reflect stimulation by EGF.

These results support the notion that EGF or an EGF-like peptide may be a natural ductal mammogen. Edery et al. (1985) have shown that EGF receptor levels in whole mammary glands vary with the physiological state of the mouse, being relatively high in the virgin animal followed

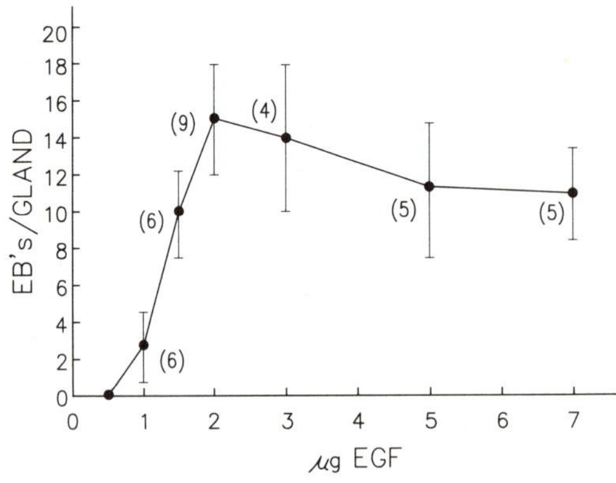

Figure 7. EGF dose–response in ovariectomized animals. Mice received a single Elvax implant containing EGF and BSA in the right No. 3 mammary gland. The left No. 3 gland received an implant containing only BSA. Numbers of treated glands are shown in parentheses. From S. Coleman, G.B. Silberstein, and C.W. Daniel (in preparation).

by a small rise during early pregnancy; levels then steadily decline through the remainder of gestation and lactation. This observation is consistent with a role for EGF in ductal development but does not establish a causal relation. To begin to establish causality, experiments akin to the classical endocrine ablation/replacement studies are required. The difficulty with the study of growth factors such as EGF is the absence of a focal source, however, and surgical ablation is impossible. Slow-release implants may prove useful here. Currently, for example, antibodies to EGF are being implanted into hormonally intact, 5-week-old animals; growth inhibition would point strongly to a natural role for EGF.

3.5. Novel Growth-Regulatory Pathways

The notion that mammary growth regulation invokes an interplay of systemic and locally produced positive and negative modulators is widely accepted (Topper and Freeman, 1980). The emerging recognition of the complexity of growth regulation and the acknowledged insufficiency of the classical ductal mammogens alone to support growth have focused attention on identifying other, possibly locally synthesized, growth regulators and the receptor-mediated pathways through which they operate. Our knowledge of this area is primitive. Evidence for *nontraditional* mammogens derives from the isolation of mitogens from tissue culture medium extracts (Howard et al.,1976; Enami et al., 1983; Kawamura, 1986), serum (Ptashne et al., 1979), milk (Bano et al., 1985), and tissue (Ikeda and Sirbasku, 1984), while our implant experiments have revealed that cAMP probably serves as an intracellular effector for as yet unidentified mammogens (Silberstein et al., 1984).

Agents that raise intracellular cAMP levels are known to stimulate mammary epithelial proliferation in vitro (Yang et al., 1980b). Implanted cholera toxin, which irreversibly activates receptor-associated adenyl cyclase, strongly stimulated end bud growth and demonstrated that a recognized intracellular effector can orchestrate all events for ductal growth (Silberstein et al., 1984). This result raises the following question: Does cAMP activate the natural pathway through which ductal growth is stimulated or is this stimulation merely fortuitous? Arguing against the latter, cAMP levels in both the mouse and rat mammary gland are known to increase during the intense cellular proliferation of pregnancy, an observation consistent with a mitogenic role for cAMP. Since none of the classical ductal mammogens is known to act through an adenyl cyclase-coupled receptor system, our observations point to an as yet unidentified, cAMP-mediated pathway.

4. Epithelial–Stromal Interactions

Epithelial–stromal or mesenchymal interactions (*mesenchyme* refers to undifferentiated stroma and is usually associated with embryonic development) are crucial to organotypic development in a variety of sex-hormone target organs (for recent review see Cunha et al., 1983). Evidence for such interactions in the postnatal mammary gland is sparse, however, and relies more on inferences drawn from observing ductal growth than on experimentation.

4.1. Stromal Requirements for Organotypic Growth

The requirement for a stromal matrix for normal ductal development is apparent from the inability of mammary epithelia to form ducts and end buds in vitro, even when cultured in a floating collagen gel which optimizes the potential for spatial organization (Yang et al., 1980a; Richards et al., 1982). In gels, the growing epithelia form thin-walled tubes and spiked culs-de-sac. It is not that cells in culture loose the capacity to undergo normal morphogenesis, however; Daniel and DeOme (1965) demonstrated that mammary epithelial cells grown in monolayer cultures could be reestablished in a parenchyma-free fat pad resulting in normal, branching growth.

Interestingly, the growth pattern seen in gel cultures was mimicked in stroma that had been artificially enriched for type I collagen. Daniel et al. (1984a) injected unpolymerized type I collagen into a fat pad and, after the bubble of collagen had polymerized, introduced a fragment of mammary duct into the center of the matrix. Histological examination of the implants after 3–6 days revealed numerous small epithelial spikes similar to those seen in cultures. When these thin-walled structures grew beyond the collagen and contacted adipose tissue, normal end buds formed.

While it is clear that fatty stroma is necessary for organotypic growth, there remains a question of whether a specific type of adipose tissue is necessary. Hoshino (1967) reported that outgrowths from ductal fragments transplanted to interscapular brown fat appeared similar to growth in the white fat of the mammary gland. Because no quantitative data were present on the extent of growth, this report is difficult to evaluate. In more recent experiments, Hoshino (1978) compared the size of ductal outgrowths after fragments of ducts were transplanted either to pararenal or mammary fat pads. Fragments in the pararenal fat pad increased up to 10-fold in length, in some cases equaling growth in the mammary fat pad. These results demonstrated that adult duct can grow in ectopic locations and argues against a requirement for specific mammary stroma.

Finally, little is known about possible metabolic cooperativity between mammary epithelium and stroma. In pregnant and lactating mouse mammary glands, Bartley et al. (1981) demonstrated that epithelium must be present to elicit regulatory changes in adipocyte glycogen and lipid metabolism, suggesting that similar reciprocity may occur in the nonpregnant animal.

4.2. Subadult Epithelium Retains Embryonic Potential

Numerous experiments have shown that the growth pattern of embryonic mammary epithelium is governed by mesenchymal influences: chimeras of salivary mesenchyme and mammary epithelium, grown in vitro (Kratochwil, 1969) or in vivo (Sakakura et al., 1976), stimulated salivary-like epithelial outgrowths. It is relevant to the understanding of postnatal growth that, in the juvenile, mammary epithelium remains responsive to embryonic mesenchyme, responding with salivary morphology to transplanted salivary mesenchyme (Sakakura, 1979b). Similar transplants of lung, pancreatic, or metanephrogenic mesenchyme had no effect, indicating that morphogenetic plasticity is partially restricted at this stage. Pregnancy results in full restriction with no response to a salivary transplant.

From the above discussion it is clear that organotypic growth is stroma/mesenchyme dependent. The persistence of embryonic potential and sensitivity to embryonic mesenchyme well into postnatal life is peculiar, but consistent with the observation that other features of postnatal development are embryonic in nature, notably, branching morphogenesis and the striking structural and molecular changes in the basal lamina and extracellular matrix accompanying duct formation (see Section 4.3 for details).

4.3. Stromal Reorganization

The region comprising the flank of the developing end bud extends from the point of maximum curvature to the point where final ductal diameter is achieved. This is a zone of intense morphogenetic activity where, in the short space of perhaps 200–300 μm, the diameter of the end bud constricts up to 10-fold as the duct is formed. In concert with these changes in epithelial form, the stroma immediately adjacent to the end bud also changes dramatically in character, becoming rich in fibrocytes which orient along the flank and subtending duct and which lace the interstitial spaces with fibrillar collagen (Williams and Daniel, 1983).

Glycosaminoglycans (GAG) are known to be important in the regulation of branching growth (Bernfield et al., 1984). Concomitant with fibrocyte infiltration, intense synthesis of sulfated GAG, primarily chondroitin sulfate, was observed in the flank region (Silberstein and Daniel, 1982a). The function of this sulfated GAG is unknown, but in other systems these molecules promote collagen fibrillogenesis (Parry et al., 1982) and are associated with cytodifferentiation and tissue stabilization (Toole and Underhill, 1983).

As described earlier in this chapter, an unusual, refolded basal lamina, approximately 1500 nm thick and rich in sulfated GAG, is synthesized by the presumptive myoepithelium (Silberstein and Daniel, 1982a; Williams and Daniel, 1983). By analogy with the salivary gland, in which GAG turnover appears to depend on action of fibrocyte-derived glycosidases (Smith and Bernfield, 1982), we speculate that the hypertrophied flank lamina may result from a local decrease in stromal-governed GAG turnover.

4.4. Stromal DNA Synthesis

In 5-week-old animals, DNA synthesis induced in unidentified stromal cells up to 250 μm distant from growing end buds has been reported by Berger and Daniel (1983), and similar observations have been made in the rat (Dulbecco et al., 1982). Analyzing thymidine autoradiographs, the heaviest concentrations of label were close to end buds and declined progressively with distance (Berger and Daniel, 1983). This response was shown to be independent of the age of the stroma since duct fragments, transplanted to growth-quiescent, parenchyma-free fat pads of mature animals, also induced labeling. Regressed ducts did not stimulate stromal DNA synthesis and senescent mammary epithelium, which had lost its proliferative potential through repeated transplantation, also failed to induce stromal DNA synthesis even in young hosts. These findings indicate that stromal DNA synthesis is a response to proliferating epithelium, and mammary parenchyma that is in static phase due to either normal processes of growth regulation or aging changes, is ineffective.

One function of this stromal response is no doubt to provide fibrocytes in the neck region of the end bud, where collagen fibrillogenesis is active. Because the stroma around end buds is rich in capillaries, it also seems reasonable to assume that endothelial cell proliferation is taking place and this angiogenesis could account for some of the observed DNA synthesis.

4.5. Receptor Induction

Epidermal growth factor is known to stimulate mammary growth in vitro and, using implants, we have shown local EGF stimulation of quiescent ducts (C. W. Daniel and G. B. Silberstein, unpublished data). EGF receptor autoradiography has revealed intense receptor aggregation in the stroma adjacent to the flank region, where fibrocytic infiltration, collagen fibrillogenesis, and sulfated GAG synthesis are taking place. Estimates of receptor number per cell, done by counting cell surface-associated silver grains, indicated that stromal cells in the end bud flank have over fivefold more receptors than stromal cells distant from end buds, strongly indicating that the growing epithelium induced localized EGE receptor activity. One other example of epithelial-induced stromal receptor activity is recorded. In the male embryo, mammary epithelium induces androgen receptors in immediately adjacent mesenchyme cells (Kratochwil, 1976). At a later time, these cells participate in androgen-induced destruction of the male mammary rudiment (Heuberger et al., 1982).

4.6. In Vitro Studies

In vitro studies provide indirect evidence for stromal involvement in epithelial growth, if not morphogenesis, specifically with respect to the acquisition of hormone sensitivity of the epithelium. McGrath (1983) isolated normal mammary epithelium from midpregnant BALB/c mice and cocultured these cells with mammary fibrocytes such that the two populations were initially separated and met to form a clear interface. At confluence, both cell types stopped growing. Addition of estradiol (10^{-8} *M*) stimulated epithelial DNA synthesis approximately 100-fold; without cell–cell contact, however, estradiol had no effect.

In a different coculture system, using growth-inhibited, irradiated 3T3-L1 cells (a line that undergoes adipocyte differentiation), Levine and Stockdale demonstrated enhanced epithelial proliferation (1984) and lactogen-induced synthesis of casein (1985). Growth stimulation may have been due to 3T3-L1-derived extracellular matrix material, since plates conditioned by these cells stimulated growth; on the other hand, hormone-induced casein synthesis required the presence of the intact feeder cells.

5. *Aging of Mammary Cells*

The question of whether normal mammalian tissue cells have a limited or unlimited growth span is of obvious significance to the fields of both aging and cancer and has intrigued generations of biologists. Most of the research on cell longevity has been carried out in tissue culture, where cells are freed from the homeostatic constraints of the organism and are free to proliferate without restriction. It is now generally accepted, following the pioneering work of Hayflick and Moorhead (1961), that nonmalignant cells from mammalian tissue display a limited potential for growth in culture, the length of which is well correlated with the lifespan of the donor species (Martin et al., 1970) and cannot be significantly extended by modifying conditions of culture (reviewed by Smith and Lincoln, 1984).

Does the mortality of cells in culture reflect an intrinsic property of the cells themselves? In vitro experiments demonstrating cell senescence, powerful as they are, must be interpreted with care because of the necessarily artificial environment of tissue culture, and it is obviously desirable to relate these findings to analogous experiments carried out in vivo. Serial transplantation of several tissue types between inbred mice has been carried out (reviewed by Daniel, 1977; Daniel et al., 1986). The mammary transplant system (DeOme et al., 1959) provides a particularly useful means for serially propagating mammary cells in young animals. Here the tissue is maintained with its normal stromal associations and growth takes place in a physiological environment. The gland-free mammary fat pad is analogous to the tissue culture flask; when filled with glandular outgrowth, samples may be transplanted into other fat pads in young hosts, and by maintaining a constant transplant interval, the extent of growth at each transfer generation provides an accurate measure of proliferative performance (Daniel et al., 1968; Daniel, 1973).

The technique of serial transplantation of mammary ductal cells into young hosts has been used to elucidate several features of cell senescence (reviewed by Daniel, 1977; Daniel et al., 1986), including the recent finding that senescent mammary cells could be stimulated to reinitiate DNA synthesis and normal morphogenesis by exposure to cAMP-active agents. These results are summarized below:

1. Mammary cells demonstrate a limited growth span even when propagated under conditions that are judged to be optimal for continued growth (Fig. 8). Growth declines an average of 15% each transfer generation; the decline is approximately linear (Fig. 9). By analogy with aging changes observed in culture and

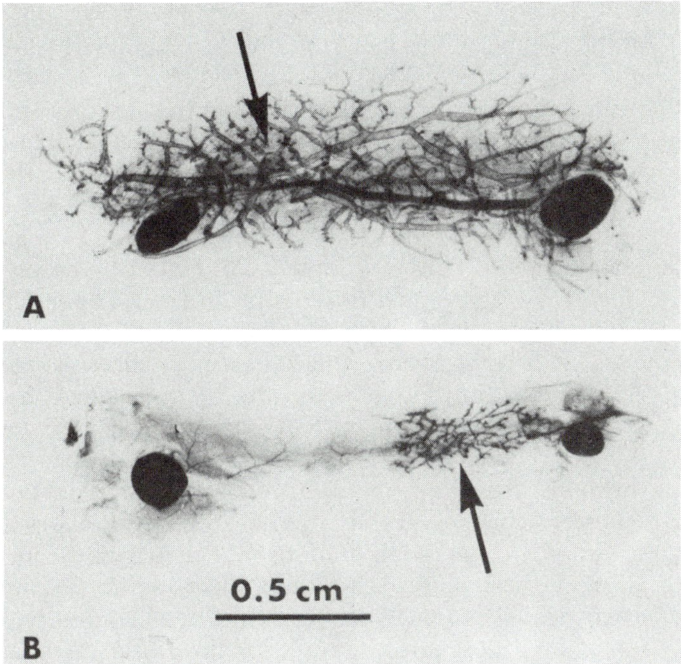

Figure 8. Representative outgrowths from serially transplanted mammary tissues, using a transplant interval of 3 months. (A) Generation 1 outgrowth showing young gland which has grown rapidly to fill the available fat. (B) Generation 4 outgrowth, tissue age 16 months, which occupies about 25% of the fat pad. Hematoxylin stain. From Daniel et al. (1975).

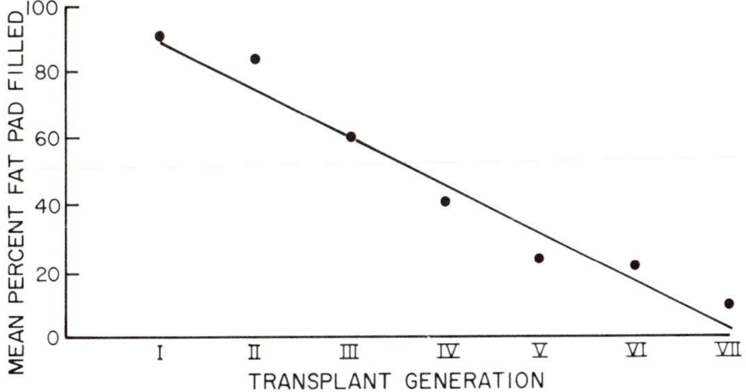

Figure 9. Decline in growth rate of mammary tissue during serial propagation. This plot summarizes the results of eight transplant experiments, and each point represents 80–100 transplants. The regression line is approximately linear, and the slope indicates a 15% loss of growth potential at each passage. From Daniel et al. (1975).

in the organism, this loss of viability is considered an expression of senescence at the cell and tissue level.

2. By maintaining the gland in static phase while control cultures were kept in continuous growth, Daniel and Young (1971) demonstrated that mammary cell senescence is related to the number of doublings experienced by the end bud cells and is not affected by the passage of chronological time.
3. Mammary cell senescence is not influenced by donor age provided the transplanted tissue is taken from virgin animals and has been in static phase during most of the animal's life. Host age does not become a factor unless transplantation takes place after reproductive involution, when the requisite hormones are not available to stimulate growth (Young et al., 1971).
4. Hyperplastic alveolar nodules (HAN), a preneoplastic lesion of the mouse mammary gland, is immortalized and does not display senescent changes. Use of precancerous tissue types allows the separation of immortalization from malignancy: That is, immortalization is an early rather than a late step in the sequence of events leading to malignancy (Daniel et al., 1968).
5. Mammary cell senescence results from a progressive inability of mammary epithelium to respond to mitogenic hormones or growth factors. Senescent tissue, which has lost its ability to pro-

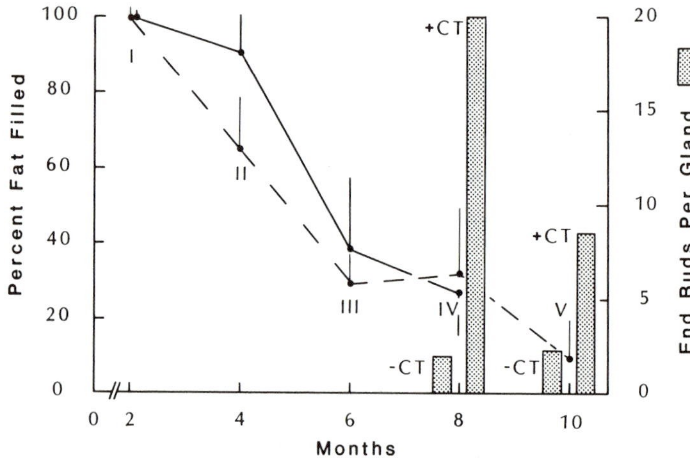

Figure 10. Growth of mammary ducts in two tissue lines. Each transplant line was initiated by tissue taken from a 3-month-old donor. End bud number, a measure of growth rate, is indicated by bars at generations 4 and 5, indicating the stimulatory effect of cholera toxin (CT). From Daniel et al. (1984b).

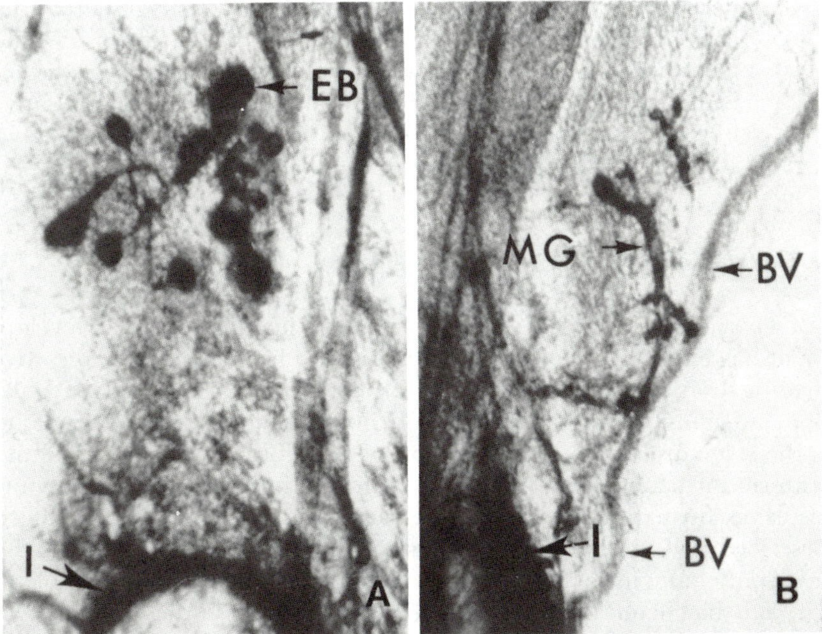

Figure 11. Stimulation of serially aged mammary outgrowths by cholera toxin. (A) Whole mount of transplant generation 5 outgrowth filling 5% of the available fat pad. Six weeks after transplantation, the gland was exposed to an Elvax implant (I) containing 4 μg of cholera toxin. Well-developed end buds (EB) are found at the tip of each duct, and their general form, size, and growth pattern appear normal. (B) Control gland whole mount showing generation 5 outgrowth from the contralateral side of the same host as (A). The Elvax implant contained no cholera toxin; the gland lacks end buds and is comparatively unstimulated. BV, blood vessel; MG, mammary gland.

liferate in virgin mice, can be stimulated to proliferate again in response to a new hormonal environment that the tissue has not experienced previously. For example, ducts that have been aged serially in virgin mice will undergo mitosis if the host becomes pregnant, but alveoli are formed rather than end buds (Daniel et al., 1971). This suggests that mammary cells lose their responsiveness to any mitogenic signals after repeated exposure and stimulation.

6. Senescent mammary cells reinitiate DNA synthesis and resume apparently normal morphogenesis in response to cholera toxin, a potent stimulator of cAMP synthesis (Figs. 10 and 11). This is the first report of partial reversal of cell aging in the absence of

neoplastic or preneoplastic transformation. It suggests that the lesion associated with aging of these cells may reside in the adenylate cyclase complex (Daniel et al., 1984b) and is consistent with other evidence mentioned above, that the limited replicative lifespan of mammary cells is linked to loss of responsiveness to systemic or local mitogens.

6. Conclusions

Over the past several years, the study of mammary ductal development has emerged from relative obscurity to become an area of active investigation by those interested in problems of developmental regulation and aging. While it has been well known that the mammary end bud is the structural focus for regulation of branching morphogenesis and pattern formation, significant new information has recently become available. Structural features of the rat and mouse end bud have been described and epithelial subpopulations, including a stem cell for the myoepithelium, have been identified using morphological, immunological, and biochemical techniques. Transplantation studies have shown that the end bud retains certain embryonic characteristics, demonstrated by its ability to respond to heterologous inductive mesenchyme even in the subadult by altering its developmental pattern.

The importance of local growth-regulatory factors, in addition to the better known systemic mammogens, is generally accepted but their identification has been difficult. The culture of mammary epithelium in collagen gel has identified substances not heretofore considered mammogens, notably epidermal growth factor and prostaglandins. In vivo, the use of slow-release plastic implants has confirmed that these growth factors are capable of stimulating local gland growth, indicating a direct effect. Additionally, slow-release implants have been used to show that stimulation of several different receptor systems can lead to local end bud growth in ovariectomized animals. The active substances fall into three catagories: steroids (estrogen), protein growth factors (EGF, prolactin, growth hormone), and direct activators of adenyl cyclase (cholera toxin, prostaglandin E). We conclude from this observation that there are multiple pathways to ductal growth.

Epithelial–stromal interactions appear to be important in the growth of mammary ducts in the subadult animal, as they are in the embryo. The fat pad is an absolute requirement for gland growth. It appears that just as the stroma determines epithelial form and function in urogenital steroid target organs, the mammary ductal tree may be similarly sensitive to stromal influences and may show a similar degree of developmental plasticity; this plasticity perhaps reflects the gland's capacity for change during the mammary growth cycle.

Epithelial influences on stromal function and development are also documented. In the embryo, epithelium has been shown to induce androgen receptors in adjacent mesenchyme. In the subadult, it has recently been shown that growing end buds induce epidermal growth factor receptors in the stroma immediately adjacent to the end bud flank. Growing end buds also stimulate stromal fibrosis around the newly formed duct as well as DNA synthesis in as yet unidentified cells ahead of the invading epithelium.

The work noted above emphasizes the embryonic character of ductal growth in the subadult animal, as evidenced in branching morphogenesis itself, changes in extracellular matrix composition, in the retention of developmental plasticity, and in the stromal fibrotic response to the developing epithelium. This progress suggests that further insights into growth regulation may come from continued investigation of mammary ductal development.

References

Bano, M., Salomon, D.S., and Kidwell, W.R., 1985, Purification of a mammary-derived growth factor from human milk and human mammary tumors, *J. Biol. Chem.* **260**(9):5745–5752.

Bartley, J.C., Emerman, J.J., and Bissell, M.J., 1981, Metabolic cooperativity between epithelial cells and adipocytes of mice, *Am. J. Physiol.* **241**(*Cell Physiol.* 10):C204–C208.

Bennett, D.C., Peachey, L.A., Durbin, H., and Rudland, P.S., 1978, A possible mammary stem cell line, *Cell* **15**:283–298.

Berger, J.J., and Daniel, C.W., 1983, Stromal DNA synthesis is stimulated by young, but not serially aged mouse mammary epithelium, *Mech. Ageing Dev.* **23**:259–264.

Bernfield, M., Banerjee, S.D., Koda, J.E., and Rapraeger, A.C., 1984, Remodeling of the basement membrane as a mechanism for morphogenetic tissue interactions, in: *The Role of the Extracellular Matrix in Development,* Alan R. Liss, New York, pp. 545–572.

Bresciani, F., 1965, Effect of ovarian hormones on duration of DNA synthesis in cells of the C3H mouse mammary gland, *Exp. Cell Res.* **38**:13–32.

Ceriani, R.I., 1970, Fetal mammary gland differentiation *in vitro* in response to hormones. II. Biochemical findings, *Dev. Biol.* **21**:530–546.

Cohn, R.M., Banerjee, S.D., and Bernfield, M.R., 1977, Basal lamina of embryonic salivary epithelia. Nature of glycosaminoglycans and organization of extracellular materials, *J. Cell Biol.* **73**:464–478.

Cowie, A.T., 1949, The relative growth of the mammary glard in normal, gonadectomized, and adrenalectomized rats, *J. Endocrinol.* **6**:147–157.

Cunha, G.R., Chung, L.W.K., Shannon, J.M., Taguchi, O., and Fujii, H., 1983 Hormone-induced morphogenesis and growth: Role of mesenchymal–epithelial interactions, *Recent Prog. Horm. Res.* **39**:559–598.

Daniel, C.W., 1973, Finite growth span of mouse mammary gland serially propagated *in vivo, Experientia* **29:**1422–1424.

Daniel, C.W., 1977, Cell longevity: *in vivo,* in: *Handbook of the Biology of Aging* (C.E. Finch and L. Hayflick, eds.), Van Nostrand Reinhold, New York, pp. 122–158.

Daniel, C.W., and DeOme, K.B., 1965, Growth of mouse mammary glands *in vivo* after monolayer culture, *Science* **149:**634–636.

Daniel, C.W., and Young, L.J.T., 1971, Lifespan of mouse mammary gland epithelium during serial propagation *in vivo:* Influence of cell division on an aging process, *Exp. Cell Res.* **65:**27–32.

Daniel, C.W., DeOme, K.B., Young, J.T., Blair, P.B., and Faulkin, L.J., 1968, The *in vivo* lifespan of normal and preneoplastic mouse mammary glands: A serial transplantation study, *Proc. Natl. Acad. Sci. USA* **61:**52–60.

Daniel, C.W., Young, L.J.T., Medina, D., and DeOme, K.B., 1971, The influence of mammogenic hormones on serially transplanted mouse mammary gland, *Exp. Gerontol.* **6:**95–101.

Daniel, C.W., Aidells, B.D., Medina, D., and Faulkin, L.J., Jr., 1975, Unlimited division potential of precancerous mouse mammary cells after spontaneous or carcinogen-induced transformation, in: *Biology of Aging and Development,* Plenum Press, New York, pp. 123–130.

Daniel, C.W., Berger, J.J., Strickland, P., and Garcia, R., 1984a, Similar growth pattern of mouse mammary cells cultivated in collagen matrix *in vivo* and *in vitro, Dev. Biol.* **104:**57–64.

Daniel, C.W., Silberstein, G.B., and Strickland, P., 1984b, Reinitiation of growth in senescent mouse mammary epithelium in response to cholera toxin, *Science* **224:**1245–1247.

Daniel, C.W., Silberstein, G.B., and Strickland, P., 1986, Mammary cells, in: *CRC Handbook of Cell Biology of Aging* (V.J. Cristofalo, ed.), CRC Press, Boca Raton, FL, pp. 289–301.

Danielson, K.G., Oborn, C.J., Durban, E.M., Butel, J.S., and Medina, D., 1984, An epithelial mouse mammary cell line exhibiting normal morphogenesis *in vivo* and functional differentiation *in vitro, Proc. Natl. Acad. Sci. USA* **81:**3756–3760.

DeOme, K.B., Faulkin, L.J. Jr., and Bern, H.A., 1959, Development of mammary tumors from hyperplastic alveolar nodules transplanted into gland-free mammary fat pads of female C3H mice, *Cancer Res.* **19:**515–520.

DuBois, M., and Elias, J.J., 1984, Subpopulations of cells in immature mouse mammary glands as detected by proliferative responses to hormones in organ culture, *Dev. Biol.* **106:**70–75.

Dulbecco, R., Henahan, M., and Armstrong, B., 1982, Cell types and morphogenesis in the mammary gland, *Proc. Natl. Acad. Sci. USA* **79:**7346–7350.

Dulbecco, R., Unger, M., Armstrong, B., Bowman, M., and Syka, P., 1983, Epithelial cell types and their evolution in the rat mammary gland determined by immunological markers, *Proc. Natl. Acad. Sci. USA* **80:**1033–1037.

Eberhard, S., Tait, L., Tay, L.K., and Russo, J., 1982, Comparative study of the cellular replication kinetics of rat mammary epithelial cells in vivo and in vitro, *Exp. Cell Res.* **141:**31–38.

Edery, M., Pang, K., Larson, L., Colosi, T., and Nandi, S., 1985, Epidermal growth factor receptor levels in mouse mammary glands in various physiological states, *Endocrinology* **117**(1)**:**405–411.

Enami, J., Enami, S., and Koga, M., 1983, Growth of normal and neoplastic mouse mammary epithelial cells in primary culture: Stimulation by conditioned medium from mouse mammary fibroblasts, *Gann* **74:**845–853.

Faulkin, L.J., Jr., and DeOme, K.B., 1960, Regulation of growth and spacing of gland elements in the mammary fat pad of the C3H mouse, *J. Natl. Cancer Inst.* **24:**953–969.

Gordon, J.R., and Bernfield, M.R., 1980, The basal lamina of the postnatal mammary epithelium contains glycosaminoglycan in a precise ultrastructural organization, *Dev. Biol.* **74:**118–135.

Haslam, S.Z., 1986, Mammary fibroblast influence on normal mouse mammary epithelial cell responses to estrogen *in vitro, Cancer Res.* **46:**310–316.

Haslam, S.Z., and Levely, M.L., 1985, Estradiol responsiveness of normal mouse mammary cells in primary cell culture: Association of mammary fibroblasts with estradiol regulation of progesterone receptors, *Endocrinology* **116:**1835–1841.

Hayflick, L., and Moorhead, P.S., 1961, The serial cultivation of a human diploid cell line, *Exp. Cell Res.* **25:**585–621.

Heuberger, B., Fitzka, I., Wasner, G., and Kratochwil, K., 1982, Induction of androgen receptor formation by epithelium–mesenchyme interaction in embryonic mouse mammary gland, *Proc. Natl. Acad. Sci. USA* **79:**2957–2961.

Hoshino, K., 1964, Regeneration and growth of quantitatively transplanted mammary glands of normal female mice, *Anat. Rec.* **150:**221–236.

Hoshino, K., 1967, Transplantability of mammary gland in brown fat pads of mice, *Nature* **213:**194–195.

Hoshino, K., 1978, Mammary transplantation and its histogenesis in mice, in: *Physiology of Mammary Glands* (A. Yokoyama, H. Mizuno, and H. Nagasawa, eds.), University Park Press, Baltimore, pp. 163–228.

Howard, E.F., Scott, D.F., and Bennett, C.E., 1976, Stimulation of thymidine uptake and cell proliferation in mouse embryo fibroblasts by conditioned medium from mammary cells in culture, *Cancer Res.* **36:**4543–4551.

Ikeda, T. and Sirbasku, D.A., 1984, Purification and properties of a mammary–uterine–pituitary tumor cell growth factor from pregnant sheep uterus, *J. Biol. Chem.* **259**(7)**:**4049–4064.

Imagawa, W., Tomooka, Y., and Nandi, S., 1982, Serum-free growth of normal and tumor mouse mammary epithelial cells in primary culture, *Proc. Natl. Acad. Sci. USA* **79:**4074–4077.

Imagawa, W., Tomooka, Y., Hamamoto, S., and Nandi, S., 1985, Stimulation of mammary epithelial cell growth *in vitro:* Interaction of epidermal growth factor and mammogenic hormones, *Endocrinology* **116**(4)**:**1514–1524.

Kawamura, K., Enami, J., Enami, S., Koezuka, M., Kohmoto, K., and Koga, M., 1986, 2. Growth and morphogenesis of mouse mammary epithelial cells cultured in collagen gels: Stimulation by hormones, epidermal growth factor and mammary fibroblast-conditioned medium factor, *Proc. Japan Acad.* **62**(Ser. B)**:**5–8.

Knight, C.H., and Peaker, M., 1982, Development of the mammary gland, *J. Reprod. Fertil.* **65:**521–536.

Kratochwil, K., 1969, Organ specificity in mesenchymal induction demonstrated in the embryonic development of the mammary gland of the mouse, *Dev. Biol.* **20:**46–71.

Kratochwil, K., 1976, Tissue interaction in androgen response of embryonic mammary rudiment of mouse: Identification of target tissue for testosterone, *Proc. Natl. Acad. Sci. USA* **73**(11)**:**4041–4044.

Levine, J.F., and Stockdale, F.E., 1984, 3T3-L1 adipocytes promote growth of mammary epithelium, *Exp. Cell Res.* **151:**112–122.

Levine, J.F., and Stockdale, F.E., 1985, Cell–cell interactions promote mammary epithelial cell differentiation, *J. Cell Biol.* **100:**1415–1422.

Lyons, W.R., 1958, Hormonal synergism in mammary growth, *Proc. R. Soc. (London) Ser. B* **149:**303–325.

Lyons, W.R., Li, C.H., and Johnson, R.E., 1958, The hormonal control of mammary growth and lactation, *Recent Prog. Horm. Res.* **14:**219–250.

Martin, G.M., Sprague, C.A., and Epstein, C.J., 1970, Replicative lifespan of cultivated human cells. Effect of Donor's age, tissue, and genotype, *Lab. Invest.* **23:**86–92.

McGrath, C.M., 1983, Augmentation of the response of normal mammary epithelial cells to estradiol by mammary stroma, *Cancer Res.* **43:**1355–1360.

Meyer, J.M., Staubli, A., and Ruch, J.V., 1981, Ruthenium red staining and tannic acid fixation of dental basement membrane, *Cell Tissue Res.* **220:**589–597.

Munford, R.E., 1964, A review of anatomical and biochemical changes in the mammary gland with particular reference to quantitative methods of assessing mammary development, *Dairy Sci. Abstr.* **26:**293–304.

Nandi, S., 1958, Endocrine control of mammary-gland development and function in the C3H/He Crgl mouse, *J. Natl. Cancer Inst.* **21:**1039–1063.

Nandi, S., 1959, Hormonal control of mammogenesis and lactogenesis in the C3H/He Crgl mouse, *Univ. Calif. Publ. Zoology* **65:**1–128.

Nandi, S., Imagawa, W., Tomooka, Y., McGrath, M.F., and Edery, M., 1984, Collagen gel culture system and analysis of estrogen effects on mammary carcinogenesis, *Arch. Toxicol.* **55:**91–96.

Parry, D.A.D., Flint, M.H., Gillard, G.C., and Craig, A.S., 1982, A role for glycosaminoglycans in the development of collagen fibrills, *FEBS Lett.* **149**(1)**:**1–7.

Pitelka, D.R., and Hamamoto, S.T., 1977, Form and function in mammary epithelium: The interpretation of ultrastructure, *J. Dairy Sci.* **60:**643–654.

Pitelka, D.R., Hamamoto, S.J., and Taggart, B.N., 1980, Basal lamina and tissue recognition in malignant mammary tumors, *Cancer Res.* **40:**1600–1611.

Ptashne, K., Hsueh, H.W., and Stockdale, F.E., 1979, Partial purification and characterization of mammary stimulating factor, a protein which promotes proliferation of mammary epithelium, *Biochemistry* **18**(16)**:**3533–3539.

Richards, J., Guzman, R., Konrad, M., Yang, J., and Nandi, S., 1982, Growth of mouse mammary end buds cultured in a collagen gel matrix, *Exp. Cell Res.* **141:**433–443.

Richards, J., Hamamoto, S., Smith, S., Pasco, D., Guzman, R., and Nandi, S., 1983, Response of end buds from immature rat mammary gland to hormones when cultured in collagen gels, *Exp. Cell Res.* **147:**95–109.

Rudland, P.S., Bennett, D.C., and Warburton, M.J., 1980a, in: *Hormones and Cancer: Proceedings of the First International Congress,* Raven Press, New York.

Rudland, P.S., Ormerod, E.J., and Paterson, F.C., 1980b, Stem cells in rat mammary development and cancer: A review, *J. R. Soc. Med.* **73:**437–442.

Rugh, R., 1968, *The Mouse: Its Reproduction and Development,* Burgess Publishing, Minneapolis.

Russo, J., and Russo, I. H., 1980, Influence of differentiation and cell kinetics on the susceptibility of the rat mammary gland to carcinogenesis, *Cancer Res.* **40:**2677–2687.

Russo, I.H., Ireland, M., Isengerg, W., and Russo, J., 1976a, Ultrastructural description of three different epithelial cell types in rat mammary gland, *Proc. Electron Microsc. Soc. Am.* **34:**146–147.

Russo, J., Isenberg, W., Ireland, M., and Russo, I.H., 1976b, Ultrastructural changes in the mammary epithelial cell population during neoplastic development induced by a chemical carcinogen, *Proc. Electron Microsc. Soc. Am.* **34:**250–251.

Russo, J., Wilgus, G., and Russo, I.H., 1979, Susceptibility of the mammary gland to carcinogenesis. I. Differentiation of the mammary gland as a determinant of tumor incidence and type of lesion, *Am. J. Pathol.* **96:**721–735.

Sakakura, T., Nishizuka, Y., and Dawe, C.J., 1976, Mesenchyme-dependent morphogenesis and epithelium-specific cytodifferentiation in mouse mammary gland, *Science* **194:**1439–1441.

Sakakura, T., Nishizuka, Y., and Dawe, C.J., 1979a, Capacity of mammary fat pads of adult C3H/HeMs mice to interact morphogenetically with fetal mammary epithelium, *J. Natl. Cancer Inst.* **63:**733–736.

Sakakura, T., Sakagami, Y., and Nishizuka, Y., 1979b, Persistence of responsiveness of adult mouse mammary gland to induction by embryonic mesenchyme, *Dev. Biol.* **72:** 201–210.

Sakakura, T., Sakagami, Y., and Nishizuki, Y., 1982, Dual origin of mesenchymal tissues participating in mouse mammary-gland embryogenesis, *Dev. Biol.* **91:**202–207.

Sekhri, K.K., Pitelka, D.R., and DeOme, K.B., 1967, Studies of mouse mammary glands. I. Cytomorphology of the normal mammary gland, *J. Natl. Cancer Inst.* **39:**459–490.

Silberstein, G.B., and Daniel, C.W., 1982a, Glycosaminoglycans in the basal lamina and extracellular matrix of the developing mouse mammary duct, *Dev. Biol.* **90:**215–222.

Silberstein, G.B., and Daniel, C.W., 1982b, Elvax 40P implants, sustained local release of bioactive molecules influencing mammary ductal development, *Dev. Biol.* **93:**272–278.

Silberstein, G.B., Strickland, P., Trumpbour, V., Coleman, S., and Daniel, C.W., 1984, *In vivo,* cAMP stimulates growth and morphogenesis of mouse mammary ducts, *Proc. Natl. Acad. Sci. USA* **81:**4950–4954.

Sinha, Y.N., and Tucker, H.A., 1966, Mammary gland growth of rats between 10 and 100 days of age, *Am. J. Physiol.* **210:**601–605.

Slavkin, H.C., Brownell, A.G., Bringas, P., Jr., MacDougall, M., and Bessem, C., 1983, Basal lamina persistence during epithelial–mesenchymal interactions in murine tooth development in vitro, *J. Cranofac. Genet. Dev. Biol.* **3:**387–407.

Smith, R.L., and Bernfield, M., 1982, Mesenchyme cells degrade epithelial basal lamina glycosaminoglycan, *Dev. Biol.* **94:**378–390.

Smith, J.R., and Lincoln, D.W. II, 1984, Aging of cells in culture, *Int. Rev. Cytol.* **89:**151–177.

Toole, B.P., and Underhill, E.B., 1983, Regulation of morphogenesis by the pericellular matrix, in: *Cell Interaction and Development: Molecular Mechanisms* (K.M. Yamada, ed.), John Wiley and Sons, New York, pp. 203–230.

Topper, Y.J. and Freeman, C.S., 1980, Multiple hormone interactions in the developmental biology of the mammary gland, *Physiol. Rev.* **60:**1049–1106.

Tucker, H.A., 1981, Physiological control of mammary growth, lactogenesis, and lactation, *J. Dairy Sci.* **64:**1403–1421.

Voytovich, A.E. and Topper, Y.J., 1967, Hormone-dependent differentiation of immature mouse mammary gland *in vitro, Science* **158:**1326–1327.

Warburton, M.J., Mitchell, D., Ormerod, E.J., and Rudland, P., 1982, Distribution of myoepithelial cells and basement membrane proteins in the resting, pregnant, lactating, and involuting rat mammary gland, *J. Histochem. Cytochem.* **30:**667–676.

Warburton, M.J., Head, L.P., Ferns, S.A., and Rudland, P.S., 1983, Induction of differentiation in a rat mammary epithelial stem cell line by dimethyl sulphoxide and mammotrophic hormones, *Eur. J. Biochem.* **133:**707–715.

Williams, J.M. and Daniel, C.W., 1983, Mammary ductal elongation: Differentiation of myoepithelium and basal lamina during branching morphogenesis, *Dev. Biol.* **97:**274–290.

Yang, J., Richards, J., Guzman, R., Imagawa, W., and Nandi, S., 1980a, Sustained growth in primary culture of normal mammary epithelial cells embedded in collagen gels, *Proc. Natl. Acad. Sci. USA* **77:**2088–2092.

Yang, J., Guzman, R., Richards, J., Imagawa, W., McCormack, K., and Nandi, S., 1980b, Growth factor- and cyclic nucleotide-induced proliferation of normal and malignant mammary epithelial cells in primary culture, *Endocrinology* **107**(1)**:**35–41.

Yang, J., Guzman, R., Richards, J., and Nandi, S., 1980c, Primary culture of mouse mammary tumor epithelial cells embedded in collagen gels, *In Vitro* **16:**502–506.

Young, L.J.T., Medina, D., DeOme, K.B., and Daniel, C.W., 1971, The influence of host and tissue age on lifespan and growth rate of serially transplanted mouse mammary gland, *Exp. Gerontol.* **6:**49–56.

2

Mammary Embryogenesis

Teruyo Sakakura

1. Introduction

The mammary gland is an organ unique to the Class Mammalia. Like other reproductive organs whose function is related to perpetuation of the species, the mammary gland grows slowly during embryonic and juvenile life and does not mature until the reproductive system begins to function at puberty. A fairly large number of studies on mammary gland embryogenesis were carried out in the 1800s and early 1900s using animals such as the echidna, duckbill, marsupial, rodent, domestic animals, and humans. Excellent reviews are available (Raynaud, 1961; Anderson, 1978). Normal morphogenesis for rat and mouse mammary glands of both male and female embryos has been described in detail by Myers (1917) and Turner and Gomez (1933). In classical textbooks of embryology, however, the mammary gland has rarely been included because interest in this organ was restricted to its phylogenetical significance and agricultural benefits. In addition, difficulties in working with the mammary gland during either in vivo or in vitro experiments and the lack of a dramatic change at embryonic stages might have contributed to its lack of popularity for developmental biology research.

The development of inbred strains of mice, particularly mammary tumor incidence strains, and the development of culture methods for the mammary gland have resulted in increased interest in this tissue. It is a target of many hormones, proliferating and involuting periodically in response to physiological changes of hormone levels. During lactation,

Teruyo Sakakura • Laboratory of Cell Biology, RIKEN, Tsukuba Life Science Center, The Institute of Physical and Chemical Research, Yatabe, Tsukuba, Ibaraki 305, Japan.

the mammary epithelium synthesizes large amounts of milk which contains specific proteins such as the caseins and α-lactalbumin. In addition, the mammary gland affords a system for analysis of pathological changes such as preneoplastic and neoplastic lesions which either develop spontaneously or are induced by carcinogenic agents. Thus, the mammary gland is now a useful tool for a variety of biological and pathological studies. Because there are a large number of excellent papers on the sequential changes of mammary gland morphogenesis based on histological observation (Myers, 1917; Turner and Gomez, 1933; Balinsky, 1950; Raynaud, 1961; Anderson, 1978), this chapter describes mammary gland embryogenesis, mainly in mice and rats, from the aspect of developmental biology.

2. *Mammary Gland Anlage*

In marsupials and monotremes, the mammary gland develops from the hair anlage. In the Placentalia, five theories have been considered as to the possible tissue of origin. The mammary glands may develop from modified sweat glands, sebaceous glands, hair anlage, or undifferentiated cutaneous glands based on similarities of morphology and certain features of each. As Raynaud (1961) pointed out, however, none of these theories of origin is entirely satisfactory. The question of origin may not be answered from morphological observations alone. In addition to the four glands mentioned above as possible tissues of origin, Rein (1882) proposed that the mammary gland is formed de novo at the expense of ectoderm and of the underlying mesenchyme. Surprisingly, the theory suggested the importance of epithelial–mesenchymal interactions in organogenesis as early as 1882.

With the progress of new technologies in the biomedical field, it is possible to study mammary gland embryogenesis at the cellular and molecular levels. This chapter describes the morphological development of mammary epithelium with special emphasis on the mesenchymal tissues of mammary gland and their interaction with the epithelium in relation to mammary gland embryogenesis.

2.1. *Mammary Epithelium*

2.1.1. *Mammary Streak*

Turner and Gomez (1933) first noted the earliest indication of mammary gland development in mice. In 10–11-day embryos (vaginal plug = 0 day), the enlargement of a single-layered ectoderm appeared

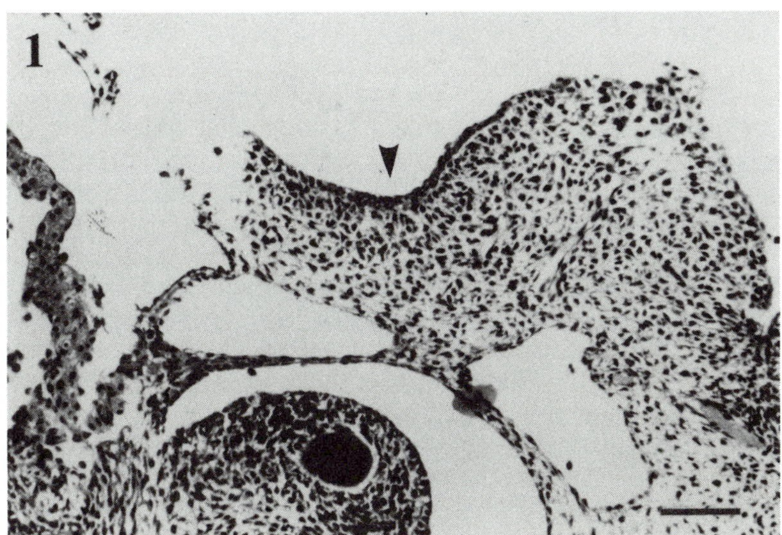

Figure 1. Mammary gland anlage of 11-day mouse embryo. The epidermal cells enlarge and form the mammary streak (arrow). Bar = 100 μm.

as a line extending from the anterior limb bud to the posterior limb bud, first on one side and then on both (Fig. 1). This was described as the mammary streak, which had been observed by others in the rat and human (Myers, 1917; Raynaud, 1961).

2.1.2. Mammary Bud

In 12-day embryos, five pairs of mammary gland anlage, three thoracic and two inguinal, are formed. Each mammary gland rudiment forms a lens-shaped structure composed of several layers of epidermal cells (Fig. 2). This is the first outwardly visible evidence of mammary gland development and clearly distinguishes the mammary bud from the surrounding tissues. Turner and Gomez (1933) described the conversion of the original mammary streak into a mammary line slightly elevated above the surface of the epidermis. Histologically, the mammary lines are formed by proliferation of the *stratum germinativum* of epidermis. The first stage in the development of the mammary bud was reported to begin with unequal proliferation of cells at intervals along the mammary lines. Between these foci of cell proliferation, the mammary lines gradually disappeared. This process was considered basically the same in many species.

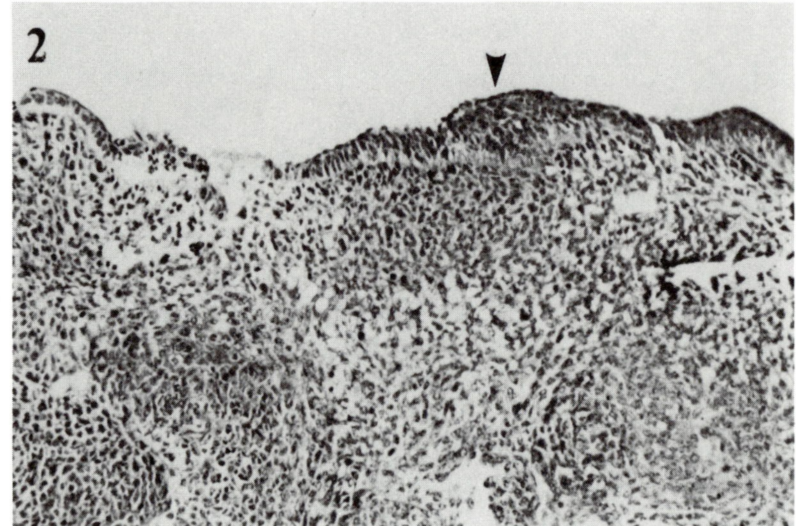

Figure 2. Mammary bud of 12-day mouse embryo. The mammary epithelium forms a lens-shaped structure (arrow).

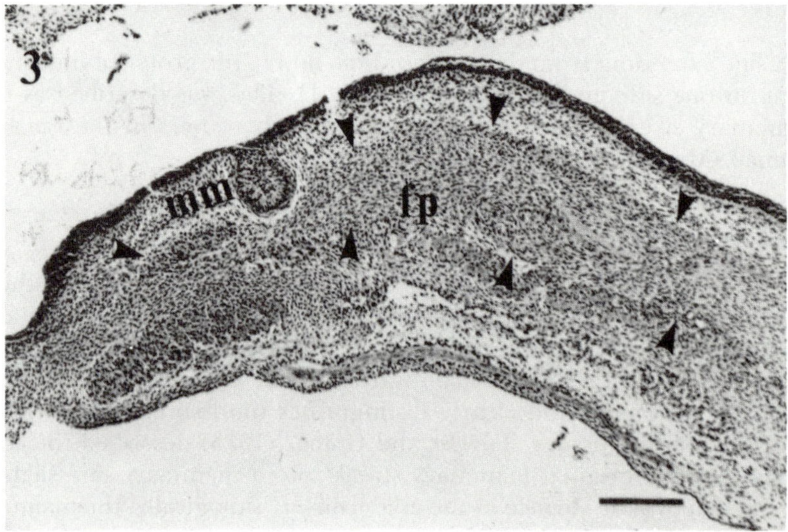

Figure 3. Mammary bud of 14-day female mouse embryo. The mammary epithelium forms a bulb-shaped structure with a narrow neck. The dense mammary mesenchyme (mm) surrounds the mammary epithelium. The first appearance of fat pad precursor tissue (fp) is recognized by a somewhat condensed tissue below the mammary rudiment (arrows). Bar = 150 μm.

This developmental process was generally accepted until 1950 when Balinsky reported quantitative experiments comparing the mitotic index in the mammary line with that of the adjacent epidermis in rabbits and mice. He found that the rate of cell proliferation in newly formed mammary buds decreased below the rate in the adjacent epidermis. This suggested that there is no growth of the mammary gland at this stage, and he postulated that the formation of a mammary line and individual mammary buds depends on displacement of cells, not on locally elevated proliferative activity in the epidermis. This hypothesis was later comfirmed by Propper (1978) who demonstrated wandering epithelial cells in the mammary line of rabbit embryos under the scanning electron microscope. These results with rabbit and mouse mammary gland suggested that the migration of epidermal cells is a fundamental process during early-stage mammary gland embryogenesis.

At the 14th day of gestation, the mammary rudiments change from lens shaped to bulb shaped with a narrow neck (Fig. 3). The inner portion of the epithelial rudiment is filled with irregular-shaped cells.

2.1.3. Mammary Sprout

In mice, sexual differentiation of the gonads occurs at the late 13th day of gestation, after which the testes start to produce androgen in male embryos. On day 14, the sexual phenotype in the mammary gland is determined.

In female embryos, very slow growth and an absence of progressive differentiation are observed from the 11th to 16th day of gestation. This interval is termed the *resting phase.* Late in the 16th day, the mammary bud elongates by rapid cellular proliferation, forming the mammary sprout (Fig. 4). At 17 days, the sprout grows rapidly downward, penetrating mammary fat pad precursor tissue which appears posterior to the mammary rudiment on day 14 (described in Section 2.1.2). The growth of epithelial elements at this stage first results in branching. Then, in the following few days until birth, the epithelium grows into the mammary fat pad precursor tissue until the mammary gland tree with about 15–20 branching ducts is formed (Fig. 5).

In male mice and rats, mammary gland development is inhibited by fetal androgen. At 14 days in mouse embryos the male mammary epithelium decreases in volume, changing from round to somewhat irregular spindle shaped. At 15 days, the epithelial stalk connecting the mammary rudiment with the epidermis becomes very narrow and finally ruptures (Fig. 6). The gland rudiment, which is detached from the epidermis and is buried in the mammary fat pad as a blind duct (Fig. 7),

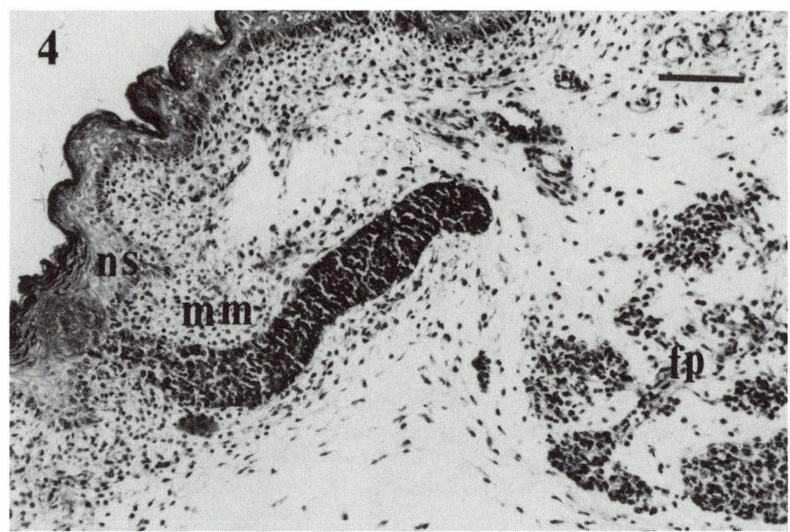

Figure 4. Mammary sprout in the late 16-day female mouse embryo. Nipple sheath (ns) is formed. Lobular structure of the fat pad precursor tissue (fp) is seen below the mammary rudiment. Dense mammary mesenchyme (mm) surrounds the mammary epithelium. Bar = 150 μm. From Sakakura et al. (1982).

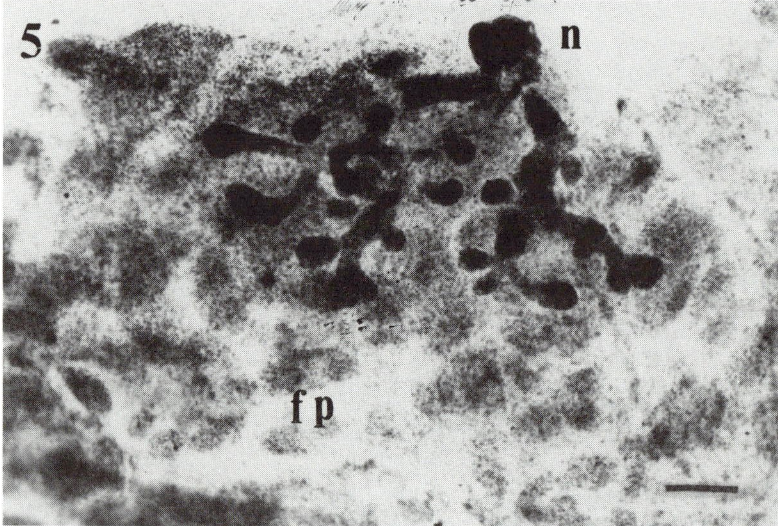

Figure 5. Whole-mount preparation of the mammary gland of newborn mouse. n = nipple, fp = fat pad precursor tissue. Bar = 200 μm.

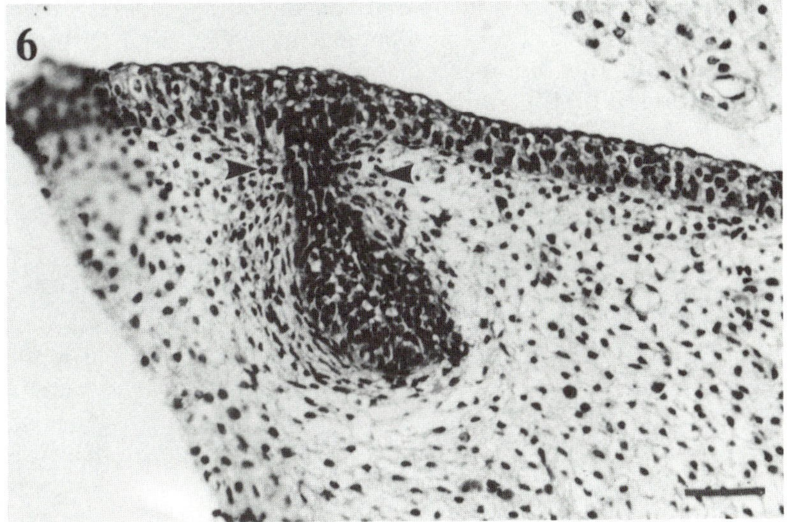

Figure 6. Mammary gland of 15-day male mouse embryo. The epithelial stalk becomes narrowed by mesenchymal cell condensation (arrows). Bar = 50 μm.

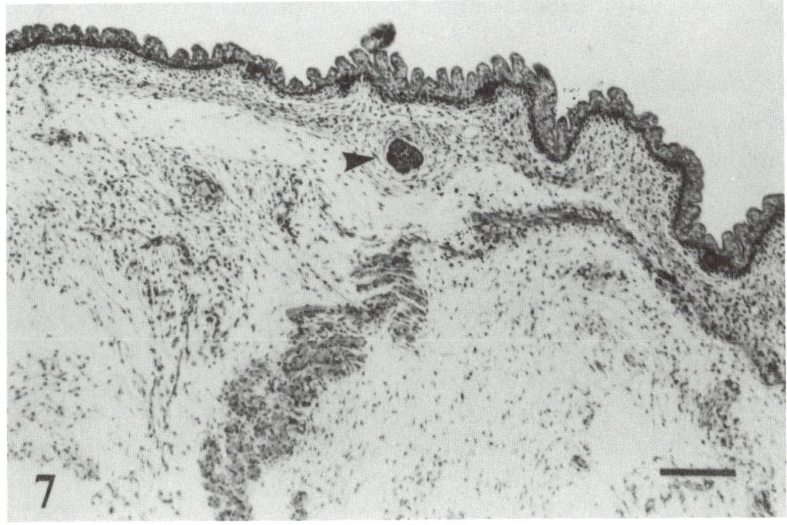

Figure 7. Mammary epithelium of 16-day male mouse embryo. The mammary gland rudiment has detached from the epidermis and becomes buried in the dermis as a blind duct (arrow). Bar = 150 μm.

then undergoes poor growth or even degeneration. There are clear strain differences in this response among mice. For instance, the epithelial rudiment often disappears completely in the mammary fat pad of male mice, and in BALB/c mice about half of the males completely lack mammary glands (Figs. 4–7). In male rats, however, the mammary glands develop as in female rats but have no external outlet.

2.1.4. *Canalization and Mammary Gland Branching*

When mammary epithelial rudiments in females start to elongate late in the 16th day, they form a more or less funnel-shaped outline. The mouth of the funnel is directed toward the surface and is partly filled with cornified cells. At the same time, several intercellular vacuoles are formed in the proximal end of the sprouts. These lumina fuse to make a canal opening to the outside through the mouth of the funnel. At approximately the same time, the primary mammary sprouts elongate by rapid cell proliferation, penetrating mammary fat pad precursor tissue with secondary and tertiary branching. The intercellular vacuolation and the fusion of those vacuoles occur in each sprout to connect its canals with those in a main milk duct. Each mammary gland averages 15–20 branched ducts at birth and retains this morphology, showing no progressive development until puberty. The mammary gland increases its volume only isometrically, in association with the growth of body size.

2.1.5. *Responsiveness to Hormones*

The question of the requirement for any particular hormone(s) in embryonic mammary morphogenesis is important. No one has been able to answer this in vivo because of the difficulties of the complete removal of the various hormones from embryos at early stages. However, as demonstrated by Ceriani (1970a,b), the 17-day embryonic rat mammary gland can respond in vitro to the hormones that induce differentiation in the adult mammary gland. Ceriani cultured 17-day rat embryo mammary anlage in the presence of various combinations of hormones including insulin, aldosterone, prolactin, progesterone, and estrogen. By morphological and biochemical analyses, 17-day embryonic mammary epithelium was shown to grow and penetrate the mesenchyme in response to insulin. Increased proliferation occurred in response to prolactin and ducts ramified into the fat pad in response to added aldosterone. Finally, casein was produced in the presence of all the hormones together. Estrogen had no positive effect but rather was toxic at higher concentrations. This indicates that embryonic mammary epithelium is already determined as real mammary cells at 17 days in utero. In fact, rat mammary epithelium can be distinguished from the epidermis histologically by using monoclonal antibodies at this stage (Dulbecco et al., 1986). A similar in vivo study has been carried out with embryonic mouse mammary epithelium (Sakakura et al., 1976). If the mammary epithelium, isolated from the surrounding mesenchyme, is recombined with salivary mesenchyme and transplanted under the kidney capsule of an adult female mouse, the epithelium undergoes morphogenesis with a typical salivary branching pattern. If the mice carrying the recombinant tissues as grafts are mated and allowed to become pregnant and lactate, the ducts of grafts proliferate and make milk. Thus, embryonic mammary epithelium can differentiate in response to lactogenic hormones.

The mammary gland is a unique organ because of its lack of function prior to lactation. Nevertheless, these experiments demonstrate that mammary epithelium has the capacity for making milk during its embryonic stages when influenced by lactogenic hormones. This would suggest that some regulatory mechanism other than the endocrine system is involved in embryonic mammary epithelial growth and differentiation.

2.2. Mammary Mesenchyme

Many organs are composed of two different tissues, epithelium and mesenchyme. Mutual interactions of these two tissues have been demonstrated to be essential for the sequential events of organogenesis, such as determination, growth, morphogenesis, and cytodifferentiation (Grobstein, 1967; Thesleff and Hurmerinta, 1981; Bissel et al., 1982). In mammary gland development, two distinct mesenchymes are also distinguished. One is dense mammary mesenchyme composed of several layers of fibroblasts immediately attached to the epithelium. The other is mammary fat pad precursor tissue which appears separately posterior to the mammary epithelium (Sakakura et al., 1982). Both the dense mammary mesenchyme and the fat pad precursor tissue participate in mammary gland development, supporting development of epithelium into ductal, lobular, and acinar complex units with structural and functional specificities unique to mammary gland.

2.2.1. Fibroblastic Dense Mammary Mesenchyme

2.2.1a. Anatomy and Histology. As may be noted from Figs. 1 and 2, the dense mammary mesenchyme is not yet a distinct tissue type at 10 and 12 days of gestation. Without specific markers, the distinction between the dense mammary mesenchyme and other surrounding tissues is very difficult. Nevertheless, the presence of a specialized mammary mesenchyme that is functionally different from the surrounding nonmammary mesenchyme has been proposed. Propper (1968) removed the mesodermal tissues from mammary and nonmammary regions of 12-day rabbit embryos and cultured them with epidermis obtained from the prospective mammary and nonmammary regions of 12-day embryos. In this experiment, when the prospective mammary epidermis was combined with nonmammary mesoderm, no mammary bud developed. On the other hand, nonmammary epidermis gave rise to mammary buds when associated with mammary mesoderm. This suggests the presence of a mesenchymal cell population in the dermis which has the capacity to induce mammary gland development.

The dense mammary mesenchyme is first recognized histologically as two to three layers of fibroblasts surrounding the mammary epithelium. This appears at 13 days in mouse embryos, concomitant with penetration of the mammary epithelium into the mammary fat pad precursor tissue. With growth of the mammary bud, fibroblasts beneath the mammary epithelium are densely packed together, forming definitive mammary mesenchyme (Fig. 3). Between the 13th and 15th day, phenotypic differentiation of male and female mammary glands occurs. In the male mammary gland at this stage, the mesenchyme condenses around the mammary bud under the influence of androgen. As a result, the epithelial cells form a stretched, narrow stalk that then degenerates and ruptures (Figs. 6 and 7). In the female mammary gland, the mesenchyme remains around the mammary epithelium without condensation (Fig. 4). However, it is not clear whether this tissue becomes a part of the general subcutaneous tissue in the nipple area, penetrates the fat pad precursor tissue as it migrates with mammary epithelium, or merely disappears.

2.2.1b. Development of Androgen Receptors. The mammary gland is a target for many hormones. In adults, the mammary epithelium proliferates and differentiates in response to hormones produced by the pituitary, adrenal glands, and ovaries. In the embryo, mammary epithelium is not influenced by hormones in vivo, although it has the capacity to respond to those hormones if the epithelium is transferred to culture or into an adult host. On the other hand, the fibroblastic dense mammary mesenchyme is responsive to androgenic hormone during the critical period of embryonic life in mice.

That endogenous androgen is responsible for the development of sexual dimorphism in mammary development in some rodents (Raynaud, 1961) was proved by experimental blockade of embryonic testosterone biosynthesis or function using inhibitors, antagonists, or antibodies (Neumann et al., 1970), or by physical gonadectomy with X-rays (Raynaud and Frilley, 1947). Kratochwil and his co-workers made a series of elegant studies on the function of testosterone in male mammary gland morphogenesis and have shown that mammary mesenchyme is the target tissue for androgen (Kratochwil, 1971; Kratochwil and Schwartz, 1976; Durnberger and Kratochwil, 1980; Heuberger et al., 1982; Wasner et al., 1983). The destruction of mammary glands occurs as a result of mammary mesenchymal condensation caused by androgen secreted by the animal's own testes. Direct evidence for this was obtained with ^{3}H-testosterone autoradiographs. When sections of embryonic mammary gland rudiments were incubated with ^{3}H-labeled androgens such as ^{3}H-testosterone or ^{3}H-5-dihydrotestosterone, the mesenchyme was the only tissue to bind the hormones (Fig. 8). A few cells possessing binding sites for ^{3}H-testosterone can be seen in sections of 12-day mammary glands, but only in those few cells closest to the epithelium. These cells increase in number to about 3000 in each mammary rudiment at day 14. They persist during the whole embryonic period and also in

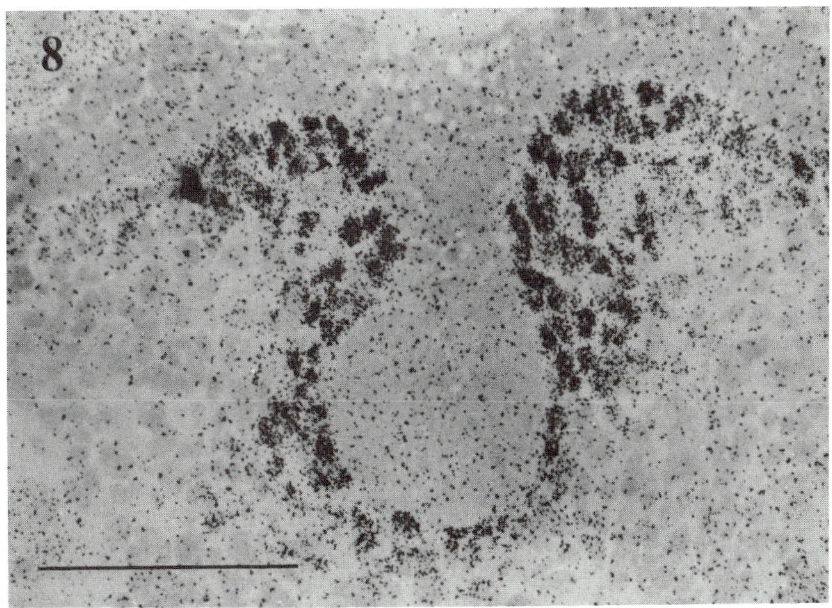

Figure 8. ^{3}H-5-Dihydrotestosterone autoradiograph of a 14-day embryonic mouse mammary rudiment. Bar = 50 μm. From Heuberger et al. (1982).

newborn mice. The location of these labeled cells is limited to the stalk area with a few cells along the invading ducts.

It has been reported that responsiveness to androgen is observed in the mammary mesenchyme only late on the 13th and 14th day of development (Kratochwil, 1977). Except during this critical period, the mammary mesenchyme does not react to androgen even though many androgen receptors are found in the mesenchymal cells and androgen is present. The mechanism by which responsiveness to androgen develops in this particular mesenchyme at such a critical and limited stage is not yet known, but it is clear that for the development of these androgen receptors, epithelial–mesenchymal interaction is necessary. In a series of tissue combinations between epithelium obtained from mammary gland (12-day), salivary gland (13-day), pancreas (11-day), and rabbit mammary epithelium and mammary mesenchyme, it was found that mammary epithelium controls the development of mesenchymal testosterone responsiveness by short-range, organ-specific and species-nonspecific induction of androgen receptor formation. Further details are given in Section 3.1.2.

2.2.1c. Function. During the development of various organs, sequential and reciprocal interactions between epithelium and mesenchyme occur. As a result of those multistep procedures, the epithelial and mesenchymal cells both acquire higher levels of differentiation. Organ development is generally divided into three phases—determination, morphogenesis, and cytodifferentiation. In mammary gland development, the chain of interactions at each developmental phase has been elucidated only partially.

In many organs including the mammary gland, the epithelium forms a characteristic structure and displays its organ-specific functions. Because the mesenchyme, on the other hand, is not a distinct tissue in structure or function, it has often been considered to be only a cell mass occupying the interepithelial spaces. Although definitive products of the specific mesenchyme have been demonstrated in only a few organs, there must be signal exchange between epithelium and mesenchyme either directly or indirectly. In lung and testis, respectively, FPF (Smith, 1979) and P-Mod-S (Skinner and Fritz, 1985) are examples of mesenchymal products stimulating epithelial differentiation. In mammary gland development, two different roles of the mesenchyme have been demonstrated so far. One is an inductive function that determines and fixes the ability of embryonic mammary epithelium to interact with the fatty stroma (Propper, 1968; Sakakura, 1983). The other is a determining factor of phenotypical sex dimorphism as described in Section 3.

2.2.2. Fat Pad Precursor Tissue

2.2.2a. Anatomy and Histology. The other mesenchymal tissue of mammary gland, that is, fatty stroma, develops as a fat pad precursor tissue in the embryonic stage. The earliest appearance of the fat pad precursor tissue in mice may be traced back to the early 14th day of gestation (Fig. 3). At this stage, a somewhat condensed tissue lies below the mammary rudiment which later becomes more visible and can be distinguished from the surrounding tissues such as skin and muscles on day 14. If this condensed tissue is isolated and transplanted under the kidney capsule, it differentiates into fatty tissue in about 2 weeks (Sakakura et al., 1982). Therefore, it appears to be the precursor of the mammary fat pad. At 15–16 days, it converts into a loose tissue (Fig. 9), and then at 16–17 days, preadipocytes form lobular structures associated with a capillary network within the loose connective tissue (Fig. 10). Fatty substances are observed by Sudan III staining in these preadipocytes (Fig. 11). The islets of preadipocytes increase in size and fuse with each other as fat cell differentiation continues. Two or three days after birth, the whole area of the fat pad precursor tissue is converted into typical white fat tissue (Fig. 12).

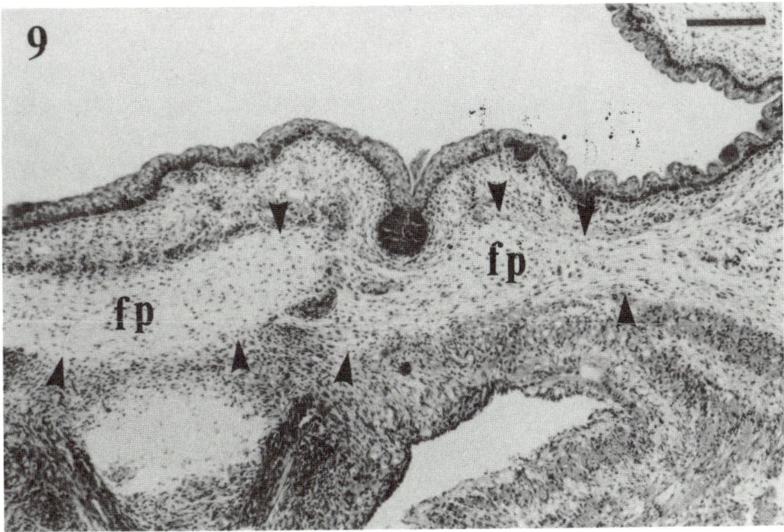

Figure 9. Mammary gland of the late 15-day female mouse embryo. Mammary fat pad precursor tissue (fp) is seen as a loose tissue at this stage (arrows). Bar = 150 μm.

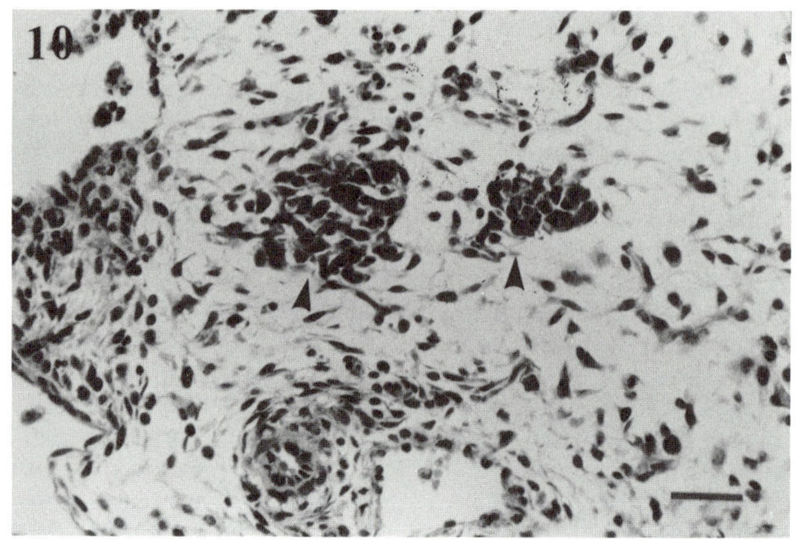

Figure 10. Preadipocyte proliferation forming islets (arrows) in the mammary fat pad precursor tissue. Bar = 30 μm.

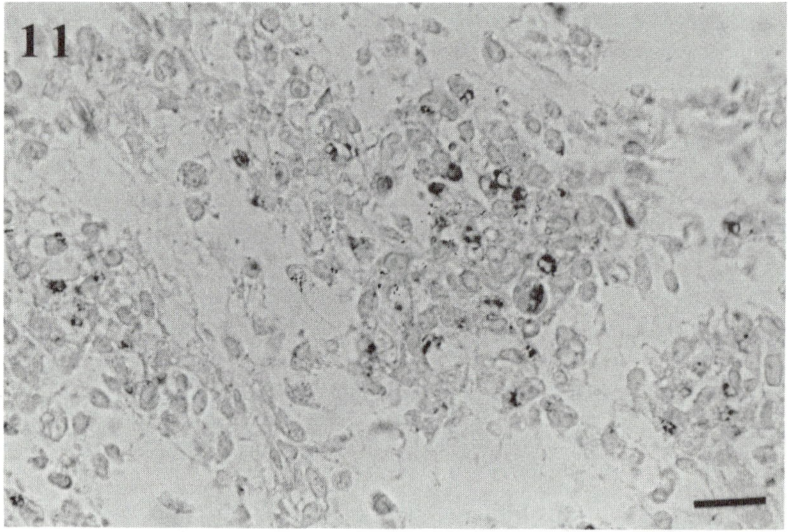

Figure 11. Section indicating the appearance of fat cells in 16-day mammary fat pad precursor tissue. Stained by Sudan III. Bar = 20 μm. From Sakakura et al. (1982).

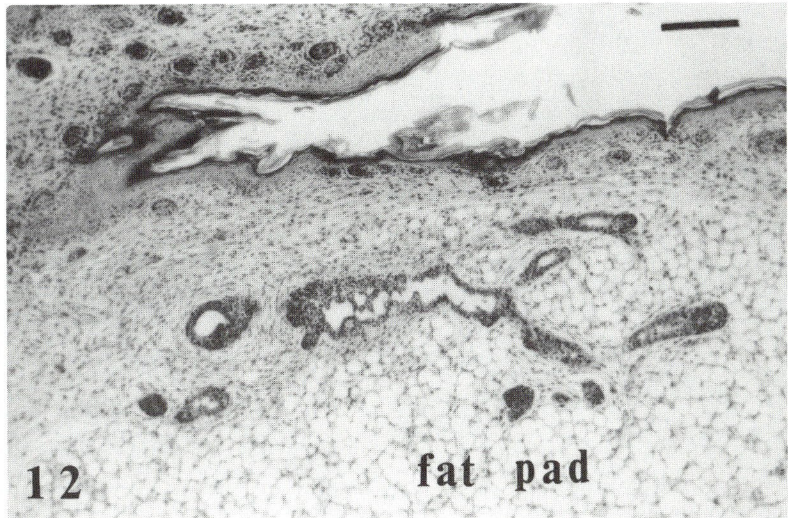

Figure 12. Mammary gland of 3-day-old female mouse neonate. Fat pad precursor tissue is converted into white fat pad. Bar = 200 μm.

2.2.2b. Fat Cell Differentiation. Fat cell differentiation in mammary gland occurs much earlier than in other fat tissue. It is first observed in the mammary gland prior to birth, whereas in other anatomical sites, such as epididymal fat pad, mesentery, and mesometrium, differentiated cells are not observed until 1–3 days postnatally (Slavin, 1979). The lipid droplets increase in size and fuse to make unilocular adipocytes in the mammary gland by 2 days after birth, but this does not happen before 7 days in the other fatty tissues. The origin of adipocytes is still mysterious. Two sources have been considered: typical or specialized fibroblasts (Green and Meuth, 1974; Slavin, 1979) and reticuloendothelial cells (Simon, 1965; Wassermann, 1965; Desnoyers and Vodovar, 1977). The 3T3-Li is a preadipocyte cell line, established by Green and Meuth (1974) from mouse 3T3 fibroblasts. This cell line is capable of making a fat pad when injected into a subcutaneous site (Green and Kehinde, 1979). This result suggested the fibroblast as a likely fat cell precursor. However, several other papers demonstrated morphological evidence of adipocytes derived from or associated with the vascular capillary network (Wassermann, 1965), reticular cells (Simon, 1965), and endothelial cells (Desnoyers and Vodovar, 1977). From these results, the reticuloendothelial cell would be suggested as a preadipocyte. It is not known whether fat cells in the mammary glands and fat cells in many other tissues such as epididymis, mesentery, mesometrium, subcutis, and bone marrow are the same in origin and function.

Enzymatic differentiation of adipocytes precedes morphological differentiation. Hausman and Thomas (1984) have classified adipose tissue differentiation into three stages: I, adipose tissue is histologically distinct from the surrounding connective tissue but does not contain lipid-laden cells or enzyme-reactive cells for lipidogenesis; II, adipocytes are not morphologically differentiated (cells are rounded and basal lamina positive) but are reactive for some enzymes; III, adipocytes are morphologically differentiated and reactive for many enzymes. According to this classification, mammary fat pad precursor tissue of 14-day embryos is in stage I, then develops to stage II at 17 days and stage III at 2–3 days after birth.

2.2.2c. Function. The mammary fat pad precursor tissue is essential for mammary gland morphogenesis at the embryonic stage. If mammary epithelium is separated from the surrounding tissue and recombined with mesenchyme from various other organs, the mammary epithelium makes a typical mammary gland with elongated ducts and end bud formation only when fat pad precursor tissue is used as the associating tissue (Sakakura et al., 1982). Dense fibroblastic mammary mesenchyme imposes a nodular proliferation on the mammary epithelium, characterized by frequent branching with many short ducts. The mechanisms involved in fat pad influence on mammary epithelial morphogenesis are not yet clear. It is well known that a fat cell has its own basement membrane. Accordingly the mammary fat pad is rich in extracellular matrix proteins including laminin, proteoheparan sulfate, and type IV collagen, which in many other tissues are produced by epithelium. This may be a possible hint at the mechanism that accounts for mammary gland morphogenesis, and extensive studies on the role of basal lamina and extracellular matrix materials in mammary morphogenesis are currently under way.

Our observations suggest that the mammary fat pad precursor tissue is an actively contributing organ itself, not merely a tissue occupying the intercellular space. This idea is compatible with the concept of the reticuloendothelial fat organ as proposed by Wassermann and McDonald (1963). If this is correct, mammary fat cells have their own precursor cells which may be called specialized fibroblasts.

2.2.3. Other Cell Types

Blood and lymph vessels and nerves are also found in the stroma. The ontogeny of these tissues has not been investigated systematically.

By histological examination, small blood vessels are observed in the embryonic mammary fat pad, forming capillary plexuses. They become apparent at 16–17 days, when the first fat droplet appears in the preadipocyte. Because of the close relation of each fat cell with the capillary, it is likely that the differentiation of adipocytes and capillaries is coordinated.

It is generally known that in adult mammary gland, a nervous network is associated with the vascular system. Furthermore, cell culture of mammary fat pad precursor tissue clearly indicates the presence of fairly large numbers of nerve cells in the tissue. These nerve cells seem to participate in mammary gland embryogenesis, but their role remains unknown.

2.3. Nipple Development

According to comparative studies of nipple morphogenesis, three main types are classified. These are the proliferation type, the epithelial ingrowth type, and the eversion type (Turner and Gomez, 1933; Anderson, 1978). The nipples of humans and many domestic animals are examples of the proliferation type. In this type, mesenchymal cell proliferation initially occurs surrounding the mammary cord. This results in an elevation of the epidermis followed by formation of nipples. In rodents such as mice, rats, and hamsters, the nipples are of the epithelial ingrowth type. In this type of development, a circular invagination of the epidermis takes place around the mammary cord, representing the nipple sheath (Fig. 4). This occurs at 18 days in the mouse and at 20 days in rat embryos. At approximately the same time, the epidermis inside the annular epidermal ingrowth at the bottom of the mammary pit is lifted, making a rounded elevated portion which is the anlage of the nipple. The formation of the nipple sheath is characteristic in the female mammary gland. Embryos of both sexes, whose gonads were destroyed by irradiation, have nipple sheaths like those of normal female embryos (Raynaud, 1961). This observation adds weight to the evidence that the testis is responsible for the absence of the nipples in male embryos and is compatible with the mechanism of sexual dimorphism in animals in general.

3. Epithelial–Mesenchymal Interactions in Mammary Gland Embryogenesis

The interactions between epithelium and mesenchyme are very important in organogenesis and organostasis in embryos and also in adults. Each process usually occurs reciprocally; the target tissue affects in turn the differentiation of the inductor tissue. Tooth development is the best example of a chain of tissue interactions finally acquiring higher differentiation levels; the mesenchyme affects the epithelium, then in turn the epithelium affects the mesenchyme, and finally the epithelium synthesizes enamel and mesenchyme synthesizes predentin (Thesleff and Hurmerinta, 1981). In mammary gland development, the entire pattern of reciprocal interactions has not yet been elucidated, but a few steps are known. First, mammary mesenchyme determines mammary epithelium and fixes the ability of embryonic mammary epithelium to interact with the fatty stroma. Second, the mammary epithelium induces androgen receptors in the mammary mesenchyme by direct cell–cell contact and thereby controls the development of androgen responsiveness in this tissue. If androgen is present at this stage, the mammary mesenchyme responds to the hormone and condenses around the mammary epithelium, causing destruction of the mammary epithelium.

3.1. Interaction between Mammary Epithelium and Fibroblastic Mammary Mesenchyme

3.1.1. Role of Fibroblastic Mesenchyme in Sexual Differentiation of Mammary Glands in Mice

As described above, male mice and rats have no nipples and mammary gland development is incomplete. In addition to the experiments already described (Raynaud and Frilley, 1947; Kratochwil, 1971), important results have been obtained from studies using androgen-insensitive X^{tfm} (testicular feminization) mutant mice (Kratochwil and Schwartz, 1976; Drews and Drews, 1977). Mammary epithelium and mesenchyme were isolated from Tfm and wild-type mouse embryos. These tissues were then recombined as Tfm epithelium/Tfm or wild-type mesenchyme and wild-type epithelium/Tfm or wild-type mesenchyme and were cultured in the presence of androgenic hormones. Male-type morphogenesis (regression of mammary gland anlage) occurred in all recombinants in which the mesenchyme was derived from wild-type mice but not when it was derived from Tfm mutants. From these studies, it is apparent that the mammary mesenchyme is the actual target and mediator of the morphogenetic effect of androgens on mammary epithelium during development.

Two questions arise concerning (1) the origin of the mesenchymal cells of characteristic condensation around the epithelial bud and (2) the specificity of the characteristics of this dense mammary mesenchyme. Durnberger and Kratochwil (1980) studied the origin of this tissue.

Mammary epithelium that retained a few layers of mesenchyme was recombined with other mammary mesenchyme; the tissues were again obtained from Tfm mutant and wild-type mice, and recombinants were cultured in the presence of testosterone. The mesenchymal cell condensation, which is responsible for the subsequent destruction of mammary epithelial rudiment, occurred only when the wild-type (androgen-responsive) mesenchyme was attached at the epithelial surface. Additionally, this happened even when these mesenchymal cells were taken from young embryos 2 days before the development of androgen receptors at 13–14 days. This demonstrates that the mesenchymal cells required for the reaction are already present at the epithelial surface at least 2 days before the hormone response occurs and that the cells do not migrate there from more distant sites. The mesenchymal competence to respond to androgen is organ specific and seems to be common to various species. If mouse mammary epithelium is cultured with mesenchyme from various sources in the presence of testosterone, the mesenchymal condensation occurs only when the mesenchyme is isolated from mammary gland, even if it is from different species such as rats and rabbits. Mesenchymal cells of nonmammary origin, including pancreatic, pulmonary, or salivary, showed no effect on the testosterone-induced condensation.

As described in Section 3.1.2, there is one molecule that is known to be present in the dense mammary mesenchyme but that is present neither in the fat pad precursor tissue nor in the general subcutis. This is a recently described glycoprotein called *tenascin* (Chiquet-Ehrismann et al., 1986). By using antibodies against tenascin, it is possible to distinguish between the dense mammary mesenchyme and the fat pad precursor tissue in sections. If tenascin is a specific biochemical marker of the dense mammary mesenchyme, an analysis of the function of this molecule may bring an answer to the second question regarding the specificity of the dense mesenchyme.

3.1.2. Role of Mammary Epithelium in the Development of Androgen Receptors in Fibroblastic Mesenchyme

Heuberger et al. (1982) have studied the interaction between mammary epithelium and mammary mesenchyme in the development of androgen responsiveness by receptor autoradiography. They made tissue recombinations similar to those in the experiment described above and examined the appearance and distribution of testosterone-binding cells as an indication of androgen responsiveness. When pure mammary epithelium was cultured with mammary mesenchyme obtained from young embryos before androgen receptors had developed, each piece of mammary epithelium was surrounded by a halo of ^{3}H-testosterone-binding mesenchymal cells. However, if mesenchyme from nonmammary sources such as pancreas and epidermis was employed, no labeled mesenchymal cells developed. From this result, they concluded that the androgen receptors are specifically induced in the adjacent mesenchyme by mammary epithelium.

3.2. Interaction between Mammary Epithelium and Fat Pad Precursor Tissue

At the beginning of mammary gland embryogenesis, the epithelium is surrounded by dense mammary mesenchyme. Then, when fat cell differentiation starts (at 16–17 days in mouse embryos and 19–20 days in rat embryos), the mammary epithelium breaks through the sheath of the dense mammary mesenchyme and penetrates fat pad precursor tissue with rapid ductal elongation and branching. At this stage, the mammary epithelium interacts with fat pad precursor tissue, an obligatory step in determining the characteristic structure of mammary gland. If embryonic mammary epithelium is recombined with the dense mammary mesenchyme and transplanted under the kidney capsule, it devel-

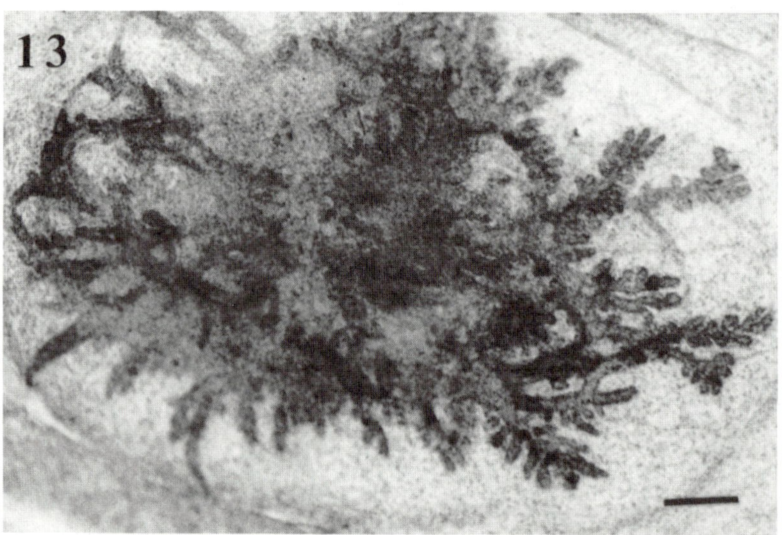

Figure 13. Whole-mount preparation of 17-day mammary epithelium recombined with dense mammary mesenchyme from 14-day embryo, 3 weeks after transplantation under the kidney capsule. The resulting gland develops a ductal hyperplasia with frequent short branching. Bar = 200 μm.

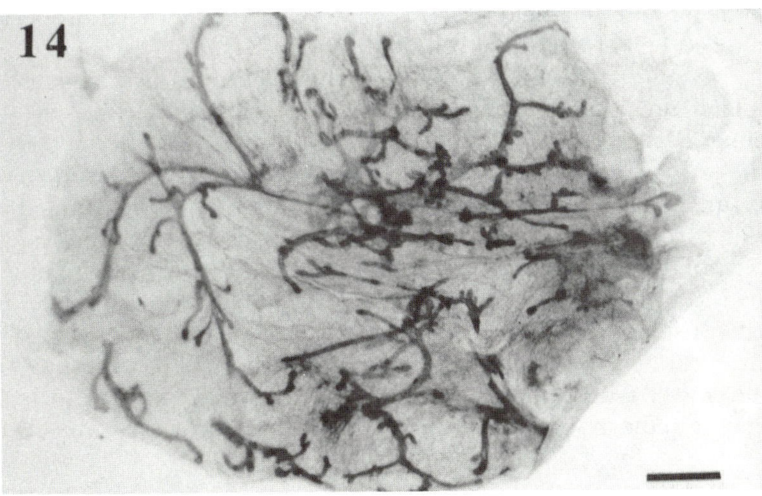

Figure 14. Whole-mount preparation of 17-day mammary epithelium recombined with fat pad precursor tissue from 14-day embryo, 3 weeks after transplantation under the kidney capsule. The resulting gland undergoes typical mammary gland morphogenesis with the "stretching out" of the ducts. Bar = 200 μm.

ops a ductal hyperplasia with frequent branching but without the "stretching out" of the ducts (Fig. 13). But if the mammary epithelium is recombined with fat pad precursor tissue, it undergoes a typical mammary gland morphogenesis with the "stretching out" of the ducts (Sakakura et al., 1982) (Fig. 14). Thus, for development of characteristic mammary morphology, fat pad precursor tissue is essential. The molecular mechanism of this interacting capacity is unclear but may be based on the stimulation by a growth-factor-like substance produced by fat pad precursor tissue.

4. Extracellular Matrix Proteins in Embryonic Mammary Gland

The interactions between two different tissues such as epithelium and mesenchyme may be mediated by one or more diffusible or nondiffusible signal substances. These include hormones, growth factors, and extracellular matrix proteins. The major groups of the extracellular matrix proteins are collagens, glycoproteins, and proteoglycans. Among these molecules, laminin, proteoheparan sulfate, and type IV collagen are synthesized by mammary epithelium (Liotta et al., 1979; Gordon and Bernfield, 1980; Silberstein and Daniel, 1982; Ormerod et al., 1983;

Rapraeger and Bernfield, 1983; Kimata et al., 1985), while fibronectin is produced by mesenchymal cells.

Even though a variety of molecules have been discovered that could mediate interactions between epithelium and mesenchyme, the total number of molecular types is small. And yet each tissue in the body has tissue-specific interactions that govern its characteristic morphogenesis and functional differentiation. The question as to how this limited variety of extracellular matrix molecular types can generate the required variety of signals and create the unique matrix necessary for organ specificity is central to the study of tissue interaction. Three possibilities have been considered: (1) differences in the molecular composition of the matrix, (2) new element(s) produced by interactions of molecules from different cell types at the molecular level, and (3) structural information inherent in the matrix architecture. To date, none of these three mecha-

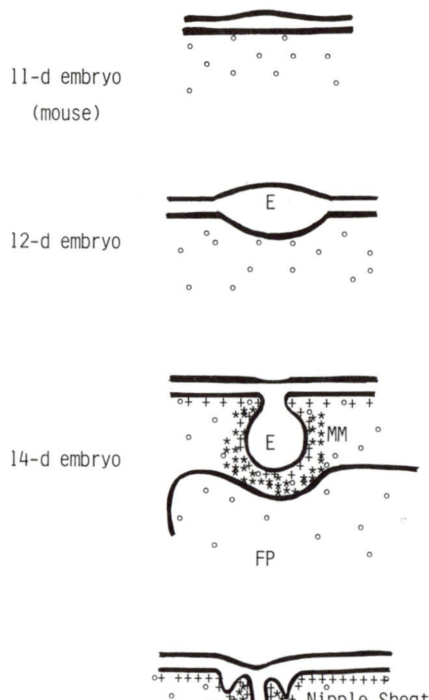

Figure 15. Distribution of extracellular matrix proteins during mouse mammary gland embryogenesis. ○, Fibronectin; +, Laminin, Proteoheparansulphate; *, Tenascin; E, Mammary epithelium; MM, dense fibroblastic mammary mesenchyme; FP, fat pad precursor tissue.

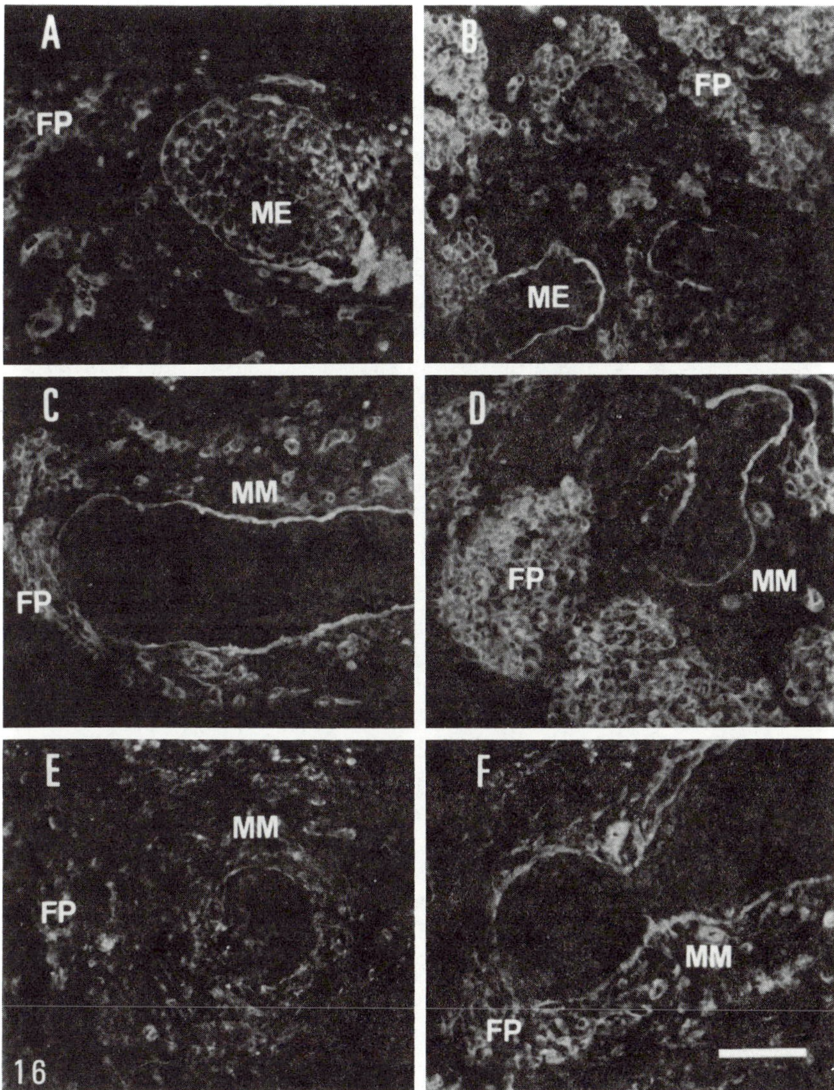

Figure 16. Immunofluorescent localization of laminin (A, B), proteoheparan sulfate (C,D), and fibronectin (E,F) in 17-day (left column) and 18-day (right column) embryonic mammary glands. ME = mammary epithelium, MM = dense mammary mesenchyme, FP = fat pad precursor tissue. Bar = 100 μm. From Kimata et al. (1985).

nisms has been shown to account for the tissue specificity in epithelial–mesenchymal interactions.

With regard to the mammary gland, there are several papers describing the development of the extracellular matrix proteins during embryogenesis in mice and rats (Kimata et al., 1985; Chiquet-Ehrismann et al., 1986). Figure 15 summarizes the results. Fibronectin is produced by both mammary mesenchyme and dermal fibroblasts throughout mammary gland embryogenesis. Laminin and proteoheparan sulfate, on the other hand, are present in the basement membrane lying between epithelium and mesenchyme at 14 days in mice. Late on the 16th day, fat pad precursor cells start to deposit fatty substance and the mammary epithelial element starts to grow, penetrating the fat pad precursor tissue. At the same time, the fat pad precursor cells initiate synthesis of laminin and proteoheparan sulfate which usually are produced by the epithelium (Fig. 16). However, there is no evidence as to how these proteins participate in the formation of basement membrane of mammary gland. An interesting observation, however, is the degradation of basement membrane at the tip of the developing mammary duct. As described in Chapter 1, the basement membrane underlying the mammary epithelium of young adult and early pregnant mice is heterogeneous in composition and structure. It is thinner or discontinuous at the tip of the growing end bud. That the same situation occurs in both embryos and adults strongly suggests the importance of extracellular matrix substances in the ductal morphogenesis of mammary gland.

Tenascin is the recently proposed name for a new extracellular matrix protein previously called *myotendinous antigen* (Chiquet and Fambrough, 1984a,b) and resembles *hexabrachion* (Erickson and Inglesias, 1984) and *J1* (Kruse et al., 1985). Tenascin was found in mammary mesenchyme closely surrounding the budding epithelial rudiment in the embryo but not in the general subcutaneous fibroblasts or the fat pad precursor tissue (Fig. 17). Interestingly, tenascin is not detected in the adult mammary gland even during pregnancy. However, it reappears in malignant tumors at the site of tumor growth and in the fibrous tissue in contact with the neoplastic epithelium. Since tenascin is specifically present in dense mammary mesenchyme, these fibroblasts must be different from other fibroblasts.

In all, there is a sufficient number of well-established but fragmental findings on epithelial–mesenchymal interactions in mammary gland embryogenesis to suggest that the embryonic mammary gland is an excellent model for the study of the regulation of growth and differentiation by tissue interactions.

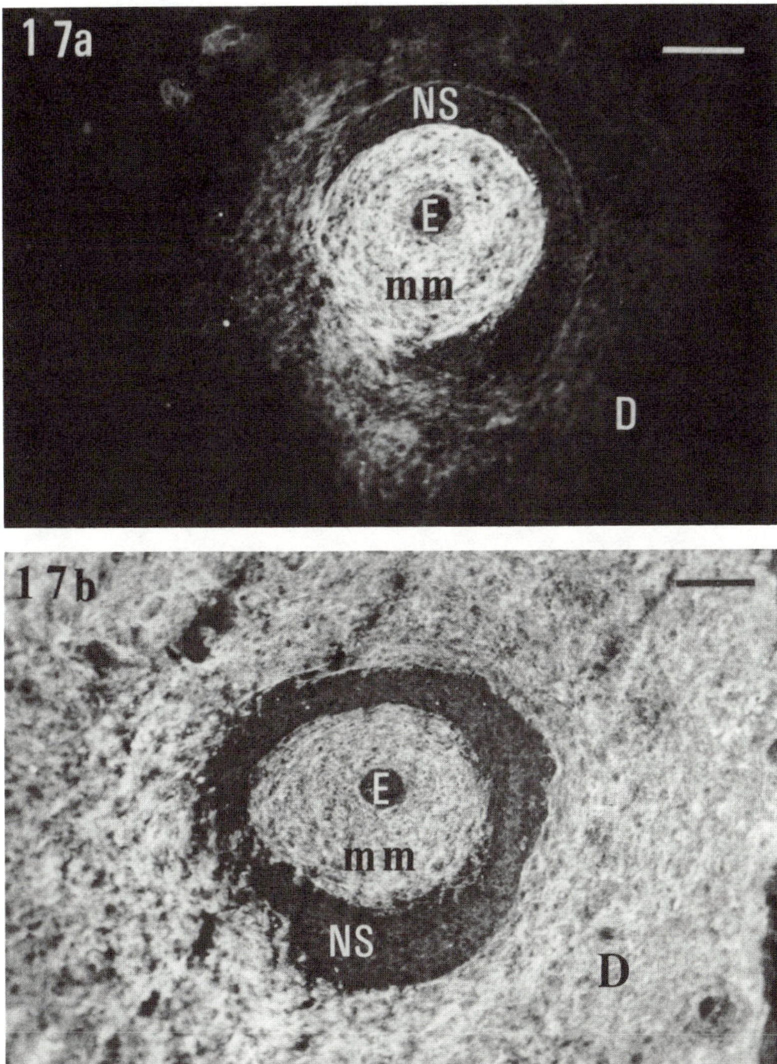

Figure 17. Indirect immunofluorescence of cryosections of 20-day embryonic rat mammary gland showing the distribution of extracellular matrix proteins. Stained with antisera to tenascin (a), fibronectin (b), and laminin (c). E = mammary epithelium, MM = dense mammary mesenchyme, D = dermis, NS = nipple sheath. Tenascin is present only in the dense mammary mesenchyme, while fibronectin and laminin are present throughout the subepithelial tissue. Bar = 50 μm. From Chiquet-Ehrismann et al. (1986).

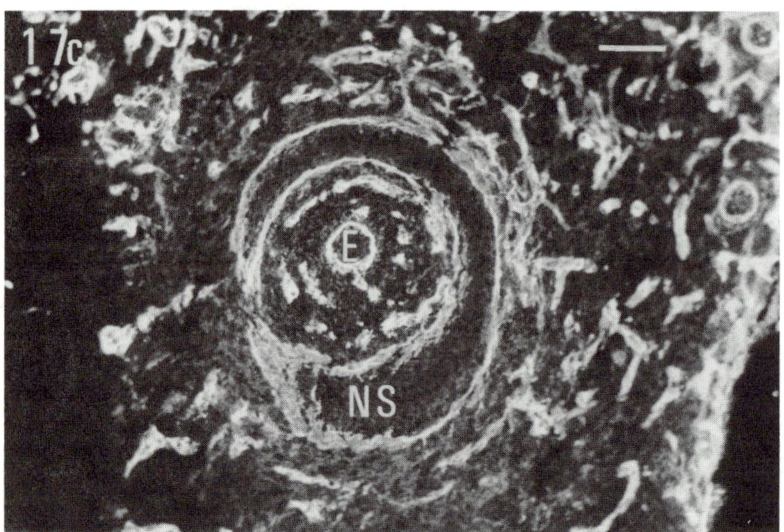

Figure 17. *(Continued)*

5. Summary

Mammary gland morphogenesis is described from the perspective of developmental biology, mainly in mice and rats.

1. Mammary epithelium first appears at 10–11 days in mouse embryos with enlargement of a single-layered ectoderm forming the mammary streak, which is a line of cells extending from the anterior limb bud to the posterior limb bud. These cells then migrate to the location where mammary glands will form, giving rise to mammary buds (five pairs in mice and six pairs in rats). The mammary bud forms a lens-shaped structure at 12 days and then changes to a bulb-shaped structure at 14 days. On day 14, the sexual phenotype is determined in the mammary gland. In female embryos, the mammary gland is in the *resting phase* during the 11th to 16th day of gestation, showing very slow or no growth. At the late 16th day, the mammary bud elongates by rapid cellular proliferation forming the mammary sprout, which penetrates mammary fat pad precursor tissue undergoing an initial branching. This then grows to form the mammary ductal tree system with about 15–20 branching ducts by birth.

2. In mammary embryogenesis, two different mesenchymes can be distinguished. One is dense mammary mesenchyme which is important for the early stages of mammary morphogenesis. The other is mammary fat pad precursor tissue which converts into white fat at the neonatal stage and is essential for typical mammary gland morphogenesis.
3. Mutual interactions between epithelium and these two mesenchymes are important in mammary gland embryogenesis. First, mammary mesenchyme determines mammary epithelium and fixes the ability of the epithelium to interact with the fatty stroma. Second, the mammary epithelium induces androgen receptors in the dense mammary mesenchyme. If androgen is present at this stage, the mammary mesenchyme responds to the hormone and condenses around the mammary epithelium, causing its destruction. As a result of this interaction, nipples are not developed in male mice and rats.
4. These two mammary mesenchymes synthesize different extracellular matrix proteins. The dense mammary mesenchyme makes fibronectin and tenascin, while the fat pad precursor tissue makes basal lamina substances such as laminin and proteoheparan sulfate.

References

Anderson, R.R., 1978, Embryonic and fetal development of the mammary apparatus, in: *Lactation: Comprehensive Treatise,* Vol. 4 (B.L. Larson, ed.), Academic Press, New York, pp. 3–40.

Balinsky, B.I., 1950, On the pre-natal growth of the mammary gland rudiment in the mouse, *J. Anat.* **84:**227–235.

Bissel, M.J., Hall, H.G., and Parry, G., 1982, How does the extracellular matrix direct gene expression? *J. Theor. Biol.* **99:**31–68.

Ceriani, R.L., 1970a, Fetal mammary gland differentiation in vitro in response to hormones. I. Morphological findings, *Dev. Biol.* **21:**506–529.

Ceriani, R.L., 1970b, Fetal mammary gland differentiation in vitro in response to hormones. II. Biochemical findings, *Dev. Biol.* **21:**530–546.

Chiquet, M., and Fambrough, D.M., 1984a, Chick myotendinous antigen. I. A monoclonal antibody as a marker for tendon and muscle morphogenesis, *J. Cell Biol.* **98:**1926–1936.

Chiquet, M., and Fambrough, D.M., 1984b, Chick myotendinous antigen. II. A novel extracellular glycoprotein complex consisting of large disulfide-linked subunits, *J. Cell Biol.* **98:**1937–1946.

Chiquet-Ehrismann, R., Mackie, E.J., Pearson, C.A., and Sakakura, T., 1986, Tenascin: An extracellular matrix protein involved in tissue interactions during fetal development and oncogenesis, *Cell* **47:**131–139.

Desnoyers, F., and Vodovar, N., 1977, Etude histocytologique comparee chez le porc et le rat du tissu adipeux perirenal au stade de son apparition, *Biol. Cell* **29:**178–182.

Drews, U., and Drews, U., 1977, Regression of mouse mammary gland anlagen in recombinants of Tfm and wild-type tissues: Testosterone acts via the mesenchyme, *Cell* **10:**401–404.

Dulbecco, R., Allen, W.R., Bologna, M., and Bowman, M., 1986, Marker evolution during the development of the rat mammary gland: Stem cells identified by markers and the role of myoepithelial cells, *Cancer Res.* **46:**2449–2456.

Durnberger, H., and Kratochwil, K., 1980, Specificity of tissue interactions and origin of mesenchymal cells in the androgen response of the embryonic mammary gland, *Cell* **19:**465–471.

Erickson, H.P., and Inglesias, J.L., 1984, A six-armed oligomer isolated from cell surface fibronectin preparations, *Nature* **311:**267–269.

Gordon, J.R., and Bernfield, M.R.M., 1980, The basal lamina of the postnatal mammary epithelium contains glycosaminoglycans in a precise ultrastructure organization, *Dev. Biol.* **74:**118–135.

Green, H., and Kehinde O., 1979, Formation of normally differentiated subcutaneous fat pads by an established preadipose cell line, *J. Cell. Physiol.* **101:**169–172.

Green, H., and Meuth, M., 1974, An established preadipose cell line and its differentiation in culture, *Cell* **3:**127–133.

Grobstein, C., 1967, Mechanisms of organogenetic tissue interaction, *Nat. Cancer Inst. Monogr.* **26:**279–299.

Hausman, G.J., and Thomas, G.B., 1984, Enzyme histochemical differentiation of white adipose tissue in the rat, *Am. J. Anat.* **169:**315–326.

Heuberger, B., Fitzka, I., Wasner, G., and Kratochwil, K., 1982, Induction of androgen receptor formation by epithelial–mesenchymal interaction in embryonic mouse mammary gland, *Proc. Natl. Acad. Sci. USA* **79:**2957–2961.

Kimata, K., Sakakura, T., Inaguma, Y., Kato, M., and Nishizuka, Y., 1985, Participation of two different mesenchymes in the developing mouse mammary gland: Synthesis of basement membrane components by fat pad precursor cells, *J. Embryol. Exp. Morphol.* **89:**243–257.

Kratochwil, K., 1971, In vitro analysis of the hormonal basis for the sexual dimorphism in the embryonic development of the mouse mammary gland, *J. Embryol. Exp. Morphol.* **25:**141–153.

Kratochwil, K., 1977, Development and loss of androgen responsiveness in the embryonic mammary rudiment of the mouse mammary gland, *Dev. Biol.* **61:**358–365.

Kratochwil, K., and Schwartz, P., 1976, Tissue interaction in androgen response of embryonic mammary rudiment of mouse: Identification of target tissue for testosterone, *Proc. Natl. Acad. Sci. USA* **73:**4041–4044.

Kruse, J., Keilhauer, G., Faissner, A., Timpl, R., and Schachner, M., 1985, The J1 glycoprotein—a novel nervous system cell adhesion molecule of the L2/HNK-1 family, *Nature* **316:**146–148.

Liotta, L.A., Wicha, M.S., Foidart, J.-M., Rennard, S.I., Garbisa, S., and Kidwell, W.R., 1979, Hormonal requirements for basement membrane collagen deposition by cultured rat mammary epithelium, *Lab. Invest.* **41:**511–518.

Myers, J.A., 1917, Studies on the mammary gland. II. The fetal development of the mammary gland on the female albino rat, *Am. J. Anat.* **22:**195–223.

Neumann, F., Berswordt-Wallrabe, von R., Elger, W., Steinbeck, H, Hahn, J.D., and Kramer, M., 1970, Aspects of androgen-dependent events as studied by antiandrogens, *Recent Prog. Horm. Res.* **26:**337–410.

Ormerod, E.J., Warburton, M.J., Hughes, C., and Rudland, P.S., 1983, Synthesis of basement membrane proteins by rat mammary epithelial cells, *Dev. Biol.* **96**:269–275.

Propper, A.Y., 1968, Relations epidermo-meseodermiques dans la differenciation de l'ebauche mammaire d'embryon de lapin, *Ann. Embryol. Morphogen.* **2**:151–160.

Propper, A.Y., 1978, Wandering epithelial cells in the rabbit embryo milk line, *Dev. Biol.* **67**:225–231.

Rapraeger, A.C., and Bernfield, M.R., 1983, Heparan sulphate proteoglycans from mouse mammary epithelial cells, *J. Biol. Chem.* **258**:3632–3636.

Raynaud, A., 1961, Morphogenesis of the mammary gland, in: *Milk: The Mammary Gland and Its Secretion,* Vol. 1 (S.K. Kon and A.T. Cowie, eds.) Academic Press, New York, pp. 3–46.

Raynaud, A., and Frilley, M., 1947, Destruction des glandes genitales, de l'embryon de souris, par une irradiation au moyen des rayons X, a l'age de treize jours, *Ann. Endocrinol. Paris* **8**:400–419.

Raynaud, A., and Raynaud, J., 1953, Les principales etapes de pa separation, d'avec l'epiderme, des ebauches mammaires des foetus males de souris; recherches sur les processus de la rupture de la tige du bourgeon mammaire, *C.R. Soc. Biol. Paris* **147**:1872–1876.

Rein, G., 1881–1882, Untersuchungen uber die embryonale Entwicklungsgeschichte der Milchdruse, *Arch. Mikr. Anat.* **20**(5.21),431,678.

Sakakura, T., 1983, Epithelial–mesenchymal interactions in mammary gland development and its perturbation in relation to tumorigenesis, in: *Understanding Breast Cancer: Clinical and Laboratory Concepts* (M.A. Rich, J.C. Hager, and P. Furmanski, eds.), Marcel Dekker, New York, pp. 261–284.

Sakakura, T., Nishizuka, Y., and Dawe, C.J., 1976, Mesenchyme-dependent morphogenesis and epithelium-specific cytodifferentiation in mouse mammary gland, *Science* **194**:1439–1441.

Sakakura, T., Sakagami, Y., and Nishizuka, Y., 1982, Dual origin of mesenchymal tissues participating in mouse mammary gland embryogenesis, *Dev. Biol.* **91**:202–207.

Silberstein, G.B., and Daniel, G.W., 1982, Glycosaminoglycans in the basal lamina and extracellular matrix of the developing mouse mammary duct, *Dev. Biol.* **90**:215–222.

Simon, G., 1965, Histogenesis, in: *Handbook of Physiology, Section 5: Adipose Tissue* (A.E. Renald and G.F. Cahill, Jr., eds.), American Physiology Society, Washington, DC, pp. 101–107.

Skinner, M.K., and Fritz, I.B., 1985, Testicular peritubular cells secrete a protein under androgen control that modulates Sertoli cell functions, *Proc. Natl. Acad. Sci. USA* **82**:114–118.

Slavin, B.G., 1979, Fine structural studies on white adipocyte differentiation, *Anat. Rec.* **195**:63–72.

Smith, B.T., 1979, Lung maturation in the fetal rat: Acceleration by injection of fibroblast-pneumonocyte factor, *Science* **204**:1094–1096.

Thesleff, I., and Hurmerinta, K., 1981, Tissue interactions in tooth development, *Differentiation* **18**:75–88.

Turner, C.W., and Gomez, E.T., 1933, The normal development of the mammary gland of the male and female albino mouse. I. Intrauterine, *Mo. Agric. Exp. Stn. Res. Bull.* **182**:3–20.

Wasner, G., Hennermann, I., and Kratochwil, K., 1983, Ontogeny of mesenchymal androgen receptors in the embryonic mouse mammary gland, *Endocrinology* **113**:1771–1780.

Wassermann, F., 1965, The development of adipose tissue, in: *Handbook of Physiology,*

Section 5: Adipose Tissue (A.E. Renald and G.F. Cahill, Jr., eds.), American Physiological Society, Washington, DC, pp. 87–100.

Wassermann, F., and McDonald, 1963, Electron microscopic study of adipose tissue (fat organs) with special reference to the transport of lipids between blood and fat cells, *Z. Zellforsch. Mikrosk. Anat. Abt. Histochem.* **59:**326.

3

Development of the Human Mammary Gland

Jose Russo and Irma H. Russo

1. Introduction

Mammary gland development is probably one of the most fascinating and puzzling biological phenomena. The most important element in this puzzle is the fact that the mammary gland seems to be the only organ that is not fully developed at birth (Dawson, 1934; Dabelow, 1957; Salazar and Tobon, 1974; Vorherr, 1974). Although immaturity at birth can be assumed in most systems, no other organ presents such dramatic changes in size, shape, and function as does the breast during growth, puberty, pregnancy, and lactation (Dawson, 1934; Geschickter, 1945; Dabelow, 1957; Ingleby and Gershon-Cohen, 1960; Tanner, 1962). Breast involution does not remain out of the picture, since it is during this period that the development of cancer becomes manifest (Leis, 1978).

This complex organ therefore has to be described in its anatomy, histology, ultrastructure, physiology, or response to hormones not as a static picture, but as a dynamic phenomenon in which each phase is transitory and heavily dependent on the age at which it is studied and the specific conditions of the host. No study of breast development, however, can depart from the morphology of the organ, since all endocrinologic, dietetic, or environmental influences have a morphologically

---

Jose Russo and Irma H. Russo • Department of Pathology, Michigan Cancer Foundation, Detroit, Michigan 48201.

observable and quantitative effect on the gland (Lyons et al., 1953, 1958; Cowie and Folley, 1961; King et al., 1983; Alvarez-Sanz et al., 1986).

The assessment of mammary development requires the use of morphometric techniques to elucidate the complex process of interaction between two embryologically different, though deeply interconnected, tissues—the parenchyma and the stroma (Dawson, 1934; Dabelow, 1957; Vorherr, 1974). The peculiar tree-like structure of the mammary gland, in which the branches of the tree are the ducts lined by epithelium, as well as the topographic localization of the areas of proliferation, requires the observation of the organ in three dimensions, such as in whole-mount preparations, to establish precisely within the tree the location of every specific structure. Using this approach, the authors have undertaken a systematic study of the gland in its different stages of development. Those stages of development in which the authors do not have original contributions are outlined briefly, and the reader is referred to the original sources.

2. Prenatal and Perinatal Development

Regarding the mammary gland's prenatal development, descriptive embryology has already demonstrated the genesis of the form and structure of the organ, since observations on the human mammary anlage date back to 1820. As reviewed by Dawson (1934) and Bassler (1970), Koelliker in 1879 and 1890, Langer in 1851, and Schmidt in 1897 carried out genuine embryological studies of the human mammary gland, and both Koelliker and Langer established that the whole mammary parenchyma arises from a single epithelial ectodermal bud.

Although in general most authors agree on the successive stages of development of the mammary gland during the embryonic and fetal stages, there are variations in nomenclature, and the exact time of appearance of each structure varies whether the authors choose to express the age of the embryo based on the estimated time of conception, the last missed menstrual period, or the length of the embryo. Because of the difficulties in establishing precisely the day of conception, we personally consider it more accurate to correlate the phases of mammary gland development with embryonal or fetal length.

There is consensus in the literature that the milk streak is first observed during the 4th week of embryonal life in the 2.5-mm-long embryo (Dawson, 1934). This becomes the mammary ridge or milk line during the 5th week, when the embryo measures 2.5–5.5 mm (Dawson, 1934; Dabelow, 1957; Vorherr, 1974). Dabelow (1957) made the most complete systematic description of mammary gland development, dividing this process into the following 10 different stages: (1) the mammary ridge stage followed by (2) the milk hill stage, with thickening of the mammary ridge (6th week, 5.5- to 11.0-mm embryo), form the early stages. When parenchymal cells start to invade the underlying stroma, the (3) mammary disc stage arises, progressing to a (4) globular stage, observed between the 7th and 8th week in the 11.0- to 25.0-mm embryos. The (5) cone stage, occurring at the 9th week, is characterized by further inward growth of the mammary parenchyma and, concomitantly, the protrusion of the overlying skin regresses. Between the 10th and 12th week (30- to 68-mm embryo), epithelial buds sprout from the invading parenchyma (6, budding stage); these newly formed buds become lobular in shape, with notching at the epithelial–stromal border, a stage known as (7) indentation, which occurs between the 12th and 13th week. Further branching into 15–25 epithelial strips or solid cords, marks the (8) branching stage, which occurs in the 15-week-old (10-cm) fetus, according to Vorherr (1974), between the 13th and 20th week of pregnancy, according to Dabelow (1957), or in the 6-month-old (20-cm) fetus according to Raynaud (1960). The solid cords become canalized by desquamation and lysis of the central epithelial cells (Dawson, 1934; Raynaud, 1960); this is the (9) canalization stage, which occurs between 20 and 32 weeks of gestation (Dabelow, 1957), although Raynaud (1960)

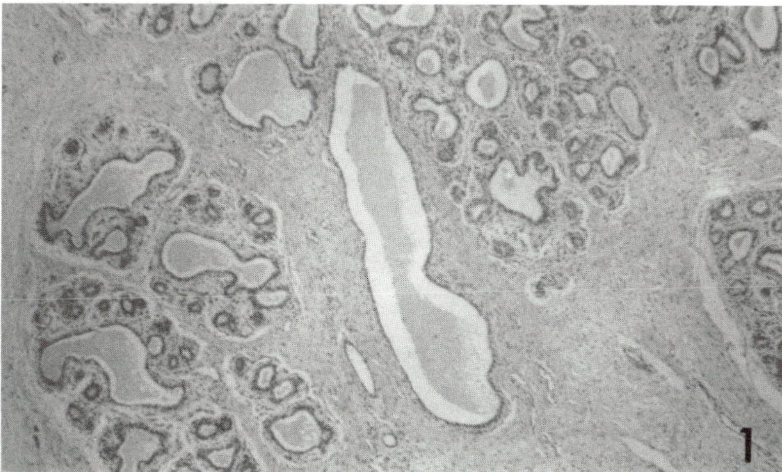

Figure 1. Mammary gland of a 2-week-old female containing a ductal structure and primitive ductolobular elements. The luminae of all structures are dilated and filled with proteinaceous fluid (hematoxylin and eosin, H&E, ×25).

considers that this process occurs simultaneously with branching, in the 22- to 25-week-old fetus (18–20 cm). A great discrepancy exists among various authors with regard to the last stage, occurring between 32 and 40 weeks of gestation; Dabelow (1957) and Vorherr (1974) described it as a process of lobuloalveolar development, the (10) end-vesicle stage, in

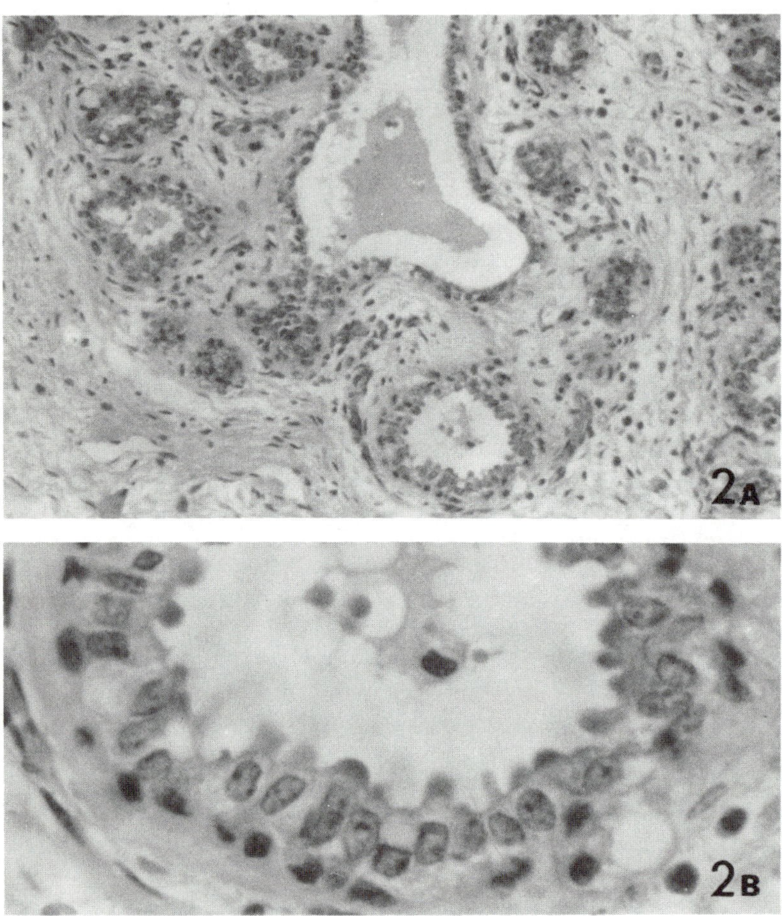

Figure 2. (A) Higher magnification of the gland shown in Fig. 1 reveals the duct and ductolobular structures to be lined by one layer of epithelial and one of myoepithelial cells. The periductal and intralobular stroma are similar and composed of fibroblasts (H&E, ×100). (B) The epithelium lining the ductolobular structures of the gland shown in Fig. 1 is low columnar and shows evidence of apocrine secretion. The cytoplasm is finely vacuolated owing to the presence of lipid droplets. The secreted material consists of proteinaceous fluid and occasional desquamated cells (H&E, ×400).

which the end vesicles are composed of a monolayer of epithelium and contain colostrum. Dawson (1934), on the other hand, considered that the canalized mammary duct is lined by two epithelial layers, and no true "secretion" occurs, but just a nipple discharge of lysed and desquamated cells. This author never observed lobules in fetal material, sustaining that lobules are not usually formed until the breast is approaching the functional development associated with the onset of puberty. Dawson (1934) refers to previous studies carried out by Berka in 1912, who mentions that the "colostrum secretion of the newborn" is not associated with the formation of secreting alveoli; Lewis and Bremer in 1927 described the "milky secretion" at birth as composed of leukocytes with or without ingested fat. It is considered that this secretion, which is commonly known as witch's milk, is equivalent to the mother's colostrom (Bloom and Fawcett, 1968; Vorherr, 1974; Hiba et al., 1977).

In our own observations, development of very primitive lobular structures (Fig. 1), composed of ducts ending in short ductules lined by one layer of epithelial and one of myoepithelial cells (Figs. 1, 2A, and 2B), was observed in the mammary gland of five newborn females. The epithelial cells have an eosinophilic cytoplasm, with typical apocrine secretion (Fig. 2B). The fine cytoplasmic vacuolization observed in the epithelial cells is due to the presence of lipid droplets, as confirmed electron microscopically (results not shown). However, secretory activity does not seem to be confined to the primitive alveolar structures, since the whole ductal system appears dilated, secretion filled, and lined by a secretory-type epithelium (Figs. 1 and 2A). These observations suggest that secretory activity is not a specialized function of the primitive lobules of the newborn, but rather, part of the generalized response of all the mammary epithelium to maternal hormonal levels (Hiba et al., 1977). The secretory activity of the newborn gland subsides within 3–4 weeks.

3. Postnatal Development

Mammary gland development during childhood does little more than keep pace with the general growth of the body until the approach of puberty (Tanner, 1962).

3.1. Adolescence

Although the main changes occurring in the mammary gland are initiated at puberty, the ulterior development of the gland varies greatly

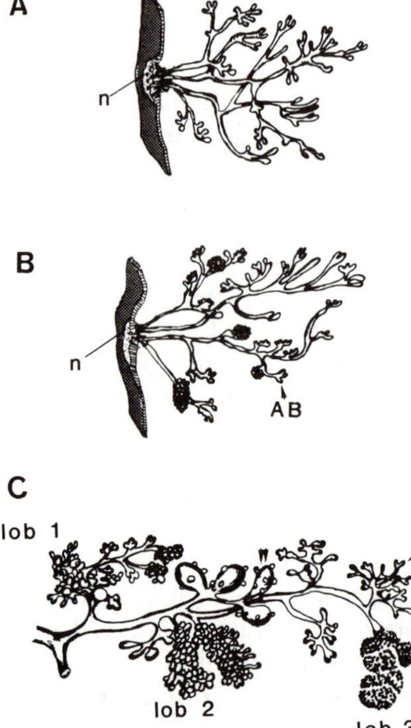

Figure 3. Schematic representation of breast development. (A) At puberty or during its onset, the ducts grow and divide in a dichotomous and sympodial basis ending in terminal end buds. (B) After the first menstruation, the first lobular structures appear (lobules type 1, see also Figs. 5–12); they are composed of alveolar buds (AB). Some branches end in terminal end buds like those depicted in Fig. 10 or terminal ducts like the one shown in Fig. 9. (C) The number of lobules increases with age and in the adult nulliparous female breast, three types of lobule may be found (lobules types 1, 2, and 3) (see Figs. 18, 22, 25, 26, and 30); n, nipple; lob, lobule.

from woman to woman, making it impossible to categorize mammary gland structure based on age (Dabelow, 1957; Dawson, 1934). Therefore, the development of the mammary gland has to be evaluated based on the architecture of the organ at each given period of time for each individual woman. Mammary gland development can be defined from the external appearance of the breast (Reynolds and Wines, 1948) or by

Figures 4–10. Whole-mount preparation of a mammary gland of an 18-year-old nulliparous woman. In Fig. 4, the mammary ductal system ends in either slender terminal ducts (arrows) or in type 1 lobules (double arrows) (see histology in Fig. 11) (×25). In Fig. 5, another area of the same gland is shown, containing typical type 1 lobules composed of alveolar buds. Sprouting of buds is observed from the duct (arrow) (×100). In Fig. 6, the appearance of the gland is variegated, being composed of lobules type 1 (inset a, Fig. 8), terminal ducts (inset b, Fig. 9), and terminal end buds (inset c, Fig. 10), level x-y, see Fig. 14 (×25). In Fig. 7, an early type 1 lobule composed of club-shaped alveolar buds is shown (×25). In Fig. 8, the same lobule type 1 is shown as in Fig. 6 (inset a) (×100). Figure 9 shows a higher magnification of the terminal ducts shown in Fig. 6 (inset b) (×100). Finally, Fig. 10 shows a higher magnification of the terminal end bud shown in Fig. 6 (inset c) (×100).

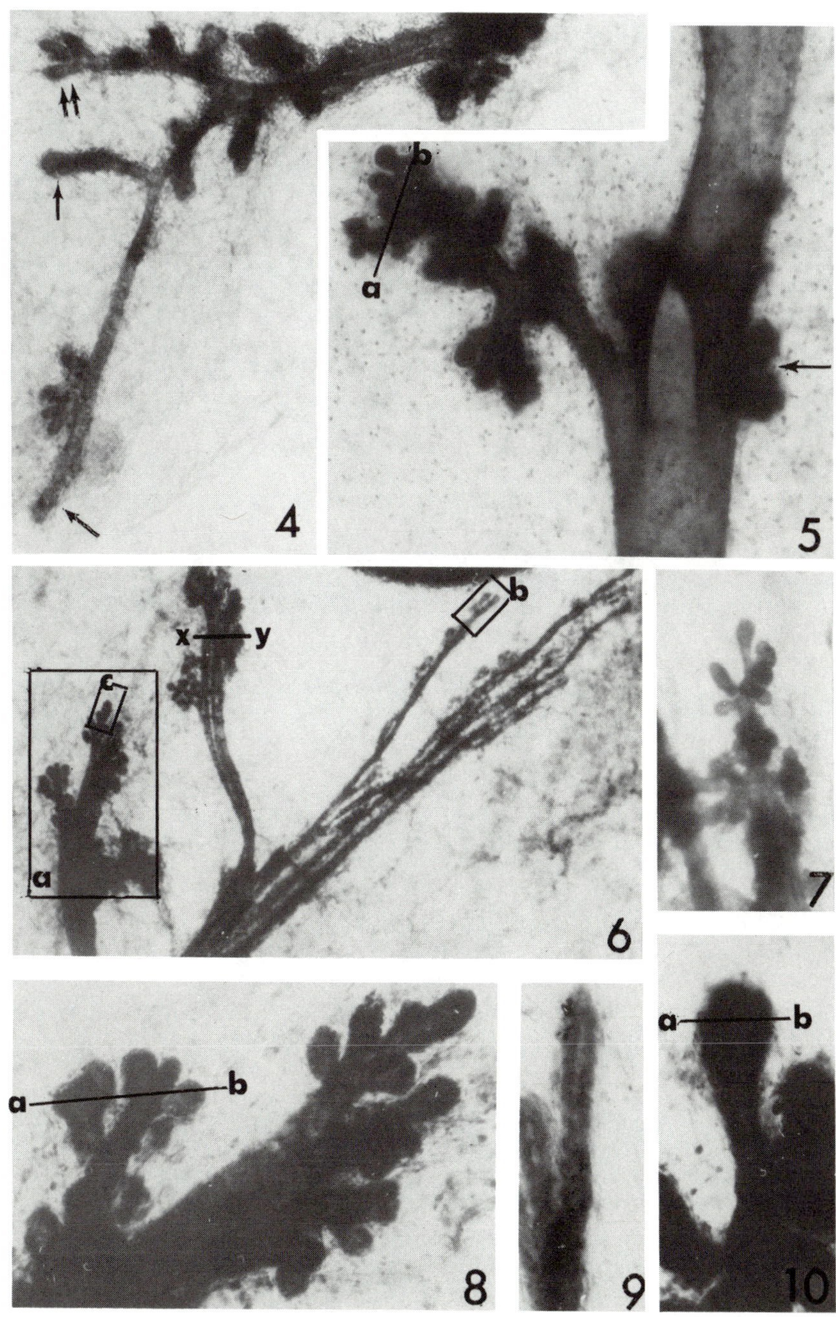
4
a
b
5
x
y
b
c
a
6
7
a
b
8
9
a
b
10

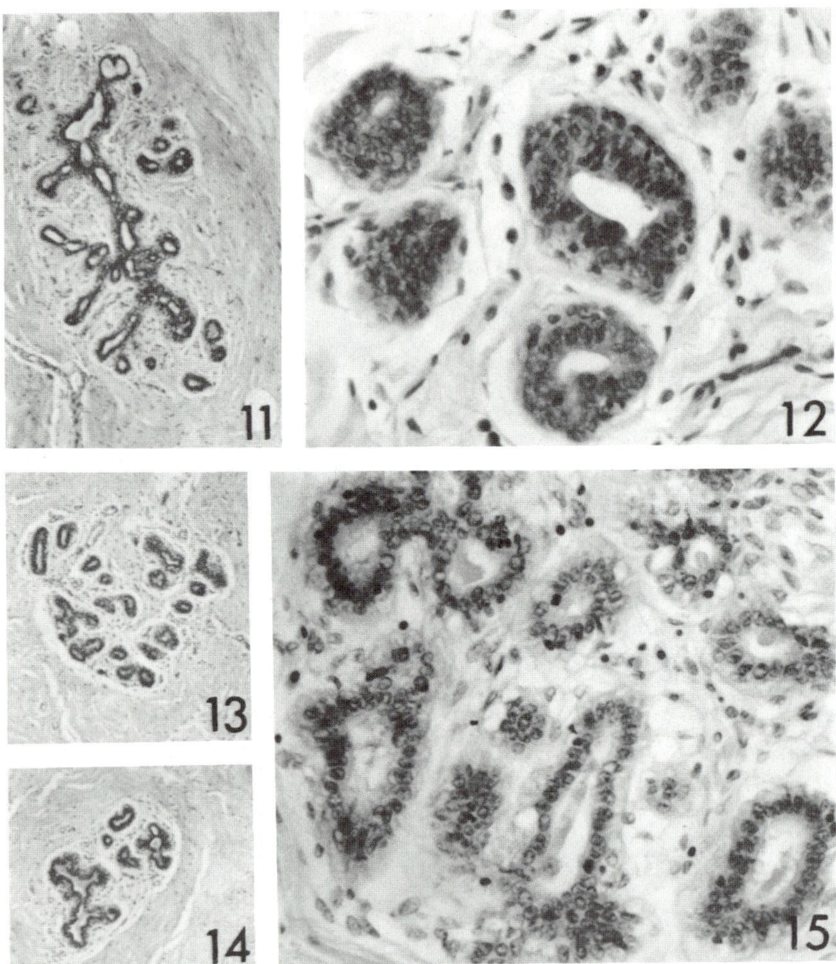

Figures 11–15. Figure 11 shows a lobule type 1 from Fig. 5, sectioned at level a-b and showing a duct sprouting alveolar buds, each one surrounded by intralobular connective tissue (H&E, ×25). Figure 12 is a cross section of the lobule type 1 shown in Fig. 8; the distal end of the alveolar buds is lined by three layers of epithelial cells (H&E, ×160). Figure 13 shows a lobule type 1 sectioned at the a-b level of Fig. 5 (H&E, ×25), while Fig. 14 shows a lobule type 1 sectioned at the x-y level of Fig. 6 (H&E, ×25). Finally, Fig. 15 shows a higher magnification of a lobule type 1 showing the double layer of cells lining the alveolar buds (H&E, ×160).

Table I. Identification Profile of the Different Compartments of Human Breast

Structure	Parameter[b]	Lob 1	Lob 2	Lob 3	Lob 4
Lobule	Area (mm^2)	0.048 ± 0.044	0.060 ± 0.026	0.129 ± 0.049	0.250 ± 0.060
AB/ductule/acinus[a]	Area (mm^2)	$0.232 \times 10^{-2} \pm 0.090 \times 10^{-2}$	$0.167 \times 10^{-2} \pm 0.035 \times 10^{-2}$	$0.125 \times 10^{-2} \pm 0.029 \times 10^{-2}$	$0.120 \times 10^{-2} \pm 0.050 \times 10^{-2}$
AB/ductule/acinus[a]	Number per lobule[c]	11.20 ± 6.34	47.0 ± 11.70	81.0 ± 16.6	180.0 ± 20.0
AB/ductule/acinus[a]	Number/mm^2 of lobule	253.8 ± 50.17	682.4 ± 169.0	560.40 ± 25.0	720.0 ± 150.0
AB/ductule/acinus[a]	Number cells/ cross section[d]	32.43 ± 14.07	13.14 ± 4.79	11.0 ± 2.0	10.0 ± 2.3

[a] AB/ductule/acinus: alveolar bud/ductule/acinus. The three nomenclatures used to identify the forming units of the lobule are cited, with AB being used only for lobules type 1, ductule for lobules type 2 and type 3, and acini for lobules type 4.

[b] Student's *t*-tests were done for all possible comparisons. Lobular areas show significant differences between lobule 1 versus 3 and 4 and between 2, 3, and 4 ($p < 0.05$). Alveolar bud areas were significant between lobules 1, 2, and 3 and between 1 and 2 versus 3 and 4 ($p > 0.001$).

[c] The number of alveolar buds per lobule was different ($p < 0.01$) in all the comparisons. The number of buds per mm^2 of lobule was significant ($p > 0.001$) between lobule 1 versus 2, 3, and 4.

[d] The number of cells per cross section was significantly different in alveolar buds of lobules 1 versus 2 and 3 ($p < 0.01$).

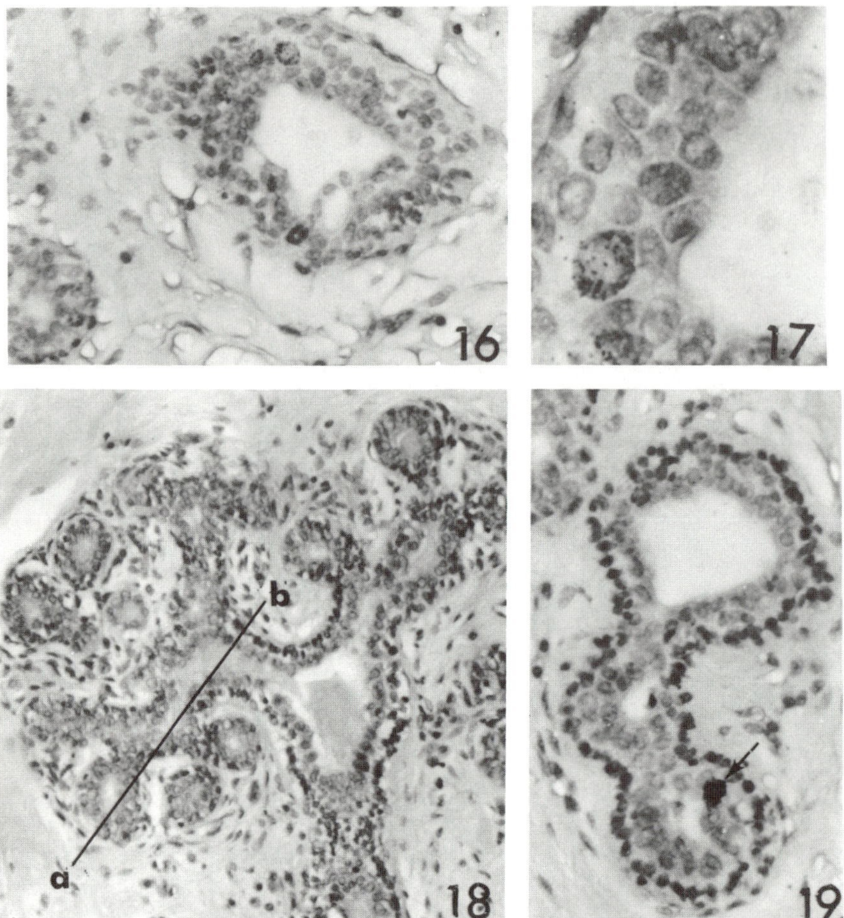

Figures 16–21. For autoradiography, tissues were incubated with 1.5 μCi ^{3}H-thymidine/ml M199 culture medium for 1 h, then fixed in Bouin's fluid and embedded in paraffin. Deparaffinized sections were coated with NTB-2 nuclear track emulsion, developed, and counterstained with hematoxylin-eosin. Figure 16 shows a terminal end bud sectioned at level a-b of Fig. 10; the epithelial layer contains labeled cells (×160). Figure 17 is a higher magnification of autoradiography of the terminal end bud of Fig. 16 showing labeled cells (×400). Figure 18 is an autoradiography of a lobule type 1 composed of alveolar buds opening into the intralobular terminal duct (H&E, ×100). Figure 19 shows a section at level a-b of Fig. 18, showing branching of the main duct, lined by an epithelial and a myoepithelial layer of cells. Observe the uptake of ^{3}H-thymidine in the epithelial layer (arrow) (×160). Figure 20 exhibits a longitudinal section of a ductal structure showing sprouts of alveolar buds all lined by two layers of cells (×100). Finally, Fig. 21 is an autoradiography of alveolar buds in a type 1 lobule, showing labeled cells (arrows) (×400).

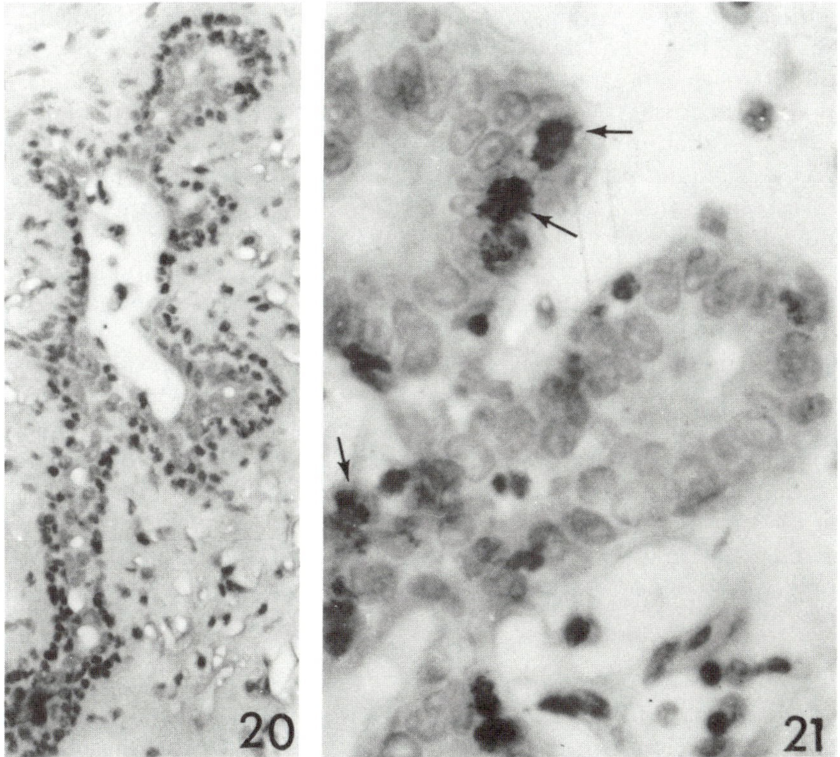

Figures 16–21. *(Continued)*

determination of mammary gland area, volume (Tanner, 1962), degree of branching, or degree of structures whose appearance indicates the level of differentiation of the gland, such as lobule formation (Dabelow, 1957; Russo and Russo, 1986).

The adolescent period begins with the first signs of sexual change at puberty and terminates with sexual maturity (Tanner, 1962). Puberty in the female sets in between the ages of 10 and 12 years. With the approach of puberty, the rudimentary mammae begin to show growth activity both in the glandular tissue and in the surrounding stroma. Glandular increase is due to the growth and division of small bundles of primary and secondary ducts (Fig. 3A). They grow and divide partly dichotomously (from the greek word *dichotomos,* or repeated bifurcation) and partly sympodially (from greek *syn* + *podion* base, involving the formation of an apparent main axis from successive secondary axes), on a dichotomous basis (Fig. 3A). The ducts grow, divide, and form club-shaped terminal end buds (Figs. 3A, 4–10). Terminal end buds give origin to new branches, twigs (Fig. 7), and small ductules or *alveolar buds* (Figs. 5, 11–14). We have coined the term alveolar bud to identify those structures that are morphologically more developed than the terminal end bud but yet more primitive than the terminal structure of the mature resting organ, which is called acinus by German pathologists or ductule by Dawson (1935). Dawson (1935) differentiates this structure from the fully secretory unit developed during pregnancy and lactation, which we prefer to call *acinus*. Alveolar buds cluster around a terminal duct, forming the lobule type 1 or virginal lobule (Figs. 11–14), each composed of approximately 11 alveolar buds (Table I). Terminal ducts (Figs. 11–15) or alveolar buds (Figs. 18–21) are lined by a two-layered epithelium, whereas terminal end buds are lined by an epithelium made up of up to four layers of cells (Figs. 16 and 17). Lobule formation is confined to the female breast and occurs within 1–2 years after the onset of the first menstrual period. The full differentiation of the mammary gland is a gradual process taking many years, and in some cases, if pregnancy does not supervene, is never attained.

3.2. Menstrual Cycle

It is acknowledged that hormonal influences play a significant role in breast development; however, the effect of their fluctuations during the menstrual cycle on parenchymal proliferation has not been definitively elucidated. Masters et al. (1977) and Meyer (1977) have shown through elegant experiments that the normal breast epithelium undergoes cyclic variations of DNA synthesis, as determined in normal breast samples cultured in the presence of ^{3}H-thymidine. These authors describe decreased DNA-labeling index (DNA-LI) in the breast epithelium during the follicular phase, with a significant increase during the luteal phase. Anderson et al. (1982) and Ferguson and Anderson (1981) also found that the lobules of the resting human breast present a peak of mitotic activity during the luteal phase (25th day of the cycle). These authors also found cyclic changes in cell deletion, or apoptosis, occurring 3 days after the peak of mitoses. Even though cell proliferation and cell death seem to balance to maintain the equilibrium of the resting breast (Ferguson and Anderson, 1981), mammary development induced by ovarian hormones during a menstrual cycle never fully returns to the starting point of the preceding cycle. Accordingly, each ovulatory cycle slightly fosters mammary development with new budding of structures which continues until about age 35 (Dabelow, 1957; Vorherr, 1974).

The study of normal breast tissue of 22 adult women ranging in age from 18 to 63 years of age (Table II) allowed us to determine that in nonpregnant glands there are two identifiable types of lobules in addition to the already described type 1. These are designated lobules type 2 (Figs. 22, 25, and 28) and type 3 (Figs. 30–36).

The transition from lobule type 1 to type 2, and of this to type 3, is a gradual process of sprouting of new alveolar buds. In lobules type 2 and type 3, these are now called *ductules;* they increase in number from approximately 11 in the lobule type 1 to 47 and 80 in lobules type 2 and type 3, respectively. The increase in number results in a concomitant increase in size of the lobules and a reduction in size of each individual structure. The alveolar buds composing a lobule type 1 (Figs. 7 and 8)

Table II. Mammary Gland Development According to Age and Reproductive History

Sample number[a]	Age[b]	Parity history[c,d]	Gland development
1	18	G0 P0	Lob[f] type 3
2	20	G0 P0	Lob type 1
3	23	G0 P0	Ducts only
4	24	G0 P0	Lob type 1 and ducts
5	30	G0 P0	Lob type 1
6	30	G1 P1	Lob types 1, 2, and ducts
7	30	G3 P3	Lob type 3
8	31	G3 P3 + Ab[e]	Lob type 1
9	31	G3 P1 + Ab[e]	Lob type 1 and ducts
10	31	G3 P3	Lob type 3
11	33	G1 P1	Lob type 3
12	34	G0 P0	Lob type 1, AB[g], ducts
13	36	G3 P3 + Ab[e]	Lob type 1
14	36	G0 P0	Lob type 1
15	39	G2 P2	Lob type 3
16	44	G5 P5	Lob types 1 and 2
17	48	G0 P0	Lob type 1 and ducts
18	50	G3 P2	Lob types 2 and 3
19	52	G1 P1	Lob types 2 and 3
20	53	G0 P0	Lob type 1 and ducts
21	60	G1 P1	Lob type 1 and ducts
22	63	G4 P4	Lob type 1 and ducts

[a]All breast samples were obtained from women undergoing reduction mammoplasty.
[b]Age in years.
[c]G, gravidity: number of pregnancies.
[d]P, parity: number of live births.
[e]Ab: pregnancies ending in abortion in addition to full-term pregnancies (P).
[f]Lob: lobule.
[g]AB: alveolar bud.

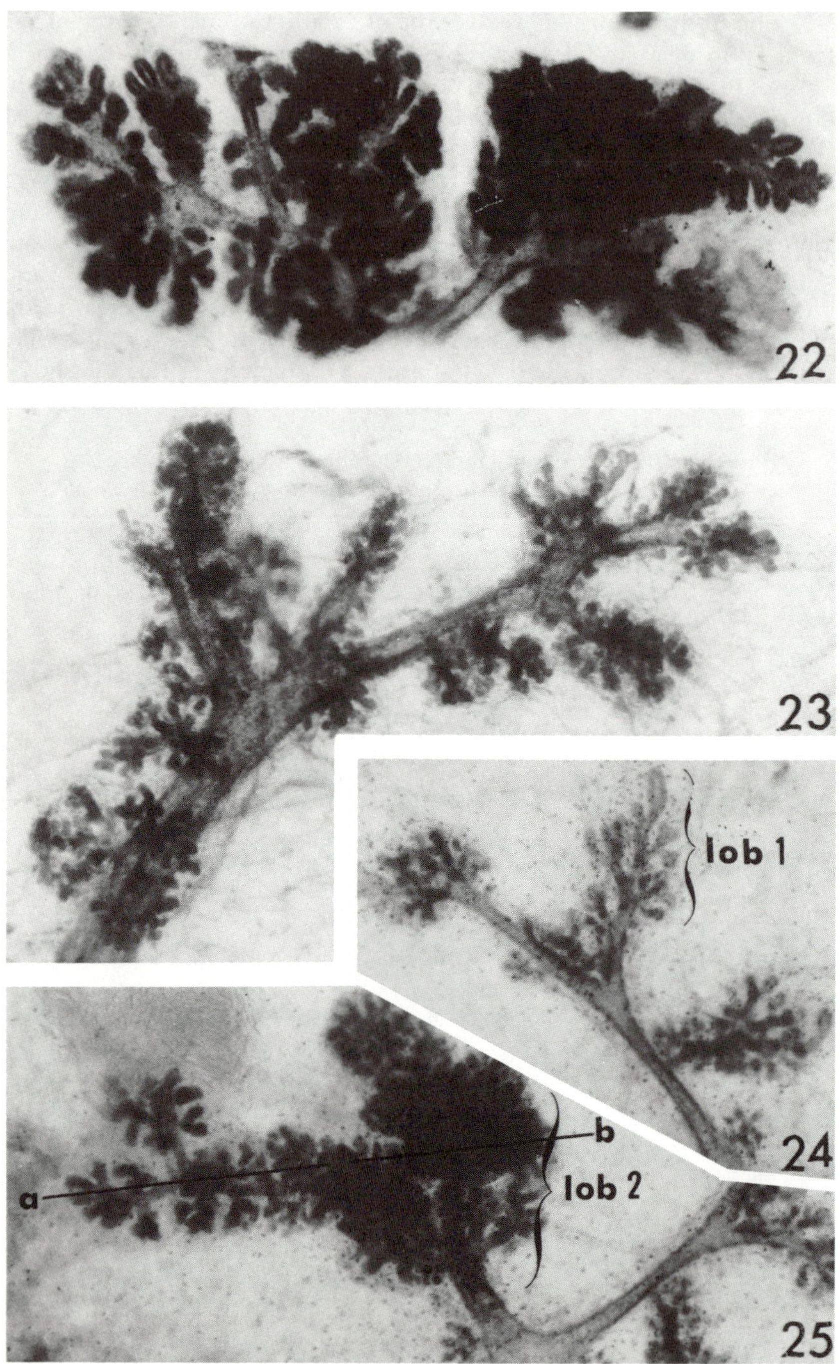
22
23
lob 1
24
b
a
lob 2
25

measure an average of 0.232×10^{-2} mm^2 (Table I), practically twice the size of the ductules composing lobules type 2 (Fig. 25), whereas the reduction in size in ductules composing lobules type 3 is less dramatic, although still significant (Table I).

Lobules type 1 are predominantly found in the breast of nulliparous young women, whereas lobules type 2 and type 3 are more frequent in the gland of parous women, although the breasts of some parous women and that of women with history of abortion also contain lobules type 1 and type 2, and they are also occasionally found in breast tissue of older women (Table II). Although these observations suggest that there is no correlation between age and gland development, the biological significance of the presence of these lobules in the breasts of women of different ages and reproductive histories has not been elucidated completely and requires further studies.

Determination of the proliferative activity (DNA-LI) of these structures by measuring the incorporation of ^{3}H-thymidine into the mammary epithelium by the technique described by Russo and Russo (1982) and Calaf et al. (1982a,b) has shown that the DNA-LI of lobules type 2 is around 0.99 and of lobules type 3 is 0.25 (Fig. 37). These values are 5 and 20 times lower than those found in lobules type 1 and up to 60 times lower than in the terminal end bud (Fig. 37). It is important to emphasize that in the study of the proliferative activity of the mammary gland, each topographic compartment has to be analyzed individually; as it is depicted in Fig. 37, there is a gradient from the terminal end bud to the lobule type 3; ductal structures have a proliferative activity intermediate between that of lobules type 1 and type 2. This gradient does not seem to be modified with aging, although in older women all proliferative activity is significantly reduced (Meyer, 1977; Russo and Russo, 1982; Russo et al., 1982).

3.3. Pregnancy

During pregnancy the breast attains its maximum development; it occurs in two distinctly dominant phases characteristic of the early and

---

Figures 22–25. Figure 22 shows the whole-mount breast tissue of a 19-year-old nulliparous woman. It is mostly composed of lobules type 1, but the increased number of alveolar buds per lobule indicates a transitional stage of lobules type 2 (toluidine blue, ×25). Figures 23 and 24 exhibit the whole-mount preparation of breast tissue of a 20-year-old nulliparous woman in which lobules types 1 (lob1) are present (toluidine blue, ×25). Finally, Fig. 25 shows the whole mount of the same breast tissue shown in Figs. 23 and 24. Lobules type 2 (lob 2) are composed of ductules, which are more abundant and smaller than the alveolar buds of type 1 lobules, which also are present (toluidine blue, ×25).

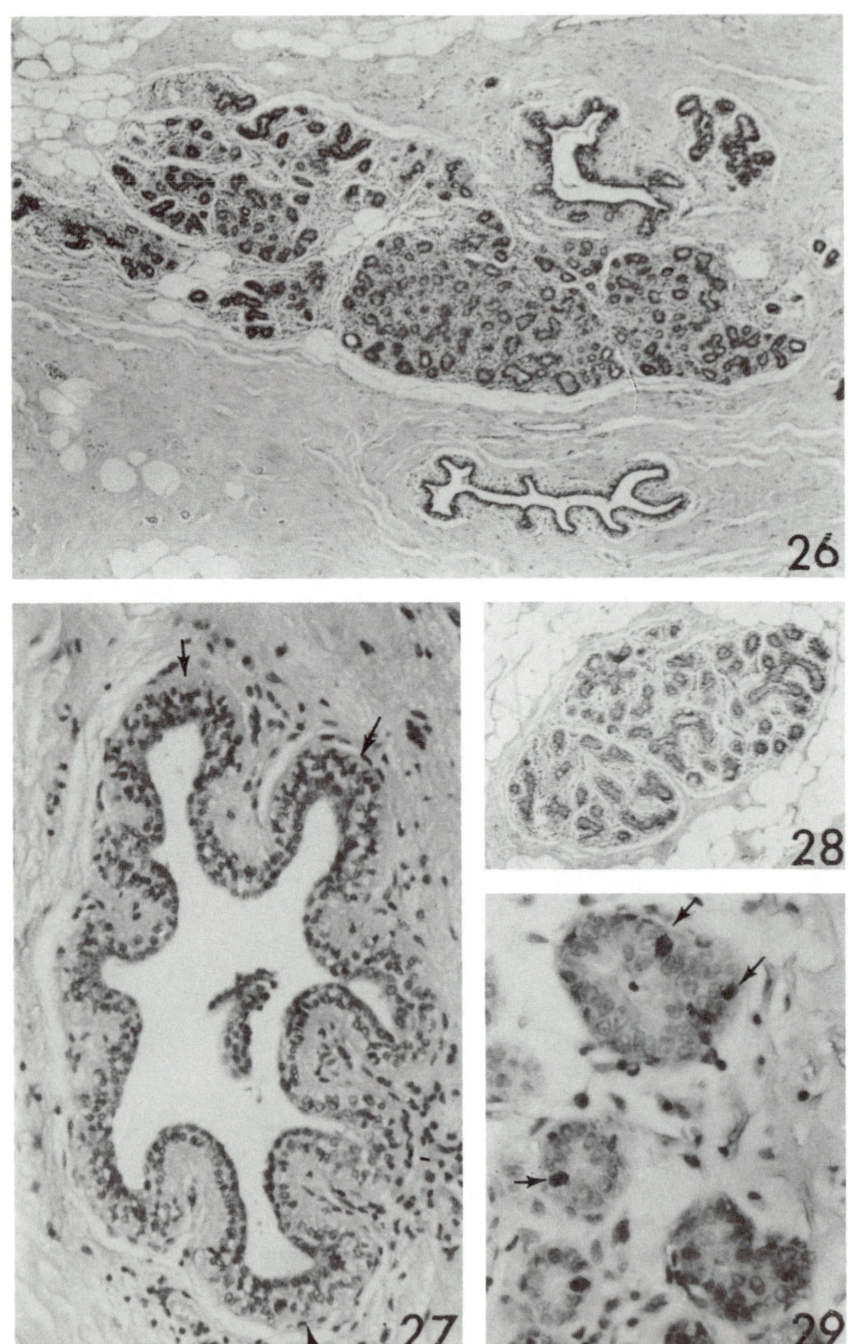
26
27
28
29

late stages of pregnancy (Dabelow, 1957; Bassler, 1970; Salazar and Tobon, 1974; Vorherr, 1974). The early stage is characterized by growth, consisting of proliferation of the distal elements of the ductal tree, resulting in the neoformation of ductules that at this stage can be called acini, thus developing a lobule type 3 into a lobule type 4 (Table I). The intensity of budding and degree of lobule formation goes beyond what has been observed in the virginal breast. In Fig. 3C, a schematic representation of the gland shows abundant budding in various stages, from short dichotomous buds up to formed lobules (Dawson, 1935; Dabelow, 1957; Vorherr, 1974). By the third month of pregnancy, the number of well-formed lobules exceeds the number of primitive budding stages; however, they are still found (Dabelow, 1957; Salazar and Tobon, 1974). In newly formed lobules, the epithelial cells composing each acinus not only increase greatly in number owing to active cell division, but they also increase in size mainly because of cytoplasmic enlargement (Salazar and Tobon, 1974).

In the middle of pregnancy, the lobules are further enlarged and increased in number. They surround the duct from which their central branch proceeds so thickly that the chief duct, the terminal duct, or intralobular terminal duct can no longer be recognized (Dabelow, 1957). The transition between the terminal ducts and the budding acinus is gradual, making the histological distinction between the two of them difficult, since both show evidence of early secretory activity (Salazar and Tobon, 1974).

Lobular development varies within a single breast (Dabelow, 1957; Salazar and Tobon, 1974) and greatly from woman to woman. Some women have well-developed glands that, around the middle of pregnancy, contain numerous lobules and more parenchyma than other poorly developed breasts at the end of pregnancy (Dabelow, 1957). The definitive structure of the ductal tree is essentially settled by the end of the first half of pregnancy; the mammary changes that characterize the second half of pregnancy are chiefly continuation and accentuation of the secretory activity (Dabelow, 1957; Salazar and Tobon, 1974; Vorherr, 1974). Further progressive branching continues with less prominent bud formation (Dabelow, 1957). At this time, the formation of true secreting

Figures 26–29. Figure 26 is a histological section of the lobules type 1 and type 2 shown in Fig. 25 (a-b level) in which the difference in size between both types of lobule can be appreciated (H&E, ×25). Figure 27 is a histological section of a duct exhibiting lateral budding of new branches; observe that the budding areas are composed of three layers of cells (arrows) (H&E, ×100). Figure 28 is a histological section of lobule type 2; compare the area occupied by this lobule with Fig. 13, taken at the same magnification (H&E, ×25). Figure 29 is an autoradiography of ductules, part of a lobule type 2, showing the uptake of ^{3}H-thymidine (arrows) (H&E, ×160).

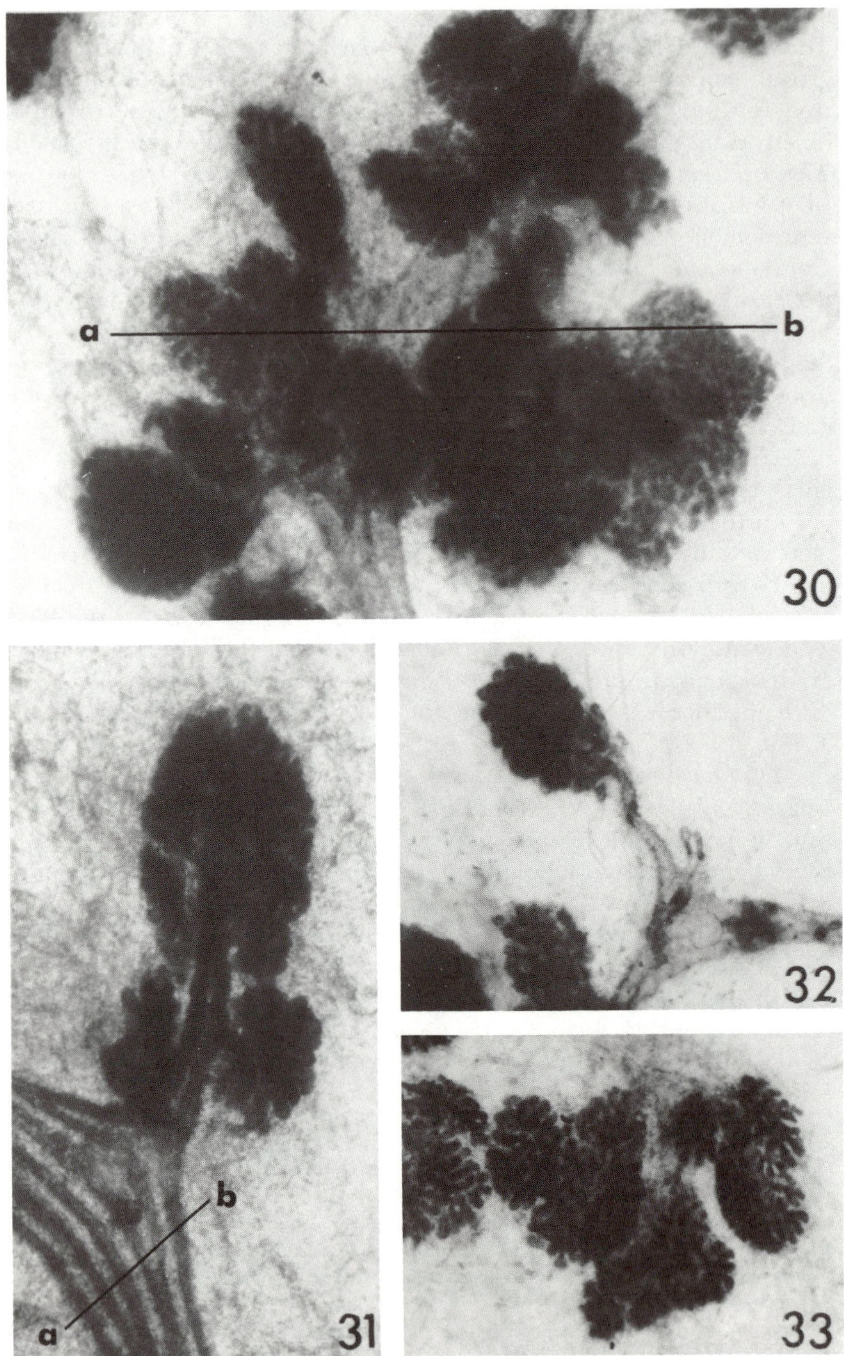
a
b
30
b
a
31
32
33

units or acini, the differentiated structures, becomes more and more evident (Salazar and Tobon, 1974; Vorherr, 1974). Proliferation of new acini is reduced to a minimum, and the luminae of those already formed become distended by accumulation of secretory material or colostrum (Salazar and Tobon, 1974; Vorherr, 1974). In addition to the process that transforms newly formed ductules into acini, there is a continued growth of the still undifferentiated glandular fields (Dabelow, 1957). Primitive stages of budding that have lagged behind the general degree of development can be found up to the time of birth. Geschickter and Lewis regarded these as virginal lobules refractory to endocrine stimuli (Dabelow, 1957), whereas Dawson (1935) considered them a reserve to replace degenerating or exhausted areas of the gland. The secretory acinus formed during pregnancy is a terminal outgrowth that marks the end of glandular differentiation. However, just before and during parturition there is a new wave of mitotic activity with an increase in the total DNA of the gland (Salazar and Tobon, 1974; Vorherr, 1974). During lactation, the process of growth and differentiation may be observed in the same lobule, side by side with the process of milk secretion.

3.4. Postlactational Changes

From midpregnancy on, a yellowish fluid containing a high protein concentration is secreted into the mammary alveoli and may be expelled from the nipple (Vorherr, 1974). After postpartum withdrawal of placental lactogen and sex steroids, which appear to prevent the action of prolactin on the mammary epithelium, lactation starts (Salazar and Tobon, 1974; Vorherr, 1974). Colostrum is secreted during the first week postpartum, followed by a 2- to 3-week period of transitional milk secretion, leading to the secretion of mature milk (Salazar and Tobon, 1974; Vorherr, 1974).

No major morphological changes of the mammary gland are observed during lactation. The mammary lobules are enlarged and the acini have a dilated lumen filled with granular, slightly basophilic material admixed with fat globules (Salazar and Tobon, 1974; Vorherr, 1974). There is a significant variation in lobular size throughout the gland, suggestive of a variation in lactogenic activity from lobule to lob-

Figures 30–33. Whole-mount preparation of breast tissue from a gravida 2, para 2, 30-year-old woman. The parenchyma is composed of numerous type 3 lobules. In the breast of parous women, even isolated branches like those depicted in Figs. 31 and 32 are well developed. Compare with Figs. 4–10 of a nulliparous woman. Lobules type 3 are composed of ductules that are smaller than the alveolar buds composing lobules type 1 (Fig. 24) (toluidine blue, ×25).

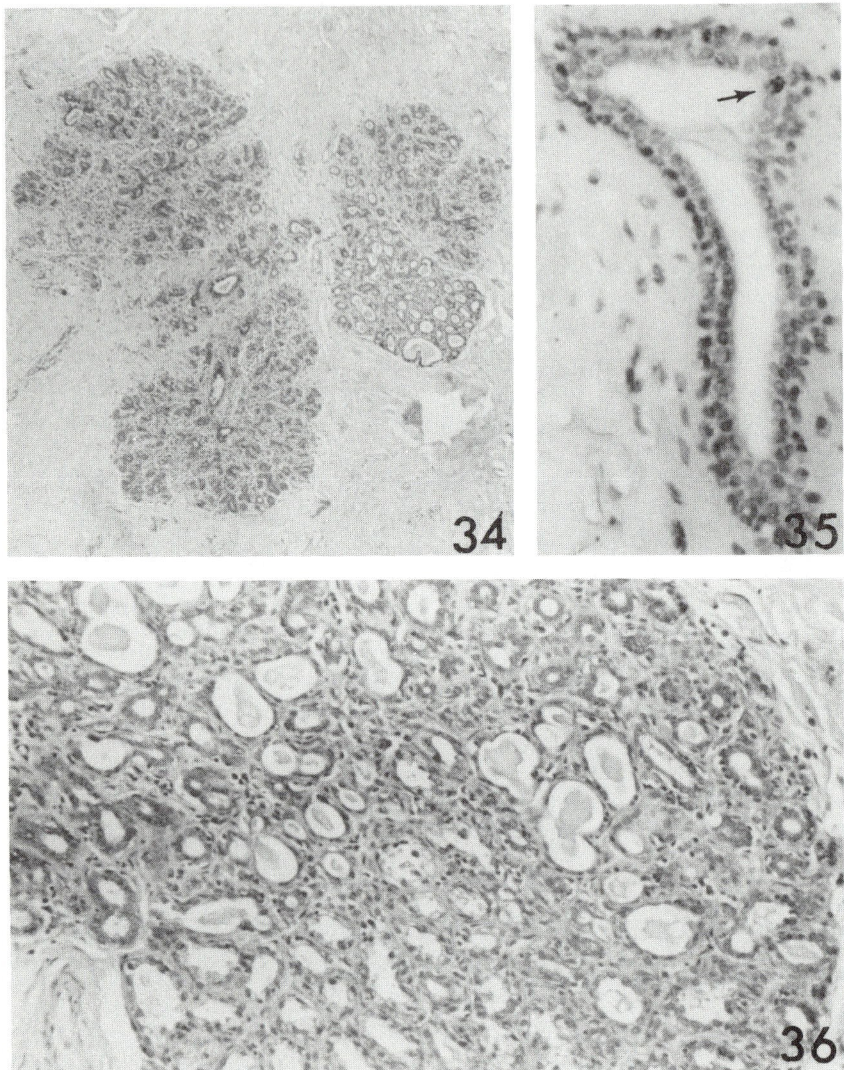

Figures 34–36. Figure 34 is a histological section of the lobules type 3 shown in Fig. 30 (level a-b) (H&E, ×25). Figure 35 is an autoradiograph of the duct shown in Fig. 31 (a-b level). It is lined by a double layer of cells. A labeled cell is observed in the lining epithelium (arrow) (H&E, ×160). Figure 36 is a higher magnification of Fig. 34 and shows the ductules composing a lobule type 3 lined by a low cuboidal epithelium. Secretory material is seen in the lumen (H&E, ×160).

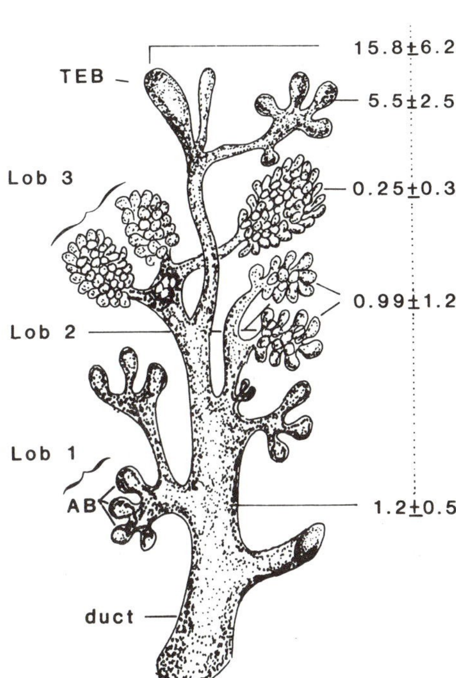

Figure 37. Schematic representation depicting the various topographic compartments of the human mammary gland: terminal end buds (TEB); alveolar buds (AB); lobules types 1, 2, and 3 (Lob 1, Lob 2, and Lob 3); and ducts. On the right-hand column is shown the DNA-LI of each structure (mean ± standard deviation) of nine women ranging in age from 18 to 62 years. A gradient in proliferative activity is observed from the TEB (15.8 ± 5.2), Lob 1 (5.5 ± 0.5), Lob 2 (0.9 ± 1.2), Lob 3 (0.25 ± 0.3), and ducts (1.2 ± 0.5).

ule (Salazar and Tobon, 1974). Milk is synthesized and released into the mammary acini and ductal system, although it can be stored for up to 48 h before the rate of milk synthesis and secretion begins to decrease (Dabelow, 1957; Vorherr, 1974). As long as milk is removed regularly from the mammary gland, the alveolar cells continue to secrete milk almost indefinitely (Vorherr, 1974).

The accumulation of milk in the ductoacinar lumina and within the cytoplasm of the lactogenic epithelial cells that occurs after weaning has an inhibitory effect on further milk synthesis (Salazar and Tobon, 1974; Vorherr, 1974). This effect is followed by a series of involutional changes in the mammary gland consisting of a multifocal asynchronous process of reduction in volume of the secretory epithelial cells and further inhibition of their secretory activity (Dawson, 1935; Salazar and Tobon, 1974).

As a consequence of these changes, mammary lobules undergo atrophy and the stroma shows a marked desmoplastic reaction and fat infiltration (Salazar and Tobon, 1974). It is considered that postlactational regression is due to two complementary mechanisms, cell autolysis, with collapse of acinar structures and narrowing of the tubules, and appearance of round cell infiltration and phagocytes in and about the disintegrating lobules, and finally, regeneration of the periductal and perilobular connective tissue with renewed budding and proliferation in the terminal tubules (Geschickter, 1945). Until the menopausal involution sets in, the parous organ shows more glandular tissue than if pregnancy or pregnancy and lactation had never occurred (Table II).

4. Involution

Mammary involution begins in premenopausal women as a consequence of a decline in ovarian function (Vorherr, 1974). Regressive changes appear both in the epithelial structures and in the stroma of the breast. The ducts and their branches remain, but the lobules shrink and collapse, although occasional acinar-like structures persist. The mammary lobules and acini, which are the last structures to appear with sexual maturity, are the first ones to regress (Vorherr, 1974).

According to Vorherr (1974), the menopausal stage of mammary involution, occurring after age 45, consists of drastic reduction in epithelial structures and fat deposition. In later stages of involution, the breast appears mainly composed of ducts with increased amount of connective tissue and fat (Dabelow, 1957; Vorherr, 1974).

5. Parenchyma–Stroma Relation

The tridimensional structure of the mammary gland requires that morphometric studies be carried out in whole-mount preparations, since this is the only method in which the architecture of the organ is preserved, thus allowing a good assessment of the parenchyma–stroma ratio. Whole mounts, prepared with the method developed in our laboratory, are excellently suited for measurement utilizing the image analysis system (Fig. 38). The study of the stroma–parenchyma ratio in 14 human breasts of puberal, post-puberal, parous, and pregnant women, showed that the relationship between parenchyma and stroma of the mammary

Figure 38. Circular percentage graph representing the proportion of parenchymal and stromal components of the breast: intralobular (ils) and interlobular (els) stroma (left-hand pie charts). The right-hand pie charts represent the proportion of parenchyma occupied by ducts and lobules types 1, 2, 3, and 4. The values were obtained using the image analysis system Zeiss MOP-Videoplan 2 and measuring total tissue area and the area of each specific structure present in 10 random sections of the breast totaling 1500–2000 mm^2/gland. Values represent the average of A—two glands of puberal age girls; B—two glands of postpuberal women; C—six parous women; D—three glands of women in their first half of pregnancy; and E—two glands of women at the end of pregnancy.

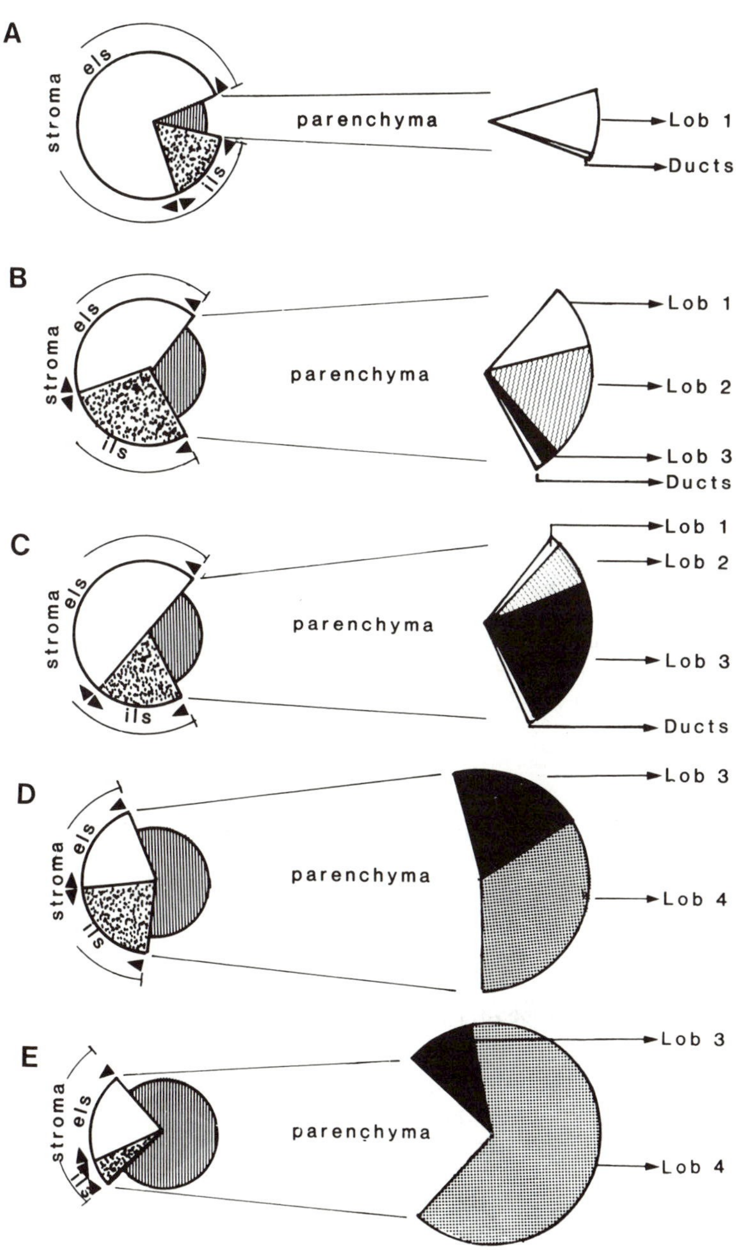
A
stroma
els
ils
parenchyma
Lob 1
Ducts
B
stroma
els
ils
parenchyma
Lob 1
Lob 2
Lob 3
Ducts
C
stroma
els
ils
parenchyma
Lob 1
Lob 2
Lob 3
Ducts
D
stroma
els
ils
parenchyma
Lob 3
Lob 4
E
stroma
els
ils
parenchyma
Lob 3
Lob 4

gland is a dynamic process. In the mammary gland of puberal women, almost 90% of the gland is made up of stroma. This can be divided into intralobular stroma, representing 17% of the total, and consisting of the connective tissue around the individual alveolar buds, and interlobular stroma, that separates one lobule from another (Fig. 38A). It is composed of fat and connective tissue. The parenchyma of these glands, representing 10% of the mammary area, is made up almost exclusively of type 1 lobules and ductal structures. In the glands of postpuberal and young nulliparous women, the parenchyma increases from 10 to 30% of the total area of the gland (0–10% is composed of lobules type 1, 10–18% lobules type 2; and 1–3% lobules type 3) (Fig. 38B). The intralobular stroma of these breasts represents about 28% of the total. Parity induces significant differences in mammary gland development. Parous women's breasts have the same percentage of parenchyma as nulliparous women; however, it is mostly composed of type 3 lobules and accounts for 24% of the total parenchyma (Fig. 38C). There is a markedly reduced proportion of type 1 and type 2 lobules.

Pregnancy induces dramatic changes in the relation of parenchyma and stroma. During the first half of pregnancy, the parenchyma area increases to 55% (Fig. 38D) and at the end of pregnancy to 73% (Fig. 38E) with a subsequent reduction in the proportion of the stroma. The proliferation of acini that results in larger lobules composed of numerous secretory units (lobules type 4, Table I) has as a consequence a marked reduction in both intralobular and interlobular stroma (Fig. 38D and E).

6. Summary and Conclusions

In summary, the human breast undergoes a complete series of changes from intrauterine life to senescence. These changes can be divided into two distinct phases: the developmental phase and the differentiation phase.

The developmental phase includes the early stages of gland morphogenesis, from nipple epithelium to lobule formation. In lobular formation, both processes, development and differentiation, take place almost simultaneously. For example, the progressive transition of lobules type 1 to types 2, 3, and 4 requires active cell proliferation, to acquire the cell mass necessary for the function of milk secretion. This latter process implies differentiation of the mammary epithelium. Therefore, the presence of lobules type 4 is the maximal expression of development and differentiation in the adult gland, whereas the presence of lobules type 3 could indicate that the gland has already been developed, but, because their lobules are not secreting milk, they are not completely differentiated. It is important to point out that the presence of proteins that are indicative of milk secretion, such as α-lactalbumin, casein, or milk fat globule membrane protein (Russo, 1985), also indicates cellular differentiation of breast epithelium. However, only when all the other components of milk are coordinately synthesized within the appropriate structure can full differentiation of the mammary gland be acknowledged.

Repeated pregnancies serve to extend lobular development. In the absence of childbearing, the size and number of lobules decline and only ductal structures and lobules type 1 and type 2 are observed. These lobule types, as previously indicated, are areas of epithelial proliferation, and they might represent the lobular irregularities or primitive lobules that Ingleby and Gershon-Cohen (1960) found in 33% of the breasts removed from women autopsied between the ages of 30 and 40 years of age who had clinically normal breasts.

The observation that lobules type 1, which we also call virginal lobules, are also found in parous women and in women with a history of abortion (Table II) suggests that this type of lobule might represent structures that have failed to respond to the influence of pregnancy and also fail to respond to lactation (Levin et al., 1964).

The meaning of the asynchronous development of the gland, even after the full stimulation of pregnancy, is not yet clear; however, based on our studies in an experimental system (Russo and Russo, 1978a,b, 1980a,b; Russo et al., 1979, 1981, 1982), the response of these structures to in vitro carcinogenesis suggests that they can be considered undifferentiated structures and possible targets for neoplastic transformation (Russo and Russo, 1986). Therefore, a better understanding of the development of the gland will further our knowledge of human diseases such as breast carcinoma.

ACKNOWLEDGMENTS: This work was supported by USPHS Grant CA 38921 from the National Cancer Institute and an Institutional Grant from the United Foundation of Greater Detroit. The authors acknowledge the technical assistance of Mr. M. Kaeck and Ms. Vivian Powell for typing the manuscript.

References

Alvarez Sanz, M.C., Liu, J.M., Huang, H.H., and Hawrylewicz, E.J., 1986, Effect of dietary protein on morphologic development of rat mammary gland, *J. Natl. Cancer Inst.* **77**:477–487.

Anderson, T.J., Ferguson, D.J.P., and Raab, G.M., 1982, Cell turnover in the "resting" human breast: Influence of parity, contraceptive pill, age and laterality, *Br. J. Cancer* **46:**376–382.

Bassler, R., 1970, The morphology of hormone induced structural changes in the female breast, *Curr. Top. Pathol.* **53:**1–89.

Bloom, W., and Fawcett, D.W. (eds.), 1968, Mammary Gland, in: *A Textbook of Histology,* Saunders, Philadelphia, pp. 767–775.

Calaf, G., Martinez, F., Russo, I.H., and Russo, J., 1982a, Age related variations in growth kinetics of primary human breast cell cultures, *Int. Res. Comm. Syst. Med. Sci.* **10:**307–308.

Calaf, G., Martinez, F., Russo, I.H., Roi, L.D., and Russo, J., 1982b, The influence of age on DNA-Labeling Index of human breast epithelium, *Int. Res. Comm. Syst. Med. Sci.* **10:**655–656.

Cowie, A.T., and Folley, S.J., 1961, The mammary gland and lactation, in: *Sex and Internal Secretion* (W.C. Young, ed.), Williams and Wilkins, Baltimore, pp. 590–642.

Dabelow, A., 1957, Die Milchdruse, in: *Handbuch der Mikroskopischen Anatomic des Menschen,* Vol. 3, Part 3, *Haut und Sinnes Organs* (W. Bargmann, ed.), Springer-Verlag, Berlin, pp. 277–485.

Dawson, E.K., 1934, A histological study of the normal mamma in relation to tumour growth. I. Early development to maturity, *Edinb. Med. J.* **41:**653–682.

Dawson, E.K., 1935, A histological study of the normal mamma in relation to tumour growth. II. The mature gland in pregnancy and lactation, *Edinb. Med. J.* **42:**569–598.

Ferguson, D.J.P., and Anderson, T.J., 1981, Morphological evaluation of cell turnover in relation to the menstrual cycle in the "resting" human breast, *Br. J. Cancer* **44:**177–181.

Geschickter, C.F. (ed.), 1945, Normal development and functional changes in the mammary gland, in: *Diseases of the Breast: Diagnosis, Pathology, Treatment,* Lippincott, Philadelphia, pp. 3–41.

Hiba, J., Del Pozo, E., Genazzani, A., Pusterla, E., Lancranjan, I., Sidiropoulos, D., and Gunti, J., 1977, Hormonal mechanism of milk secretion in the newborn, *J. Clin. Endocrinol. Metab.* **44:**973–976.

Ingleby, H., and Gershon-Cohen, J. (eds.), 1960, The normal breast, in: *Comparative Anatomy, Pathology and Roentgenology of the Breast,* University of Pennsylvania Press, Philadelphia. pp. 3–119.

King, M.M., McCoy, P., and Russo, I.H., 1983, Dietary fat may influence DMBA-initiated mammary gland carcinogenesis by modification of mammary gland development, in: *Current Topics on Nutrition and Disease* (D.A. Roe, ed.), Alan R. Liss, New York, pp. 61–69.

Leis, H.P. Jr., 1978, Epidemiology of breast cancer: Identification of high risk women, in: *The Breast,* Chapter 4 (H.S. Gallager, H.P. Leis, R.K. Snyderman, and J. Urban, eds.) Mosby, St. Louis, pp. 37–48.

Levin, M.L., Sheehe, P.R., Graham, S., and Glidewell, O., 1964, Lactation and menstrual function as related to cancer of the breast, *Am. J. Public Health* **54:**580–587.

Lyons, W.R., Li, C.H., and Johnson, R.E., 1953, Some of the hormones required by the mammary gland in its development and functions, *J. Clin. Endocrinol.* **13:**836–837.

Lyons, W.R., Li, C.H., and Johnson, R.E., 1958, The hormonal control of mammary growth and lactation, *Recent Prog. Horm. Res.* **14:**219–254.

Masters, J.R.W., Drife, J.O., and Scarisbrick, J.J., 1977, Cyclic variations of DNA synthesis in human breast epithelium, *J. Natl. Cancer Inst.* **58:**1263–1265.

Meyer, S.J., 1977, Cell proliferation in normal human breast ducts, fibroadenomas, and other ductal hyperplasias as measured by tritiated thymidine, effects of menstrual phase, age and oral contraceptive hormones, *Human Pathol.* **8:**67–81.

Raynaud, A., 1960, Morphogenesis of the mammary gland, in: *Milk: The Mammary Gland and its Secretions* (S.K. Kou and A.T. Cowie, eds.), Academic Press, New York, pp. 3–45.

Reynolds, E.L., and Wines, J.V., 1948, Individual differences in physical changes associated with adolescence in girls, *Am. J. Dis. Child* **75:**329–350.

Russo, I.H., and Russo, J., 1978a, Developmental stage of the rat mammary gland as determinant of its susceptibility to 7,12-dimethylbenz(a)anthracene, *J. Natl. Cancer Inst.* **61:**1439–1449.

Russo, J., and Russo, I.H., 1978b, DNA-Labeling Index and structure of the rat mammary gland as determinants of its susceptibility to carcinogenesis, *J. Natl. Cancer Inst.* **61:**1451–1459.

Russo, J., Wilgus, G., and Russo, I.H., 1979, Susceptibility of the mammary gland to carcinogenesis. I. Differentiation of the mammary gland as determinant of tumor incidence and type of lesion, *Am. J. Pathol.* **96:**721–736.

Russo, J., and Russo, I.H., 1980a, Influence of differentiation and cell kinetics on the susceptibility of the rat mammary gland to carcinogenesis, *Cancer Res.* **40:**2677–2687.

Russo, J., and Russo, I.H., 1980b, Susceptibility of the mammary gland to carcinogenesis. II. Pregnancy interruption as a risk factor in tumor incidence, *Am. J. Pathol.* **100:**497–511.

Russo, J., Wilgus, G., Tait, L., and Russo, I.H., 1981, Influence of age and parity on the susceptibility of rat mammary gland epithelial cells in primary cultures to 7,12-dimethylbenz(a)anthracene, *In Vitro* **17:**877–884.

Russo, J., and Russo, I.H., 1982, Is differentiation the answer in breast cancer prevention? *Int. Res. Comm. Syst. Med. Sci.* **10:**935–941.

Russo, J., Tay, L.K., and Russo, I.H., 1982, Differentiation of the mammary gland and susceptibility to carcinogenesis, *Breast Cancer Res. Treat.* **2:**5–73.

Russo, J., 1985, Immunocytochemical markers in breast cancer, in: *Immunocytochemistry in Tumor Diagnosis* (J. Russo, ed.), Martinus Nijhoff Publishing, Boston, pp. 207–232.

Russo, J., and Russo, I.H., 1986, Role of differentiation on transformation of human breast epithelial cells, in: *Cellular and Molecular Biology of Experimental Mammary Cancer* (D. Medina, W. Kidwell, G. Heppner, and E. Anderson, eds.), Plenum Press, New York.

Salazar, H., and Tobon, H., 1974, Morphologic changes of the mammary gland during development, pregnancy and lactation, in: *Lactogenic Hormones, Fetal Nutrition and Lactation* (J. Josimovich, ed.), Wiley, New York, pp. 221–277.

Tanner, J.M. (ed.), 1962, The development of the reproductive system, in: *Growth at Adolescence,* Blackwell Scientific, Oxford, pp. 28–39.

Vorherr, H. (ed.), 1974, Development of the female breast, in: *The Breast,* Academic Press, New York, pp. 1–18.

II

Cell Biology of the Mammary Gland

4

Form and Function in the Mammary Gland

The Role of Extracellular Matrix

Mina J. Bissell and H. Glenn Hall

In the days of seemingly unlimited funding and personnel, the shotgun approach to biology yielded substantial knowledge. Today more taste must be displayed. Because a question can be asked at the molecular level does not mean it is worth asking, any more than just another histological or electron microscopic study of a developing tissue or cell is justifiable. . . . Our knowledge of tissue interactions [and cell–ECM interactions] in embryos [as in adults] is still so primitive that investigations at all levels are necessary if we are to fully explain these processes and their consequences in mechanistic terms.

Norman K. Wessells (1977) (reproduced with permission)

1. Introduction: Extracellular Matrix as an Inducer

Two fundamental and as yet unresolved questions continue to intrigue biologists of diverse background: How are tissues generated? How is

Mina J. Bissell and H. Glenn Hall • Laboratory of Cell Biology, Division of Biology and Medicine, Lawrence Berkeley Laboratory, University of California, Berkeley, California 94720.

tissue specificity maintained? To answer the first question, developmental biologists long ago evoked the concept of *embryonic induction*—the exact nature of which is poorly understood. Nevertheless, inductive interactions have been postulated and demonstrated between ectoderm and mesoderm or epithelium and mesenchyme in many systems (for a general review see Wessells, 1977).

The classical studies of Kratochwil (1969) indicated that isolated mammary epithelium recombined with its own mesenchyme develops a typical mammary pattern. When recombined with salivary mesenchyme, however, it resembles a salivary gland. Later studies (Kratochwil and Schwartz, 1976; Sakakura et al., 1976; Drews and Drews, 1977; Kratochwil, 1977; Hoshino, 1978) confirmed and expanded the role of mesenchyme in morphogenesis and in hormonal response of the mammary gland (see Chapters 1 and 2 in this volume).

The mechanism by which the mesenchyme brings about these profound responses remains obscure. Recent advances in our understanding of the structure and biochemistry of the extracellular matrix (ECM) have focused attention on the inductive capability of the ECM. Although a cause-and-effect relation in development is less clear for ECM than for mesenchyme, the phenomenon is easily demonstrable in culture in terms of maintenance of expression of tissue-specific functions. This appears to be true for many tissues, but the mammary gland has provided a versatile model system for studying the dramatic effect of ECM on gene expression. (For general reviews see Hay, 1981; Bissell et al., 1982; MacKenzie and Fusenig, 1983; Porter and Whelan, 1984; Trelstad, 1984; Cunha et al., 1985.)

The operational framework of this chapter is based on three premises:

1. A unit of function in higher organisms in general, and in the mammary gland in particular, is larger than the cell. At the least, the unit includes the cell plus its extracellular matrix; in a larger context, the unit is the organ itself.
2. The ECM on which the cells sit is an extension of the cells and an active participant in regulation of their function; that is, the ECM is an *informational* entity in the sense that it receives, imparts, and integrates structural and functional signals.

Abbreviations: ECM, Extracellular matrix; EHS, Engelbreth–Holm–Swarm tumor; HSPG, heparan sulfate proteoglycan; PMME, primary mouse mammary epithelium. We have adopted the nomenclature used by Henninghausen and Sippel for the mouse milk proteins (1982a,b). The recommendation of the Committee on the Nomenclature and Methodology of Milk Proteins (Eigel et al., 1984) cannot be followed easily for mouse proteins since these have not been sequenced as yet. It is expected that a consensus will emerge on further purification and characterization of these proteins.

3. ECM-induced functional differentiation in the mammary gland is mediated through changes in cell shape; that is, form and function are intimately related.

The extensive literature on the structure and function of the mammary gland and milk protein composition is not reviewed in this chapter. Instead, we focus on recent literature directly related to the influence of extracellular matrix on mammary-specific gene expression. Because this is a new and rapidly expanding field, we are including recent data—some of which are in press or as yet unpublished (both from our own laboratory and those of others). An indication of how recent some of these concepts are is the fact that neither *extracellular matrix* nor *basal lamina* appears in the index of recent books on regulation of lactation (Mepham, 1983; Neville and Neifert, 1983; Larson, 1985) or in otherwise excellent books on development (Slack, 1983). There is older literature, however, that indirectly relates to the subject of this chapter, and we have tried to include those references of which we are aware.

2. *Mammary Model Systems: How Relevant?*

The choice of culture system for studies of gene expression bears a fundamental and direct relation to the relevance of the results obtained. The early literature of cell culture, where growth and survival were the primary concerns of the investigators, is replete with statements and conclusions that may have little relevance to the physiological state (for a review of earlier data in this area see Bissell, 1981). Studies on mammary epithelial cells bring this point home. Here the choice is not only whether organ culture, primary culture, or established cell lines retain epithelial characteristics, but also under which conditions organ or primary cultures have appropriate functional activity. For example, it is clear that cells on plastic retain their epithelial characteristics and furthermore that they reveal their sensitivity to prolactin by increasing the level of specific mRNA upon prolactin addition (Lee et al., 1985). Yet, based on their inability to secrete β-casein after 8 days in culture, one might conclude that these cells either have lost the prolactin receptor or have lost the ability to transcribe β-casein message—both wrong conclusions. We know that mRNA for β-casein is indeed induced after prolactin addition even on plastic (Lee et al., 1985). Once the cells are placed on an appropriate substratum (floating collagen gels or reconstituted basal lamina, see below), β-casein is processed and secreted. Thus, mammary epithelial cells of many species respond optimally to prolactin by producing and secreting β-casein *only if* the cells are placed on a "correct" substratum or if the cells are placed in high enough density to make their own ECM (Shannon and Pitelka, 1981; Haeuptle et al., 1983; Ringo and Rocha, 1983; Wilde et al., 1984; Lee et al., 1984, 1985; Durban et al., 1985; Levine and Stockdale, 1985; Rocha et al., 1985; Bissell et al., 1986a,b; Li et al., 1987).

Tissue heterogeneity is yet another consideration when employing model systems for studies of cell–hormone–ECM interactions and gene expression. For example, DuBois and Elias (1984) using organ culture of immature mouse mammary gland demonstrated that different regions of the gland require different hormonal combinations for proliferation and maintenance. In culture, this regional heterogeneity would be disrupted, giving rise to random mixing with some populations possibly being predominant. The information obtained about hormone susceptibility from such cultures may not be applicable to the entire population. Such cell culture heterogeneity has been described by McGrath et al. (1985) for normal rat mammary cells where one subpopulation responds to EGF and another to prolactin and progesterone.

Cell lines derived from mammary tissue may retain epithelial morphology but usually lose their functional differentiation, a general process observed for all cells in culture(Bissell, 1981). The pathologists have always known that maintenance of tissue cytostructure is important for retention of tissue-specific functions, but this is a more recent recognition for cell and, especially, molecular biologists. Thus, loss of cell–cell and cell–matrix interactions through repeated trypsinizations undoubtedly is instrumental in irreversible loss of function. Indeed, the only functional mammary cell strain isolated to date (COMMA-1D isolated from pregnant mice by Danielson et al., 1984) is quite heterogeneous and produces large amounts of matrix proteins (unpublished data), findings that may explain COMMA-1D's functionality. Once individual COMMA-1D cells are cloned, they basically lose their ability to respond to lactogenic hormones and substrata (D. Medina et al., 1987). It should be noted that "normal" mammary cell strains have been isolated and characterized from rat (Bennett et al., 1979), mouse (Danielson et al., 1984; Ehrmann et al., 1984), and human (Stampfer et al., 1980; Hammond et al., 1984). Much interesting literature has been generated with cloned rat cell lines from investigation into the possible existence of stem cell populations, the conversion of one cell type to another, pattern of synthesized and secreted proteins, and so on (Warburton et al., 1981; Barraclough et al., 1984; Ormerod and Rudland, 1985; Paterson and Rudland, 1985; Paterson et al., 1985). The level of functional differentiation in these cell strains and lines in terms of milk protein production, however, has not been reported (with the exception of COMMA-1D cells, see Section 4.2.2a).

Organ cultures of the mammary gland (Juergens et al., 1965; Banerjee, 1976) have produced valuable information on regulation of functional differentiation, yet this model system poses a different problem. The most important function of the mammary gland is to secrete milk; hence, the definition of functional differentiation for the gland must include synthesis and secretion of milk proteins as well as other specific milk components such as lactose and medium-chain fatty acids. In organ culture, the ducts seal after a few days. Since it is well known that synthesis and secretion of milk proteins are coupled processes, cessation of the latter most probably will feed-back, reducing the rate of synthesis and/or increasing internal degradation—undoubtedly altering normal regulatory mechanisms. Nevertheless, the organ culture has the advantages of including all the cell types in their "correct" relation, containing the basal lamina, and maintaining an appropriate cytostructure.

It is clear from the above that for the mammary gland no single system is ideal and the choice has to depend on the questions being asked. The advantages and disadvantages of using the whole animal are well known and are not reiterated. For studies of cell–ECM interaction and functional differentiation, the use of primary cultures cultivated in defined media on various substrata appears most promising. The hope, of course, is to reassemble a "normal" secretory gland from the sum of its component parts. This will necessitate learning much more about the cellular heterogeneity of the gland, the role of the stroma, the composition of ECM, and the mechanisms of hormone action in the mammary gland.

3. Operational Definition of ECM

ECM is defined in many ways by different investigators. For the purpose of this chapter, we define it as the acellular materials that connect cells within tissues. In the case of epithelial cells, ECM includes the basement membrane (Kefalides et al., 1979). The latter contains a basal lamina, "a nearly uniformly thick (thin) layer closely associated with and derived from the parenchymal cells," and a reticular lamina, "an adjacent layer of variable thickness derived from the connective tissue cells"—the two acting as a functional unit (Bernfield, 1984). The basal lamina typically contains laminin, type IV collagen, proteoglycans (usually heparan sulfate proteoglycan, HSPG), and glycoproteins such as entactin (Table I).

Despite substantial recent advances in understanding the biochemistry of ECM components, little is known about the supramolecular

Table I. Major Basal Lamina Proteins

Protein	Molecular properties	Selected references
Collagen IV[a]	1(IV) and 2(IV) chains; M_r = 550,000–600,000	Kefalides et al. (1979)
Laminin	Light (200K) and heavy (400K) chains: M_r= 1,000,000	Chung et al. (1977); Timpl et al. (1979)
Fibronectin	M_r = 450,000; two similar chains	Semanoff et al. (1982)
Heparan sulfate proteoglycan	M_r = 130,000; 10% protein	Gordon and Bernfield (1980); Hogan et al. (1982); Laurie et al. (1986)
Entactin	M_r = 150,000; single chain	Carlin et al (1981); Hogan et al. (1982)

[a]Type V is also known to be a component of basal lamina. However, it has not been studied as extensively as the components listed above.

organization and tissue-specific composition of ECM. The availability of a mouse tumor (Englebreth–Holm–Swarm tumor, EHS; Orkin et al., 1977) that produces a substantial amount of basal lamina in vivo has made it possible to isolate individual components and to determine their structure (Kleinman et al., 1986). Most biochemical studies of basal lamina composition have used this tumor with the realization that it may not represent accurately a "normal" basement membrane. In addition, immunocytochemistry has shown that basement membranes evolve during development and that different organs have basal lamina with different compositions (Wan et al., 1984). It is also important to keep in mind that slight changes in composition could lead to substantial changes in the three-dimensional organization, which, as we will argue below, is undoubtedly important in maintenance and modulation of function.

4. *Influences of the ECM on Mammary Differentiation*

The mammary gland provides a versatile and attractive model for studying the relation of shape to function. Studies with cultured cells are aided by the fact that milk composition provides a convenient reference point for in vivo studies. The success of culture conditions can therefore be measured against synthetic and secretory activities that match the pattern observed for milk (see Section 4.2.2a).

Attempts to culture mammary epithelium started as early as 1924 (Maximow). These and other early attempts led to overgrowth of stroma or complete loss of function, raising the question of whether epithelial cells were lost or were irreversibly altered in culture. A classic experiment performed by Daniel and DeOme (1965), however, indicated clearly that cultured mammary cells of mice, when injected into gland-free mammary fat pads in situ, were largely capable of reforming normal ductal morphology and producing milk after the animal gave birth. Thus, the importance of cellular environment (stroma and/or unknown host factors, in addition to lactogenic hormones) in regulation of mammary-specific function was indicated more than 20 years ago. Interestingly, initial successes in achieving some functional activity in culture came either with mixed populations (Lasfargues, 1957) or under crowded conditions (Ceriani, 1976)—situations that may promote production of a higher level of ECM components (our unpublished studies on COMMA-1D, and Schwarz and Bissell, 1977).

Reconstituted rat tail collagen was introduced as a substratum for cultured cells in 1956 (Ehrman and Gey). Since then, collagen has been shown to be essential for differentiation, as well as for maintenance or induction of tissue-specific functions in numerous systems, and that literature is not reviewed here. The turning point for culturing the epithelial cells from the mammary gland, however, came only when Emerman and Pitelka (1977), following the examples of Elsdale and Bard (1972) and Michaelopoulos and Pitot (1975), placed mouse cells on the top of rat tail collagen gels. A new chapter in our understanding and appreciation of the role of substrata and shape was written when these investigators used a spatula to release the gel to float. Sometimes, the most simple experiments have the most profound consequences! These are detailed in Sections 4.1 and 4.2.

4.1. Morphological Consequences of Cell–ECM Interactions

The formation of the mammary gland, like most developmental events, is a complex process involving changes in cellular shape, proliferation, and morphogenetic organization. The process entails the extension of growing cords of epithelial cells from the nipple area into the fatty stroma to form elongated branching ducts. Concurrent with growth is differentiation of cell types, establishment of their relative spatial relations, and their organization into ducts and terminal alveoli (for more detail see Chapters 1–3 this volume).

4.1.1. Morphology at the Cellular Level

The profound changes that occur when secretory mammary epithelial cells are taken from the gland and plated in isolation on plastic surfaces, as well as the reestablishment of morphological differentiation when the same cells are placed on floating gels have been well documented (Emerman and Pitelka, 1977; Emerman et al., 1977; Burwen et al., 1980; Shannon and Pitelka, 1981; MacKenzie et al., 1982; Foster et al., 1983; Haeuptle et al., 1983). Viewed by transmission electron microscopy, primary mouse mammary epithelial cells on plastic or on attached collagen gels have a high nuclear : cytoplasmic ratio, lack internal polarization and secretory apparatus, and have short, stubby microvilli on their apical surfaces. By contrast, within 2–5 days after the gel is released, cells become polar and columnar and contain an extensive network of distended rough endoplasmic reticulum, Golgi apparati, secretory vesicles, and fat droplets. After a visible and continuous basal lamina separates the epithelium from the gel, cells have tight junctions and extensive microvilli on their apical surface (Emerman and Pitelka, 1977). A dramatic example of changes in cell shape, cytostructure, and surface activity of primary mouse mammary epithelial cells when placed on EHS-reconstituted matrix is shown in Fig. 1. These changes are not peculiar to primary cells. COMMA-1D cells on floating gels or on plastic coated with reconstituted basal lamina from EHS tumor show similar morphological changes. These morphological metamorphoses are not culture artifacts and have functional correlates in vivo (Fig. 2; Pitelka et al., 1973). There are striking differences in the luminal surface of an alveolus of a lactating mouse gland fixed in the engorged (Fig. 2a) versus the depleted state (Fig. 2b). The morphology and secretory capability of cells on plastic or flat gels, and those on floating gels or EHS, mimic the engorged and emptied states of the alveoli in the lactating gland.

The absence of surface activity and the flat morphology of cells on plastic do not imply a takeover by nonepithelial cells. These cells are capable of forming large and small domes as a result of active transport across the epithelial sheet (Misfeldt et al., 1976; Fig. 3 and Lee et al., 1985) depending on age and culture density, synthesize low levels of mRNA for some of the milk proteins, and secrete transferrin (see Section 5.2). While it would be too simplistic to correlate all functional changes with morphology, a striking correlation nevertheless is apparent. As we shall see in Section 4.2.2b, cells on EHS-reconstituted basal lamina and HSPG-coated dishes have elevated levels of β-casein mRNA. Yet both their secretory capabilities and their morphologies are quite different (Li et al., 1987). Whether secretory changes are a direct consequence of the cell's cytostructure, or whether each of these parameters is the consequence of other regulatory steps is an intriguing and important problem in mammary gland biology.

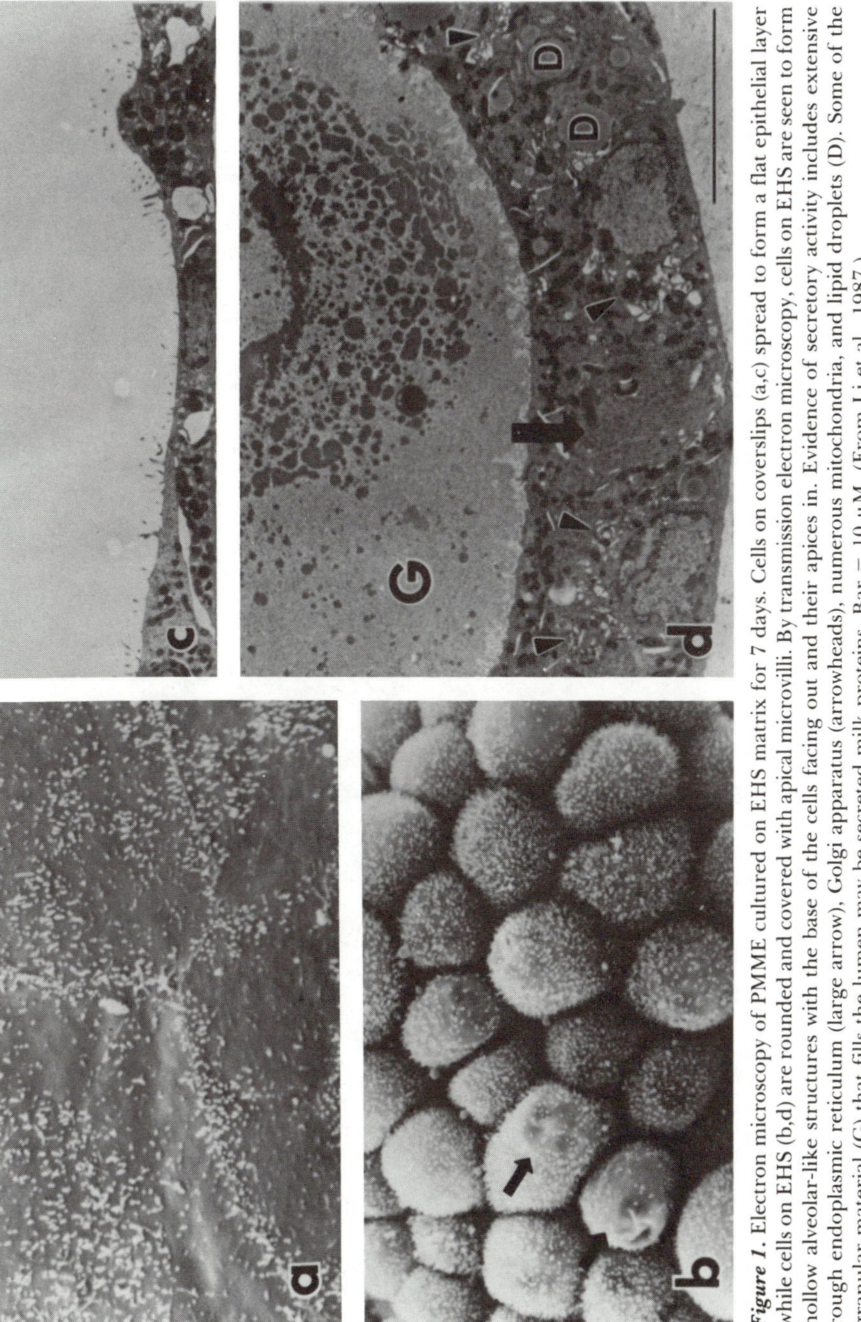

Figure 1. Electron microscopy of PMME cultured on EHS matrix for 7 days. Cells on coverslips (a,c) spread to form a flat epithelial layer while cells on EHS (b,d) are rounded and covered with apical microvilli. By transmission electron microscopy, cells on EHS are seen to form hollow alveolar-like structures with the base of the cells facing out and their apices in. Evidence of secretory activity includes extensive rough endoplasmic reticulum (large arrow), Golgi apparatus (arrowheads), numerous mitochondria, and lipid droplets (D). Some of the granular material (G) that fills the lumen may be secreted milk proteins. Bar = 10 μM. (From Li et al., 1987.)

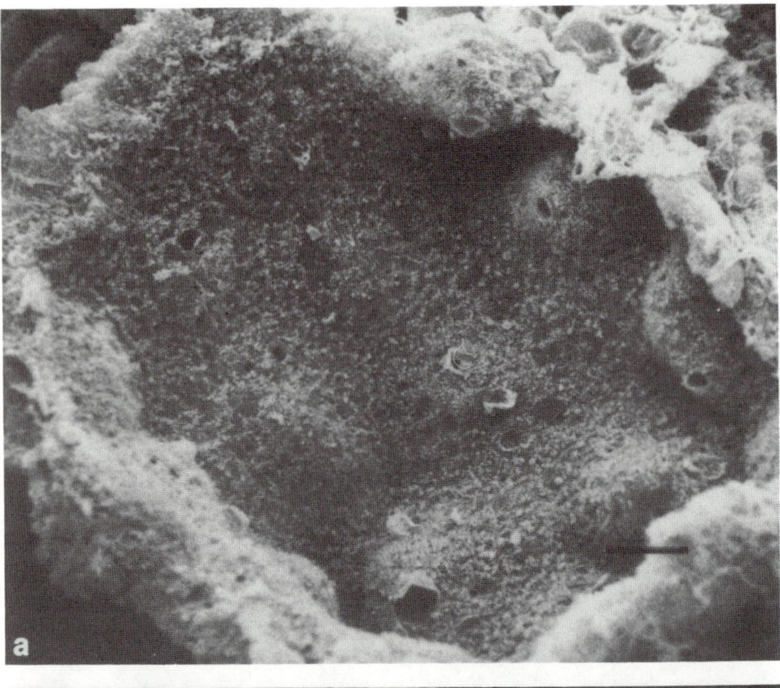
a

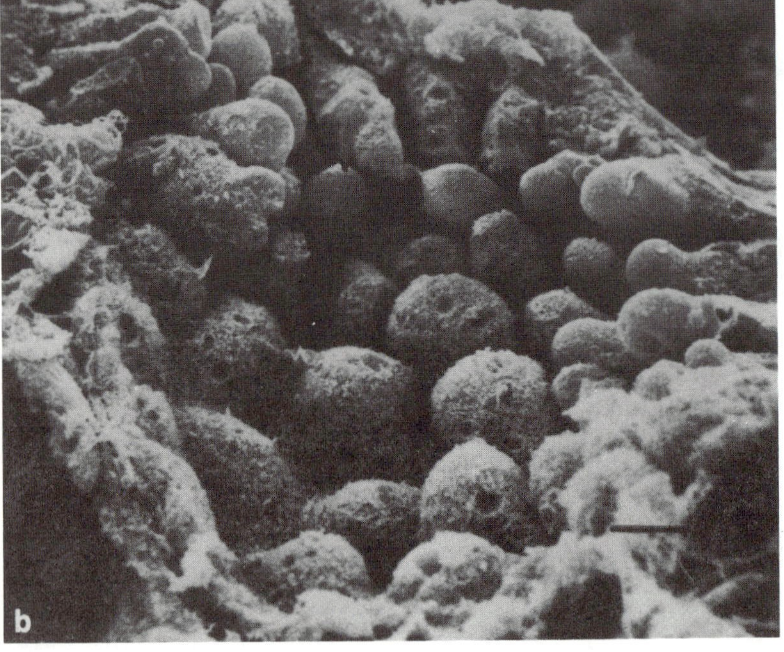
b

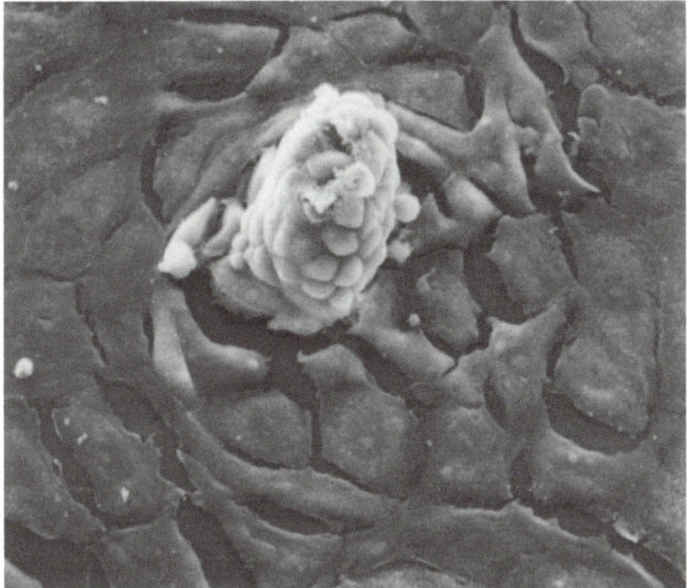

Figure 3. Appearance of a small dome on primary mammary epithelial cells grown on a glass coverslip. Magnification about ×1500. J. Aggeler and M.J. Bissell (unpublished).

4.1.2. Establishing of the Tissue: Growth and Morphogenesis

Regenerating tissues, culture systems, and theoretical models have been employed in an attempt to separate the processes of cellular growth and rearrangement in morphogenesis and to identify the regulatory factors. These systems have revealed the central role of ECM not only in affecting the form of individual cells but also in the development of the tissue as a whole.

Figure 2. Scanning electron micrograph of the luminal surface of part of an alveolus. Cells fixed in the inflated state (a) are flat or only slightly convex. Cells surfaces are irregularly covered with microvilli, and several small craters left by extracted fat droplets are visible. The luminal area seen here includes about 11 cells in full face view. Cells fixed in the contracted state (b) appear to bulge deeply into the lumen. Most cell apices are irregularly covered with microvilli and small fat craters, but several are smooth where they are distended over large fat droplets. Compare the number and shapes of cells visible here with those in (a). Magnifications ×1000. Original photos courtesy of Dr. Dorothy Pitelka (Pitelka et al., 1973; reproduced with permission).

4.1.2a. Attachment and Growth. The use of cleared mammary fat pads (once the epithelial rudiment is removed from fat pad of 3-week-old female) as an environment to promote the growth of mammary epithelial cells (DeOme et al., 1959) suggests that the mammary stroma including the adipose tissue provides the substratum and other necessary factors for growth. However, mesenchyme from other tissues, such as the salivary gland, also promotes proliferation (Sakakura et al., 1976). While there is an increasing recognition that ECM may act as a "sink" to retain growth factors (Matsuda et al., 1984), there is also evidence that some growth-inducing factors can be attributed to the ECM molecules themselves. The growth of primary mammary cells is sustained by embedding the cells in type I collagen gels (Yang et al., 1979; Foster et al., 1983; Haeuptle et al., 1983; Suard et al., 1983). Substratum-attached material from 3T3 fibroblast lines, with or without differentiation into adipocytes, promotes the growth of mouse mammary epithelium (Levine and Stockdale, 1984). ECM from whole rat mammary glands promotes the growth of rat mammary epithelial cells when compared to growth on plastic, but growth on collagen substrata was not assessed in that study (Wicha et al., 1982). The basement membrane components produced by the mammary cells, such as type IV collagen, appear to be involved in attachment as well as growth. Mammary cells appear to attach faster and grow better on type IV collagen than on type I (Wicha et al., 1979).

An interrelation may exist between the growth-promoting effect of soluble hormones, growth factors, and the ECM. The growth response of rat mammary epithelial cells to hormones is dependent on the substratum on which the cells are placed (McGrath et al., 1985). Again, this response may be mediated by the synthesis of type IV collagen: EGF stimulates the synthesis of type IV collagen, and hydrocortisone suppresses its degradation (Salomon et al., 1981). The embedding of mammary cells in collagen, in the studies mentioned above, appears to be permissive for cell response to hormones and growth factors so that, along with the use of defined medium, the effect of the individual factors can be studied (Nandi et al., 1984; Imagawa et al., 1985; McGrath et al., 1985). In other systems, components of the ECM can either substitute for growth factors or modulate the cellular response to them (Gospodarowicz et al., 1982; Gatmaitan et al., 1983). A cell line that differentiates into adipocytes (3T3-L1), in addition to producing an ECM, produces soluble factors that appear to promote further the growth of the epithelial cells (Levine and Stockdale, 1984).

4.1.2b. Morphogenesis. Adult mammary epithelium is capable of proliferating in response to either salivary or mammary mesenchyme but the resulting morphology is characteristic of the type of mesenchyme (Sakakura et al., 1979a). Mouse mammary fat pads of any age can support the growth and morphogenesis of mammary epithelial cells but not of other epithelial cell types except hair follicles (Sakakura et al., 1979b). In addition, separate specificities for morphological determination exist within the mammary mesenchyme, resulting in different epithelial morphologies (Sakakura et al., 1982).

The mesenchymal factors that determine the morphology of the glands are not well defined, but they may well be components of, or specifically associated with, the ECM. In many systems, ECM components have been shown to serve as a guiding substratum for migratory cells (Dunn and Ebendal, 1978; Couchman et al., 1980; Greenberg et al., 1981; Erickson and Turley, 1983; Boucaut et al., 1984a,b; Bronner-Fraser, 1984; Schor et al., 1985a,b). In the mammary gland, the penetration of the growing bud probably involves a dynamic interaction between the contractile myoepithelial cells and/or their progenitor cap cells and the ECM (see Chapter 1 in this volume; Williams and Daniel, 1983; Ormerod and Rudland, 1985). For example, both human (Yang et al., 1979) and rabbit (Haeuptle et al., 1983) mammary cells embedded in collagen gels form spike-like structures penetrating the gel. Similar structures were also formed by a tumor-derived cloned cell strain, Rama 25, which has the characteristics of a stem cell (Bennett, 1980). Subsequent clones of this strain indicated that it consisted of two cell types, a cuboidal and an elongated cell type (Bennett et al., 1981) believed to be similar to myoepithelial and ductal epithelial cells, both of which were necessary for penetration of the cells into collagen. While the authors conclude in both these reports that intrinsic characteristics of these cells alone are sufficient for formation of the tubules in collagen gels, they fail to note that the provided collagen (plus a small amount of other ECM components undoubtedly present as contaminants) *is* a mesenchymal component and that in vivo a mesenchymal cell type producing collagen would thus be necessary.

Continuing differentiation of the mammary gland involves establishment of polarity of the epithelial cells and the formation of lumina which serve to collect and route the secreted milk. Lumina are formed starting as small cavities between cells which fuse to form the larger cavities. Cells are recruited into the developing lumen structure. The signals that initiate lumen formation are not known, but it has been hypothesized that the determinant of polarity comes from the basal side, perhaps as a result of changes in composition of the basal lamina (Hogg et al., 1983). Support for the involvement of ECM in lumen formation comes from our earlier work using a mammary cell strain (NMuMG) in culture. When these cells were grown as a monolayer on a collagen gel and overlaid with additional collagen, they reorganized to form lumina (Hall et al., 1982). The process of lumen formation in culture had many similarities to the process observed in vivo. For example, the lumina started out as small cavities that tended to fuse into larger cavities with the recruitment of more cells into the structure. The similarity of the morphology of lumina formed in culture (mouse) and in vivo (human) can be seen in Fig. 4.

Lumen formation in the spike-like structures formed by cells embedded in a collagen gel has not been studied in detail. The collagen gel in which normal human mammary epithelial cells were embedded needed to be released for lumen formation to take place (Foster et al., 1983). The contraction of the gels allowed further organization of cells into cord-like tubules. This may have depended on the ability of the cells to orient the collagen fibers that then could orient the cells (*dynamic reciprocity*; see Section 5.3.) Because the spike-like structures in collagen gels do not correlate well with the more rounded and organized end buds in vivo, experiments were conducted to determine what determinants may be responsible for the normal morphology in vivo (Daniel et al., 1984). Collagen gels containing embedded mouse mammary cells were placed in cleared mammary fat pads. The embedded cells continued to form the spike-like structures when in contact with the collagen gel or in contact with fibrillar material in the fat pad. However, those cells that contacted adipocytes formed normal end bud structures, indicating that collagen gels alone did not contain all the necessary information for proper end bud formation. More recently, we have found a relation between cortisol and collagen-induced lumen morphogenesis by NMuMG cells, pointing to interactions between hormones and ECM. In serum-free medium supplemented with transferrin, prostaglandin E, insulin, and triiodothryonine, lumen formation was initiated but regressed unless cortisol was present (Bissell et al., 1986a; H. G. Hall and M. J. Bissell, unpublished data).

Figure 4. Electron micrographs of lumen formed by mammary epithelial cells. (a) Tip of an epithelial cord at 17 days shows advanced stage of lumen formation with well-developed junctional complexes linking neighboring epithelial cells whose free surfaces now bear numerous microvilli. (b) NMuMG cells sandwiched between two layers of rat-tail collagen (type I) form a lumen that is completely enclosed and contains electron-dense material. The upper collagen gel is at the top, the lower gel at the bottom. Microvilli project into the lumen. Magnification ×7000. Note similarities between the lumen formed in vivo to that in culture. Photo (a) courtesy of Dr. C. Tickle (Hogg et al., 1983); reproduced with permission. Photo (b) H.G. Hall (unpublished).

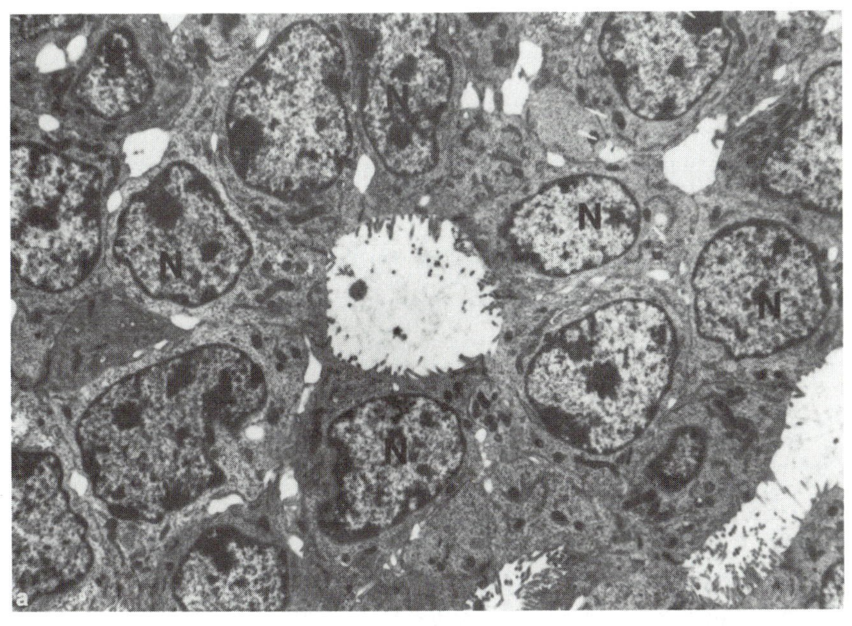
N
N
N
N
N
a

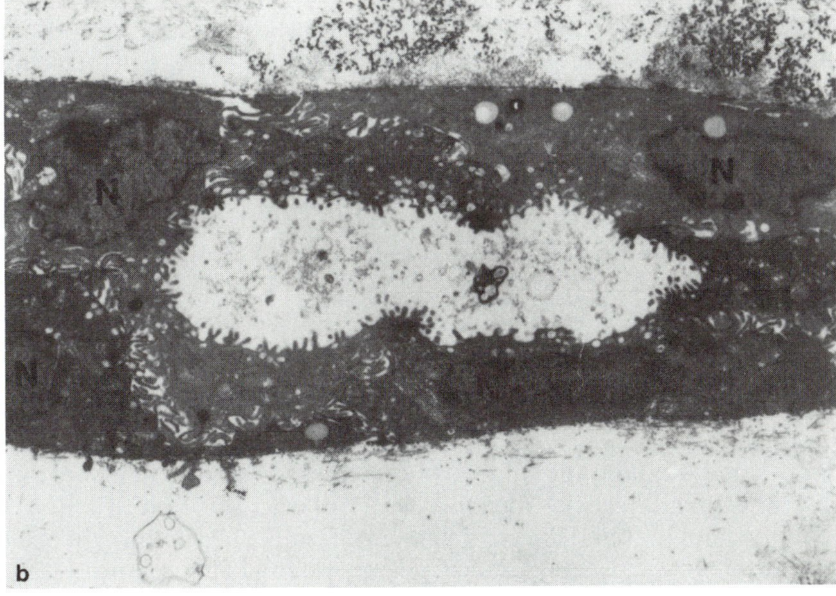
N
N
N
b

4.2. Functional Consequences of Cell–ECM Interactions

4.2.1. Metabolism

Mammary epithelial cells are among the most metabolically active cells found in nature (Collier, 1985). Profound metabolic alterations occur in the mammary gland in preparation for lactation. There is an enormous literature on metabolic regulation in the gland of various species (for comprehensive reviews see Larson and Smith, 1974; Larson, 1978, 1985; Mepham, 1983; Neville and Neifert, 1983). Here, we summarize changes in metabolic pattern only as a function of the mammary cell's interaction with the extracellular matrix, the literature on which is limited.

Glucose is a major substrate for the synthesis of organ-specific products in the gland of nonruminant animals. The pattern of glucose use changes during the transition from the pregnant to the lactating state. Using high specific activity ^{14}C-glucose and two-dimensional paper chromatography we showed that the glucose metabolites generated by freshly isolated epithelial cells from virgin, pregnant, and lactating glands were strikingly different, especially in the ability of the cells to synthesize glycogen (Emerman et al., 1980, 1981). If cells maintained on floating gels were analogous to cells in vivo, it would follow that the glucose metabolite pattern should modulate when cells are placed on different substrata. This indeed was the case: Cells from pregnant gland maintained on floating collagen gel were similar to pregnant gland in terms of glycogen and lactose synthesis and were very different from the same cells on plastic where lactose could not be detected at all (Emerman et al., 1981). Cells from lactating glands, however, resembled the pregnant gland when maintained on floating gels, indicating that some "lactogenic" factors were missing in culture. Since milk components are not removed by suckling (as is the case in the lactating gland), it is possible that a feedback mechanism prevents the lactating cells from expressing their full potential, leading to reversion to the pregnant state on floating gels. It would be interesting to design experiments to test this possibility. Recent studies with human mammary cell strains indicate that the glucose metabolite pattern in these cells modulates with different media composition. Under some culture conditions, the pattern is similar to the pattern of mouse cells on floating gels (J. Bartley, G. Levine, and M. Stampfer, unpublished data). Preliminary results indicate that the metabolite pattern changes as a function of growth on ECM, and on at least one type of biomatrix the cells express some β-casein and α-lactalbumin (J. Bartley et al., personal communication).

Enzymes involved in other metabolic pathways, such as nucleic acid degradation, have also been shown to modulate as a function of both the reproductive cycle and the substratum. Ringo and Rocha (1983) measured xanthine oxidase in the glands of virgin, pregnant, and lactating mice and showed it to be highest in the lactating tissue. The level increased appreciably (24-fold) in primary mouse mammary epithelial cells when cultured on released gels as compared to attached gels. While the exact role of xanthine oxidase remains obscure, the enzyme can be used as another indicator of the functional activity of the mammary gland.

4.2.2. *Milk Protein Gene Expression*

> *"The principal problems encountered in our laboratory are not the result of limitations of recombinant DNA technology, but rather those of cell biology, i.e. cell–cell and cell–substratum interactions as well as cell shape are critical factors regulating milk protein gene expression"*
> Rosen et al., 1986.

The dramatic morphological changes observed when mammary cells are seeded onto collagen gels and floated are accompanied by multiple and complex functional changes. Modulations in mRNA levels are not necessarily coordinated with changes in synthesis and secretion of individual milk proteins.

4.2.2a. Synthesis and Secretion. The lactation literature has been reviewed extensively (Mepham, 1983; Neville and Neifert, 1983; Nickerson and Akers, 1984; Larson, 1985) and is not further reviewed here.

Emerman et al. (1977) and Shannon and Pitelka (1981) measured γ-casein levels in primary mouse mammary epithelial cells in the presence and absence of prolactin on floating collagen gels and showed that it was modulated as a function of hormones and substrata. Suard et al. (1983) measured β-casein, α-lactalbumin, and transferrin in the medium of rabbit mammary epithelial cells grown on collagen gels and demonstrated dependence on substrata, shape, and hormones. Interestingly, transferrin secretion appears to be insensitive to prolactin but is modulated by substrata (Bissell et al., 1986a; Lee et al., 1987). Wilde et al. (1984), working also with rabbit mammary cells, confirmed the findings of Suard et al (1983). In addition, they compared collagen gels with mammary biomatrices and essentially found little difference between the two, although floating gels appeared to be slightly more effective than biomatrices. Wicha et al. (1982) reported that α-lactalbumin secretion in rat mammary cells was much more responsive to mammary biomatrix than to floating gels, indicating that there may be species differences in response to biomatrix. Nevertheless, the similarities in response to substrata by different species are much greater than the differences. By and large, floating collagenous substrata, homologous and even heterologous biomatrices, and reconstituted basement membrane from various sources lead to changes in morphology and increased milk protein synthesis and secretion in all species tested so far.

Using the two-dimensional pattern of mouse skim milk proteins as a reference (Fig. 5), we analyzed the secreted proteins of primary mouse mammary epithelial cells maintained on plastic (P), on attached collagen type I gels (G), or on released gels (RG). The pattern of secreted proteins is more complex than that of milk under all three conditions. Furthermore, there are both substratum- and shape-specific changes (Fig. 6). The secreted proteins fall into at least four categories: (1) Milk proteins, such as transferrin, are present under all culture conditions. Transferrin modulates as a function of substratum but is less sensitive to lactogenic hormones. (2) Milk proteins, such as caseins, are extremely hormone, substratum, and shape dependent. Caseins are not usually secreted by cells cultured on plastic but appear in larger quantities in the medium of cells on attached gels (Fig. 6b) and are fully "induced" in medium from the floating gel cultures (Fig. 6c). (3) A few proteins are present in culture medium but are not detected in skim milk. Some of these are related to milk fat globule proteins which are routinely removed in the process of skimming the milk (e.g., "f", which is probably butyrophilin, modulates as a function of substratum and can be detected in freshly isolated cells (Lee et al., 1984). Others are unknown proteins that are not present in either milk or in medium from freshly isolated cells (e.g., "e" proteins in Fig. 6 which appear to be substrata insensitive). It would be of great interest to identify these proteins, because their presence indicates that either a repressor has been removed or an inducer is present in culture to allow such high level of expression. (4) Milk proteins, such as whey acidic protein (WAP) and possibly α-lactalbumin, are essentially absent even in medium from floating gel cultures. To determine whether proteins were synthesized but retained intracellularly, we immunoprecipitated cellular proteins with a broad spectrum polyclonal antibody to skim milk proteins. These experiments showed that, with the exception of β-casein in cells on plastic where a small intracellular pool was detected in the absence of secretion, secretion was a reasonably good measure of protein synthetic rate (data not shown, Lee et al., 1985). Pulse chase experiments clearly indicated that the intracellular pool of β-casein in cells on plastic was rapidly degraded, suggesting that a change in cell shape and possibly establishment of cell–cell interactions may be

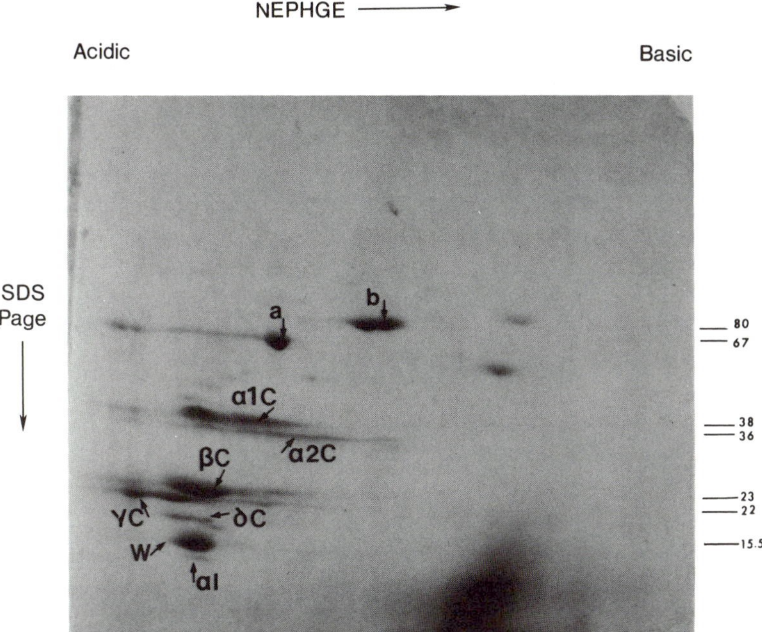

Figure 5. Two-dimensional gel electrophoresis of mouse skim milk. The 300 μg of milk protein was precipitated with trichloroacetic acid (TCA), washed with acetone, and dissolved in lysis buffer containing 9.5*M* urea, 2.0% NP-40, 5% β-mercaptoethanol, 1.6% pH 5–7, and 0.4% pH 3.5–10 ampholines. First dimension was nonequilibrium pH gradient electrophoresis (NEPHGE) with acidic end on the left and basic end on the right. Second dimension was SDS 6–15% PAGE. The gel was stained with Coomassie Blue to visualize the spots. A, albumin; b, transferrin; αlc, α-casein; α2c, α-casein; βc, β-casein; γc, γ-casein; δc, δ-casein; W, whey acidic protein; αl, α-lactalbumin. From Lee et al. (1984); reproduced with permission.

essential for secretion of β-casein but not transferrin. Recent experiments with individual components of the basement membrane support this notion. When primary mouse mammary epithelial cells are grown on EHS-derived basement membrane, they form closed secretory structures (Fig. 1) that contain a high concentration of milk proteins (our unpublished data). Culturing cells on the individual components of the basal lamina (type IV collagen, laminin, and HSPG), however, does not lead to much increase in secretory activity. Indeed, cells on HSPG ap-

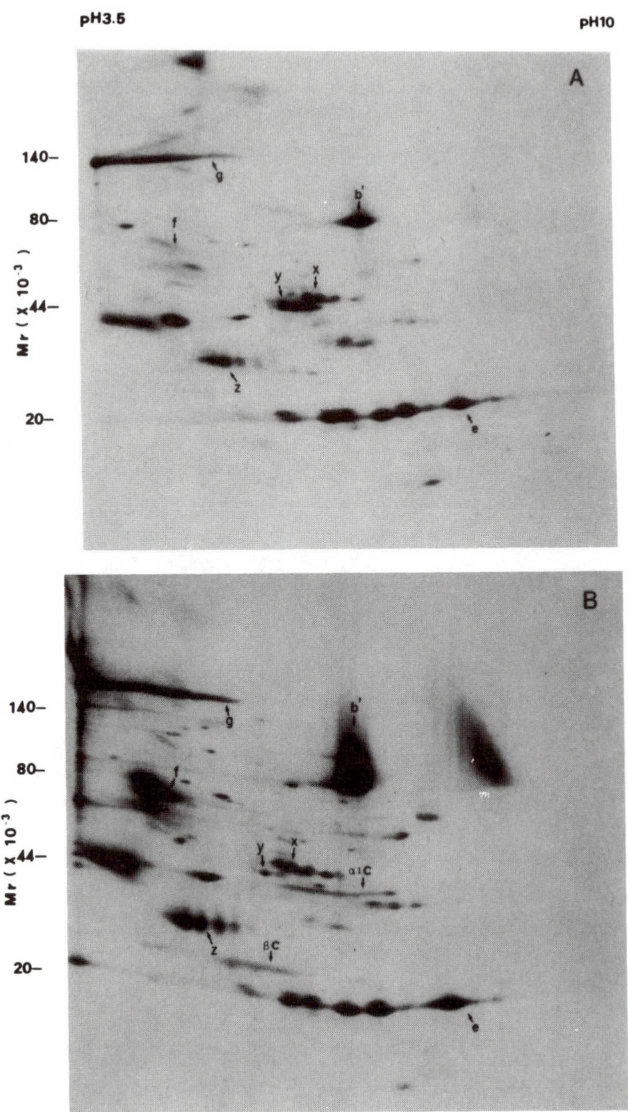

Figure 6. Two-dimensional pattern of [^{35}S]methionine-labeled proteins secreted by cultured PMME cells. Cells cultured for 1 week on (A) plastic, (B) attached gel, and (C) floating gel were labeled with 100 μCi of [^{35}S] methionine/plate in medium 199. Media were collected 24 h later and processed for two-dimensional electrophoresis. Then 2×10^5 dpm of each sample was loaded. Legend is the same as in Fig. 8, except that gels were exposed for 5 days. g, x, y, and z are unknown proteins not found in skim milk (see text for discussion of e and f). From Lee et al. (1984); reproduced with permission.

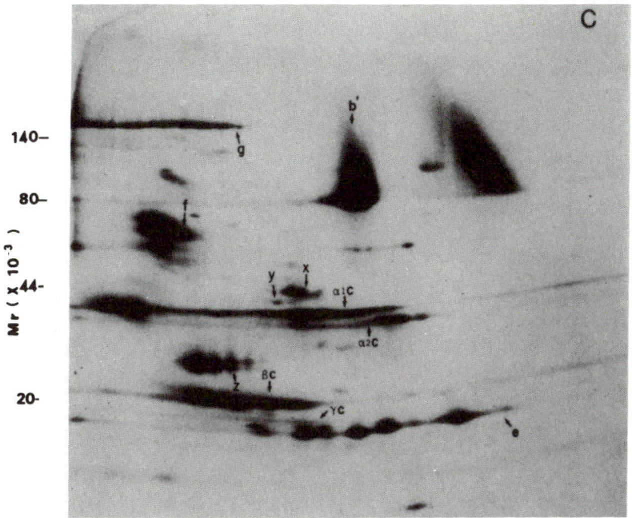

Figure 6. *(Continued)*

pear to be inhibited selectively for β-casein secretion despite an appreciable increase in β-casein mRNA levels (Fig. 7 and Section 4.2.2b).

4.2.2b. Milk Protein mRNA Levels. Messenger RNAs for milk proteins change gradually as the animal prepares for parturition. Reminiscent of other aspects of mammary gland development, there are more similarities than differences between species in the response of the gland to changes in hormonal levels. All species studied in some detail in organ and cell culture (mouse, rat, guinea pig, and rabbit) respond to prolactin by increasing casein mRNA. Cortisol and insulin were reported to amplify prolactin action but to be ineffective by themselves in several species (Devinoy et al., 1978; Matusik and Rosen, 1978; Takemoto et al., 1980; Teyssot and Houdebine, 1980; also see reviews mentioned above). Mehta et al. (1980) and Nagaiah et al. (1981) had reported that glucocorticoid is essential for casein gene expression in explanted mouse mammary tissue. Later, Kulski et al. (1983) showed that accumulation of the caseins in rat mammary explants derived from adrenalectomized rats is virtually dependent on administration of exogenous hydrocortisone. For a brief summary of studies on mRNA levels in the mammary gland see Mercier and Gaye (1983); for more in depth analysis see Rosen et al. (1980, 1985, 1986) and Houdebine et al. (1983). Here, we concentrate again only on the influence of substrata on mRNA levels. Preliminary

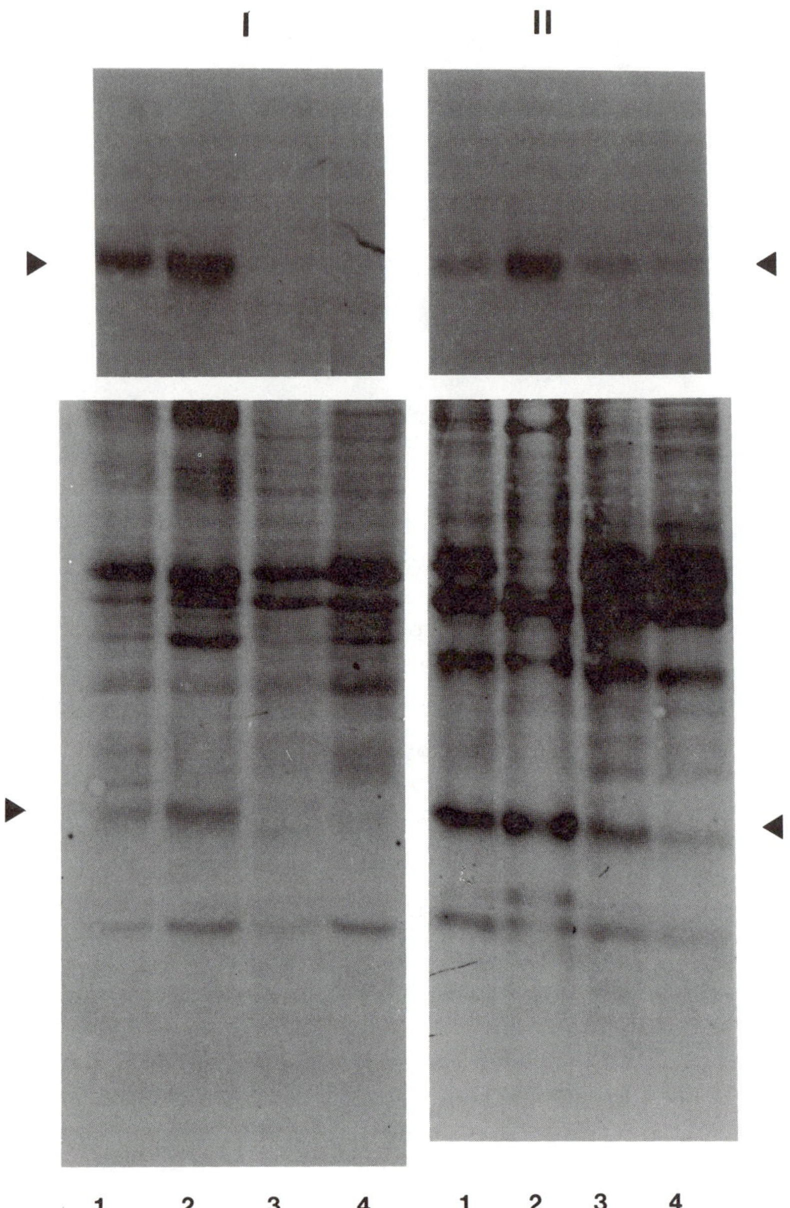
I
II
1
2
3
4
1
2
3
4

data by Supowit et al. (1981) indicated a twofold increase of β-casein mRNA level on released gels in comparison to attached gels. We took this observation further by showing that (1) the increase in β-casein mRNA could be anywhere from two- to eightfold; (2) while cells on plastic responded to prolactin by increasing β-casein mRNA, cells on floating collagen gels were at least five times as responsive (a 50-fold as opposed to a 10-fold induction after 36 h of prolactin treatment); and (3) whey acidic protein mRNA (WAP) was not present under any of the conditions tested (Lee et al., 1985).

Recent studies with COMMA-1D cells indicate that β-casein expression in early passages of these cells is responsive to both hormones and substrata, with the magnitude of response being similar to primary mammary epithelial cells (Fig. 8a; Bissell et al., 1986a). Cells in their ninth passage on plastic did not contain detectable levels of mRNA for β-casein in the absence of prolactin. A transfer onto floating gels in the next passage (10th) produced a 60-fold induction in mRNA levels in the presence of prolactin. The 10th passage cells on plastic again contained negligible β-casein mRNA. This experiment with COMMA-1D indicates clearly that the substratum effect is not due to the selection of a particular subpopulation; that is, the cells indeed are functionally reversible. The WAP message, as expected from our previous data, was totally absent under all conditions. Recently, Rosen and his colleagues (1986) have shown similar data for β-casein in COMMA-1D cells grown on floating collagen gels. Interestingly, transferrin mRNA level is not affected by prolactin levels (as is the case with transferrin protein) but is greatly modulated by substratum in COMMA-1D (Fig. 8b). There is, however, some hormonal sensitivity in PMME cells (L. H. Chen & M. J. Bissell, submitted).

The best substratum tried so far, at least for the mouse cells, is the EHS-reconstituted matrix. Primary mouse mammary cells and COMMA-1D cells on EHS form either tight spheres that appear to have many secretory granules, or ducts, ductules, and ridges (not shown; Bissell et al., 1986b; Li et al., 1987). In either case, the level of β-casein mRNA is dramatically increased compared to plastic and even to floating gels (Fig. 9). The individual ECM components (laminin, fibronectin, type IV collagen) or glycosaminoglycans (heparin, heparan sulfate, hyaluronic acid)

Figure 7. Equivalent amounts of secreted proteins from two separate experiments are shown. *Bottom,* autoradiograms; *top,* β-casein immunoblot performed on identical samples. Experiment I, lane 1, plastic; 2, released gel; 3, HSPG, 5 μg/cm^2; 4, HSPG, 2 μg/cm^2. Experiment II, lane 1, plastic; 2, released gel; 3, HSPG, 10 μg/ml medium; 4, HSPG, 2 μg/cm^2. Arrow indicates the β-casein band. (From Li et al., 1987.)

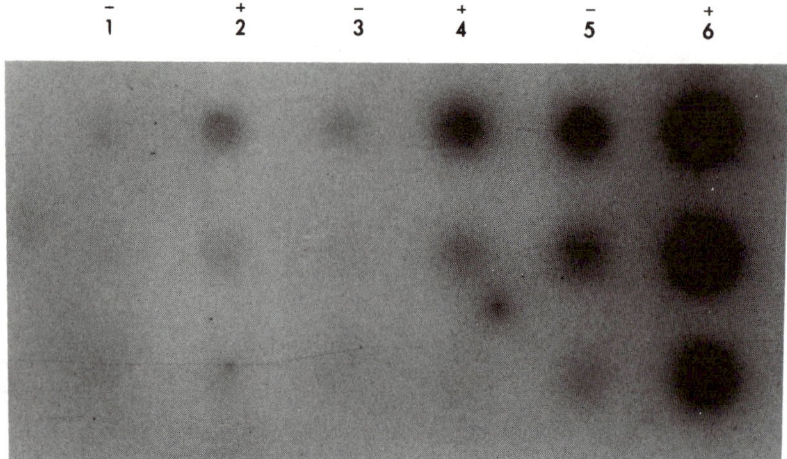

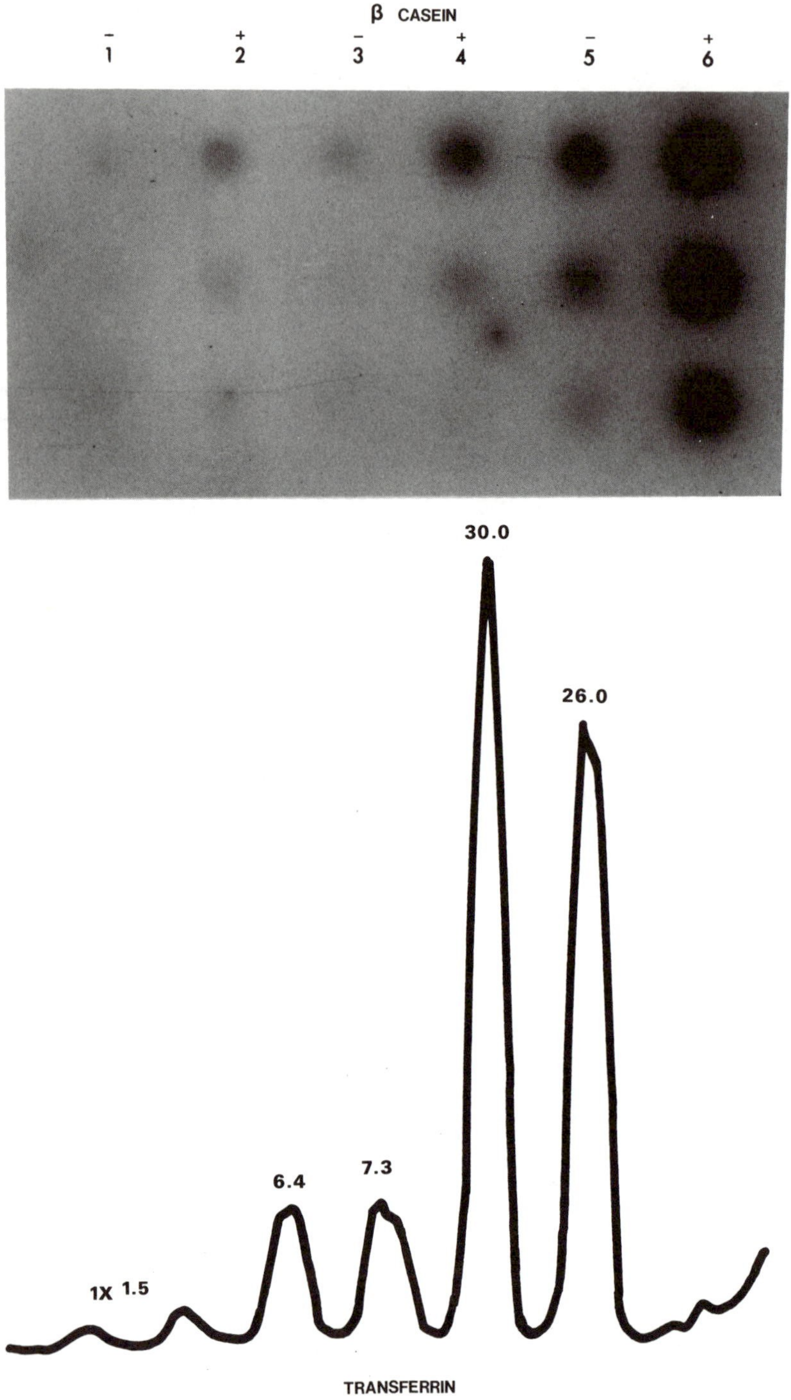

30.0
26.0
6.4
7.3
1X 1.5

TRANSFERRIN

were tested with COMMA-1D and were not much better than type I collagen. When EHS, as well as these components, were used to coat type I collagen gels, which were then floated, β-casein message level was increased three- to fourfold over EHS alone in all cases (Bissell et al., 1986a; Medina et al., 1987), indicating an additional role for changes associated with flotation; most notably, cell shape changes. Individual ECM components were more effective with primary mammary epithelial cells. Laminin increased β-casein mRNA two- to threefold in some experiments (Fig. 9, lane 3) and HSPG was even more effective (Fig. 9, lane 4). The HSPG effect is complex; coated on plastic dishes by itself, the compound is toxic to cells, possibly because of its charge density. Its effect on mRNA levels is therefore difficult to quantify. It can nevertheless be concluded that increases in β-casein mRNA levels do not correlate with β-casein protein levels in the medium. Other proteins are secreted at levels comparable to cells on other substrata, indicating that the process of secretion in general is not impaired (Fig. 7; Li et al., 1987). As mentioned above (Section 4.1), this may be a cell-shape related effect on milk protein secretion and may provide a means of studying translational and secretory processes as distinct from processes that regulate mRNA levels.

5. *How Does the ECM Influence Form and Function?*

Every cell in an organism has a history of prior events that defines its developmental status. Nevertheless, at any given state the ability of a cell either to remain where it is or to change identity in one direction or the other will be influenced by its environment. This includes both the soluble factors (nutrients, hormones, growth factors) and the extracellular physicochemical environment (the ECM and surfaces of other

---

Figure 8. Quantification of β-casein and transferrin mRNA in COMMA-1D cells. (a) β-casein: RNA was extracted and processed from cultures grown for 4 days with (+) or without (−) prolactin on plastic (1,2), on flat gels (3,4), and on released gels (5,6). All cultures contained insulin and cortisol. RNA equivalent to 15 μg of DNA was dotted (*top*). Second and third dots are 1/2 dilutions. From Medina et al. (1987); reproduced with permission. (b) Transferrin: RNA was extracted and processed from cultures as described in part (a). Cultures 2, 4, and 6 contained 3 μg/ml prolactin. All cultures contained insulin and cortisol. Nick-translated cDNA for mouse transferrin (L.-H. Chen and M.J. Bissell, submitted) was used as a probe and RNA equivalent to 5 μg of DNA was dotted. This figure shows a graph of optical density of the dots measured on a LKB densitometer. Relative concentrations were determined by comparison to a standard two-fold serial dilution curve (data not shown), where plastic minus prolactin equals 1×. L.-H. Chen, M. Li, and M. J. Bissell (unpublished).

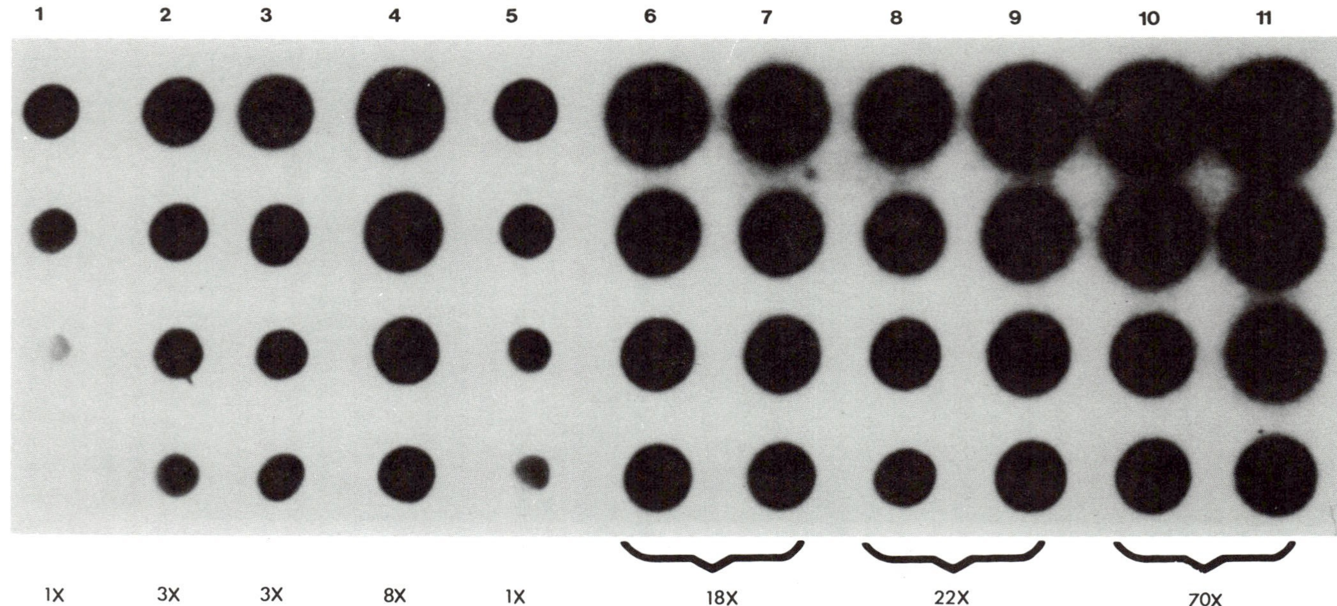

Figure 9. β-casein mRNA levels on different substrata. Cytoplasmic RNA was extracted as described in Li et al. (1986) 6 days postseeding, dotted onto nitrocellulose, and hybridized with nick-translated β-casein probe. Top dot: 4 μg RNA; other dots are 1/2 dilutions. Lane 1, plastic; 2, released gel; 3, laminin; 4, HSPG; 5, type IV collagen; 6 and 7, EHS on plastic; 8 and 9, EHS on flat gel; 10 and 11, EHS on released gel (Li et al., 1987).

cells). In vivo, the environment will also be the normal consequence of a history of events evolving sequentially and serving to coax the cell along its developmental path. Cells themselves undoubtedly modify their environment so as to pull (or push) themselves to the next stage of differentiation. Such a mechanism may be accomplished through the synthesis and restructuring of the ECM. That this mechanism must be operative in vivo is indicated by the fact that cells placed in culture in an environment without an appropriate ECM change their behavior and function radically until they either produce their own appropriate environment (a critical mass of ECM and/or crowding to ensure cell–cell interactions) or are given an appropriate ECM.

Almost 6 years ago we presented a model that described the minimum required unit for tissue-specific functions as the cell plus its ECM (Fig. 10; Bissell et al., 1982). The many inductive interactions between mesenchyme and epithelium responsible for developmental processes,

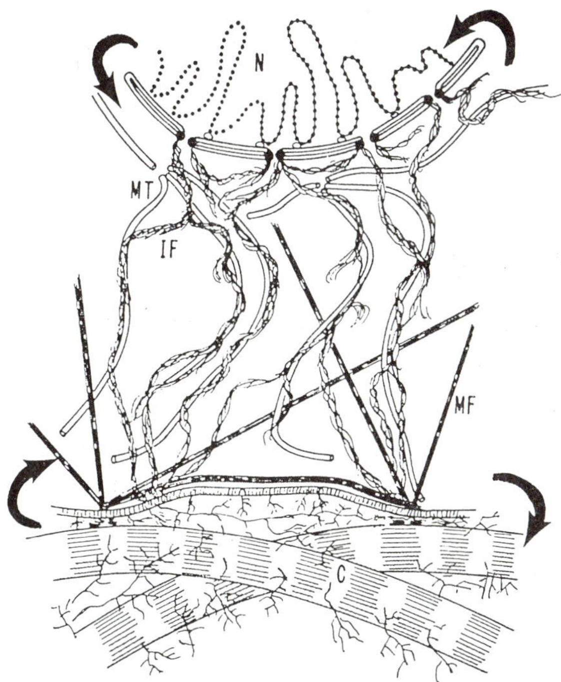

Figure 10. Model of dynamic reciprocity: This is the postulated minimum required unit for tissue-specific function (cell plus its ECM). From Bissell et al. (1982); reproduced with permission. N, nucleus; C, collagen; MT, IF, and MF, cytoskeletal components.

which may be mediated through the ECM, were outlined. We hypothesized that the influence of the ECM is communicated through the organization of the cytoskeleton (itself with connections to the nuclear matrix), possibly mediated by shape changes resulting in regulation of gene expression at all levels: transcription, mRNA processing, translation, posttranslational modifications, secretion, and extracellular organization. Long before our proposal, the ECM had been recognized by anatomists, histologists, and embryologists to be an essential mediator in the spatial arrangements of cells in tissues, and visible changes in structures of the ECM had been noted to accompany differentiation and morphogenesis (Wessells, 1977). The role of the ECM in inductive interactions had been hypothesized and debated. Aspects of ECM construction were recognized with the major biochemical components known but with important components, such as laminin, discovered just a few years earlier. Evidence for functional cellular responses to ECM was just beginning to emerge, underscoring the potential residing in ECM as proposed in the model. ECM influenced the attachment of cells and allowed a permissive response to growth factors. Collagen as a substratum allowed the cell to assume different shapes (with a possible change in the cytoskeleton) resulting in expression of tissue-specific phenotype, and collagen affected cell polarity and tissue organization. Preliminary evidence of transmembrane connections of the ECM to the cytoskeleton and of translatable mRNA association with the cytoskeleton provided a circumstantial basis for the hypothetical mechanism of control at different levels.

Since that time, considerable evidence has accumulated either to establish firmly or to implicate strongly the ECM in both developmental events and tissue-specific gene expression. The studies with the mammary gland described in this chapter along with studies on hepatocytes (Reid et al., 1986) have contributed significantly to deciphering the effect of the ECM in maintenance of eukaryotic function and to establish that the ECM is an essential component of tissue specificity. It is now known that individual components of the ECM are specific for certain cell types and states of differentiation in mediating attachment, growth, and morphology. More importantly, as described in this chapter, ECM is shown to affect the mRNAs for many tissue-specific gene products. Among the products affected by the ECM are the mRNAs of the newly synthesized ECM components themselves, allowing for the postulated dynamic reciprocity and the cascade of developmental events.

5.1. ECM Effects on ECM Synthesis

During embryological development of the mammary gland, a basement membrane is formed between the epithelium and the mesenchyme, the composition of which changes during the growth of mammary gland and as a function of the reproductive cycle. The differentiation of *cap* cells to myoepithelial cells is accompanied by changes in the appearance of the basal lamina. This process is also associated with changes in the stroma with fibrocyte accumulation involved in collagen synthesis (Williams and Daniel, 1983). Wicha et al. (1980) reported that an inhibitor of collagen synthesis, *cis*-hydroxy proline, caused involution-like structural alterations of the mammary glands in rats in vivo. Wakimoto and Oka (1983), using another collagen inhibitor, L-azatidine-2-carboxylic acid (LACA), showed that functional differentiation was disrupted in organ culture but not when cells were grown on floating collagen gels. Despite the fact that inhibitors cause toxicity and their use is subject to artifacts, these and other studies (Liotta et al., 1980) suggest that basal lamina synthesis may be required for a functional mammary gland.

Many studies have described production of basal lamina components by mammary cells in culture (Martinez-Hernandez et al., 1976; Liotta et al., 1979; Warburton et al., 1981, 1982, 1984; Ormerod et al., 1983). Studies with these and other cell types have shown that ECM and its components can cause both positive and negative changes in the level and composition of ECM molecules themselves (Meier and Hay, 1975; Emerman and Pitelka, 1977; Dessau et al., 1978; David et al., 1981; Parry et al., 1982, 1985; Kato and Gospodarowicz, 1985; Majack and Bornstein, 1985). This *dynamic reciprocity* in effect establishes a feedback loop, the disruption of which can lead to overproduction (Robinson and Gospodarowicz, 1983), involution (Liotta et al., 1979; Wicha et al., 1980), and quite possibly abnormal growth and differentiation and eventually cancer and metastasis (Liotta and Hart, 1982). We recently measured mRNA levels for ECM components in the mammary gland and in primary mammary epithelial cells in culture and observed significant modulations as a function of the reproductive cycle and culture substrata for types I, III, and IV collagens, laminin, and fibronectin (Fig. 11; Park and Bissell, 1986). It is interesting that mammary epithelial cells make a considerable amount of fibronectin mRNA and that its level is modulated as a function of substratum. Similar changes for laminin and type IV collagen mRNA are also observed (preliminary unpublished data).

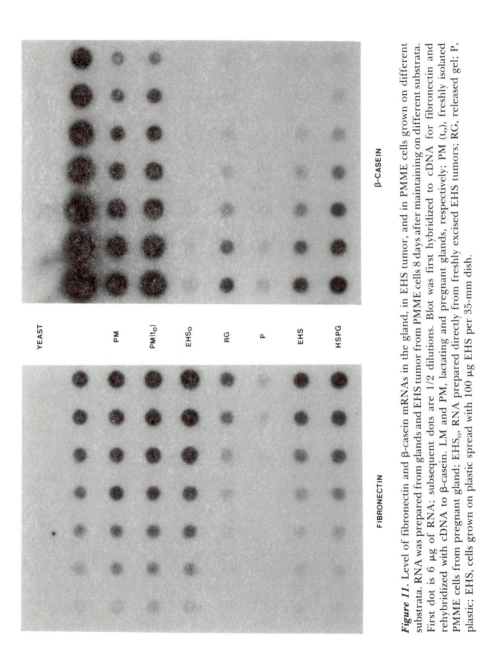

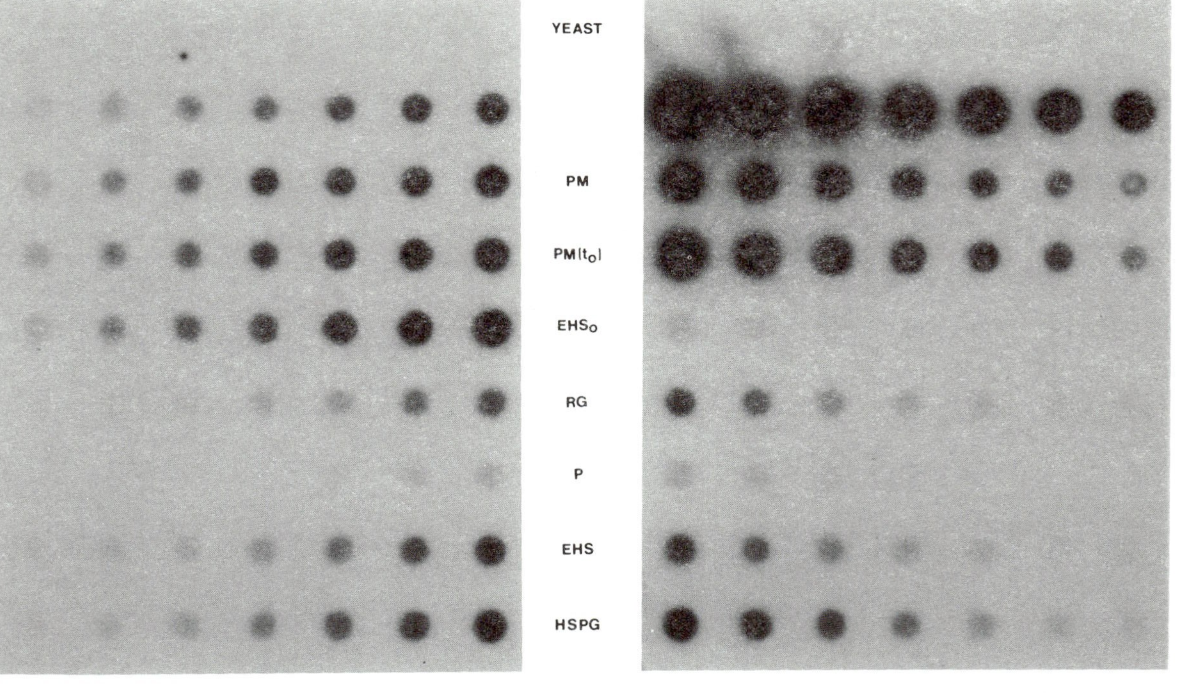

Figure 11. Level of fibronectin and β-casein mRNAs in the gland, in EHS tumor, and in PMME cells grown on different substrata. RNA was prepared from glands and EHS tumor from PMME cells 8 days after maintaining on different substrata. First dot is 6 μg of RNA; subsequent dots are 1/2 dilutions. Blot was first hybridized to cDNA for fibronectin and rehybridized with cDNA to β-casein. LM and PM, lactating and pregnant glands, respectively; PM (t_o), freshly isolated PMME cells from pregnant gland; EHS_o, RNA prepared directly from freshly excised EHS tumors; RG, released gel; P, plastic; EHS, cells grown on plastic spread with 100 μg EHS per 35-mm dish.

5.2. ECM Effect on Shape

The pioneering studies of Folkman and his collaborators on the effect of shape on cellular growth (Folkman and Greenspan, 1975; Folkman and Moscona, 1978), studies of Emerman and Pitelka (1977) mentioned earlier on shape-related mammary functions, and our own early data on the influence of shape on transport of small molecules (Bissell et al., 1977) suggest that the geometry of the cell may be intimately involved in regulation of its function. There are now numerous studies from other systems where changes in cell shape are shown to have profound (but not necessarily the same) functional consequences: When some cells were mechanically stretched, they proliferated (Brunette, 1984). The degree of individual cell spreading in a new elegant study correlated with the degree of DNA synthesis (O'Neill et al., 1986). Hybrids between Friend cells and fibroblasts synthesized hemoglobin only in suspension (Allan and Harrison, 1980). When chondrocytes were grown on plastic and allowed to spread, they lost their ability to synthesize cartilage-specific (type II) collagen. When returned to suspension culture, they redifferentiated (Benya and Shaffer, 1982; Glowacki et al., 1983). Fibronectin modulation of cell shape in 3T3-preadipocytes prevented their differentiation (Spiegelman and Ginty, 1983) and "rounding" by any means led to elaboration of large quantities of degradative enzymes not previously expressed in rabbit synovial fibroblasts (Aggeler et al., 1984). The kinetics of adhesion and the final cell shape were strikingly different when hepatocytes were plated on type IV collagen compared to fibronectin and laminin (D. M. Bissell et al., 1986). Basement membranes not only influenced normal epithelial morphology but also could profoundly influence the behavior and morphology of tumor cells (Ingber et al., 1981). Ingber and Jamieson (1985) postulate that histodifferentiation is regulated by physical forces transduced over basement membranes (*tensegrity*), a concept worthy of serious consideration.

That the ECM influences mammary morphology at both the cellular and tissue levels was discussed in Section 4. The striking changes in size and shape of the mammary gland as a whole and of fat cells (Elias et al., 1973) and especially of myoepithelial cells (Emerman and Vogl, 1986; see Fig. 12 where a probe for actin highlights the myoepithelial component of the gland) as a function of the reproductive cycle have been well documented. Whether the ECM changes are related to shape changes in vivo or whether the observed shape changes are achieved by other mechanisms is not known. The exact relation of functional change to these spectacular changes in shape (Figs. 1, 2, and 12) is difficult to pursue in vivo. It is clear from the above discussion, however, that signif-

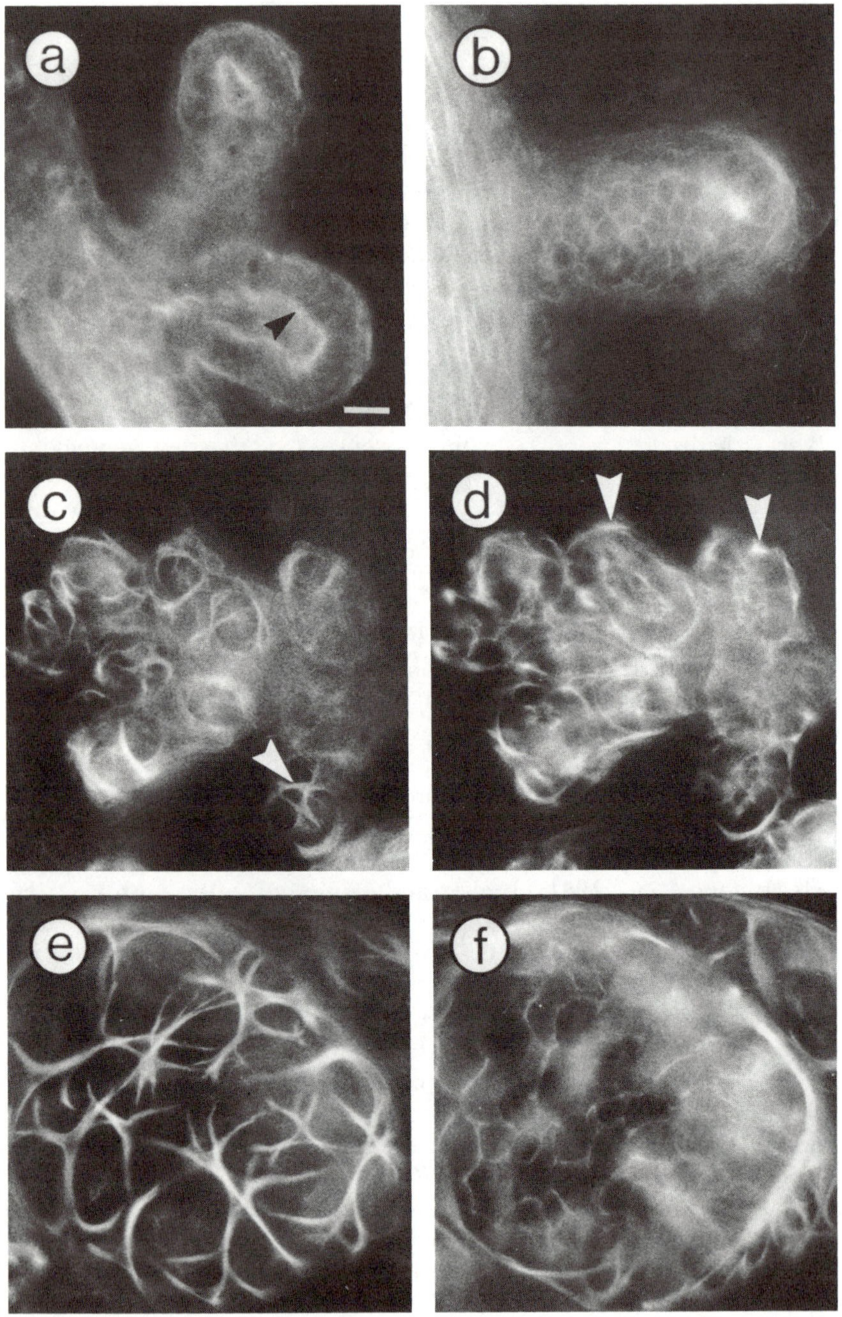
a
b
c
d
e
f

icant functional changes accompany shape changes in culture. Indeed, when gel contraction and thus cell-shape change are prevented by growing primary mammary epithelial cells on glutaraldehyde-fixed collagen gels (the cells in this case cannot contract the gel), the functional changes described in Section 5 will not occur even when the gel is released to float (Shannon and Pitelka, 1981; Lee et al., 1984).

5.3. ECM Effects on Cytoskeleton Synthesis and Organization

As tissues develop, specialization is also manifested in the intermediate filament composition, particularly in the cytokeratins of epithelial cells, including mammary cells (see Chapter 6 in this volume). Tubulin content and microtubular organization are also known to vary in the mammary gland during the reproductive cycle (Guerin and Loizzi, 1980) and the disruption of microtubules with colchicine is known to disrupt milk synthesis and secretion (see Chapter 5 in this volume; Nickerson et al., 1980). Changes in cell morphology that coincide with ECM-induced changes in gene expression should be manifested in cytoskeletal reorganization. Such ECM-induced reorganization is expected to be mediated through transmembrane association of ECM and cytoskeleton (reviewed in Bissell et al., 1982). In NMuMG cells, a heparan sulfate transmembrane component with an internal actin-binding domain has been isolated (Rapraeger and Bernfield, 1983), indicating that the connection may be even more direct than previously assumed. Figure 13 illustrates the close connection between NMuMG cells and the collagen fibers in the ECM; thus, the structural orientation of the cytoskeleton

Figure 12. The distribution of actin in epithelial and myoepithelial cells in murine mammary gland at different stages of the reproductive cycle. Panels (a) and (b) are of lateral buds in a gland from a virgin animal. In (a), the plane of focus is at the center of the bud's longitudinal axis. Very little staining is present at the base of the epithelium while the apex is heavily labeled (arrowhead). The apical staining is interpreted as originating from the highly concentrated microvilli present at this stage. In the bud shown in (b), the plane of focus is through the apex of the epithelium. Actin associated with junctional complexes is clearly evident (arrowhead). The gland shown in (c) and (d) is from a late pregnant mouse. In (c), myoepithelial cells are visible (arrowhead). In (d), the plane of focus has been adjusted to cross-section the secretory elements. Note that myoepithelial labeling (arrowheads) is evident at the base of the epithelium. Also note that the staining of the apices of epithelial cells is less than in (a). Panels (e) and (f) are of an alveolus from a lactating gland. In (e), entire myoepithelial cells are shown. In (f), the plane of focus has been adjusted to resolve actin patterns associated with junctions between secretory epithelial cells (arrowhead). Bar = 10 μm. (a–f) ×470. Original courtesy of Emerman and Vogl (1986); reproduced with permission.

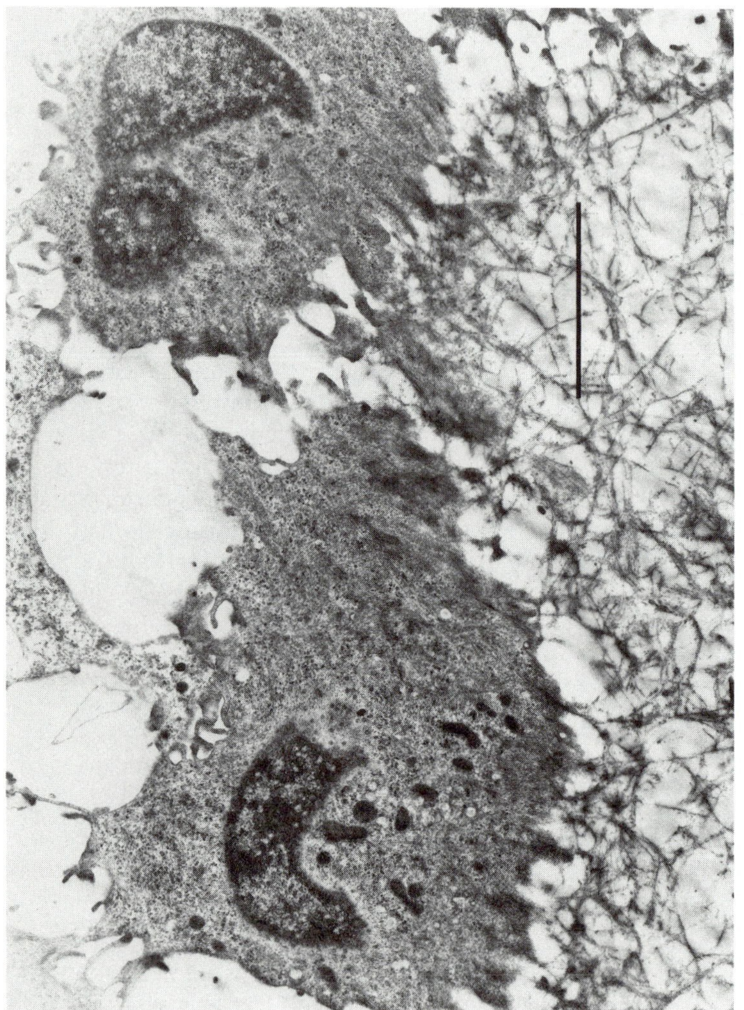

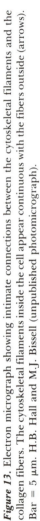

Figure 13. Electron micrograph showing intimate connections between the cytoskeletal filaments and the collagen fibers. The cytoskeletal filaments inside the cell appear continuous with the fibers outside (arrows). Bar = 5 μm. H.B. Hall and M.J. Bissell (unpublished photomicrograph).

effectively extends across the cell boundary through the orientation of the collagen fibers. It is therefore not surprising to find that the cytoskeletal elements themselves may be among the components whose synthesis is influenced by cytoskeletal reorganization (Laszlo and Bissell, 1983; Ben Ze'ev, 1985).

In a number of different systems, synthesis of cytoskeletal elements has been correlated with cell morphology or influenced by ECM. Cytokeratin synthesis in Madin-Darby bovine kidney epithelial cells coincides with the degree of cell–cell contact, presumably as a consequence of increased desmosome construction (and associated tonofilaments) (Ben Ze'ev, 1984). Synthesis of vimentin in some, but not all, epithelial and fibroblastic cells correlates with the cells spreading onto a substratum and functioning as individual units (Lane et al., 1982; Rheinwald et al., 1984; Ben Ze'ev, 1984; Asch and Asch, 1985). In fibroblasts, vinculin synthesis increases with cell–cell contact (also requiring cell–substratum contact) as a result of increased focal contacts and zonula adherens type junctions (Ungar et al., 1986) as well as after disruption of the cytoskeleton by tumor promoters (Laszlo and Bissell, 1983). Tumor promoters also affect the rate of synthesis of ECM components such as collagen and fibronectin (Blumberg et al., 1976; Bissell et al., 1979; Driedger and Blumberg, 1980). Growth of granulosa cells plated on bovine epithelial cell-derived ECM results in a reduction of actin stress cables and synthesis of actin, α-actinin, vinculin, and actin mRNA (Ben Ze'ev and Amsterdam, 1986). We have shown that NMuMG cells respond to collagen substrata with increased synthesis of an intermediate filament protein, probably a cytokeratin (Hall and Bissell, 1986). Integration of these and other as yet isolated findings into a general mechanistic model relating ECM to organization and synthesis of cytoskeleton awaits further experimentation.

5.4. Summary: A Possible Mechanism Relating Form to Function

The concept that shape per se regulates function is difficult to translate into a mechanism largely because *shape* is too general a term. To be fruitful, shape needs to be translated into specific cellular structures and even molecules, and we are far from being able to accomplish this feat. Nonetheless, one could argue that the structure itself is the message, and indeed we have presented evidence for just that in this chapter (see Pitelka and Hamamoto, 1983, and also Ingber and Jamieson, 1985, for how the structure could be set up and maintained). The examination of whole mounts of cells by Wolosewick and Porter (1976) revealed such a wealth and complexity of intracellular structure that our view of the cell cytoplasm has had to change radically. Undoubtedly, much more will come to light as more powerful and yet gentler techniques are devised for the electron microscope. A recent view of detergent-extracted cytoskeletons of mouse mammary epithelial cells shows a complex array of fibrillar structures associated both with cellular membrane and with the nuclear cage (Fig. 14A and B). A comparable view of another mammary cell suspected to be myoepithelial reveals a different cytoskeletal organization with prominent microfilament bundles (Fig. 14C and D). Association of polyribosomes (of unknown specificity) with the cytoskeletons of these cells can easily be visualized in these preparations.

There is increasing evidence that mRNA is associated not only with membranes but also with cytoskeletal structures (for a brief review see Nielsen et al., 1983). In many cell types 70–80% of the poly(A)$^+$mRNA is found in the cytoskeletal fraction (Lenk et al., 1977; van Venrooij et al., 1981; Jeffery, 1982). The association of mRNA with the cytoskeleton is also indirectly suggested by the finding that mRNA in oocytes and embryos and in single cells is not uniformly distributed (Ernst et al., 1980; Fulton et al., 1980; Capco and Jäckle, 1982; Capco and Jeffery, 1982; Jeffery, 1982; Lawrence and Singer, 1986). Our preliminary results indicate that more than 90% of β-casein and transferrin mRNA are associated with the Triton-extracted cytoskeleton of mouse mammary epithelial cells (L. H. Chen and M. J. Bissell, unpublished data). Furthermore, it has been known for a number of years that colchicine and other microtubule-disrupting drugs inhibit milk protein synthesis and secretion as well as decreasing mRNA levels for β-casein (Ollivier-Bousquet, 1979; Houdebine and Djiane, 1980; Nickerson et al., 1980). How could cytoskeleton and extracellular matrix regulate the level of mRNA? We postulate that modulation of mRNA levels as a function of substratum (and hence shape) is due to increases in mRNA half-life, most probably in the cytoplasm as the result of polysome–cytoskeleton interactions (Neilsen et al., 1983). Studies with EHS matrix, some of which were cited above, may shed light on at least one aspect of this regulation. EHS-reconstituted matrix restores mammary function only to mammary cells (our data), liver function only to liver cells (D. M. Bissell, personal communication), and Sertoli cell function only to Sertoli cells (Hadley et al., 1985). EHS does not induce β-casein in hepatocytes or bestow mammary cells with the ability to synthesize and secrete albumin. Based on studies with rare and moderately abundant mRNA in mouse L cells, it has been argued previously that posttranscriptional regulation may be the prevalent control in eukaryotic cells to determine the level of individual mRNAs (Carneiro and Schibler, 1984). If tissue-specific mRNA were indeed synthesized at all times after functional commitment, but sta-

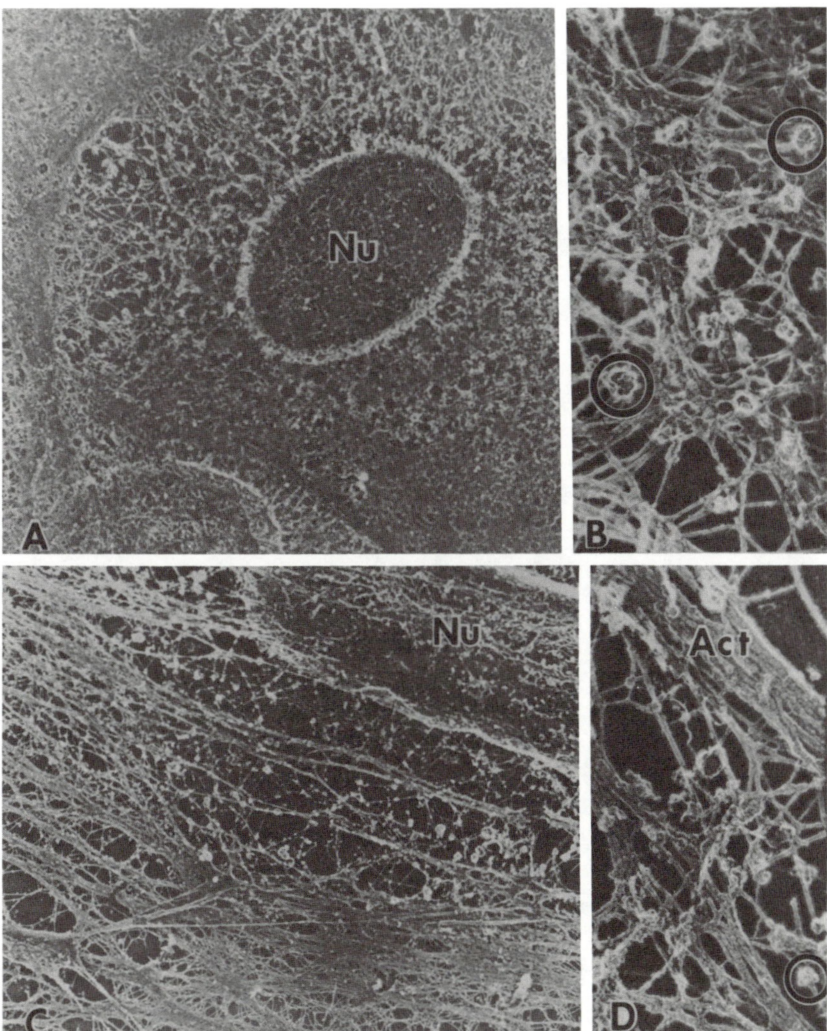

Figure 14. Mouse mammary epithelial cell cytoskeletons. Primary mammary epithelial cells cultured on glass coverslips were subjected to extraction with Triton-X-100 and fixed; rotary platinum replicas of the cytoskeletons were prepared for high-resolution transmission electron microscopy. In A and B, low and high magnification views of a typical epithelial cell are shown. The nuclear lamina (Nu) and cell borders are easily visualized. At high magnification, polyribosomes (circles) are observed attached to the filamentous cytoskeletal mesh. In C and D, comparable views of myoepithelial cell (or a mammary fibroblast) are seen. Magnification ×5000 (A,C); ×890,000 (B,D). Original courtesy of J. Aggeler and M. J. Bissell (unpublished).

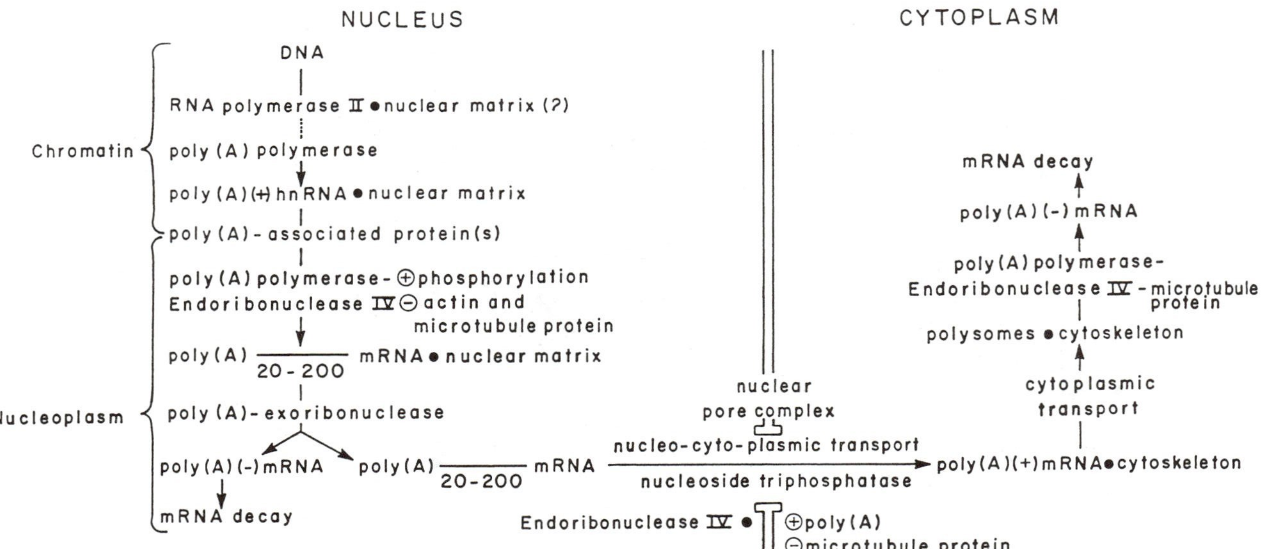

Figure 15. Diagram illustrating mechanisms hypothesized for intranuclear and intracytoplasmic transport and metabolism of mRNA and its precursors, guided by nuclear and cytoplasmic structural elements. The scheme is reproduced here to emphasize the number of steps involved between transcription and the final level of mRNA in the cytoplasm and the intimate role played by nuclear matrix and cytoskeletal structures in many of these steps. From Müller et al. (1983); reproduced with permission.

bilized or processed only in the presence of a correct environment (correct hormones and shape), then the tissue specificity of EHS action could be explained. The hypothesis that EHS acts post-transcriptionally by stabilizing the already-transcribed tissue-specific mRNA does not preclude the possibility that it may also act at the transcriptional level. This is only to emphasize that one aspect of basement membrane function is its ability to alter mRNA stability in the nucleus or in the cytoplasm. It appears from our current data that lactogenic hormones are active participants in this association (Bissell and Aggeler, 1987).

There is evidence that mRNA for cytoskeletal proteins themselves change as a function of shape (Fulton et al., 1980; Farmer et al., 1983; Ben Ze'ev, 1984). There is additional evidence, some of which has been reviewed (Nielsen et al., 1983), that the cytoskeleton is involved in protein synthesis. Equally intriguing, however, are findings to support the notion that cytoskeletal proteins may also be involved in nuclear regulation of mRNA processing (Müller et al., 1983). In our preoccupation with DNA sequences and transcriptional events, we often overlook other, and possibly equally important, rate-limiting steps after transcription (for a review see Müller et al., 1983, 1985). In the scheme depicted in Fig. 15, many steps in mRNA processing (both intranuclear and cytoplasmic) involve interaction with the cytoskeletal elements. The systematic analysis of the nonchromatin substructure of the nucleus (Fey et al., 1986) and the recent findings showing lamin's (nuclear membrane proteins) homology to intermediate filaments (Aebi et al., 1986; McKeon et al., 1986) add additional credence to the earlier postulates on the role of nuclear matrix in gene expression (e.g., see Cook et al., 1982) and to the validity of our model of dynamic reciprocity (Bissell et al. 1982).

The cytoskeleton, not unexpectedly, thus emerges as the structure most likely to integrate form into function. We have come a long way in a short time toward appreciating that the cytoplasm is not simply a bag of enzymes and toward respecting the central role of the cytoskeleton in gene regulation. We have a long way to go before we can clearly delineate which cytoskeletal structure is associated with which mRNA, how cytoskeletal components could participate in mRNA processing in the nucleus, and whether the ECM affects both processes.

ACKNOWLEDGMENTS: We thank Judy Aggeler, Jack Bartley, and Dorothy Pitelka for critical reading of this chapter, our co-workers and colleagues for providing us with unpublished data and original photographs (as acknowledged in the text), Debbie Farson and Jill Hatier for help with the unpublished experiments cited, Debbie Farson, Lance

Gee, and Ross Ramos for additional help with figures and references, and Lucinda Olney and Sally Tubach for expert secretarial assistance. Acknowledgments for cDNA clones, antibodies, and other reagents are given in the original publications. The work from the authors' laboratories was supported by the Health Effects Research Division, Office of Health and Environmental Research, U.S. Department of Energy, Contract DE-AC-03- 76SF00098, an NIH Biomedical Research Support Grant RR05918, and a gift for research from the Monsanto Company, St. Louis, to M.J.B. and in part by an NIH grant, HD17892, to H.G.H.

References

Aebi, U., Cohn, J., Buhle, L., and Gerace, L., 1986, The nuclear lamina is a meshwork of intermediate-type filaments, *Nature* **323:**560–562.

Aggeler, J., Frisch, S.M., and Werb, A., 1984, Changes in cell shape correlate with collagenase gene expression in rabbit synovial fibroblasts, *J. Cell Biol.* **98:**1662–1671.

Allan, M., and Harrison, P., 1980, Co-expression of differentiation markers in hybrids between Friend cells and lymphoid cells and the influence of the cell shape, *Cell* **19:**437–447.

Asch, H.L., and Asch, B.B., 1985, Expression of keratins and other cytoskeletal proteins in mouse mammary epithelium during the normal development cycle and primary culture, *Dev. Biol.* **107:**470–482.

Banerjee, M.R., 1976, Responses of mammary cells to hormones, *Int. Rev. Cytol.* **47:**1–97.

Barraclough, R., Kimbell, R., and Rudland, P.S., 1984, Increased abundance of a normal cell mRNA sequence accompanies the conversion of rat mammary cuboidal epithelial cells to elongated myoepithelial-like cells in culture, *Nucleic Acid Res.* **12:**8097–8114.

Bennett, D.C., 1980, Morphogenesis of branching tubules in cultures of cloned mammary epithelial cells, *Nature* **285:**657–659.

Bennett, D.C., Peachey, L.A., Durbin, H., and Rudland, P.S., 1979, A possible mammary stem cell line, *Cell* **15:**283–298.

Bennett, D.C., Armstrong, B.L., and Okado, S.M., 1981, Reconstitution of branching tubules from two cloned mammary cell types in culture, *Dev. Biol.* **87:**193–199.

Benya, P.D., and Shaffer, J.D., 1982, Dedifferentiated chondrocytes reexpress the differentiated collagen phenotype when cultured in agarose gels, *Cell* **30:**215–224.

Ben Ze'ev, A., 1984, Differential control of cytokeratins and vimentin synthesis by cell–cell contact and cell spreading in cultured epithelial cells, *J. Cell Biol.* **99:**1424–1433.

Ben Ze'ev, A., 1985, in: *Cell and Muscle Motility* (J.W. Shay, ed.), Plenum Press, New York, pp. 23–53.

Ben Ze'ev, A., and Amsterdam, A., 1986, Regulation of cytoskeletal proteins involved in cell contact formation during differentiation of granulosa cells on extracellular matrix, *Proc. Natl. Acad. Sci. USA* **83:**2894–2898.

Bernfield, M., 1984, Basement membrane and cell movement, *Ciba Found. Symp.* **108:**1–5.

Bissell, D.M., Stamatoglov, S.C., Nermat, M.V., and Hughes, R.C., 1986, Interactions of rat hepatocytes with type IV collagen, fibronectin and laminin matrices. Distinct matrix-controlled modes of attachment and spreading, *Eur. J. Cell Biol.* **40:**72–78.

Bissell, M.J., 1981, The differentiated state of normal and malignant cells or how to define a "normal" cell in culture, *Int. Rev. Cytol.* **70:**27–100.

Bissell, M.J., and Aggeler, J., 1987, Dynamic reciprocity: How do extracellular matrix and hormones direct gene expression? in: *Mechanisms of Signal Transduction by Hormones and Growth Factors* (M. Cabot, ed.), Alan Liss, New York, in press.

Bissell, M.J., Farson, D., and Tung, A.S.C., 1977, Cell shape and hexose transport in normal and virus-transformed cells in culture. *J. Supramolecular Structure* **6:**1–12.

Bissell, M.J., Hatie, C., and Calvin, M., 1979, Is the product of the *src* gene a promoter? *Proc. Natl. Acad. Sci. USA* **76:**348–352.

Bissell, M.J., Hall, H.G., and Parry, G., 1982, How does the extracellular matrix direct gene expression? *J. Theor. Biol.* **99:**31–68.

Bissell, M.J., Lee, E.Y-H., Li, M., and Hall, G., 1986a, The role of the matrix in regulating differentiation of endocrine sensitive cells, in: *Proceedings, The Second NIADDK Symposium on the Study of Benign Prostatic Hyperplasia,* U.S. Government Printing Office, Washington, DC.

Bissell, M.J., Li, M.L., Chen, L.-H., and Lee, E.Y-H., 1986b, Regulation of milk proteins in the mouse mammary epithelial cells by extracellular matrix and hormones, in: *Growth and Differentiation of Mammary Epithelial Cells in Culture* (J. Enami and R. Ham, eds.), Japan Scientific Society, Tokyo, Japan.

Blumberg, P.M., Driedger, P.E., and Rossow, P.W., 1976, Effect of phorbol ester on a transformation-sensitive surface protein of chick fibroblasts, *Nature* **264:**446–447.

Boucaut, J.C., Darribère, T., Boulekbache, H., and Thiery, J.P., 1984a, Prevention of gastrulation but not neurulation by antibodies to fibronectin in amphibian embryos, *Nature* **307:**364–367.

Boucaut, J.C., Darribère, T., Poole, T.J., Aoyama, H., Yamada, R.M., and Thiery, J.P., 1984b, Biologically active synthetic peptides as probes of embryonic development: A competitive peptide inhibitor of fibronectin function inhibits gastrulation in amphibian embryos and neural crest cell migration in avian embryos, *J. Cell Biol.* **99:**1822–1830.

Bronner-Fraser, M., 1984, Latex beads as probes of a neural crest pathway: Effects of laminin, collagen, and surface charge on bead translocation, *J. Cell Biol.* **98:**1947–1950.

Brunette, D.M., 1984, Mechanical stretching increases the number of epithelial cells synthesizing DNA in culture, *J. Cell Sci.* **69:**35–45.

Burwen, S.J., and Pitelka, D.R., 1980, Secretory function of lactating mouse mammary epithelial cells cultured on collagen gels, *Exp. Cell Res.* **126:**249–262.

Capco, D.G., and Jäckle, H., 1982, Localized protein synthesis during oogenesis of *Xenopus laevis.* Analysis by *in situ* hybridization, *Dev. Biol.* **94:**41–50.

Capco, D.G., and Jeffery, W.R., 1982, Transient localizations or messenger RNA in *Xenopus laevis* oocytes, *Dev. Biol.* **89:**1–12.

Carlin, B., Jaffe, R., Bender, B., and Chung, A.E., 1981, Enactin, a novel basal lamina-associated sulfated glycoprotein, *J. Biol. Chem.* **256:**5209–5214.

Carneiro, M., and Schibler, U., 1984, Accumulation of rare and moderately abundant mRNAs in mouse L-cells is mainly post-transcriptionally regulated, *J. Mol. Biol.* **178:**869–880.

Ceriani, R.K., 1976, Hormone induction of specific protein synthesis in midpregnancy mouse mammary cell culture, *J. Exp. Zool.* **196:**1–12.

Chung, A.E., Freeman, I.L., and Braginski, J.E., 1977, A novel extracellular membrane elaborated by a mouse embryonal-carcinoma-derived cell line, *Biochem. Biophys. Res. Commun.* **79:**859–868.

Collier, R.J., 1985, Nutritional, metabolic, and environmental aspects of lactation, in: *Lactation* (B.L. Larson, ed.), Academic Press, New York, pp. 80–128.

Cook, P.R., Wang, J., Hayday, A., Lania, L., Fried, M., Chiswell, D.J., and Wyke, J.A.,

1982, Active viral genes in transformed cells lie close to the nuclear cage, *EMBO J.* **1**:447–452.

Couchman, J.R., Green, M.R., and Rees, D.A., 1980, Membrane–matrix interactions in cell movement and growth, *Cell Biol. Int. Rep.* **4**:804.

Cunha, G.R., Bigsby, R.M., Cooke, P.S., and Sugimura, Y., 1985, Stromal–epithelial interactions in adult organs, *Cell Differ.* **17**:137–148.

Daniel, C.W., and DeOme, K.B., 1965, Growth of mouse mammary glands *in vivo* after monolayer culture, *Science* **149**:634–636.

Daniel, C.W., Berger, J.J., Stricklang, P., and Garcia, R., 1984, Similar growth patterns of mouse mammary cells cultivated in collagen matrix in vivo and in vitro, *Dev. Biol.* **104**:57–64.

Danielson, K.G., Oborn, C.J., Durban, E.M., Butel, J.S., and Medina, D., 1984, Epithelial mouse mammary cell line exhibiting normal morphological genesis *in vivo* and functional differentiation *in vitro, Proc. Natl. Acad. Sci. USA* **81**:3756–3760.

David, G., Van der Schueren, B., and Bernfield, M., 1981, Basal lamina formation by normal and transformed mouse mammary epithelial cells duplicated in vitro, *J. Natl. Cancer Inst.* **67**:719–728.

DeOme, K.B., Faulkin, L.J., Bern, H.A., and Blair, P.B., 1959, Development of mammary tumors fom hyperplastic alveolar nodules transplanted into gland-free mammary fat pads of female C3H mice, *Cancer Res.* **19**:515–520.

Dessau, W., Sasse, Joachim, Timpl, R., Jilek, F., and Mark, K.v.d., 1978, Synthesis and extracellular deposition of fibronectin in chondrocyte cultures, *J. Cell Biol.* **79**:342–355.

Devinoy, E., Houdebine, L.M., and Delouis, C., 1978, Role of prolactin and glucocorticoids in the expression of casein genes in rabbit mammary gland organ culture, *Biochim. Biophys. Acta* **517**:360–366.

Drews, U., and Drews, U., 1977, Regression of mouse mammary gland anlagen in recombinants of Tfm and wild-type tissues: Testosterone acts via the mesenchyme, *Cell* **10**:401–404.

Driedger, P.E., and Blumberg, P.M., 1980, Structure–activity relationships in chick embryo fibroblasts for phorbol-related diterpene esters showing anomalous activities *in vivo, Cancer Res.* **40**:339–346.

DuBois, M., and Elias, J.J., 1984, Subpopulations of cells in immature mouse mammary gland as detected by proliferative responses to hormones in organ culture, *Dev. Biol.* **106**:70–75.

Dulbecco, R., Allen, W.R., and Bowman, M., 1984, Lumen formation and redistribution of inframembranous proteins during differentiation of ducts in the rat mammary gland, *Proc. Natl. Acad. Sci. USA* **81**:5763–5766.

Dunn, G.A., and Ebendal, T., 1978, Contact guidance on oriented collagen gels, *Exp. Cell Res.* **111**:475–479.

Durban, E.M., Medina, D., and Butel, J.S., 1985, Comparative analysis of casein synthesis during mammary cell differentiation in collagen and mammary gland development *in vivo, Dev. Biol.* **109**:288–298.

Ehrman, R.L., and Gey, G.O., 1956, The growth of cells on a transparent gel of reconstituted rat-tail collagen, *J. Natl. Cancer Inst.* **16**:1375–1403.

Ehrmann, U.K., Peterson, W.D. Jr., and Misfeldt, D.S., 1984, To grow mouse mammary epithelial cells in culture, *J. Cell Biol.* **98**:1026–1032.

Eigel, W.N., Butler, J.E., Ernstrom, C.A., Farrell, H.M. Jr., Harwalkar, V.R., Jenness, R., and Whitney, R. McL., 1984, Nomenclature of proteins of cow's milk: Fifth revision, *J. Dairy Sci.* **67**:1599–1631.

Elias, J.J., Pitelka, D.R., and Armstrong, R.C., 1973, Changes in fat cell morphology during lactation in the mouse, *Anat. Rec.* **177:**533–548.

Elsdale, T., and Bard, J., 1972, Collagen substrata for studies on cell behavior, *J. Cell Biol.* **54:**626–637.

Emerman, J.T., and Pitelka, D.R., 1977, Maintenance and identification of morphological differentiation in dissociated mammary epithelium on floating collagen membranes, *In Vitro* **13:**316–328.

Emerman, J.T., and Vogl, A.W., 1986, Cell size and shape changes in the myoepithelium of the mammary gland during differentiation, *Anat. Rec.* **216:**405–415.

Emerman, J.T., Enami, J., Pitelka, D., and Nandi, S., 1977, Hormonal effects on intracellular and secreted casein in cultures of mouse mammary epithelial cells on floating collagen membranes, *Proc. Natl. Acad. Sci. USA* **74:**4466–4470.

Emerman, J.T., Bartley, J.C., and Bissell, M.J., 1980, Interrelationship of glycogen metabolism and lactose synthesis in mammary epithelial cells of mice, *Biochem. J.* **192:**695–702.

Emerman, J.T., Bartley, J.C., and Bissell, M.J., 1981, Glucose metabolite patterns as markers of functional differentiation in freshly isolated and cultured mouse mammary epithelial cells, *Exp. Cell Res.* **134:**241–250.

Erickson, C.A., and Turley, E.A., 1983, Substrata formed by combinations of extracellular matrix components alter neural crest cell motility in vitro, *J. Cell Sci.* **61:**299–323.

Ernst, S.G., Hough-Evans, B.R., Britten, R.J., and Davidson, E.H., 1980, Limited complexity of the RNA in micromeres of sixteen-cell sea urchin embryo, *Dev. Biol.* **79:**119–127.

Farmer, S.R., Wan, K.M., Ben-Ze'ev, A., and Penman, S., 1983, Regulation of actin mRNA levels and translation responds to changes in cell configuration, *Mol. Cell Biol.* **3:**182–189.

Fey, E.G., Krochmalnic, G., and Penman, S., 1986, The nonchromatin substructures of the nucleus the ribonucleoprotein (RNP)-containing and RNP-depleted matrices analyzed by sequential fractionation and resinless section electron microscopy, *J. Cell Biol.* **102:**1654–1665.

Folkman, J., and Greenspan, H.P., 1975, Influence of geometry on control of cell growth, *Biochim. Biophys. Acta* **417:**211–236.

Folkman, J., and Moscona, A., 1978, Role of cell shape in growth control, *Nature* **273:**345–349.

Foster, C.S., Smith, C.A., Dinsdale, E.A., Monaghan, P., and Neville, A.M., 1983, Human mammary gland morphogenesis *in vitro:* The growth and differentiation of normal breast epithelium in collagen gel cultures defined by electron microscopy, monoclonal antibodies, and autoradiography, *Dev. Biol.* **96:**197–216.

Fulton, A.B., Wan, K.M., and Penman, S., 1980, The spatial distribution of polyribosomes in 3T3 cells and the associated assembly of proteins into the skeletal framework, *Cell* **20:**849–857.

Gatmaitan, Z., Jefferson, D.M., Ruiz-Opazo, N., Biempica, L., Arias, I.M., Dudas, G., Leinwand, L.A., and Reid, L.M., 1983, Regulation of growth and differentiation of a rat hepatoma cell line by the synergistic interactions of hormones and collagenous substrata, *J. Cell Biol.* **97:**1179–1190.

Glowacki, J., Trepman, E., and Folkman, J., 1983, Cell shape and phenotypic expression in chondrocytes, *Proc. Soc. Exp. Biol. Med.* **172:**93–98.

Gordon, J.R., and Bernfield, M.R., 1980, The basal lamina of the postnatal mammary epithelium contains glycosaminoglycans in a precise ultrastructural organization, *Dev. Biol.* **74:**118–135.

Gospodarowicz, D., Cohen, D., and Fujii, D.K., 1982, Regulation of cell growth by the basal lamina and plasma factors: Relevance to embryonic control of cell proliferation and differentiation, *Cold Spring Harbor Conf. Cell Proliferation* **9:**95–124.

Greenberg, J.H., Seppa, S., Seppa, H., and Hewitt, A.T., 1981, Role of collagen and fibronectin in neural crest cell adhesion and migration, *Dev. Biol.* **87:**259–266.

Guerin, M.A., and Loizzi, R.F., 1980, Tubulin content and assembly in guinea pig mammary gland during pregnancy, lactation and weaning (40932), *Proc. Soc. Exp. Biol. Med.* **165:**50–54.

Hadley, M.A., Byers, S.W., Suarez-Quian, C.A., Kleinman, H., and Dym, M., 1985, Extracellular matrix regulates Sertoli cell differentiation, testicular cord formation, and germ cell development *in vitro, J. Cell Biol.* **101:**1511–1522.

Hall, H.G., and Bissell, M.J., 1986, Characterization of the intermediate filament proteins of murine mammary gland epithelial cells, *Exp. Cell Res.* **162:**379–389.

Hall, H.G., Farson, D.A., and Bissell, M.J., 1982, Lumen formation by epithelial cell lines in response to collagen overlay: A morphogenetic model in culture, *Proc. Natl. Acad. Sci. USA* **79:**4672–4676.

Hammond, S.L., Ham, R.G., and Stampfer, M.R., 1984, Serum-free growth of human mammary epithelial cells: Rapid clonal growth in defined medium and extended serial passage with pituitary extract, *Proc. Natl. Acad. Sci. USA* **81:**5435–5439.

Hay, E.D. (ed.), 1981, *Cell Biology of Extracellular Matrix,* Plenum Press, New York.

Haeuptle, M-T., Suard, Y.L.M., Bogenmann, E., Reggio, H., Racine, L., and Kraehenbuhl, J-P., 1983, Effect of cell shape change on the function and differentiation of rabbit mammary cells in culture, *J. Cell Biol.* **96:**1425–1434.

Henninghausen, L.G., and Sippel, A.E., 1982a, Characterization and cloning of the mRNAs specific for the lactating mouse mammary gland, *Eur. J. Biochem.* **125:**131–141.

Henninghausen, L.G., and Sippel, A.E., 1982b, Mouse whey acidic protein is a novel member of the family of "four disulfide core" proteins, *Nucleic Acid Res.* **10:**2677–2684.

Hogan, B.L.M., Taylor, A., and Cooper, A.R., 1982, Murine parietal endoderm cells synthesize heparan sulphate and 170K and 145K sulphated glycoproteins as components of Reichart's membrane, *Dev. Biol.* **90:**210–214.

Hogg, N.A.S., Harrison, C.J., and Tickle, C., 1983, Lumen formation in the developing mouse mammary gland, *J. Embryol. Exp. Morphol.* **73:**39–57.

Hoshino, K., 1978, Mammary transplantation and its histogenesis in mice, in: *Physiology of Mammary Gland* (A. Yokoyama, H. Mizuno, and H. Nagasawa, eds.), Japan Scientific Societies Press, Tokyo, pp. 163–228.

Houdebine, L.M., and Djiane, J., 1980, Effects of lysosomotropic agents and of microfilament and microtubule disrupting drugs on the activation of casein-gene expression by prolactin in the mammary gland, *Mol. Cell. Endocrinol.* **17:**1–15.

Houdebine, L-M., Djiane, J., Teyssot, B., Servely, J-L., Kelly, P.A., Delouis, C., Ollivier-Bousguet, M., and Devinoy, E., 1983, Prolactin and casein gene expression in the mammary cell, in: *Regulation of Gene Expression by Hormones* (K.W. McKerns, ed.), pp. 71–92.

Imagawa, W., Tomooka, Y., Hamamoto, S., and Nandi, S., 1985. Stimulation of mammary epithelial cell growth in vitro: Interaction of epidermal growth factor and mammogenic hormones, *Endocrinology* **116:**1514–1524.

Ingber, D.E., and Jamieson, J.D., 1985, Cells as tensegrity structures: Architectural regulation of histodifferentiation by physical forces transduced over basement membrane, in: *Gene Expression During Normal and Malignant Differentiation* (L.C. Anderson, C.G. Gahmberg, and P. Ekblom, eds.) Academic Press, Orlando, FL, pp. 13–32.

Ingber, D.E., Madri, J.A., and Jamieson, J.D., 1981, Role of basal laminin neoplastic disorganization of tissue architecture, *Proc. Natl. Acad. Sci. USA* **78:**3901–3905.

Jeffery, W.R., 1982, Messenger RNA in the cytoskeletal framework: Analysis by in situ hybridization, *J. Cell Biol.* **95:**1–7.

Juergens, W.G., Stockdale, F.E., Topper, Y.J., and Elias, J.J., 1965, Hormone-dependent differentiation of mammary gland in vitro, *Proc. Natl. Acad. Sci. USA* **54:**629–634.

Kato, Y., and Gospodarowicz, D., 1985, Effect of exogenous extracellular matrices on proteoglycan synthesis by cultured rabbit costal chondrocytes, *J. Cell Biol.* **100:**486–495.

Kefalides, N.A., Alper, R., and Clark. C.C., 1979, Biochemistry and metabolism of basement membranes, *Int. Rev. Cytol.* **61:**167–228.

Kleinman, H.K., McGarvey, M.L., Hassell, J.R., Star, V.L., Cannon, F.B., Laurie, G.W., and Martin, G.R., 1986, Basement membrane complexes with biological activity, *Biochemistry* **25:**312–318.

Kratochwil, K., 1969, Organ specificity in mesenchymal induction demonstrated in the embryonic development of the mammary gland of the mouse, *Dev. Biol.* **20:**46–71.

Kratochwil, K., 1977, Development and loss of androgen responsiveness in the embryonic rudiment of the mouse mammary gland, *Dev. Biol.* **61:**358–365.

Kratochwil, K., and Schwartz, P., 1976, Tissue interactions in androgen response of embryonic mammary rudiment of mouse: Identification of target tissue for testosterone, *Proc. Natl. Acad. Sci. USA* **73:**4041–4044.

Kulski, J.K., Topper, Y.J., Chomczynski, P., and Qasba, P., 1983, An essential role for glucocorticoid in casein gene expression in rat mammary explants, *Biochem. Biophys. Res. Commun.* **114:**380–387.

Lane, E.B., 1982, Monoclonal antibodies provide specific intramolecular markers for the study of epithelial tonofilament organization, *J. Cell Biol.* **92:**665–673.

Larson, B.L. (ed.), 1978, *Lactation, A Comprehensive Treatise,* Vol. IV, Academic Press, New York.

Larson, B.L. (ed.), 1985, *Lactation,* Iowa State University Press, Ames, IA.

Larson, B.L., and Smith, V.R. (eds.), 1974, *Lactation, A Comprehensive Treatise,* Vols. I, II, and III, Academic Press, New York.

Lasfargues, E.Y., 1957, Cultivation and behavior *in vitro* of the normal mammary epithelium of the adult mouse, *Exp. Cell Res.* **13:**553–562.

Laszlo, A., and Bissell, M.J., 1983, TPA induces simultaneous alterations in the synthesis and organization of olmentin, *Exp. Cell Res.* **148:**221–234.

Laurie, G.W., Bing, J.T., Kleinman, H.K., Hassell, J.R., Aumailley, M., Martin, G.R., and Feldman, R.J., 1986, Localization of binding sites for laminin, heparan sulfate proteoglycan and fibronectin on basement membrane (Type IV) collagen, *J. Mol. Biol.* **189:**205–216.

Lawrence, J.B., and Singer, R.H., 1986, Intracellular localization of messenger RNAs for cytoskeletal proteins, *Cell* **45:**407–415.

Lee, E.Y-H., Parry, G., and Bissell, M.J., 1984, Modulation of secreted proteins of mouse mammary epithelial cells by the extracellular matrix, *J. Cell Biol.* **98:**146–155.

Lee, E.Y-H., Lee, W.-H., Kaetzel, C.S., Parry, G., and Bissell, M.J., 1985, Interaction of mouse mammary epithelial cells with collagenous substrata: Regulation of casein gene expression and secretion, *Proc. Natl. Acad. Sci. USA* **82:**1419–1423.

Lee, E.Y.-H., Barcellos-Hoff, M.H., Li, H.-C., Parry, G., and Bissell, M.J., 1987, Transferrin is a major mouse milk protein and is synthesized by mammary epithelial cells, *In Vitro Cell Develop. Biol.* **23:**221–226.

Lenk, R., Ransom, L., Kaufmann, Y., and Penman, S., 1977, A cytoskeletal structure with associated polyribosomes obtained from HeLa cells, *Cell* **10:**67–78.

Levine, J.F., and Stockdale, F.E., 1984, 3T3-L1 Adipocytes promote the growth of mammary epithelium, *Exp. Cell Res.* **151:**112–122.

Levine, J.F., and Stockdale, F.E., 1985, Cell–cell interactions promote mammary epithelial cell differentiation, *J. Cell Biol.* **100:**1415–1422.

Li, M.-L., Aggeler, J., Farson, D.A., Hatier, C., Hassell, J., and Bissell, M.J., 1987, Influence of a reconstituted basement membrane and its components on casein gene expression and secretion in mouse mammary epithelial cells, *Proc. Natl. Acad. Sci. USA* **84:**136–140.

Liotta, L.A., and Hart, I.R. (eds.), 1982, Tumor invasion and metastasis, in: *Developments in Oncology,* Vol. 7, Martinus Nijhoff Publishers, Amsterdam.

Liotta, L.A., Wicha, M.S., Foidart, J.M., Rennard, S.I., Garbisa, S., and Kidwell, W.R., 1979, Hormonal requirements for basement membrane collagen deposition by cultured rat mammary epithelium, *Lab. Invest.* **41:**511–518.

MacKenzie, I.C., and Fusenig, N.E., 1983, Regeneration of organized epithelial structure, *J. Invest. Dermatol.* **81:**189s–194s.

MacKenzie, D.D.S., Forsyth, I.A., Brooker, B.E., and Turvey, A., 1982, Culture of bovine mammary epithelial cells on collagen gels, *Tissue Cell* **14:**231–241.

Majack, R.A., and Bornstein, P., 1985, Heparin regulates the collagen phenotype of vascular smooth muscle cells: Induced synthesis of an Mr 60,000 collagen, *J. Cell Biol.* **100:**613–619.

Martinez-Hernandez, A., Fink, L.M., and Pierce, G.B., 1976, Removal of basement membrane in the involuting breast, *Lab. Invest.* **34:**455–462.

Matsuda, R., Spector, D., and Strohman, R.C., 1984, There is selective accumulation of a growth factor in chicken skeletal muscle, *Dev. Biol.* **103:**267–275.

Matusik, R.J., and Rosen, J.M., 1978, Prolactin induction of casein mRNA in organ culture: A model system for studying peptide hormone regulation of gene expression, *J. Biol. Chem.* **253:**2343–2347.

Maximow, A., 1924, Tissue cultures of mammary gland, *Anat. Rec.* **27:**210.

McGrath, M., Palmer, S., and Nandi, S., 1985, Differential response of normal rat mammary epithelial cells to mammogenic hormones and EGF, *J. Cell Physiol.* **125:**182–191.

McKeon, F.D., Kirschner, M.W., and Caput, D., 1986, Homologies in both primary and secondary structure between nuclear envelope and intermediate filament proteins, *Nature* **319:**463–468.

Medina, D., Oborn, C.J., Kittrell, F.S., and Ulrich, R.J., 1986, Properties of mouse mammary epithelial cell lines characterized by *in vivo* transplantation and *in vitro* immunocytochemical methods, *J. Natl. Cancer Inst.* **76:**1143–1156.

Medina, D., Li, M. L., Oborn, C. J., and Bissell, M. J., 1987, Casein gene expression in mouse mammary epithelial cell lines: Dependence upon extracellular matrix and cell type, *Exp. Cell Res.* (in press).

Mehta, N.W., Ganguly, N., Ganguly, R., and Banerjee, M.R., 1980, Hormonal modulation of the casein gene expression in a mammogenesis–lactogenesis culture model of the whole mammary gland of the mouse, *J. Biol. Chem.* **255:**4430–4434.

Meier, S., and Hay, E.D., 1975, Control of corneal differentiation *in vitro* by extracellular matrix, in: *Extracellular Matrix Influences on Gene Expression* (H.C. Slavrin and R.C. Greulich, eds.), Academic Press, New York, pp. 185–196.

Mepham, T.B. (ed.), 1983, *Biochemistry of Lactation,* Elsevier, Amsterdam.

Mercier, J.-C., and Gaye, P., 1983, Milk protein synthesis, in: *Biochemistry of Lactation* (T.B. Mepham, ed.), Elsevier, Amsterdam, p. 177.

Michaelopoulos, G., and Pitot, H.C., 1975, Primary culture of parenchymal liver cells on collagen membranes, *Exp. Cell Res.* **94:**70–78.

Misfeldt, D.S., Hamamoto, S.T., and Pitelka, D.R., 1976, Transepithelial transport in cell culture, *Proc. Natl. Acad. Sci. USA* **73:**1212–1216.

Müller, W.E.G., Bernd, A., and Schroder, H.C., 1983, Modulation of poly(A) (+)mRNA-metabolizing and transporting systems under special consideration of microtubule protein and actin, *Mol. Cell. Biochem.* **53/54:**197–220.

Müller, W.E.G., Agutter, P.S., Bernd, A., Bachmann, M., and Schroder, H.C., 1985, Role of post-transcriptional events in aging: Consequences for gene expression in eukaryotic cells, in: *Thresholds in Aging* (M. Bergener and H.B. Stahelin, eds.), Academic Press, London, pp. 21–56.

Nagaiah, K., Bolander, F.F., Nicholas, K.R., Takemoto, T., and Topper, Y.J., 1981, Prolactin-induced accumulation of casein mRNA in mouse mammary explants: A selective role or glucocorticoid, *Biochem. Biophys. Res. Commun.* **98:**380–387.

Nandi, S., Imagawa, W., Tomooka, Y., McGrath, M.F., and Edery, M., 1984, Collagen gel culture system and analysis of estrogen effects on mammary carcinogenesis, *Arch. Toxicol.* **55:**91–96.

Neville, M.C., and Neifert, M.R. (eds.), 1983, *Lactation: Physiology, Nutrition, and Breast-Feeding,* Plenum Press, New York.

Nickerson, S.C., and Akers, R.M., 1984, Biochemical and ultrastructural aspects of milk synthesis and secretion, *Int. J. Biochem.* **16:**855–865.

Nickerson, S.C., Smith, J.J., and Keenan, T.W., 1980, Role of microtubules in milk secretion—action of colchicine on microtubules and exocytosis of secretory vesicles in rat mammary epithelial cells, *Cell Tissue Res.* **207:**361–376.

Nielsen, P., Goelz, S., and Trachsel, H., 1983, The role of the cytoskeleton in eukaryotic protein synthesis, *Cell Biol. Int. Rep.* **7:**245–254.

Ollivier-Bousquet, M., 1979, Effets de la cytochalasine B et de la colchicine sur l'action rapide de la prolactine dans la glande mammaire de lapine en lactation, *Eur. J. Cell Biol.* **19:**168–174.

O'Neill, C., Jordan, P., and Ireland, G., 1986, Evidence for two distinct mechanisms of anchorage stimulation in freshly explanted and 3T3 Swiss mouse fibroblasts, *Cell* **44:**489–496.

Orkin, R.W., Gehron, P., McGoodwin, E.B., Martin, G.R., Valentine, T., and Swarm, R., 1977, A murine tumor producing a matrix of basement membrane, *J. Exp. Med.* **145:**204–220.

Ormerod, E.J., and Rudland, P.S., 1985, Isolation and differentiation of cloned epithelial cell lines form normal rat mammary glands, *In Vitro Cell Dev. Biol.* **21:**143–153.

Ormerod, E.J., Warburton, M.J., Hughes, C., and Rudland, P.S., 1983, Synthesis of basement membrane proteins by rat mammary epithelial cells, *Dev. Biol.* **96:**269–275.

Park, C., and Bissell, M.J., 1986, Messenger RNA for basement membrane components in the mouse mammary gland and in cells in culture, *J. Cell Biol.* **103:**101a.

Parry, G., Lee, E.Y-H., and Bissell, M.J., 1982, Modulation of the differentiated phenotype of cultured mouse mammary epithelial cells by collagen substrata, in: *The Extracellular Matrix* (S.P. Hawkes and J. Wang, eds.), Academic Press, New York, pp. 303–308.

Parry, G., Lee, E.Y-H., Farson, D., Koval, M., and Bissell, M.J., 1985, Collagenous substrata regulate the nature and distribution of glycosaminoglycans produced by differentiated cultures of mouse mammary epithelial cells, *Exp. Cell Res.* **156:**487–499.

Paterson, F.C., and Rudland, P.S., 1985, Identification of novel, stage-specific polypeptides associated with the differentiation of mammary epithelial stem cells to alveolar-like cells in culture, *J. Cell Physiol.* **124:**525–538.

Paterson, F.C., Warburton, M.J., and Rudland, P.S., 1985, Differentiation of mammary epithelial stem cells to alveolar-like cells in culture: Cellular pathways and kinetics of the conversion process, *Dev. Biol.* **107:**301–313.

Pitelka, D.R., and Hamamoto, S.T., 1983, Ultrastructure of the mammary secretory cell, in: *Biochemistry of Lactation* (T.B. Mepham, ed.), Elsevier, Amsterdam, pp. 29–78.

Pitelka, D.R., Hamamoto, S.T., Duafala, J.G., and Nemanic, M.K., 1973, Cell contacts in the mouse mammary gland, *J. Cell Biol.* **56:**797–818.

Porter, R., and Whelan, J. (eds.), 1984, *Ciba Foundation Symposium 108: Basement Membranes and Cell Movement,* Pitman, London.

Rapraeger, A.C., and Bernfield, M., 1983, Heparan sulfate proteoglycans from mouse mammary epithelial cells. A putative membrane proteoglycan associates quantitatively with lipid vesicles, *J. Biol. Chem.* **258:**3632–3636.

Reid, L.M., Narita, M., Fujita, M., Murray, Z., Liverpool, C., and Rosenberg, L., 1986, Matrix and hormonal regulation of differentiation in liver cultures, in: *Liver Cells in Culture* (A. Guillouza and C. Guillouza, eds.), John Libbey, Eurotext, INSERM, pp. 225–258.

Rheinwald, T.G., O'Connell, T.M., Connell, N.D., Ryback, S.M., Allen-Hoffmann, B.L., LaRocca, Y-J.W., and Rehwoldt, S.M., 1984, Expression of specific keratin subsets and vimentin in normal human epithelial cells: A function of cell type and conditions of growth during serial culture, in: *Cancer Cells 1* (A.J. Levine, G.F. Cande Woude, W.C. Topp, and J.D. Watson, eds.), Cold Spring Harbor Laboratory, Cold Spring Harbor, NY, pp. 217–227.

Ringo, D.L., and Rocha, V., 1983, Xanthine oxidase, an indicator of secretory differentiation in mammary cells, *Exp. Cell Res.* **147:**216–220.

Robinson, J., and Gospodarowicz, D., 1983, Effect of *p*-nitrophenyl β-*d*-xyloside on proteoglycan synthesis and extracellular matrix formation by bovine corneal endothelial cell cultures, *J. Biol. Chem.* **259:**3818–3824.

Rocha, V., Ringo, D.L., and Read, D.B., 1985, Casein production during differentiation of mammary epithelial cells in collagen gel culture, *Exp. Cell Res.* **159:**201–210.

Rosen, J.M., Matusik, R.J., Richards, D.A., Gupt, P., and Rodgers, J.R., 1980, Multihormonal regulation of casein gene expression at the transcriptional and post-transcriptional levels in the mammary gland, *Recent Prog. Horm. Res.* **36:**157–193.

Rosen, J.M., Jones, W.K., Campbell, S.M., Bisbee, C.A., and Yu-Lee, L.-Y., 1985, Structure and regulation of peptide hormone-responsive genes, in: *Proceedings of the UCLA Symposium on Membrane Receptors and Cellular Regulation* (C.R. Kahn and M. Czech, eds.), Alan R. Liss, New York, pp. 385–396.

Rosen, J.M., Rodgers, J.R., Couch, C.H., Bisbee, C.A., David-Inouye, Y., Campbell, S.M., and Yu-Lee, L.-Y., 1986, Multihormonal regulation of milk protein gene expression, in: *Metabolic Regulation: Application of Recombinant DNA Techniques* (R. Hanson and A. Goodridge, eds.), New York Academy of Science, New York **478:**63–76.

Sakakura, T., Nishizuka, Y., and Dawe, C.J., 1976, Mesenchyme-dependent morphogenesis and epithelium-specific cytodifferentiation in mouse mammary gland, *Science* **194:**1439–1441.

Sakakura, T., Sakagami, Y., and Nishizuka, Y., 1979a, Persistence of responsiveness of adult mouse mammary gland to induction by embryonic mesenchyme, *Dev. Biol.* **72:**201–210.

Sakakura, T., Nishizuka, Y., and Dawe, C.J., 1979b, Capacity of mammary fat pads of adult C3H/HeMs mice to interact morphogenetically with fetal mammary epithelium, *J. Natl. Cancer Inst.* **63:**733–736.

Sakakura, T., Sakagami, Y., and Nishizuka, Y., 1982, Dual origin of mesenchymal tissues participating in mouse mammary gland embryogenesis, *Dev. Biol.* **91:**202–207.

Salomon, D.S., Liotta, L.A., and Kidwell, W.R., 1981, Differential response to growth factor by rat mammary epithelium plated on different collagen substrata in serum-free medium, *Proc. Natl. Acad. Sci. USA* **78:**382–386.

Schor, S.L., Shor, A.M., Rushton, G., and Smith, L., 1985a, Adult, foetal and transformed fibroblasts display different migratory phenotypes on collagen gels: Evidence for an isoformic transition during foetal development, *J. Cell Sci.* **73:**221–234.

Schor, S.L., Schor, A.M., Durning, P., and Rushton, G., 1985b, Skin fibroblasts obtained from cancer patients display foetal-like migratory behavior on collagen gels, *J. Cell Sci.* **73:**235–244.

Schwarz R.I., and Bissell, M.J., 1977, Dependence of the differentiated state on the cellular environment: Modulation of collagen synthesis in tendon cells, *Proc. Natl. Acad. Sci. USA* **74:**4453–4457.

Semanoff, S., Hogan, B.L.M., and Hopkins, C.R., 1982, Localization of fibronectin, laminin-entactin, and entactin in Reichert's membrane by immunoelectron microscopy, *EMBO J.* **1:**1171–1175.

Shannon, J.M., and Pitelka, D.R., 1981, The influence of cell shape on the induction of functional differentiation in mouse mammary cells in vitro, *In Vitro* **17:**1016–1028.

Slack, J.M.W., 1983, *From Egg to Embryo: Determining Events in Early Development,* Cambridge University Press, London.

Spiegelman, B.M., and Ginty, C.A., 1983, Fibronectin modulation of cell shape and lipogenic gene expression in 3T3-adipocytes, *Cell* **35:**657–666.

Stampfer, M.R., Hallowes, R.C., and Hackett. A.J., 1980, Growth of normal human mammary epithelial cells in culture, *In Vitro* **16:**415–425.

Suard, Y.M.L., Haeuptle, M-T., Farinon, E., and Kraehenbuhl, J-P., 1983, Cell proliferation and milk protein gene expression in rabbit mammary cell cultures, *J. Cell Biol.* **96:**1435–1442.

Supowit, S.C., Asch, B.B., and Rosen, J.M., 1981, Casein gene expression in normal and neoplastic mammary tissue, in: *Cell Biology of Breast Cancer* (C. McGrath, M. Brennon, and M. Rich, eds.), Academic Press, New York, pp. 247–263.

Takemoto, T., Nagamatsu, Y., and Oka, T., 1980, Casein and α-lactalbumin messenger RNAs during the development of mouse mammary gland, *Dev. Biol.* **78:**247–257.

Teyssot, B., and Houdebine, L.M., 1980, Effects of colchicine on the transcription rate of β-casein and 28S-ribosomal RNA genes in the rabbit mammary gland, *Biochem. Biophys. Res. Commun.* **97:**463–473.

Timpl, R., Rohde, H., Robey, P.G., Rennard, S.I., Foidart, J.-M., and Martin, G.R., 1979, Laminin, a glycoprotein from basement membranes, *J. Biol. Chem.* **254:**9933–9937.

Trelstad, R.L. (ed.), 1984, *The Role of Extracellular Matrix in Development,* Alan R. Liss, New York.

Ungar, F., Geiger, B., and Ben Ze'ev, A., 1986, Cell contact- and shape-dependent regulation of vinculin synthesis in cultured fibroblasts, *Nature* **319:**787–791.

van Venrooij, W.J., Sillekens, P.T.G., van Ekelen, C.A.G., and Reinders, R.J., 1981, On the association of mRNA with the cytoskeleton in uninfected and adenovirus-infected human KB cells, *Exp. Cell Res.* **135:**79–91.

Wakimoto, H., and Oka, T., 1983, Involvement of collagen formation in the hormonally induced functional differentiation of mouse mammary gland in organ culture, *J. Biol. Chem.* **258:**3775–3779.

Wan, Y-J., Wu, T-C., Chung, A.E., and Damjanov, I., 1984, Monoclonal antibodies to laminin reveal the heterogeneity of basement membranes in the developing and adult mouse tissues, *J. Cell Biol.* **98:**971–979.

Warburton, M.J., Ormerod, E.J., Monaghan, P., Ferns, S., and Rudland, P.S., 1981, Characterization of a myoepithelial cell line derived from a neonatal rat mammary gland, *J. Cell Biol.* **91:**827–836.

Warburton, M.J., Ferns, S.A., and Rudland, P.S., 1982, Enhanced synthesis of basement membrane proteins during the differentiation of rat mammary tumour epithelial cells in myoepithelial-like cells in vitro, *Exp. Cell Res.* **137:**373–380.

Warburton, M.J., Monaghan, P., Ferns, S.A., Rudland, P.S., Perusinghe, N., and Chung, A.E., 1984, Distribution of entactin in the basement membrane of the rat mammary gland, *Exp. Cell Res.* **152:**240–254.

Wessells, N.K., 1977, *Tissue Interactions and Development,* Benjamin-Cummings, Menlo Park, CA.

Wicha, M.S., Liotta, L.A., Garbisa, S., and Kidwell, W.R., 1979, Basement membrane collagen requirements for attachment and growth of mammary epithelium, *Exp. Cell Res.* **124:**181–190.

Wicha, M.S., Liotta, L.A., Vonderhaar, B.K., and Kidwell, W.R., 1980, Effects of inhibition of basement membrane collagen deposition on rat mammary gland development, *Dev. Biol.* **80:**253–266.

Wicha, M.S., Lowrie, G., Kohn, E., Bagavandon, P., and Mahn, T., 1982, Extracellular matrix promotes mammary epithelial growth and differentiation in vitro, *Proc. Natl. Acad. Sci. USA* **79:**3213–3217.

Wilde, C.J., Hasan, H.R., and Mayer, R.J., 1984, Comparison of collagen gels and mammary extracellular matrix as substrata for study of terminal differentiation in rabbit mammary epithelial cells, *Exp. Cell Res.* **151:**519–532.

Williams, J.M., and Daniel, C.W., 1983, Mammary ductal elongation: Differentiation of myoepithelium and basal lamina during branching morphogenesis, *Dev. Biol.* **97:**274–290.

Wolosewick, J.J., and Porter, K.R., 1976, Stereo high-voltage electron microscopy of whole cells of the human diploid line WI-38, *Am. J. Anat.* **147:**303–324.

Yang, J., Richards, J., Bowman, P., Guzman, R., Enami, J., McCormick, K., Hamamoto, S., Pitelka, D., and Nandi, S., 1979, Sustained growth and three-dimensional organization of primary mammary tumor epithelial cells embedded in collagen gels, *Proc. Natl. Acad. Sci. USA* **76:**3401–3405.

5

Mammary Cytoskeleton and the Regulation of Microtubules

Robert F. Loizzi

1. Introduction

Cytoskeletal elements, which constitute the fibrillar infrastructure of all cells, have been implicated in many types of bulk movements including secretion and intracellular organelle transport. In mammary gland epithelial cells, drugs such as colchicine and cytochalasin B alter the integrity of microtubules and microfilaments, respectively, and also interfere with the production and/or secretion of milk components. Colchicine, for example, inhibits milk secretion both in vitro and in vivo, while cytochalasin B inhibits lactose synthesis. These observations, discussed more fully in Section 3, associate regulation of milk secretion with cytoskeletal integrity and lactose production and suggest that regulation of lactose release would also regulate milk flow. Since these earlier studies, new questions have arisen. Are synthesis and release coupled or separately controlled? Do cytoskeletal elements function in endocytosis as well? What regulates microtubule formation and tubulin synthesis? Does dimeric tubulin have a role?

The major portion of this chapter focuses on microtubules in mammary epithelium, especially the correlation of their integrity with alveolar cell function and differentiation in lactogenesis and lactation, and some evidence is reviewed that this correlation reflects hormonal regulation of microtubule assembly and disassembly related to milk production

Robert F. Loizzi • Research Resources Center and the Department of Physiology and Biophysics, University of Illinois at Chicago, Chicago, Illinois 60680.

and secretion. First, however, a brief description of the various filamentous proteins and associated molecules making up the cytoskeleton is presented to help maintain the perspective that microtubules are but one element of a complex, dynamic, and multifunctional system. A number of reviews and symposia volumes provide extensive information on the cytoskeleton and its elements (Kirschner, 1978; Poste and Nicolson, 1981; *Cold Spring Harbor Laboratory Symposia on Quantitative Biology*, Vol. 46, 1981, Parts 1 and 2; Hall, 1982; Hill and Kirschner, 1983; Bourguignon and Bourguignon, 1984; Borisy et al., 1984; Wang et al., 1985; Soifer, 1986).

1.1. Components of the Cytoskeleton

At least three cytoskeletal systems have been identified using immunocytochemical light and electron microscopic techniques. These have been named according to three different filamentous structures observed: microfilaments, 6 nm in diameter; intermediate filaments, 7–11 nm; and microtubules, 22 nm. Since these structures are assembled from subunits and associated molecules, the complete system includes the visible filaments plus the soluble components. Together, these systems most probably determine cellular shape and are directly involved in axonal transport, chromosome movements in mitosis, organelle movements, modulation of surface receptors, and bulk transport including both uptake into cells, endocytosis, and secretion or exocytosis.

1.1.1. Microfilaments

Microfilaments use actin as their primary protein. Regulation of actin polymerization (i.e., globular or G-actin → filamentous or F-actin), as well as the association of microfilaments in the cell, depends on a large group of actin-binding proteins or factors causing capping, severing, stabilizing, sequestering, spacing, bundling, and so on. In enteric cells, for example, each of the highly geometric luminal microvilli contains a core bundle of microfilaments held in place by the bundling factors fimbrin and villin. Microfilaments form a meshwork just beneath the plasmalemma to which a variety of other molecules such as protein kinases may attach and carry out specific functions. Microfilaments also are found in short, straight bundles running parallel to and just under the plasmalemma in *stress fibers*. In the presence of myosin, parallel microfilaments of opposite polarity can be made to slide past each other, thus effecting a shortening of the filament pair. If each is attached at its opposite end to a membranous structure (e.g., a vesicle or two plasmalemma sites), the "contraction" results in movement of the two structures toward each other. When microfilaments of living cells are exposed to antiactin or the microfilament-disrupting drug cytochalasin B, both cell motility and intracellular shortening are interrupted. Talin and other proteins have been proposed to provide transmembrane linkages between actin filaments and cell surface fibronectin for a variety of cell–matrix interactions (Horwitz et al., 1986).

1.1.2. Intermediate Filaments

Intermediate filaments take several forms. A lacy network can be demonstrated in most cultured cells with its filamentous ends attached to the outer membrane of the nuclear envelope and extending to the plasmalemma. Intermediate filaments are also concentrated in various, filament-rich regions such as the terminal web in the apical region of many lining-type epithelial cells and extending into the cytoplasm from desmosomes, structures connecting adjacent cells laterally. The function of intermediate filaments is largely unknown; by default, they are usually assigned a structural role in the cell, often providing tensile strength, although intracellular communication is another possibility. In human red cell ghosts, for example, desmin, spectrin, and actin form a complex, filamentous network anchored to the membrane by yet another protein, ankyrin (Langley and Cohen, 1986). The primary protein in the intermediate filaments of a particular cell depends on the embryological origin of that cell. There are five types of filament: keratin, neurofilaments, glial, desmin, and vimentin. Epithelial cells contain immunologically distinguishable keratin filaments that can be differentiated further into more than 30 subtypes (see Chapter 6 in this volume). Neurofilaments are found in neurons, glial filaments in glial cells, desmin in muscle, and vimentin in cells of mesenchymal origin such as fibroblasts. Immunofluorescent typing of intermediate filaments is sufficiently specific and reproducible to identify the cellular origin of tumors, for example, keratins in carcinomas, vimentin in lymphomas, and desmin in rhabdomyosarcomas. Intermediate filaments present in bovine mammary gland epithelial cells contain polypeptides immunologically identical to those in prekeratin isolated from cow hooves (Franke et al., 1978). Desmosomes in cultured mammary cells contain keratin-type intermediate filaments (Bologna et al., 1986). Contractile myoepithelial cells stain positively for prekeratin but not desmin, thus confirming their epithelial rather than muscle origin (Franke et al., 1980). Monoclonal antikeratin antibodies have been used to distinguish preneoplastic and neoplastic mouse mammary epithelial cells from normal cells (Asch and Asch,

1986). Finally, as suggested earlier, intermediate filaments appear to have a special relation with extracellular matrix materials such as basement membrane proteins, laminin, and type IV collagen (Warburton et al., 1985) including apparent connections of intermediate filaments and extracellular collagen fibers observable with electron microscopy (Hall and Bissell, 1986).

1.1.3. Microtubules

The third filamentous member of the cytoskeletal family is the microtubule. Commonly observed in the mitotic spindle and in the cores of cilia and flagella, microtubules appear as long, fairly straight, apparently hollow cylinders in virtually all cell types with the exception of mammalian red blood cells. They have been described in lactating mammary epithelial cells by several investigators (Sandborn et al., 1964; Nickerson and Keenan, 1979; Nickerson et al., 1982). Microtubules are assembled from two similar but immunologically distinct globular peptides, α- and β-tubulin, usually coupled as an α-β dimer, which are the basic subunits of microtubules and which use GTP during polymerization. In Sections 2.2 and 2.3, the process of polymerization and its regulation are treated in detail. For comparison with microfilaments and intermediate filaments, however, immunofluorescent staining of tubulin in spread cells growing in culture yields a complex of gently curving lines radiating from a point of concentration near the nucleus toward the periphery (Asch et al., 1979). The densely stained point of origin or cell center consists of the paired centrosomes arranged perpendicular to each other. These organelles are nucleating sites for microtubule growth, both in the interphase cell just described and for the spindle formation in mitotic cells.

Various types of intracellular transport and exocytosis have been associated with microtubules, and evidence for this role is discussed in relation to milk secretion (Section 3.1). The most dramatic evidence, however, comes from reconstituted axoplasmic flow systems in which organelles and even latex beads are moved along microtubules simulating axonal transport (Schroer and Kelly, 1985; Vale et al., 1985a). A protein purified from squid axoplasm, kinesin, has been shown to cause both unidirectional and bidirectional movement along microtubules (Vale et al., 1985b).

Like the other two filamentous structures, microtubules appear also to have structural functions in cells. Treatment with microtubule-altering drugs causes a loss of intracellular organization, particularly on membranous organelles such as the Golgi apparatus and rough endoplasmic reticulum which undergo random changes from their normal location and separation of component elements.

2. Tubulin and Microtubules

2.1. Cellular Localization

A significant amount of ^{3}H-colchicine binding activity is associated with the final pellet in the tubulin assay (cf. Section 3.2), even after extraction of free tubulin and solubilization of microtubules (Jeanrenaud et al., 1977; Guerin and Loizzi, 1980). This activity probably includes molecular tubulin, which is incorporated into various cell membranes, as well as some adsorbed tubulin and small, microtubule fragments. Dustin (1978a) has reviewed reports of tubulin localization in the plasmalemma and other cell membranes as well as the association of microtubules with these structures. Using a variety of techniques, tubulin has been observed in brain cells and synaptosomal membrane preparations from brain and avian erythrocytes, as well as the leukocytes mentioned above. Tubulin was isolated from guinea pig brain plasmalemma fractions, which electron microscopic examination had shown to be microtubule-free, and then polymerized into microtubules (Bhattacharyya and Wolff, 1976). Zisapel et al. (1980) used gel electrophoresis and peptide mapping to identify tubulin in synaptic vesicle membrane and concluded that this membrane contains more α subunit than β and that the α is an integral vesicle membrane protein while the β is peripherally attached and easily dissociated from the membrane. Intracellularly, tubulin has also been associated with a variety of cell organelles, particularly the Golgi vesicles and the pores of nuclear membranes (reviewed by Dustin, 1978a).

Membrane tubulin may function as nucleating sites for microtubule formation or it may have a more physiological, regulatory function. One proposed role of plasmalemmal tubulin is to regulate the association of subunits within membrane-bound receptor–enzyme complexes such as adenylate cyclase (Peters, 1956; Zor, 1983). Binding of a hormone to its receptor in the cell membrane is thought to promote binding of guanyl nucleotide with the GTP regulatory protein or G-unit, followed by a coupling of the G-unit (Spiegel and Downs, 1981) with the catalytic moiety of adenylate cyclase. Microtubule-altering agents such as colchicine increase the interaction of the G-unit with the catalytic moiety (Rasenick et al., 1981). The explanation for this effect is that the ability of the G-unit to diffuse laterally within the membrane is a limiting factor in cyclase activation and that colchicine and agents that increase membrane fluidity, such as free fatty acids and certain local anesthetics, all increase protein mobility within the membrane and thus lead to cyclase activation. Evidence with a variety of tubulin-binding agents, such as vincristine, suggests that whether they act on microtubules attached to the membrane or on nonpolymerized tubulin molecules within it, either action increases planar mobility of subunits within the plasmalemma. These effects have been observed in cell-free preparations of cerebral cortex (Rasenick et al., 1981) and in cultured S49 lymphoma cells in which adrenergic- and PGE_1-stimulated accumulation of cyclic AMP is enhanced by colchicine and vinblastine (Kennedy and Insel, 1979).

The incorporation of tubulin within secretory vesicle membranes may offer an alternate explanation for the inhibitory effects of microtubule-altering drugs on secretion. Precisely this suggestion has been raised by Patton and his group for mammary gland (Patton et al., 1977; Sokka and Patton, 1983) and by Busson-Mabillot et al. (1982) regarding secretion by lacrimal glands. Some experimental support for the notion exists: When tubulin was incorporated into liposomal membrane consisting of bilayers of dipalmitoyl phosphatidylcholine and vesicles were held at a temperature below phase transition for 10–20 min, in this case 28–30°C, the vesicles has a tendency to aggregate and fuse (Kumar et al., 1982). Addition of calcium also caused vesicles to fuse into larger structures. Microtubule-altering drugs, however, had no effect on liposomal aggregation or fusion nor did vesicle-bound tubulin associate with microtubules when tubulin was assembled in vitro.

2.2. Assembly and Disassembly

Many of the proposed cytoskeletal and transport functions of microtubules use the ability of 6S dimeric tubulin, MW 110,000, to polymerize reversibly into microtubules under physiological conditions (Soifer, 1975; Sloboda et al., 1976; Dustin, 1978a). Studies of this phenomenon were facilitated by Weisenberg's observations that tubulin isolated from brain formed microtubules in vitro when tubulin and calcium concentrations, ionic strength, and temperature (Weisenberg, 1975; Tash et al., 1980) were controlled. Purified tubulin was found to have the following minimal requirements for polymerization: maintenance of low calcium concentration with a chelator such as EGTA; a temperature close to 37°C; 1 m*M* GTP; and a critical tubulin concentration estimated at 0.2 mg/ml. Microtubule formation in vitro also depends critically on the buffers employed, preferring zwitterionic buffers, such as MES, PIPES, and glutamate, which are preferred over buffers such as phosphate (Foster and Rosemeyer, 1986). Disassembly results from the opposite conditions, namely, cold temperature, elevated calcium, and lack of GTP. Under certain conditions, ATP will substitute for GTP in inducing tubulin polymerization through the exchangeable GTP site (Duanmo et al., 1986). The binding and hydrolysis of GTP during assembly may serve to stabilize tubulin subunits within the microtubule (Caplow and Reid, 1985). (For a review of tubulin binding sites and structural domains see Maccioni et al., 1985.)

Studies with brain tubulin have shown that polymerization is aided by a family of microtubule-associated proteins or MAPs which copurify with tubulin and which constitute about 10–15% of the weight of tubulin (purified with several successive polymerization–depolymerization cycles and separation by ultracentrifugation). The MAPs include both low molecular weight proteins, such as tau proteins (Weingarten et al., 1975), which have molecular weights of about 70,000, and also proteins with molecular weights of about 300,000–350,000 (reviewed by Sloboda et al., 1976; Wiche, 1985). Separation of MAPs from tubulin uses their adherence to a phosphocellulose column and release by the addition of KCl to the elution buffer. Electron micrographs of microtubules polymerized in the presence of MAPs reveal the latter as regularly spaced, short, filamentous projections extending laterally from the microtubules. Sloboda et al. (1976) reported that polymerization of brain tubulin involves phosphorylation of one of the high molecular weight MAPs, MAP-2. In rat brain, a Ca^{2+}/phospholipid-dependent kinase appears responsible for phosphorylating 30 sites of the MAP-2 molecule (Tsuyama et al., 1986). In turn, axonal MAPs appear to be influenced by linkages with actin–microfilaments and subsequent phosphorylation of a 200-kDa subunit of the neurofilament (Minami and Sakai, 1985, 1986) and by Ca^{2+}/calmodulin (Sobue et al., 1985). Association between MAPs and microfilaments is further suggested by the decoration of stress fibers in cultured mammalian cells using a monoclonal antibody to bovine brain MAP-1 (Asai et al., 1985) and by MAP–neurofilament cross-reactivity (Luca et al., 1986). These observations indicate that MAPs may serve to integrate various elements of the cytoskeleton as well as promote microtubule formation.

Microtubule-altering drugs such as colchicine are thought to inhibit spindle formation and disrupt "labile" forms of polymerized tubulin by binding to the tubulin dimer at the growing end of the potential microtubule and thus blocking addition of the next dimer. The "capped" microtubules, however, continue to disassemble at the opposite end and gradually shorten until only molecular tubulin remains. Interestingly, colchicine in vitro at substoichiometric concentrations with tubulin also inhibits depolymerization at the disassembly or minus end of the microtubule (Bergen and Borisy, 1986). Margolis and Wilson (1978) tested this concept by pulse labeling bovine brain microtubules in vitro with ^{3}H-GTP. They observed that, under steady-state conditions, microtubules maintained a constant length by adding tubulin dimers to one end (indicated by GTP binding) and removing dimers at the other end (GTP release) at equal rates. Since, in this steady-state situation, the GTP pulse label "traveled" down the length of microtubules from the assembly to the disassembly ends, the concept was termed *treadmilling* and forms the basis for one theory of how microtubules affect transport within cells. Recent studies in intact cells, however, using other tubulin labeling methods, such as biotinylated subunits (Kristofferson et al., 1986; Schulze and Kirschner, 1986) and fluorescence photobleaching using a laser microbeam (Wadsworth and Salmon, 1986) suggest a much more heterogeneous system in which some microtubules are more stable than others and in which some subunit addition or subtraction may occur at both ends.

2.3. Factors in Regulation

Physiologically, intracellular regulation of microtubule assembly and disassembly is only poorly understood. It appears to involve a growing list of factors and processes that include—in addition to MAPs and GTP—the dynamic equilibrium between free (dimeric) and polymerized tubulin, cytosolic calcium concentration, tubulin synthesis, microtubule opposite ends assembly–disassembly, calmodulin, cyclic nucleotides, special nucleating sites for assembly, and cytoplasmic proteins with regulatory activity.

A state of dynamic equilibrium between free tubulin dimers and microtubules exists in the cytoplasm in which, under certain physiological conditions, shifts in the direction of polymerized tubulin result in either longer or increased numbers of microtubules or both. Thus, physiological regulation of polymerization is determined to some extent by the level of unpolymerized tubulin available for assembly into microtubules and by the factors governing tubulin synthesis. When microtubules in cultured fibrobasts were depolymerized with colchicine or nocadazole, there was a rapid inhibition of tubulin synthesis and a reduction in the level of translatable tubulin mRNA (Ben-Ze'ev et al., 1979). Vinblastine, which disrupts microtubules by aggregating tubulin into large paracrystals without increasing free tubulin, results in an enchancement of tubulin synthesis rather than an inhibition.

Microtubule assembly in vivo involves special nucleating sites or microtubule organizing centers, MTOCs (Pickett-Heaps, 1975), which are associated with a variety of cell organelles such as membranes, the kinetochores of chromosomes, centrioles, or existing microtubules.

Microtubule assembly and disassembly are very sensitive to calcium concentrations. Microtubules in detergent-extracted monkey cells (Schliwa et al., 1981) were completely stable when calcium concentrations were below 1 μM but underwent disassembly in concentrations greater than 1–4 μM which began in the cell periphery and proceeded toward the cell center. The pattern and time course of disassembly were not markedly altered at calcium concentrations up to 500 μM, suggesting that, within this concentration range, the effects are catalytic rather than stoichiometric. Calcium in the millimolar range causes rapid destruction of microtubules. The status of cytoplasmic microtubules is therefore sensitive to variations in physiological concentrations of calcium. Cytosolic calcium levels are lowered by calcium pumps in the plasmalemma and various organelles. Mitochondrial uptake of calcium, for example, stimulated tubulin polymerization in an in vitro system (Fuller et al., 1975). The Golgi complex in mammary gland alveolar cells contains a Ca^{2+}–ATPase system that transports calcium from the cytosol into Golgi vesicles (Baumrucker and Keenan, 1975; Neville et al., 1981; West, 1981; Virk et al., 1985). This system reduces cytosolic calcium levels, particularly in the region of the Golgi complex, and also packages calcium into secretory vesicles containing milk proteins.

Calmodulin or calcium-dependent regulator protein is a major calcium binding protein in nonmuscle cells analogous to troponin in muscle cells (Marcum et al., 1978; Kumagai and Nishida, 1980). In its presence, the ability of calcium to inhibit microtubule formation is increased significantly. Observations suggesting that calmodulin may have a physiological role in regulating microtubule assembly and disassembly include its localization on the mitotic spindle (Anderson et al., 1978; Welsch et al., 1978, 1979; Watanabe and West, 1982), the copurification of both cAMP- and calmodulin-dependent kinases in brain microtubule preparations (Vallano et al., 1985), and the binding of calmodulin to both tau and MAP-2 in vitro and resultant microtubule assembly (Kumagai et al., 1986). Calmodulin plays a role in stimulus–secretion coupling by calcium in a wide variety of exocrine and endocrine secreting cells (Means and Dedman, 1980; Means et al., 1982a, 1982b; Schubart et al., 1982). Calcium stimulates secretion in mammary gland (Smith et al., 1982a) and most other secretory cells (Cantin, 1984). Calmodulin concentration in mammary gland varies with the lactation cycle. Riss and Baumrucker (1982) reported that purified calmodulin from bovine tissue approximately doubled 1 week prepartum. Similarly, calmodulin activity in rat mammary glands undergoes a sharp rise from days 15 through 20 of pregnancy with the levels during lactation approximately double those of early pregnancy (Pizarro et al., 1981). While these studies do not reveal whether the increased calmodulin activity functions in microtubule assembly–disassembly, nevertheless, the coincident calmodulin increase with the prepartum increase in prolactin secretion, as well as tubulin polymerization (cf. Section 3.2), at least in the rat (reviewed by Cowie et al., 1980), indicates temporal linkage of these activities during lactogenesis.

Similar changes occur in mammary gland cyclic nucleotides and related enzymes, suggesting that they also have important regulatory roles in lactogenesis and lactation. Mammary cAMP levels in rats (Louis and Baldwin, 1975; Sapag-Hagar and Greenbaum, 1973, 1984), mice (Rillema, 1976a), and guinea pigs (Loizzi, 1983a) increase progressively during late pregnancy to a prepartum peak, then drop abruptly at parturition, are maintained at low levels during lactation, and then rise again during weaning. Cyclic GMP levels undergo the reverse changes. These are accompanied by changes in the activities of their respective cyclases and phosphodiesterases, which could explain the fluctuations of the nucleotides, while in vitro studies with cAMP indicate it inhibited synthesis of nucleic acid and fatty acid synthesis (Sapag-Hagar et al., 1974), casein synthesis (Rillema, 1976b), and lactose synthesis (Loizzi et al., 1975; Loizzi, 1978). Methyl xanthines and other phosphodiesterases inhibited lactose synthesis in guinea pig mammary gland slices up to 100% in dose–response studies, while inhibition with cAMP and various analogues usually reached a plateau at 30–40%. Similar inconsistent inhibition of lactose synthesis and glucose uptake by isolated mammary gland acini were observed by Wilde and Kuhn (1981). In explant cultures of midpregnant mouse mammary glands, raising intracellular cAMP levels by a variety of means resulted in greater inhibition of hormonally induced synthesis of α-lactalbumin than casein, also suggesting a negative regulatory role for cAMP in milk protein synthesis (Perry and Oka, 1980). Cyclic AMP is also excreted in milk (Sapag-Hagar and Greenbaum, 1974). The content of cAMP in guinea pig milk is highest in early lactation when lactose production is maximal; that is, lactose synthesis is highest when cAMP removal is greatest (Loizzi, 1983). Conversely, cAMP stimulated intracellular protein transport and exocytosis in rabbit (Ollivier-Bousquet and Denamur, 1975) and bovine (Park et al., 1979) mammary gland slices. Nevertheless, the postpartum decrease of cAMP combined with its in vitro inhibitory effects suggested a physiological, inhibitory role for this nucleotide with respect to synthesis of milk constituents.

With respect to tubulin polymerization, evidence seems to favor the concept that cAMP promotes microtubule assembly under certain conditions, although conflicting observations have resulted in considerable confusion. As cells in culture reached confluency, growth slowed and cAMP levels rose while exogenous cAMP or its analogues decreased cell proliferation (Hsie and Puck, 1971; Johnson et al., 1971; Prasad and Hsie, 1971) and increased cell differentiation including greater numbers and organization of microtubules (DiPasquale et al., 1976). In transformed cells this response was termed *reverse transformation* (Puck et al., 1972). The opposite concept, that cAMP depolymerizes microtubules, arose partly from observations that induced lysosomal enzyme secretion by polymorphonuclear leukocytes was inhibited by colchicine and cAMP and stimulated by cGMP (Zurier et al., 1973; Weissman et al., 1975). However, in several types of secretory cell, cAMP stabilized microtubules and/or increased the rate of secretion (reviewed by Dustin, 1978b). Garland (1979) observed that cAMP inhibited assembly of microtubules in vitro when using "crude" 100,000*g* supernatant tubulin but not twice cycle-purified tubulin. Among the various proteins that copurify with tubulin during repeated depolymerization–polymerization cycling are MAPs, described above, and protein kinases, both cAMP-dependent and independent. Similarly, cAMP-dependent phosphorylation of MAPs has been reported to promote (Sloboda et al., 1976), have no effect on (Rappaport et al., 1976), or inhibit (Jameson et al., 1980) tubulin polymerization.

Brinkley et al. (1980) devised a lysed cell system for measuring microtubule growth in situ. Cultured cells grown on coverslips and that have been stabilized and permeabilized can serve as templates for initiating microtubule assembly when soluble, exogenous factors such as 6S tubulin and nucleotides are added. This system was used to quantitate the number of organizing centers (MTOCs), and the number and length of microtubules using antitubulin immunofluorescence. A difference was found between 3T3 and SV-3T3 cells in their ability to initiate microtubule assembly; specifically, while both cell types had the same number of organizing centers, the number of microtubules growing from each center in SV-3T3 cells was about half that in 3T3 cells. This difference could be eliminated by adding cAMP, which stimulated assembly in SV-3T3 but not 3T3 cells. These results suggested that an unknown substrate capable of cAMP-stimulated protein phosphorylation was involved in tubulin assembly and that the process may be inhibited in SV-3T3 cells owing to lack of a required factor (Tash et al., 1980, 1981). Extensive investigation is currently directed at the mechanism and sites of protein phosphorylation in tubulin polymerization and its regulation. Two phosphorylated polypeptides were isolated from extracted cytoskeletal material with molecular weights of 69 and 80 kDa (Pallas and Solomon, 1982). Soifer et al. (1982) photoaffinity labeled cAMP binding proteins to localize the regulatory subunit for the cAMP-dependent protein kinase which copurifies with tubulin. The major cAMP binding protein was distinct from activity associated with both the high molecular weight MAPs and tubulin.

Finally, a recent finding opens the possibility of cytoplasmic proteins that regulate microtubule formation. While cold temperatures are usually employed to depolymerize microtubules, a portion of them remain intact. Margolis et al. (1986) recently isolated a 145-kDa protein factor from cold-resistant microtubules. They named the protein *stable tubule only polypeptide* or STOP protein and believe that it physiologically stabilizes microtubules against disassembly.

3. Mammary Gland Microtubules and Tubulin

3.1. Effects of Microtubule-Altering Drugs on Milk Secretion

Colchicine and other microtubule-altering drugs inhibit the secretion of milk components both in vitro in incubating tissue fragments and cells and in vivo in lactating animals. Ollivier-Bousquet and Denamur (1973), using electron microscopic autoradiography, showed that colchicine inhibits exocytosis of milk protein in incubated mammary gland fragments. Patton (1974) found that the microtubule-altering drugs, colchicine and vincristine, suppressed milk flow up to 70% when administered to goats via retrograde infusion through the teat canal. In a later study, Knudson et al. (1978), using this technique with rats and goats, found that inhibition was associated with cytoplasmic disorganization, loss of cell polarity, and an intracellular accumulation of secretory vesicles and large lipid droplets suggesting interference with exocytosis. Infusion in prepartum lactating goats does not cause these effects (Sordillo et al., 1984). In addition to suppression of milk flow, infusion of colchicine into lactating goats results in the secretion of new milk proteins, one of which has been postulated to have a regulatory effect on the immune system (Groves and Farrell, 1985). However, the known solubility of colchicine in lipids coupled with small numbers of observable microtubules in alveolar cells and their lack of association with vesicles raises an alternate explanation for the suppressive action of these drugs, that is, interference with vesicular membrane fusion and cytoplasmic organization rather than a direct role of microtubules in exocytosis.

We observed that colchicine decreased lactose secretion by guinea pig mammary gland slices (Loizzi et al., 1975) and that vincristine but not lumicolchicine caused similar inhibition (Guerin and Loizzi, 1978). Inhibition of lactose secretion into the media was not accompanied by an equivalent suppression of synthesis. However, cytochalasin B, which alters microfilaments and inhibits glucose transport, inhibited lactose synthesis in guinea pig slices (Amato and Loizzi, 1979, 1981). Since glucose uptake could be normalized by increasing extracellular glucose without increasing lactose synthesis, cytochalasin B may be blocking precursors from the Golgi complex where lactose is synthesized, possibly via microfilaments. Both drugs inhibit prolactin-stimulated endocytosis in rabbit mammary gland slices but cytochalasin B stimulates casein secretion (Ollivier-Bousquet, 1979). Nikerson et al. (1980a) and Akers and Nickerson (1983) reported that colchicine, both in vivo and in vitro, produced cytoplasmic disorganization and loss of microtubules in rat mammary gland. Vinblastine caused similar morphological changes that were accompanied by decreased protein synthesis as well as secretion (Nickerson et al., 1980b). The same workers further differentiated the actions of these drugs in isolated mammary gland acini (Smith et al., 1982b,c). Colchicine caused intracellular accumulation of protein and presumably lactose; the synthesis of both was inhibited by cytochalasin B and vinblastine, and the latter interfered with protein transport from the rough endoplasmic reticulum. In view of the multiple actions of these drugs as well as an increasing understanding of the interaction among cytoskeletal elements and the physiology of cell membranes, it is best to take a cautious approach regarding the roles of microtubules and microfilaments based on drug actions.

3.2. Tubulin Synthesis and Polymerization During Pregnancy and Lactation

3.2.1. Whole Gland Changes

Colchicine and other microtubule-altering drugs have toxic effects on cells often unrelated to microtubules, which may explain their inhibition of secretion in mammary and other cells. While morphometric analysis of microtubules from electron micrographs showed a vectorial cytoplasmic gradient, thus supporting a secretory role, and a good correlation with mammary gland function and drug treatment (Nickerson et al., 1980a,b, 1982), microtubules in alveolar cells are often not well preserved and their appearance in micrographs prevents meaningful quantitative analysis.

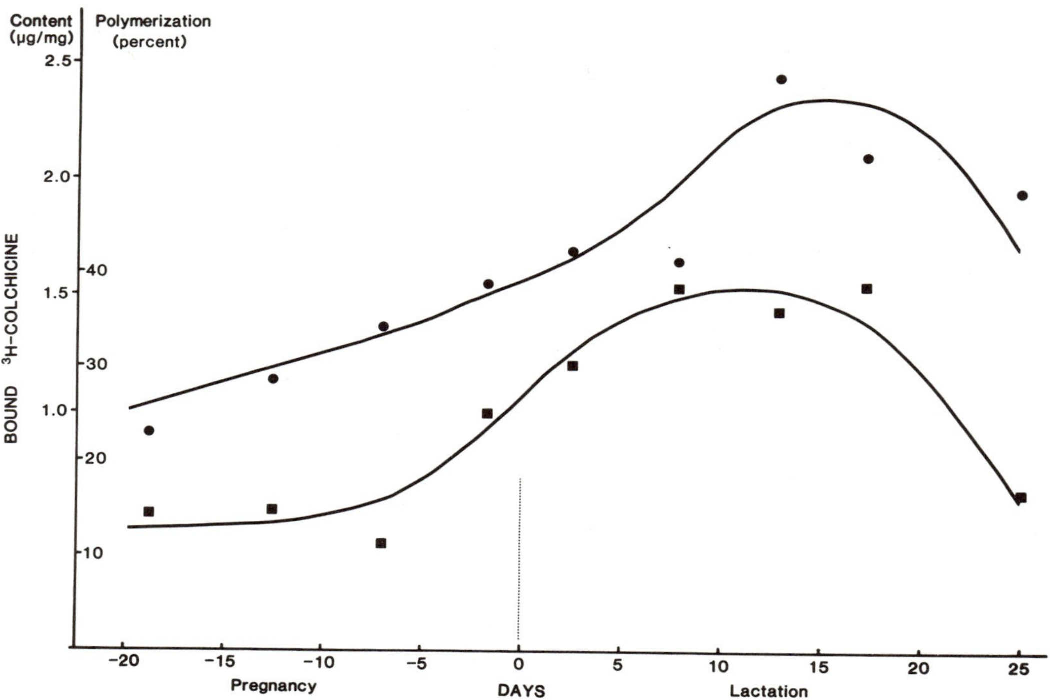

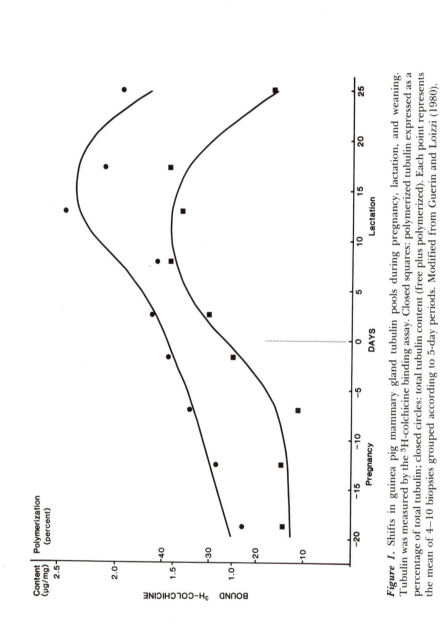

Figure 1. Shifts in guinea pig mammary gland tubulin pools during pregnancy, lactation, and weaning. Tubulin was measured by the ^{3}H-colchicine binding assay. Closed squares: polymerized tubulin expressed as a percentage of total tubulin; closed circles: total tubulin content (free plus polymerized). Each point represents the mean of 4–10 biopsies grouped according to 5-day periods. Modified from Guerin and Loizzi (1980).

For these reasons, we decided to quantitate microtubules biochemically using a colchicine binding assay based on several sources (Sherline et al., 1974; Rappaport et al., 1975; Pipeleers et al., 1977a,b; Sherline and Mundy, 1977) that allows separation of the free and polymerized tubulin pools. Following measurement of ^{3}H-colchicine binding by each, the size of the polymerized tubulin pool is expressed as a percentage of the total, that is, free plus polymerized, tubulin-bound colchicine measurements. The colchicine binding assay, with some variations, has been used to measure dimeric and polymerized tubulin in a wide variety of tissues (Pipeleers et al., 1975; Rappaport et al., 1975; Montague et al., 1976; Pipeleers et al., 1977a,b; Sherline and Mundy, 1977; Beertsen et al., 1982), including mammary gland (Nickerson and Keenan, 1979; Guerin and Loizzi, 1980; Loizzi, 1983b).

Free and polymerized tubulin pools were measured in guinea pig mammary gland biopsies from 3 weeks prepartum through weaning and the biopsy tubulin values combined into 5-day interval groups (Guerin and Loizzi, 1980). Note in Fig. 1 that the relative size of the polymerized pool remains low, 9–15% of the total, through 1 week prepartum at which time it gradually increases to a peak of 35–40% during midlactation, and then returns to low levels at weaning. The increase in absolute polymerized tubulin content is approximately sevenfold; however, since total tubulin content itself increases nearly threefold, indicating net tubulin synthesis, this results in a smaller change in percentage polymerization. A similar increase was observed in rat mammary gland in which tubulin polymerization increased from 6.0% on day 20 of pregnancy to 21.8% on day 9 of lactation (Loizzi, 1983b). Glands from lactating rats had twice as much total tubulin as those from pregnant rats.

3.2.2. Alveolar Cell Changes

One explanation for the observed increases in polymerized tubulin in mammary gland tissue with the onset and maintenance of lactation is a greater proportion of microtubule-rich cells (e.g., changes in relative contributions of acinar, duct, stromal, leucocyte, and adipocyte cell populations) rather than more microtubules per alveolar cell. Therefore, we examined tubulin changes in the alveolar cells themselves using immunofluorescent localization and biochemical quantitation of tubulin pools in isolated mammary gland cell populations. In the first approach (Loizzi, 1980), tubulin was localized using antibody raised in rabbits against guinea pig brain tubulin which had been purified by three cycles of polymerization–depolymerization followed by polyacrylamide gel electrophoresis. Antiserum or affinity column-purified antitubulin followed by fluorescein-labeled goat anti-rabbit IgG was used to stain cryostat sections of mammary glands from late pregnant (1 week prepartum), early lactating (2–3 days postpartum), and peak lactating guinea pigs. Glands from pregnant animals contained small alveoli, composed of nonsecreting cuboidal acinar cells surrounding a lumen and myoepithelial cells, capillaries, and sparse connective tissue. Cytoplasm of those acinar cells was diffusely fluorescent, while myoepithelial cells fluoresced brightly, even in control sections stained with nonimmune serum, possibly because of the presence of endogenous, fluorescent neurotransmitters. In glands from early lactation, scattered concentrations of bright fluorescence started appearing in the apical regions of some acinar cells but not in other cell types. By peak lactation (Fig. 2), nearly every acinar cell contained a bright, sometimes punctate layer directly below the apical membrane and surrounding lipid droplets and other inclusions in this region. The immunofluorescence results therefore suggest a developmental change in tubulin distribution from pregnancy to lactation in which tubulin becomes more concentrated in the apical portions of alveolar secretory cells but does not change or even appear to be present in appreciable quantities in other cell types. While these fluorescent images of antitubulin in sections of in situ tissues differ from the usual lacy network seen in relatively flat, cultured cell preparations in which microtubules are easily identified (Weber et al., 1975; Asch et al., 1979), they suggest a tubulin distribution that corresponds to electron microscopic descriptions of apically concentrated microtubules in mammary gland cells (Baumrucker and Keenan, 1975; Nickerson and Keenan, 1979). Finally, the developmental changes suggest that the increases in total and polymerized tubulin observed in the biopsy study during lactogenesis and lactation actually reflect changes within the alveolar cells.

Further verification of this idea was obtained from measurements of tubulin pools in cell populations isolated from mammary glands of late pregnant (1 week or less prepartum) and peak lactating guinea pigs on albumin density gradients (Kraehenbuhl, 1977; Pencek and Loizzi, 1981). Pregnant and lactating animals usually yielded about seven bands of mammary gland cells which were examined by light and electron microscopy (Loizzi and Pencek, 1982; Turner-Pencek and Loizzi, 1982), including L.M. morphometric analyses of cross-sectional areas and other parameters. A variety of cell types were observed with secretory alveolar cells concentrated in the intermediate bands. When tubulin assays were done on each band, bands 4 and 5, which were richest in alveolar secretory cells, contained twice as much tubulin as the two extreme bands 1 and 7 (8–11 pmol/10^6 cells versus 2–5 pmol in cells from lactating ani-

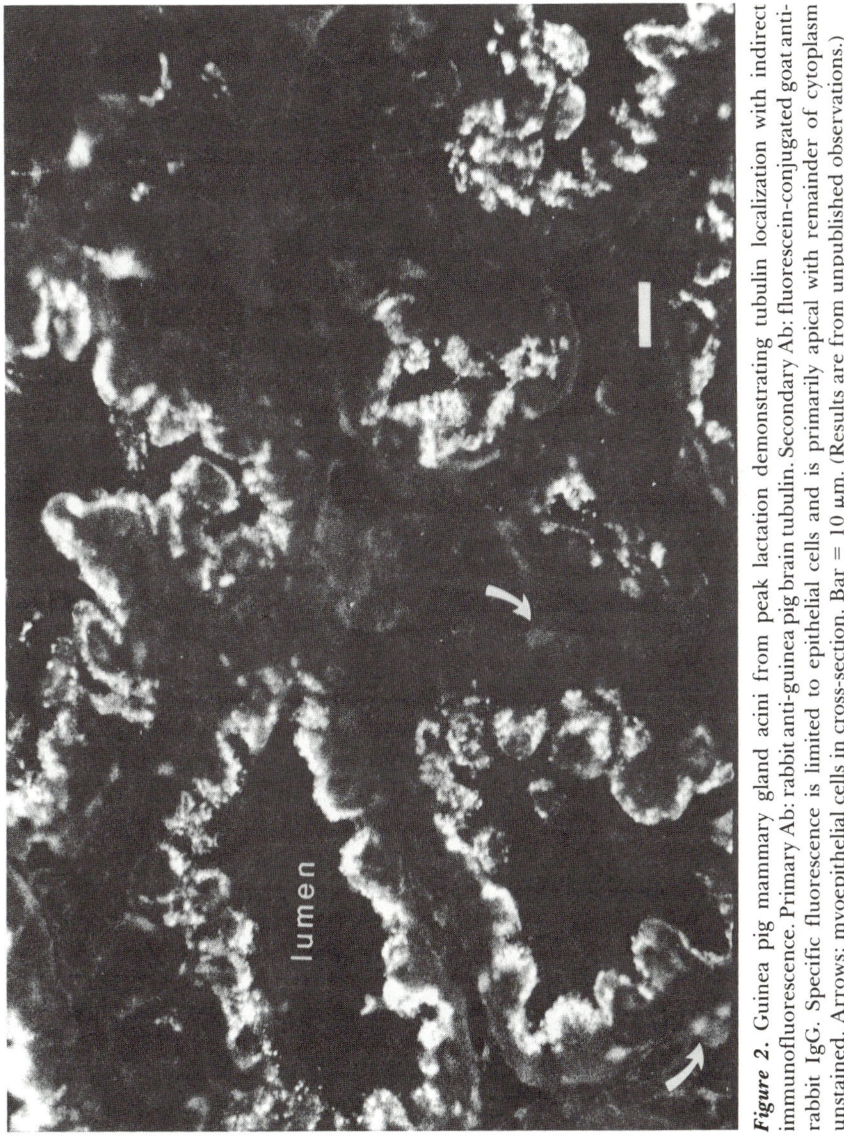

Figure 2. Guinea pig mammary gland acini from peak lactation demonstrating tubulin localization with indirect immunofluorescence. Primary Ab: rabbit anti-guinea pig brain tubulin. Secondary Ab: fluorescein-conjugated goat anti-rabbit IgG. Specific fluorescence is limited to epithelial cells and is primarily apical with remainder of cytoplasm unstained. Arrows: myoepithelial cells in cross-section. Bar = 10 μm. (Results are from unpublished observations.)

mals) and more than twice as much of it in the polymerized state (16–24% versus 55%). Tubulin differences between lactating and pregnant animals were less than expected but still significant (32% more tubulin per cell in the lactating and 17% greater polymerization). Two factors may account for this. First, lactogenesis-related differentiation in guinea pig mammary gland begins much earlier in pregnancy than in many other rodents such as rat and mouse. Thus, glands of animals in this study, 1 week prepartum, had already undergone significant alveolar cell differentiation. Second, it is likely that the largest secretory cells, those swollen with secretory vesicles and lipid droplets, were the most fragile and the least likely to survive enzymatic treatment and repeated centrifugation. The results of this study indicated that alveolar secretory cells are considerably richer in tubulin than other cell types in mammary gland and contain a much larger polymerized pool as well. Thus, the isolated cell study also supports the concept that the increased polymerization with lactation observed in the biopsy study described earlier is due primarily to intra-alveolar cell increases. This does not preclude an increase in the number of these cells within the gland which would raise the average percentage polymerization as well as tubulin content.

3.3. Tubulin Polymerization and Synthesis in Vitro

The effects of drugs and hormones on tubulin polymerization were studied in 2-h incubated mammary gland slices from 18-day pregnant and peak lactating rats (Loizzi, 1984) using the ^{3}H-colchicine binding assay to measure free and polymerized tubulin pools. In tissues from both the pregnant and lactating rats DB-cAMP, cGMP, both in micromolar quantities, and taxol increased the size of the polymerized tubulin pool significantly. Since net tubulin content did not change, stimulation of tubulin synthesis probably did not occur in this short time interval. The basal polymerized pool in lactating tissue was about four times that in the pregnant, but the absolute increases in polymerized tubulin due to the drugs were approximately the same in the two groups. Ultrastructurally, microtubules were observed mainly beneath the apical membrane in close proximity to secretory vesicles and lipid droplets undergoing exocytosis.

In vitro effects of drugs and hormones were also studied in mammary cells isolated from 15-day pregnant rats and cultured for 1 week on floating collagen gel membranes (Loizzi, 1984) according to the methods of Emerman and Pitelka (1977) and Emerman et al. (1977) with treatment during the last 5 days. The results indicated that the polymerized pool in control cultures was about double that in control lactating slices (above), which agrees with the extensive microtubule complex observed by immunofluorescence in normal, cultured cells. All three steroid hormones used, hydrocortisone, estradiol-17β, and progesterone, significantly increased relative polymerization beyond the control values. In addition, the steroids markedly increased total tubulin concentration. Taxol and hydrocortisone dose–response studies yielded maximal increases, two- to threefold, in both polymerization and tubulin content. Additivity did not occur when the hormones were used in combination, suggesting that each was maximally stimulating tubulin through generalized protein synthesis. Ultrastructurally, taxol treatment caused bundling of microtubules, especially in the peripheral cytoplasm adjacent to the plasmalemma between the RER and Golgi complex [cf. Tokunaka et al. (1983) re. taxol-induced microtubules associated with RER]. The increases in polymerization observed in the two types of in vitro study may have been due to different causes. In slices, cyclic nucleotides may directly stimulate polymerization via microtubule-associated protein kinase. Taxol stimulation probably occurred via decreasing the microtubular pool by forming taxol complexes (Manfredi et al., 1982), thus shifting the equilibrium toward polymerization. In cultured cells, apparently the resulting decrease in free tubulin then induced tubulin synthesis resulting in an increased total tubulin. Finally, the steroids, all of which are known to induce mammary cell development, would be expected to stimulate directly tubulin synthesis as well as that of other proteins. This would result, first, in an increase in the free tubulin pool followed by increased polymerization owing to the equilibrium between free tubulin and microtubules. Similarly, polymerization may also have been stimulated directly by the steroids, perhaps reflecting a mitogenic effect. The results caution against direct application of tissue culture observations to in situ cells. The large pool of polymerized tubulin in cultured cells compared to that in slices may reflect the large microtubule complex observed in cultured cells with immunofluorescence and electron microscopy and may be related to the flat shape of these cells and contact with the substratum.

3.4. Tubulin Polymerization in Induced Lactogenesis

3.4.1. Roles of Estrogen and Progesterone

The increases in mammary gland tubulin polymerization observed in the biopsy studies can also be produced by artificially stimulating lactogenesis in the intact animal (Loizzi, 1983b). Eighteen-day pregnant rats were ovariectomized using the procedures described by Kuhn (1969) and others (Vermouth and Deis, 1974; Nicholas and Hartman,

1981a,b; Deis and DeLouis, 1983), and mammary glands were examined for lactose and tubulin at intervals over the following 48 h (Fig. 3). Lactose content rose about 700% between 18 and 24 h, indicating the onset of induced lactogenesis. Intact rat mammary glands contained 10.4 pmol tubulin/mg protein of which 3.6% was polymerized. Eighteen hours following surgery, the average size of the polymerized pools for the ovariectomized and sham-operated groups were similar at 5.4 and 4.7% of the total tubulin, respectively. Between 18 and 24 h, however, that of the ovariectomized group increased 2.4-fold. Lactating rats had a much larger polymerized pool, about 22%. While total tubulin content did not change in ovariectomized rats, it doubled in mammary glands of lactating rats. The results indicate that during induced lactogenesis in rats, the increase in the size of the polymerized tubulin pool in mammary gland and the initiation of lactose synthesis occur simultaneously.

How does ovariectomy stimulate tubulin polymerization? Kuhn observed that in the rat OVX-induced lactogenesis results from progesterone withdrawal (Kuhn, 1969; Kuhn et al., 1980). Raising prolactin

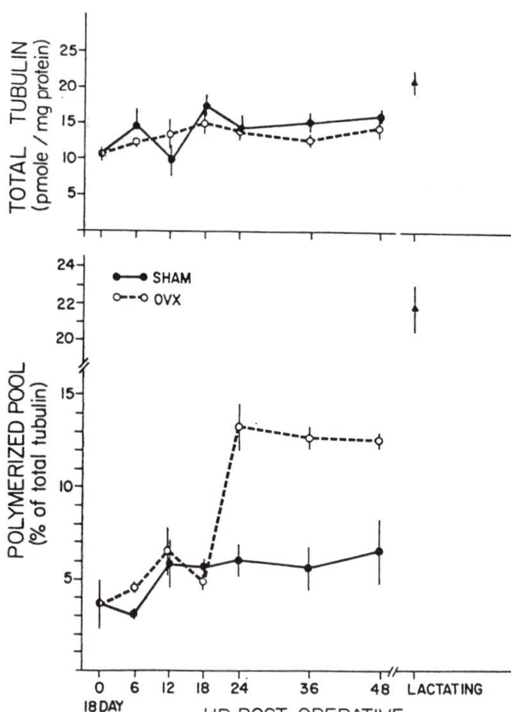

Figure 3. Changes in mammary gland tubulin following bilateral ovariectomy (OVX) in 18-day pregnant rats. *Upper graph:* total (free + polymerized) tubulin content based on ^{3}H-colchicine binding assay. *Lower graph:* fraction of total tubulin in polymerized state. OVX values are compared to sham-operated and 9-day lactating (▲) values. Usually, each point is the mean plus or minus SEM of six or more animals (three at 48 h). From Loizzi (1983b).

levels in late pregnant rats with perphenazine alone does not induce lactogenesis (Simpson et al., 1973). In the above study, progesterone levels had substantially decreased by 6 h following surgery, and 18 h preceding the rise in tubulin polymerization. In cannulated rats, ovariectomy increased prolactin levels 16–18 h following ovariectomy (Nicholas and Hartman, 1981a,b). Intact rats undergoing normal lactogenesis have increased prolactin 1–2 days prior to parturition (Amenomori et al., 1970). To answer the question of whether the increase in polymerization was also the result of progesterone withdrawal, a second ablation study (Loizzi, 1985) was carried out examining the effects of estrogen and progesterone replacement on OVX-induced changes. Silastic implants containing estradiol-17β, progesterone, or both were inserted subcutaneously at the time of ovariectomy in 18-day pregnant rats and mammary glands were collected 24 h later (Fig. 4). Again, the polymerized pool approximately doubled in ovariectomized rats compared to the sham-operated, which was concomitant with initiation of lactose synthesis, while total tubulin did not change. However, in rats fitted with implants containing progesterone or progesterone plus estradiol, the

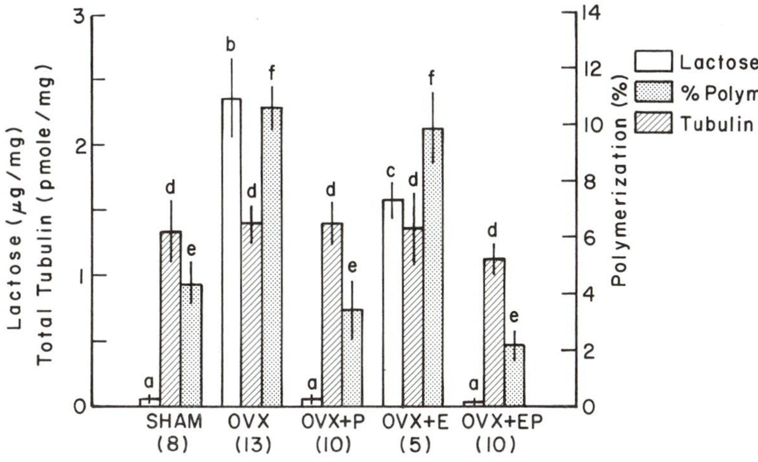

Figure 4. Effects of estrogen and progesterone replacement on the ovariectomy-induced increase in mammary gland polymerized tubulin. Silastic implants filled with progesterone (P) and estrogen (E) were inserted at the time of surgery. Mammary gland samples were obtained 24 h after surgery. Bars indicate the mean plus or minus SEM; the number of animals in each condition is indicated in parentheses. Within each of the three parameters (lactose, tubulin content, and percentage polymerization), bars with the same letters indicate treatment groups that are not significantly different from each other ($p<0.05$). From Loizzi (1985).

increases in both relative tubulin polymerization and lactose content were blocked. Estradiol alone did not block polymerization but it slightly reduced lactose content compared to ovariectomized alone. Hormone replacements did not affect total tubulin content. Thus, ovariectomy-induced stimulation of polymerization as well as lactose synthesis in the mammary glands of these animals were related to progesterone withdrawal. The possibility exists that steroid hormones may directly affect tubulin polymerization in cells. Sharp and Parry (1985) found that tubulin isolated from hamster brain bound the synthetic estrogen diethylstilbesterol competitively with colchicine. While at high doses (10^{-5} *M*), diethylstilbesterol inhibited tubulin polymerization into intact microtubules, at lower doses (10^{-7}–10^{-6} *M*), diethylstilbesterol enhanced polymerization and also inhibited cold-induced depolymerization of existing microtubules.

3.4.2. Prolactin and Placental Lactogen

Mammary gland differentiation following ovariectomy may be influenced by placental lactogen and/or prolactin. In the rat, low molecular weight placental lactogen peaks in late pregnancy at 17–21 days (Kelly et al., 1975) and binds equally well to mammary gland and ovarian prolactin receptors (Glaser et al., 1984). An ablation study was carried out in which administration of the prolactin secretion inhibitor CB-154 was combined with a complete hysterectomy to reduce or prevent a rise in the plasma levels of both prolactin and placental lactogen.

Figure 5 demonstrates the values for lactose, total tubulin, and percentage polymerization. It can be seen that hysterectomy plus CB-154 blocks the fivefold increase in lactose content owing to ovariectomy but has no effect on the increase in polymerized tubulin. Total tubulin contents in all four treatment groups are approximately equal.

Since we had shown that in peak lactation both the polymerized pool and total tubulin in mammary gland are two to three times that in lactogenesis, a study was carried out with lactating animals to determine if CB-154 administration (0 time, 24 h, and 78 h) would have an effect on microtubule polymerization. The results indicated that lactose content remained high through 48 h but decreased significantly at 96 h. The percentage polymerization in lactating animals was about 35% in both the controls and the 24-h animals after which polymerization decreased to 18%. Total tubulin content remained stable at about three times the content of the 19-day pregnant animals. These data suggest that maintenance of the very large polymerized pool in peak lactation may be prolactin dependent.

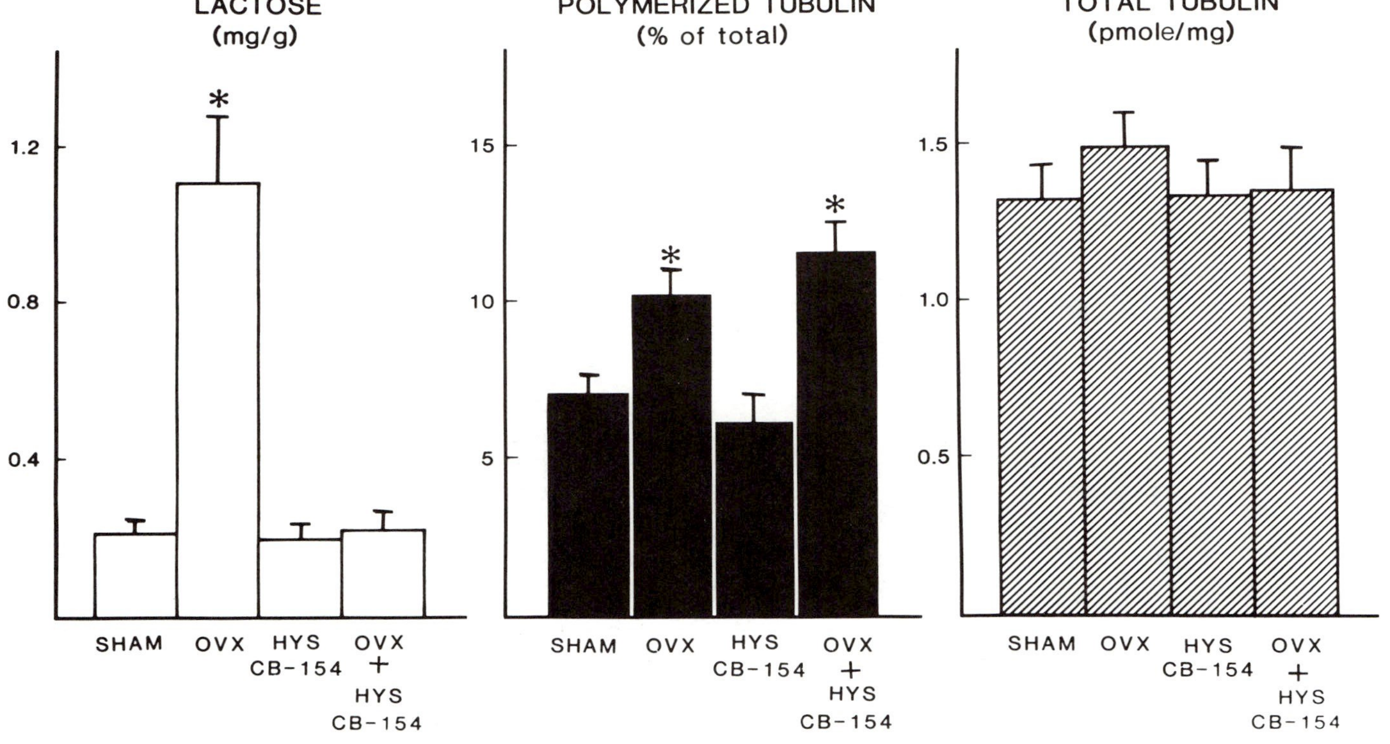

Figure 5. The effects of hysterectomy and prolactin secretion inhibitor, (HYS) + CB-154, on the ovariectomy-induced (OVX) stimulation of lactose production and tubulin polymerization in mammary glands of 19-day pregnant rats. Surgery and CB-154 administration was carried out 24 h previously. Asterisks indicate significant difference ($p<0.05$) from respective SHAM values. From Loizzi (in preparation).

3.5. Conclusions from Whole Animal Studies

Our whole animal studies have shown, first, that the polymerized pool of tubulin, which most likely represents the microtubular fraction, increases in guinea pig and rat mammary glands during late pregnancy with the onset of lactogenesis and continues to increase until peak lactation: and second, that these increases take place within the alveolar cells themselves. In addition, using the rat as a model, we observed that ovariectomy in late pregnancy stimulates tubulin polymerization coincident with lactogenesis. Moreover, replacement of progesterone with implants in ovariectomized animals blocks this stimulation. Thus, in the rat, the stimulus that triggers lactogenesis, progesterone withdrawal, also appears to stimulate an increase in microtubule formation.

The question then arises as to the degree of coupling between regulation of microtubule formation and lactogenesis in mammary gland. Since it is known that several hormones have roles in the initiation of lactogenesis and maintenance of lactation, we next examined whether preventing a rise in serum prolactin with CB-154 and reducing placental lactogen with hysterectomy prevented the ovariectomy-stimulated increase in lactose production and the increase in tubulin polymerization. The observation that stimulation of tubulin polymerization was not blocked in the same mammary glands where lactose synthesis was inhibited suggested that while prolactin and/or placental lactogen are required for lactogenesis to take place, neither appeared to be requisite for increased tubulin polymerization in the late pregnant rat. This uncoupling of two lactogenic phenomena on the basis of hormonal requirements indicates that, beyond the progesterone withdrawal stimulus for both, tubulin polymerization is not an obligatory accompaniment to lactogenesis but may be regulated, at least in part, by a separate mechanism. Since in none of the present studies was net tubulin content altered by ablation or drug treatment, control of polymerization appears to take place during assembly of tubulin into microtubules rather than tubulin synthesis, possibly via synthesis of cofactors such as MAPs.

4. Summary

The cytoskeletal system in mammary gland epithelial cells serves such diverse functions as maintenance of structural integrity, intracellular transport, motility, and communication. It consists of microfilaments, intermediate filaments, and microtubules and several associated proteins. The constituent proteins of some of these elements exist in equilibrium between free and polymerized forms. Earlier studies using microtubule-altering drugs such as colchicine indicated that microtubules were required for milk secretion. While this may be true, the role of membrane-bound tubulin, as well as other effects of these drugs, provides additional explanations for secretory inhibition. Microfilament-disrupting drugs inhibit lactose synthesis, which appears due to both an inhibition of glucose uptake by the cell as well as a more direct effect on lactose synthesis itself. The sizes of the free and polymerized tubulin pools in mammary gland undergo changes in relation to the lactational state of the gland. During late pregnancy and associated with lactogenesis, either natural or induced, the equilibrium shifts toward the polymerized fraction doubling it from approximately 5 to 10%. Net tubulin content does not change. In lactation, the lactogenic pool doubles or triples again, this time accompanied by a net tubulin synthesis. That these changes are related to the epithelial cells can be shown both with fluorescent antibody labeling as well as tubulin analysis of isolated cell populations. In vitro studies with slices and cultured cells indicate that tubulin polymerization and synthesis can be promoted with cyclic nucleotides and mammogenic steroid hormones. Endocrine ablation and hormone replacement studies indicate that the increased tubulin polymerization, following ovariectomy, like lactose synthesis, is stimulated by progesterone withdrawal. While both processes are associated with lactogenesis, tubulin polymerization does not appear to have the same dependency on prolactin and/or placental lactogen as does lactose synthesis. Three conclusions from these studies are that, first, regulation of tubulin polymerization, such as in lactogenesis, may occur independently from tubulin synthesis and is likely to involve MAPs, alterations in calcium concentrations, calmodulin, cAMP, and the removal of polymerized tubulin from equilibrium such as in microtubule bundling; second, the decoupling of lactogenesis and increased tubulin polymerization suggests, at least in part, separate regulatory mechanisms for the two; and, third, parturition adds a new element, net tubulin synthesis, along with further increases in polymerization, suggesting yet another control mechanism. Future research might be directed at each of these regulatory mechanisms, the interaction of the various cytoskeletal elements, regulation of assembly and disassembly in the system as a whole, and its role(s) in milk synthesis and secretion.

ACKNOWLEDGMENT: This research is supported by NIH grant HD 11601.

References

Akers, R.M., and Nickerson, S.C., 1983, Effect of prepartum blockade of microtubule formation on milk production and biochemical differentiation of the mammary epithelium in Holstein heifers, *Eur. J. Biochem.* **15:**771–775.

Amato, P.A., and Loizzi, R.F., 1979, The effects of cytochalasin B on glucose transport and lactose synthesis in lactating mammary gland slices, *Eur. J. Cell Biol.* **20:**150–155.

Amato, P.A., and Loizzi, R.F., 1981, The identification and localization of actin and actin-like filaments in lactating guinea pig mammary gland alveolar cells, *Cell Motility* **1:**329–347.

Amenomori, Y., Chen, C.L., and Meites, J., 1970, Serum prolactin levels in rats during different reproductive states, *Endocrinology* **86:**506–510.

Anderson, B.M., Osborn, M., and Weber, K., 1978, Specific visualization of the distribution of the calcium dependent regulatory protein of cyclic nucleotide phosphodiesterase (modulator protein) in tissue culture cells by immunofluorescence microscopy: Mitosis and intercellular bridge, *Eur. J. Cell Biol.* **17:**354–364.

Asai, D.J., Thompson, W.C., Wilson, L., Dresden, C.F., Schulman, H., and Purich, D.L., 1985, Microtubule-associated proteins (MAPs): A monoclonal antibody to MAP-1 decorates microtubules in vitro but stains stress fibers and not microtubules in vivo, *PNAS (USA)* **82:**1434–1438.

Asch, B.B., and Asch, H.L., 1986, A keratin epitope that is exposed in a subpopulation of preneoplastic and neoplastic mouse mammary epithelial cells but not in normal cells, *Cancer Res.* **46:**1255–1262.

Asch, B.B., Medina, D., and Brinkley, B.R., 1979, Microtubules and actin containing filaments of normal, preneoplastic, and neoplastic mouse mammary epithelial cells, *Cancer Res.* **39:**893–907.

Baumrucker, C.R., and Keenan, T.W., 1975, Membranes of mammary gland. X. Adenosine triphosphate dependent calcium accumulation by Golgi apparatus rich fractions from bovine mammary gland, *Exp. Cell Res.* **90:**253–260.

Beertsen, W., Heersche, J.N.M., and Aubin, J.E., 1982, Free and polymerized tubulin in cultured bone cells and Chinese hamster ovary cells: The influence of cold and hormones, *J. Cell Biol.* **95:**387–393.

Ben-Ze'ev, A., Farmer, S.R., and Penman, S., 1979, Mechanisms of regulating tubulin synthesis in cultured mammalian cells, *Cell* **17:**319–325.

Bergen, L.G., and Borisy, G.G., 1986, Tubulin-colchicine complex (TC) inhibits microtubule depolymerization by a capping reaction exerted preferentially at the minus end, *J. Cell. Biochem.* **30:**11–18.

Bhattacharyya, B., and Wolff, J., 1976, Polymerisation of membrane tubulin, *Nature* **264:**576–577.

Bologna, M., Allen, R., and Dulbecco, R., 1986, Organization of cytokeratin bundles by desmosomes in rat mammary cells, *J. Cell Biol.* **102:**560–567.

Borisy, G.G., Cleveland, D.W., and Murphy, D.B. (eds.), 1984, *Molecular Biology of the Cytoskeleton,* Cold Spring Harbor Laboratory, Cold Spring Harbor, NY.

Bourguignon, L.Y.W., and Bourguignon, G.J., 1984, Capping and the cytoskeleton, *Int. Rev. Cytol.* **87:**195–224.

Brinkley, B.R., Pepper, D.A., Cox, S.M., Fistel, S., Brenner, K.S.L., Wible, L.J., and Pardue, R.L., 1980, Characteristics of centriole- and kinetochore-associated microtubule assembly in mammalian cells, in: *Microtubules and Microtubule Inhibitors 1980* (M. De-Brabander and J. DeMay, eds.), Elsevier/North-Holland, Amsterdam, pp. 281–296.

Busson-Mabillot, S., Chambaut-Guerin, A.M., Ovtracht, L., and Muller, P., 1982, Microtubules and protein secretion in rat lacrimal glands: Localization of short-term effects of colchicine on the secretory process, *J. Cell Biol.* **95:**105–117.

Cantin, M.D., 1984, *Cell Biology of the Secretory Process,* Karger, New York.

Caplow, M., and Reid, R., 1985, Directed elongation model for microtubule GTP hydrolysis, *PNAS (USA)* **42:**3267–3271.

Cold Spring Harbor Laboratory Symposia on Quantitative Biology, Vol. 46, 1981, Parts 1 and 2.

Cowie, A.T., Forsyth, I.A., and Hart, I.C., 1980, *Hormonal Control of Lactation,* Springer-Verlag, New York.

Deis, R.P., and DeLouis, C., 1983, Lactogenesis induced by ovariectomy in pregnant rats and its regulation by oestrogen and progesterone, *J. Steroid Biochem.* **18:**687–690.

DiPasquale, A.M., McGuire, J., Moellmann, G., and Wasserman, S., 1976, Microtubule assembly in cultivated Greene melanoma cells is stimulated by dibutyryl adenosine 3′:5′-cyclic monophosphate or cholera toxin, *J. Cell Biol.* **71:**735–748.

Duanmu, C., Lin, C., and Hamel, E., 1986, Tubulin polymerization with ATP is mediated through the exchangeable GTP site, *Biochim. Biophys. Acta* **881:**113–123.

Dustin, P., 1978a, *Microtubules,* Springer-Verlag, New York.

Dustin, P., 1978b, Secretion, exo- and endocytosis, in: *Microtubules,* Springer-Verlag, New York, pp. 284–307.

Emerman, J.T., and Pitelka, D.R., 1977, Maintenance and induction of morphological differentiation in dissociated mammary epithelium on floating collagen membranes, *In Vitro* **13:**316–378.

Emerman, J.T., Enami, J., Pitelka, D.R., and Nandi, S., 1977, Hormonal effects on intracellular and secreted casein in cultures of mouse mammary epithelial cells on floating collagen membranes, *Proc. Natl. Acad. Sci. USA* **74:**4466–4470.

Foster, K., and Rosemeyer, M., 1986, Microtubule formation and the initial association of tubulin dimmers, *FEBS Lett* **194:**78–84.

Franke, W.W., Weber, K., Osborn, M., Schmid, E., and Freudenstein, C., 1978, Antibody to prekeratin, *Exp. Cell Res.* **116:**429–445.

Franke, W.W., Schmid, E., Freudenstein, C., Appelhans, B., Osborn, M., Weber, K., and Keenan, T.W., 1980, Intermediate-sized filaments of the prekeratin type in myoepithelial cells, *J. Cell Biol.* **84:**633–645.

Fuller, G.M., Ellison, J., McGill, M., and Brinkley, B.R., 1975, The involvement of mitochondria and calcium in regulating microtubule assembly *in vitro, J. Cell Biol.* **67:**126a.

Garland, D.L., 1979, cAMP inhibits the *in vitro* assembly of microtubules, *Arch. Biochem. Biophys.* **198:**335–337.

Glaser, L.A., Kelly, P.A., and Gibori, G., 1984, Differential action and secretion of rat placental lactogens, *Endocrinology* **115:**969–976.

Groves, M.L., and Farrell, H.M. Jr., 1985, Isolation and characterization of new proteins produced by the infusion of colchicine in goat mammary gland, *Biochim. Biophys. Acta* **844:**105–112.

Guerin, M.A., and Loizzi, R.F., 1978, Inhibition of mammary gland lactose secretion by colchicine and vincristine, *Am. J. Physiol. (Cell Physiol.)* **234:**C177–180.

Guerin, M.A., and Loizzi, R.F., 1980, Tubulin content and assembly states in guinea pig mammary gland during pregnancy, lactation, and weaning, *Proc. Soc. Exp. Biol. Med.* **165:**50–54.

Hall, G., and Bissell, M., 1986, Characterization of the intermediate filament proteins of murine mammary gland epithelial cells, *Exp. Cell Res.* **162:**379–389.

Hall, P.F., 1982, The role of the cytoskeleton in endocrine function, in: *Cellular Regulation of Secretion and Release* (P. Michael Conn, ed.), Academic Press, New York, Chap. 6, pp. 195–222.

Hill, T.L., and Kirschner, M.W., 1983, Regulation of microtubule and actin filament assembly–disassembly by associated small and large molecules, *Int. Rev. Cytol.* **84:**185–234.

Horwitz, A., Duggan, C.B., Berkerle, M.C., and Burridge, K., 1986, Interaction of plasma membrane fibronectin receptor with talin—a transmembrane linkage, *Nature* **320**(10):531–533.

Hsie, A.W., and Puck, T.T., 1971, Morphological transformation of Chinese hamster cells by dibutyryl adenosine cyclic 3′:5′-monophosphate and testosterone, *Proc. Natl. Acad. Sci. USA* **68:**358–361.

Jameson, L., Frey, T., Zeeberg, B., Dalldorf, F., and Caplow, M., 1980, Inhibition of microtubule assembly by phosphorylation of microtubule-associated proteins, *Biochemistry* **19:**2472–2479.

Jeanrenaud, B., Le Marchand, Y., and Patzelt, C., 1977, Role of microtubules in hepatic secretory processes, in: *Membrane Alterations as Basis of Liver Injury* (M. Pepper, L. Bianchi, and U. Reutter, eds.), University Park Press, Baltimore, pp. 247–255.

Johnson, G.S., Friedman, R.M., and Pastan, I., 1971, Restoration of several morphological characteristics of normal fibroblasts in sarcoma cells treated with adenosine 3′:5′-cyclic monophosphate and its derivatives, *Proc. Natl. Acad. Sci. USA* **68:**425–429.

Kelly, P.A., Shiu, R.P.C., Robertson, M.C., and Friesen, H.G., 1975, Characterization of rat chorionic mammotropin, *Endocrinology* **96:**1187–1195.

Kennedy, M.S., and Insel, P.A., 1979, Inhibitors of microtubule assembly enhance beta-adrenergic and prostaglandin El-stimulated cyclic AMP accumulation in S49 lymphoma cells, *Mol. Pharmacol.* **16:**215–223.

Kirschner, M.W., 1978, Microtubule assembly and nucleation, *Int. Rev. Cytol.* **54:**1–71.

Knudson, C.M., Stemberger, B.H, and Patton, S., 1978, Effects of colchicine on ultrastructure of the lactating mammary cell: Membrane involvement and stress on the Golgi apparatus, *Cell Tissue Res.* **195:**169–181.

Kraehenbuhl, J.P., 1977, Dispersed mammary gland epithelial cells. I. Isolation and separation procedures, *J. Cell Biol.* **72:**390–405.

Kristofferson, D., Mitchison, T., and Kirschner, M., 1986, Direct observation of steady-state microtubule dynamics, *J. Cell Biol.* **102:**1007–1019.

Kuhn, N.J., 1969, Progesterone withdrawal as the lactogenic trigger in the rat, *J. Endocrinol.* **44:**39–54.

Kuhn, N.J., Carrick, D.T., and Wilde, C.J., 1980, Lactose synthesis: The possibilities of regulation, *J. Dairy Sci.* **63:**328–336.

Kumagai, H., and Nishida, E., 1980, The interactions between calcium-dependent regulatory protein (calmodulin) and microtubule proteins. Further studies on the mechanism of microtubule assembly inhibition by calmodulin, *Biomed. Res.* **1:**223–229.

Kumagai, H., Nishida, E., Kotane, S., and Sakai, H., 1986, On the mechanism of calmodulin-induced microtubule assembly in vitro, *J. Biochem.* **99:**521–525.

Kumar, N., Blumenthal, R., Henkart, M., Weinstein, J.N., and Klausner, R.D., 1982, Aggregation and calcium-induced fusion of phosphatidylcholine vesicle–tubulin complexes, *J. Biol. Chem.* **257:**15137–15144.

Langley, R.C., Jr., and Cohan, C.M., 1986, Association of spectrin with desmin intermediate filaments, *J. Cell. Biochem.* **30:**101–109.

Loizzi, R.F., 1978, Cyclic AMP inhibition of mammary gland lactose synthesis: Specificity and potentiation by 1-methyl-3-isobutyl xanthine, *Horm. Metab. Res.* **10:**415–419.

Loizzi, R.F., 1980, Immunofluorescent localization of tubulin in mammary gland from lactating and pregnant guinea pig, *J. Cell Biol.* **87:**245a.

Loizzi, R.F., 1983a, Cyclic AMP changes in guinea pig mammary gland and milk, *Am. J. Physiol. (Endocrinol. Metab. 8)* **245:**E549–E554.

Loizzi, R.F., 1983b, Ovariectomy-induced tubulin polymerization in pregnant rat mammary gland, *Proc. Soc. Exp. Biol. Med.* **173:**252–255.

Loizzi, R.F., 1984, Tubulin polymerization in rat mammary gland cells, *J. Cell Biol.* **99:**42a.

Loizzi, R.F., 1985, Progesterone withdrawal stimulates mammary gland tubulin polymerization in pregnant rats, *Endocrinology* **116:**2543–2547.

Loizzi, R.F., de Pont, J.J., and Bonting, S.L., 1975, Inhibition by cyclic AMP of lactose production in lactating guinea pig mammary gland slices, *Biochim. Biophys. Acta* **392:**20–25.

Loizzi, R.F., and Pencek, P.F., 1982, Ultrastructure of cell populations isolated from pregnant and lactating mammary gland, *J. Cell Biol.* **95:**55a.

Louis, S.L., and Baldwin, R.L., 1975, Changes in the cyclic 3′:5′-adenosine monophosphate system of rat mammary gland during the lactation cycle, *J. Dairy Sci.* **58:**861–869.

Luca, F., Bloom, G., and Vallee, R.B., 1986, A monoclonal antibody that cross-reacts with phosphorylated epitopes on two microtubule-associated proteins and two neurofilament polypeptides, *PNAS (USA)* **83:**1006–1010.

Maccione, R.B., Serrano, L., and Avila, J., 1985, Structural and functional domains of tubulin, *BioEssays* **2:**88–92.

Manfredi, J.J., Parness, J., and Horwitz, S.B., 1982, Taxol binds to cellular microtubules, *J. Cell Biol.* **94:**688.

Marcum, J.M., Dedman, J.R., Brinkley, B.R., and Means, A.R., 1978, Control of microtubule assembly–disassembly by calcium-dependent regulator protein, *Proc. Natl. Acad. Sci. USA* **75:**3771–3775.

Margolis, R.L., and Wilson, L., 1978, Opposite end assembly and disassembly of microtubules at steady state *in vitro, Cell* **13:**1–80.

Margolis, R.L., Rauch, C.T., and Job, D., 1986, Purification and assay of a 145-kDa protein (STOP-145) with microtubule-stabilizing and motility behavior, *Proc. Natl. Acad. Sci. USA* **83:**639–643.

Means, A.R., and Dedman, J.R., 1980, Calmodulin in endocrine cells and its multiple roles in hormone action, *Mol. Cell. Endocrinol.* **19:**215–227.

Means, A., Tash, J.S., and Chafouleas, J.G., 1982a, Physiological implications of the presence, distribution, and regulation of calmodulin in eukaryotic cells, *Physiol. Rev.* **62:**1–39.

Means, A.R., Tash, J.S., Chafouleas, J.G., Lagace, L., and Guerriero, V., 1982b, Regulation of the cytoskeleton by Ca^{2+} calmodulin and cAMP. Part II. Endocytosis and cytoskeleton, *Ann. N.Y. Acad. Sci.* **383:**69–84.

Minami, Y., and Sakai, H., 1985, Dephosphorylation suppresses the activity of neurofilament to promote tubulin polymerization, *FEBS Lett* **185**(2):239–242.

Minami, Y., and Sakai, H., 1986, Effects of microtubule-associated proteins on network formation by neurofilament-induced polymerization of tubulin, *FEBS Lett* **195:**68–72.

Montague, W., Howell, S.L., and Green, I.C., 1976, Insulin release and the microtubular system of the islets of Langerhans: Effects of insulin secretagogues on microtubule subunit pool size, *Horm. Metab. Res.* **8:**166–169.

Neville, M.C., Selker, F., Semple, K., and Watters, C., 1981, ATP-dependent calcium transport by a Golgi-enriched fraction from mouse mammary gland, *J. Membrane Biol.* **61:**97–105.

Nicholas, K.R., and Hartman, P.E., 1981a, Progesterone control of the initiation of lactose synthesis in the rat, *Aust. J. Biol. Sci.* **34:**435–443.

Nicholas, K.R., and Hartman, P.E., 1981b, Progressive changes in plasma progesterone, prolactin and corticosteroid levels during late pregnancy and the initiation of lactose synthesis in the rat, *Aust. J. Biol. Sci.* **34:**445–454.

Nickerson, S.C., and Keenan, T.W., 1979, Distribution and orientation of microtubules in milk secreting epithelial cells of rat mammary gland, *Cell Tissue Res.* **202:**303–312.

Nickerson, S.C., Smith, J.J., and Keenan, T.W., 1980a, Ultrastructural and biochemical response of rat mammary epithelial cells to vinblastine sulfate, *Eur. J. Cell Biol.* **23:**115–121.

Nickerson, S.C., Smith, J.J., and Keenan, T.W., 1980b, Role of microtubules in milk secretion—Action of colchicine on microtubules and exocytosis of secretory vesicles in rat mammary epithelial cells, *Cell Tissue Res.* **207:**361–376.

Nickerson, S.C., Akers, R.M., and Weinland, B.T., 1982, Cytoplasmic organization and quantitation of microtubules in bovine mammary epithelial cells during lactation and involution, *Cell Tissue Res.* **223:**421–430.

Ollivier-Bousquet, M., 1979, Effects de la cytochalasine B et de la colchicine sur l'action rapide de la prolactine dans la glande mammaire de lapine en lactation, *Eur. J. Cell Biol.* **19:**168.

Ollivier-Bousquet, M., and Denamur, M.R.D., 1973, Inhibition par la colchicine de la secretion des proteines du lait, *C.R. Acad. Sci. Paris* **276:**2183–2186.

Ollivier-Bousquet, M., and Denamur, R., 1975, Effect de l'etat physiologique et du 3′5′ adenosine monophosphate cyclique sur le transit intracellulars et l'excretion des proteines du lait. Etude autoradiographique en microscopie electronique, *J. Microsc. Biol. Cell.* **23:**63–82.

Pallas, P., and Solomon, F., 1982, Cytoplasmic microtubule-associated proteins: Phosphorylation at novel sites is correlated with their incorporation into assembled microtubules, *Cell* **30:**407–414.

Park, C.S., Smith, J.J., Eigel, W.N., and Keenan, T.W., 1979, Selected hormonal effects on protein secretion and amino acid uptake by acini from bovine mammary gland, *Int. J. Biochem.* **10:**889–894.

Patton, S., 1974, Reversible suppression of lactation by colchicine, *FEBS Lett.* **48:**85–87.

Patton, S., Stemberger, B.H., and Knudson, C.M., 1977, The suppression of milk fat globulin secretion by colchicine: An effect coupled to inhibition of exocytosis, *Biochim. Biophys. Acta* **499:**404–410.

Pencek, P.F., and Loizzi, R.F., 1981, Morphological characterization and tubulin status of several populations of alveolar cells isolated from lactating guinea pig mammary gland, *J. Cell Biol.* **91:**325a.

Perry, J.W., and Oka, T., 1980, Cyclic AMP as a negative regulator of hormonally induced lactogenesis in mouse mammary gland organ culture, *Proc. Natl. Acad. Sci. USA* **77:**2093–2097.

Peters, R., 1956, Hormones and the cytoskeleton, *Nature* **177:**426.

Pickett-Heaps, J.D., 1975, Aspects of spindle evolution, *Ann. N.Y. Acad. Sci.* **253:**352–361.

Pipeleers, D.G., Pipeleers-Marichal, M.A., and Kipnis, D.M., 1975, Microtubule assembly and the intracellular transport of secretory granules in pancreatic islets, *Science* **191:**88–90.

Pipeleers, D.G., Pipeleers-Marichal, M.A., Sherline, P., and Kipnis, D.M., 1977a, A sensitive method for measuring polymerized and depolymerized forms of tubulin in tissues, *J. Cell Biol.* **74:**341–350.

Pipeleers, D.G., Pipeleers-Marichal, M.A.P., and Kipnis, D.M., 1977b, Physiological regulation of total tubulin and polymerized tubulin in tissues, *J. Cell Biol.* **74:**351–357.

Pizarro, M., Puente, J., and Sapag-Hagar, M., 1981, Calmodulin and cyclic nucleotide-phosphodiesterase activities in rat mammary gland during the lactogenic cycle, *FEBS Lett.* **136:**127–130.

Poste, G., and Nicolson, G.L. (eds.), 1981, *Cytoskeletal Elements and Plasma Membrane Organization,* North-Holland Publishing, New York.

Prasad, K.N., and Hsie, A.W., 1971, Morphological differentiation of mouse neuroblastoma cells induced *in vitro* by dibutyryl adenosine 3′:5′-cyclic monophosphate, *Nature New Biol.* **233:**141–142.

Puck, T.T., Waldren, C.A., and Hsie, A.W., 1972, Membrane dynamics in the action of dibutyryl adenosine 3′:5′-cyclic monophosphate and testosterone on mammalian cells, *Proc. Natl. Acad. Sci. USA* **69:**1943–1947.

Rappaport, L., Leterrier, J.F., Virion, A., and Nunez, J., 1976, Phosphorylation of microtubule-associated proteins, *Eur. J. Biochem.* **62:**539–549.

Rappaport, E., Berkley, P.D., and Bucher, N.L.R., 1975, Charcoal adsorption assay for measurement of colchicine binding and tubulin content of crude tissue extracts, *Anal. Biochem.* **69:**92–99.

Rasenick, M.M., Stein, P.J., and Bitensky, M.W., 1981, The regulatory subunit of adenylate cyclase interacts with cytoskeletal components, *Nature* **294:**560–562.

Rillema, J.A., 1976a, Cyclic nucleotides, adenylate cyclase, and cyclic AMP phosphodiesterase in mammary glands from pregnant and lactating mice, *Proc. Soc. Exp. Biol. Med.* **151:**748–751.

Rillema, J.A., 1976b, Possible interaction of cyclic nucleotides with the prolactin stimulation of casein synthesis in mouse mammary gland explants, *Biochim. Biophys. Acta* **432:**348–352.

Riss, T.L., and Baumrucker, C.R., 1982, Calmodulin purification and quantitation from bovine mammary tissue, *J. Dairy Sci.* **65:**1722.

Sandborn, E., Koen, P.F., McNabb, J.D., and Moore, G., 1964, Cytoplasmic microtubules in mammalian cells, *J. Ultrastructure Res.* **11:**123–138.

Sapag-Hagar, M., and Greenbaum, A.L., 1973, Changes in the activities of adenylcyclase and cAMP phosphodiesterase and of the level of 3′:5′-cyclic adenosine monophosphate in rat mammary gland during pregnancy and lactation, *Biochem. Biophys. Res. Commun.* **53:**982–987.

Sapag-Hagar, M., and Greenbaum, A.L., 1974, The role of cyclic nucleotides in the development and function of rat mammary tissue, *FEBS Lett.* **46:**180–183.

Sapag-Hagar, M., Greenbaum, A.L., Lewis, D.J., and Hallowes, R.C., 1974, The effects of dibutyryl cAMP on enzymatic and metabolic changes in explants of rat mammary tissue, *Biochem. Biophys. Res. Commun.* **59:**261–268.

Schliwa, M., Euteneuer, U., Bulinski, J.C., and Izant, J.G., 1981, Calcium lability of cytoplasmic microtubules and its modulation by microtubule-associated proteins, *Proc. Natl. Acad. Sci. USA* **78:**1037–1041.

Schroer, T.A., and Kelly, R.B., 1985, In vitro translocation of organelles along microtubules, *Cell* **40:**729–730.

Schubart, U.K., Erlichman, J., and Fleischer, N., 1982, Insulin release and protein phosphorylation: Possible role of calmodulin, *Fed. Proc.* **41:**2278–2282.

Schulze, E., and Kirschner, M., 1986, Microtubule dynamics in interphase cells, *J. Cell Biol.* **102:**1020–1031.

Sharp, D.C., and Parry, J.M., 1985, Diethylstilboesterol: The binding and effects of diethylstilboesterol upon the polymerisation and depolymerisation of purified microtubule protein in vitro, *Carcinogenesis* **6:**865–885.

Sherline, P., Bodwin, C.K., and Kipnis, D.M., 1974, A new colchicine binding assay to tubulin, *Anal. Biochem.* **62:**400–407.

Sherline, P., and Mundy, G.R., 1977, Role of the tubulin-microtubule system in lymphocyte activation, *J. Cell Biol.* **74:**371–376.

Simpson, A.A., Simpson, M.H.W., and Kulkarni, P.N., 1973, Effect of perphenazine during late pregnancy on prolactin production and lactogenesis in the rat, *J. Endocrinol.* **57:**431–436.

Sloboda, R.D., Dentler, W.L., Bloodgood, R.A., Telzer, B.R., Granett, S., and Rosenbaum, J.L., 1976, Microtubule-associate proteins (MAPs) and the assembly of microtubules *in vitro*, *Cell Motility* **3:**1171–1212.

Smith, J.J., Park, C.S., and Keenan, T.W., 1982a, Calcium and calcium ionophore A23187 alter protein synthesis and secretion by acini from rat mammary gland, *Int. J. Biochem.* **14:**573–576.

Smith, J.J., Nickerson, S.C., and Keenan, T.W., 1982b, Metabolic energy and cytoskeletal requirements for synthesis and secretion by acini from rat mammary gland. I. Ultrastructural and biochemical aspects of synthesis and release of milk proteins, *Int. J. Biochem.* **14:**87–98.

Smith, J.J., Nickerson, S.C., and Keenan, T.W., 1982c, Metabolic energy and cytoskeletal requirements for synthesis and secretion by acini from rat mammary gland. II. Intracellular transport and secretion of protein and lactose, *Int. J. Biochem.* **14:**99–109.

Sobue, K., Tanaka, T., Ashino, N., and Kakiuchi, S., 1985, Calcium and calmodulin regulate microtubule-associated protein–actin filament interaction in a flip-flop switch, *Biochim. Biophys. Acta* **845:**366–372.

Soifer, D.D. (ed.), 1975, The biology of cytoplasmic microtubules, *Ann. N.Y. Acad. Sci.* **253:**1.

Soifer, D., Mack, K., and Chambers, D.A., 1982, Photoaffinity labelling of a microtubule-associated cyclic AMP-binding protein, *Arch. Biochem. Biophys.* **219:**388–393.

Soifer, D. (ed.), 1986, *Dynamic Aspects of Microtubule Biology,* Vol. 466, New York Academy of Science, New York.

Sokka, T.K., and Patton, S., 1983, In vivo effects of colchicine on milk fat globule membrane, *Biochim. Biophys. Acta* **731:**1–8.

Sordillo, L.M., Oliver, S.P., and Nickerson, S.C., 1984, Carprine mammary differentation and initiation of lactation following prepartum colchicine infusion, *Int. J. Biochem.* **16:**1265–1272.

Spiegel, A.M., and Downs. R.W., 1981, Guanine nucleotides: Key regulators of hormone receptor–adenylate cyclase interaction, *Endocr. Rev.* **2:**275–305.

Tash, J.S., Means, A.R., Brinkley, B.R., Dedman, J.R., and Cox, S.M., 1980, Cyclic nucleotide and Ca^{2+}-regulation of microtubule initiation and elongation, in: *Microtubules and Microtubule Inhibitors 1980* (M. DeBrabander and J. DeMay, eds.), Elsevier/North-Holland, Amsterdam, pp. 281–296.

Tash, J.S., Lagace, L., Lynch, D.R., Cox, S.M., Brinkley, B.R., and Means, A.R., 1981, Role of cAMP-dependent protein phosphorylation in microtubule assembly and function, in: *Protein Phosphorylation* (O.M. Rosen and E.G. Krebs, eds.), Cold Spring Harbor Laboratory, Cold Spring Harbor, NY, pp. 1171–1181.

Tokunaka, S., Friedman, T.M., Toyama, Y., Pacifici, M., and Holtzer, H., 1983, Taxol induces microtubule-rough endoplasmic reticulum complexes and microtubule-bundles in cultured chondroblasts, *Differentiation* **24:**39–47.

Tsuyama, S., Bramblett, G.T., Huang, K.P., and Flavin, M., 1986, Calcium/phospholipid-dependent kinase recognizes sites in microtubule-associated Protein 2 which are phosphorylated in living brain and are not accessible to other kinases, *J. Biol. Chem.* **261**(9)**:**4110–4116.

Turner-Pencek, P.F., and Loizzi, R.F., 1982, A morphometric study of isolated cell populations from pregnant and lactating guinea pig mammary gland, *J. Cell Biol.* **95:**39a.

Vale, R.D., Schnapp, B.J., Reese, T.S., and Sheetz, M.P., 1985a, Organelle, bead and microtubule translocations promoted by soluble factors from the squid giant axon, *Cell* **40:**559–569.

Vale, R.D., Schnapp, B.J., Mitchison, T., Steuer, E., Reese, T.S., and Sheetz, M.P., 1985b,

Different axoplasmic proteins generate movement in opposite directions along microtubules in vitro, *Cell* **43:**623–632.

Vallano, M.L., Goldring, J.R., Buckholz, T.M., Larson, R.E., and DeLorenzo, R.J., 1985, Separation of endogenous calmodulin and cAMP-dependent kinases from microtubule preparations, *Proc. Natl. Acad. Sci. USA* **82:**3202–3206.

Vermouth, N.T., and Deis, R.P., 1974, Prolactin release and lactogenesis after ovariectomy in pregnant rats: Effect of ovarian hormones, *J. Endocrinol.* **63:**13–20.

Virk, S.S., Kirk, C.J., and Shears, S.B., 1985, Ca^{+2} transport and Ca^{+2}-independent ATP hydrolysis by Golgi vesicles from lacating rat mammary glands, *Biochem. J.* **226:**741–748.

Wadsworth, P., and Salmon, E.D., 1986, Analysis of the treadmilling model during metaphase of mitosis using fluorescence redistribution after photo bleaching, *J. Cell Biol.* **102:**1032–1038.

Wang, E., Fischman, D., Liem, R.K.H., and Sun, T.-T. (eds.), *Intermediate Filaments*, Vol. 455, New York Academy of Science, New York.

Warburton, M.J., Ferns, S.A., Hughes, C.M., and Rudland, P.S., 1985, Characterization of rat mammary cell types in primary culture: Lectins and antisera to basement membrane and intermediate filament proteins as indicators of cellular heterogeneity, *J. Cell Sci.* **79:**287–304.

Watanabe, K., and West, W., 1982, Calmodulin, activated cyclic nucleotide phosphodiesterase, microtubules, and vinca alkaloids, *Fed. Proc.* **41:**2292.

Weber, K., Bibring, Th., and Osborn, M., 1975, Specific visualization of tubulin-containing structures in tissue culture cells by immunofluorescence. Cytoplasmic microtubules, vinblastine-induced paracrystals, and mitotic figures, *Exp. Cell Res.* **95:**111–120.

Weingarten, M.D., Lockwood, A.H., Hwo, S.-Y., and Kirscher, M.W., 1975, A protein factor essential for microtubule assembly, *Proc. Natl. Acad. Sci. USA* **72:**1858–1862.

Weisenberg, R., 1975, The role of nucleotides in microtubule assembly, *Ann. N.Y. Acad. Sci.* **253:**573–576.

Weissman, G., Goldstein, I., Hoffstein, S., and Tsung, P.K., 1975, Reciprocal effects of cAMP and cGMP on microtubule-dependent release of lysosomal enzymes, *Ann. N.Y. Acad. Sci.* **253:**750–762.

Welsch, M.J., Dedman, R., and Brinkley, B.R., 1978, Calcium-dependent regulator protein: Localization in mitotic apparatus of eukaryotic cells, *Proc. Natl. Acad. Sci. USA* **75:**1867–1871.

Welsch, M.J., Dedman, J.R., Brinkley, B.R., and Means, A.R., 1979, Tubulin and calmodulin. Effects of microtubule and microfilament inhibitors on localization in the mitotic apparatus, *J. Cell Biol.* **81:**624–684.

West, D.W., 1981, Energy-dependent calcium sequestration activity in a Golgi apparatus fraction derived from lactating rat mammary glands, *Biochim. Biophys. Acta* **673:**374–386.

Wiche, G., 1985, High-molecular-weight microtubule associated proteins (MAPs): A ubiquitous family of cytoskeletal connecting links, *Trends Biochem. Sci.* **10**(2):67–70.

Wilde, C.J., and Kuhn, N.J., 1981, Lactose synthesis and the utilization of glucose by rat mammary acini, *Eur. J. Biochem.* **13:**311–316.

Zor, U., 1983, Role of cytoskeletal organization in the regulation of adenylate cyclase–cyclic adenosine monophosphate by hormones, *Endocr. Rev.* **4:**1–21.

Zisapel, N., Levi, M., and Gozes, I., 1980, Tubulin: An integral protein of mammalian synaptic vesicle membranes, *J. Neurochem.* **34:**26–32.

Zurier, R.B., Hoffstein, S., and Weissman, G., 1973, Mechanisms of lysosomal enzyme release from human leukocytes. I. Effect of cyclic nucleotide and colchicine, *J. Cell Biol.* **58:**27–41.

6

Keratin Expression in the Mammary Gland

Joyce Taylor-Papadimitriou and E. Birgitte Lane

1. Intermediate Filaments and (Cyto)keratins

The term *cytoskeleton* was first used by Joseph Needham to describe the then undefined cellular network thought to be involved in coordinating the enzyme activities of cells and in relaying messages from the cell membrane to the nucleus (Peters, 1956). Since then, three filament systems have been identified that could provide the basic components for such a cytoskeleton. These are the microtubules (25-nm diameter), the actin filaments (4–6 nm), and the intermediate filaments (10 nm). The first two systems are highly conserved, ubiquitous, and by now quite well-defined in both structure and function. They may indeed be considered to fulfill some of the functions Needham anticipated. The third system is by contrast highly tissue specific in its biochemistry, and while suggestions of enzymic or membrane-associated functions are at this stage still controversial, intermediate filaments do at least in some tissues appear to perform a structural role and in that sense may be seen as the closest of the three systems to a (literal) cell cytoskeleton. Yet the significance of the heterogeneity of intermediate filament proteins remains an unsolved puzzle.

Originally, five classes of intermediate filaments were described immunologically and biochemically (see Lazarides, 1980), which were expressed in five different categories of tissue. Recently, this classification

Joyce Taylor-Papadimitriou and E. Birgitte Lane • Imperial Cancer Research Fund, Lincoln's Inn Fields, London WC2A 3PX, United Kingdom.

has become revised to types I–IV intermediate filament proteins in the light of cDNA and protein sequence data that have become available (see Steinert and Parry, 1985, for a discussion of this). The essential elements of this classification are listed in Table I. Epithelial cells normally express equimolar amounts of type I and type II keratin proteins, but under certain circumstances (such as in tissue culture) they can be induced to express vimentin type III filaments as well.

The keratins appear to be the most fundamental intermediate filaments of the vertebrate body. They are the first to appear in embryogenesis, and keratin-containing epithelium is the primary tissue type from which all organs and tissues develop. The terms prekeratin and cytokeratin were coined to distinguish the intermediate filament proteins from the filament-plus-matrix complex product of terminally differentiated keratinocytes, but as the subject of intermediate filaments becomes more widely familiar, the prefixes are being dispensed with in current literature: see, for example, the recent symposium report cited under Lane et al. (1985).

The framework on which our current understanding of keratin expression is organized is substantially based on two pieces of work published in the last few years. First, Moll et al. (1982a) cataloged the major keratins of the human body tissues and identified them numerically as keratins 1–19 by their relative size (migration in SDS polyacrylamide gels) and charge (by isoelectric focusing). This numerical classification means it is no longer necessary to describe these proteins in terms of molecular weight estimates, which will be calculated differently by different laboratories. Thus, keratins 1–8 in the type II group are larger and neutral-to-basic in charge, while the type I keratins 9–19 are smaller and acidic. Type I and type II keratins will only form filaments in combination with each other, so that it is believed that any individual epithelial cell will contain at least one type I and one type II keratin, and some may contain as many as 10 different keratins.

Table I. Intermediate Filament Types

Gene family	Filament proteins	Tissue type
Type I	Keratins: Small, acidic	Epithelia
Type II	Keratins: Neutral to basic	Epithelia
Type III	Vimentin	Mesenchyme
	Desmin	Muscle
	Glial fibrillary acidic protein	Astroglia
Type IV	Neurofilaments	Neurones

Second, Sun and colleagues drew attention to the emerging pattern of coexpression of keratins in pairs, ranking the pairs from the small type I with small type II keratins to large type Is with large type IIs, and presented a predictive hypothesis linking the differentiated state of an epithelium with the expression of defined keratin pairs (Sun et al., 1984). As more information becomes available on tissue expression of keratins, the details of this hypothesis are constantly under revision, but the idea has provided the field with a very constructive conceptual framework, and several predictions are still upheld. For example, keratins 5 and 14 are found in all keratinocytes (Nelson et al., 1984); keratinocytes additionally express another pair of keratins as they differentiate, such as 1 and 10 in cornifying epidermis, 4 and 13 in noncornifying mucosal stratified epithelium (Van Muijen et al., 1986), and 6 and 16 in hyperproliferative situations (Sun et al., 1984) such as tissue culture and certain skin diseases (Weiss et al., 1984). Keratins 8 and 18 are characteristic of the simple, nonstratifying epithelium phenotype. The basic structural phenotypes of epithelia with respect to their characteristic keratin profiles in human are illustrated diagrammatically in Fig. 1.

Thus, the keratins provide unique and specific markers for studies on epithelial differentiation and for classification of cell types in com-

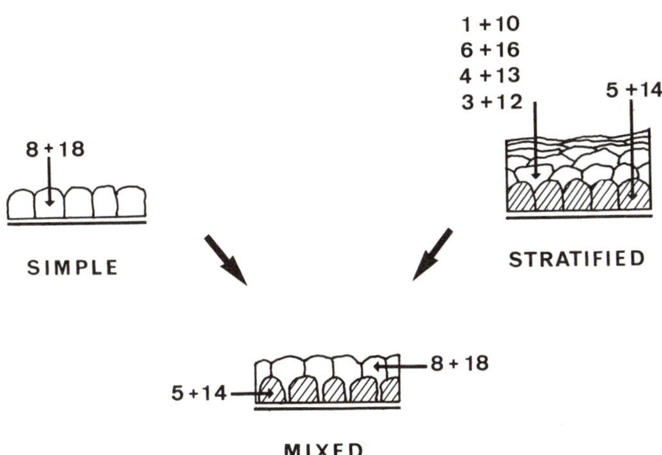

Figure 1. Structural types of epithelium, showing the characteristic major (human) keratins which they express. Many simple epithelia including the mammary gland also express keratins 7 and 19, but not all do. Keratin 19 is also found in fetal but not adult basal epidermal cells and is heterogeneously expressed in basal cells of nonkeratinizing stratified epithelia. The "mixed" epithelial type like the mammary gland may represent an evolutionary intermediate between simple and stratified epithelia (see Section 7).

plex tissues such as the mammary gland. In this chapter, we emphasize studies on keratin expression in the human mammary gland, primarily because the human keratins are the best characterized and because several antibodies with defined specificity exist that recognize these keratins. Some data relating to the rodent system are also discussed since certain developmental stages are more readily accessible.

2. *Methods for Detecting Keratins*

2.1. *Biochemical Methods*

The most direct and unequivocal way of determining whether a particular keratin is expressed in a tissue is to analyze the detergent-insoluble extract of the tissue by two-dimensional gel electrophoresis and relate the spots on the stained gel (defined by apparent molecular weight in SDS and by isolectric point) to the standard keratins that have been described by several laboratories and numerically cataloged, for the human species, by Moll et al. (1982a). A numerical system for rodent keratins and cow keratins has been put forward by Schiller et al. (1982), although it is likely that the final standard version of such nomenclature will ultimately be one that reflects the relation of each protein to the human system, based on protein sequence analysis. Analysis by one-dimensional SDS gel electrophoresis alone is insufficient characterization since many of the keratins have similar molecular weights. The use of the numerical catalog to refer to the keratins, once they have been identified, is extremely important for comparing results from different laboratories. The keratins expressed by a large number of human tissues have now been characterized in this way, and the results have been recently summarized by Quinlan et al. (1985).

2.2. *In Situ Identification of Keratins*

Where tissues are composed of several epithelial cell types that cannot easily be separated, the biochemical approach is limited to defining the sum total of keratins expressed by the tissue as a whole. Keratins that are only expressed by a small subset of cells may go undetected. To analyze keratin expression at the cellular level, in situ analysis is required, and antibodies reacting with defined single keratins provide the best tools for such analysis, since they allow a direct visual approach. Antibodies to a (defined) group of keratins may also be useful if used in conjunction with biochemical analysis and such pleurispecific monoclonal antibodies have been used effectively on a number of occasions (e.g., Nelson et al., 1984; Weiss et al., 1984; Nagle et al., 1986) to identify keratins in tissues. However, since we do not as yet have the technology to determine directly which of its several immunoblotting targets a pleurispecific antibody is seeing in native tissue sections, staining using such antibodies can only be interpreted with the help of parallel biochemical studies.

Monospecific antibodies to keratins are clearly the instruments of choice for in situ identification of keratins, and these are now gradually becoming available (Debus et al., 1982; Lane, 1982; Ramaekers et al., 1983a, 1985; Bartek et al., 1985a,b; Van Muijen et al., 1986). Monoclonal antibodies are undoubtedly more specific in their reaction profile than polyclonal antisera and a positive staining reaction given by a monoclonal antibody shown to react with a single keratin (by immunoblotting) can be taken as a definite indication that the keratin is indeed expressed in the positively staining cell. The converse, however, is not necessarily true, and a cell that does not stain with the same monoclonal antibody could still be expressing the keratin but for some reason the specific epitope could be masked. For example, conformationally determined epitopes may only be available when a certain combination of keratins are expressed and copolymerized. However, if several monoclonal antibodies and/or a polyclonal antiserum of similar biochemical specificity show the same lack of reaction, it is likely to be because the keratin is in fact not expressed. In practice, a differential staining pattern of two cell types pragmatically distinguishes them, and a subclassification is possible even if it may not be clear whether the differences are due to actual keratin expression or to conformational differences. Conformational differences could also reflect variations in physiology or biological function. Indeed, an analysis of the more subtle differences in keratin expression detectable by monoclonal antibodies may in the future help to define the changes that occur in epithelial cells as they progress from one functional phenotype to another.

The cloning of several genes coding for keratins has produced another set of tools for looking at keratin expression. The use of cDNA to detect mRNA in mixed tissues is subject to the same criticisms that apply to the biochemical approaches; namely, the method discriminates against rare species and gives no positional information. In situ hybridization would allow a more detailed analysis at the cellular level, but as yet such techniques do not appear to be as sensitive as the best antibody methods. The successful use of in situ hybridization to monitor protein expression depends on the absence of posttranscriptional regulation of the keratin genes. Moreover, of the keratins detected biochemically in human mammary epithelia, the sequences of only some have been published, that is, keratin 1 (Johnson et al., 1985), keratin 6 (Hanukoglu and Fuchs, 1983), keratin 14 (Hanukoglu and Fuchs, 1982), and keratin 17 (Raychaudury et al., 1986). At present, the methods used for monitoring keratin expression in the mammary gland are predominantly biochemical or immunological.

3. Structural Origin of the Mammary Gland

As with all eccrine or exterior-secreting glands, the mammary gland is derived from the epidermis during fetal life. In its final structural form, as well as in its patterns of development, it belongs to the same tissue type as sweat glands, salivary glands, and lachrymal glands. Not surprisingly, therefore, the mammary gland also exhibits a similar keratin phenotype to that of sweat glands and salivary glands.

As might be predicted from the study of adult tissues, changes in keratin expression during embryogenesis are correlated with changes in tissue differentiation. Keratins are present from the earliest stages of vertebrate embryogenesis and are even detectable in the oocyte (Lehtonen et al., 1983; Godsave et al., 1984). Oocyte levels, however, are very low. A surge of keratin synthesis was described for the early blastocyst stage (day 4 in mouse embryos: Jackson et al., 1981) and keratin synthesis has been detected even earlier at the 4–8 cell stage (Oshima et al., 1983), when cells first begin to be committed to trophectoderm differentiation as structured epithelium. These first keratins are the mouse keratins A (Endo A) and D (Endo B), equivalent to human keratins 8 and 18, respectively, that is, the keratins characteristic of simple epithelia. The third keratin to appear (day 6) is the equivalent of human keratin 19 just after implantation and at a time that is very close to the appearance of vimentin filaments in the primary mesenchyme cells (Jackson et al., 1980, 1981). The appearance of the mesenchyme cells marks the first event of nonepithelial tissue differentiation, and until this point all the cells in the developing embryo in both embryonic ectoderm and embryonic endoderm express simple epithelial keratins. All tissues of the adult body therefore are derived from cells that originally expressed keratins. It is not unreasonable to suppose that the same is true for the first stages of human development.

The embryonic ectoderm begins to give rise to presumptive keratinocytes when a second layer of cells forms at 4–5 weeks gestational age in the human (Holbrook, 1979), and the outer layer now becomes known as the periderm. The monolayer of periderm cells with its simple epithelial keratin phenotype persists long after the epidermis develops to its full thickness and expresses adult keratins (Holbrook, 1979; Dale et al., 1985). It is finally lost at about 24–26 weeks gestational age in human embryos, but mice are born with remnants still attached. Periderm expresses keratins 8 and 18 as detected histochemically (Moll et al., 1982b; Dale et al., 1985; Lane et al., 1985), and thus retains its status as simple epithelium in spite of the keratinocytes developing underneath; periderm also expresses keratin 19, as do the basal keratinocytes at this stage (Lane et al., 1985). The keratinocytes themselves are recognizable by their keratins as early as samples have been examined, and even when the human epidermis under the periderm is only two cells thick a distinct basal/suprabasal compartmentalization can be seen by histochemistry that parallels that of the adult (Moll et al., 1982b; Dale et al., 1985; Lane et al., 1985), and biochemical analysis confirms the presence of keratins 5 + 14 and 1 + 10.

Studies on the mouse have shown that soon after the epidermis begins to stratify, the development of the mammary gland commences. Mammary gland buds can be seen in 12-day-old mouse embryos as epidermal knobs, which begin to push downward and invade the mesenchyme at 15 days in mouse (Hogg et al., 1983) and around 6 weeks in human (Moore, 1982). In the human, the epidermis at this time consists of periderm plus one layer of keratinocyte precursors, so the suprabasal keratins are not yet expressed. The peg-like appendages become elongated and penetrate and branch into the connective tissue as solid chords of cells. Once most of the invasion of the mesenchyme has been accomplished, vertical slits develop within the chord of cells, probably because of reduced adhesion between the cells in the center, which eventually coalesce to form the gland lumen (Hogg et al., 1983). A degree of extension and branching takes place but by birth this has become arrested with only the major ducts formed, until puberty, pregnancy, and lactation induce further degrees of developmental maturation at appropriate times. Thus, the mammary gland arises from a developing epidermis that consists of two cell types, that is, the keratinocyte precursors expressing epidermal-type keratins (human 5 and 14) and keratin 19, and the periderm expressing simple epithelial keratins 8 and 18 as well as 19.

In the adult mammary gland, the epithelium in the larger ducts superficially appears to be a bilayered stratified epithelium, but on closer examination the luminal cells can be seen to extend thin processes down to the basal laminae; this is particularly noticeable in tissue sections stained for immunofluorescence with any keratin antibody that stains only the luminal cells (see Figure 2B). Both cell types are therefore in contact with the basal laminae. The basal or myoepithelial cell type is never exposed to the lumen of the gland and is always covered by luminal or secretory cells, while the luminal cells have a free surface. In the smaller ducts and lobules, which begin to appear at puberty, there are fewer basal cells and in sections the basal layer appears to be discontinuous. One of the questions that remains but that can be approached using immunological markers is whether the phenotype of each of the two fundamental cell types in the adult is the same throughout the mammary tree.

4. Keratins Present in Mammary Epithelial Cells

4.1. Keratins Detected Biochemically in the Human Mammary Gland

Ultrastructural studies on human material showed that both major epithelial cell types in the mammary gland contained intermediate filaments (Tannenbaum et al., 1979) before it was demonstrated that these filaments were composed of keratin (Franke et al., 1980). On the basis of biochemical analysis, Moll and colleagues have reported the presence of keratins 5, 7, 8, 14, 15, 17, 18, and 19 in the human mammary gland ducts (Moll et al., 1982a). Of these, keratins 7, 8, 18, and 19 are commonly found in simple epithelia (nonstratifying) with 8 and 18 probably "diagnostic" of simple epithelia. Keratins 5, 14, 17, and 19 are found in stratified squamous epithelia, with 5 and 14 regarded as diagnostic of the stratified squamous cell types such as the keratinocyte (Nelson et al., 1984; Gusterson et al., 1985). There is no biochemical evidence for the presence of the suprabasal keratinocyte differentiation keratins (i.e., 4 + 13, 6 + 16, and 1, 2 + 10) in mammary gland, but we have recently started to obtain evidence that low levels of keratin 10 at least may be present in luminal cells of the ducts (unpublished immunohistochemical results).

4.2. Differences between Basal (Myoepithelial) and Luminal Cells

It is clear from a number of immunohistochemical studies that basal and luminal cells express different keratin phenotypes, and the mammary gland was one of the first sites where differences in keratin expression between subpopulations of epithelial cells are demonstrated (Franke et al., 1980). The monoclonal antibodies that we and others have used to try to define keratin expression by different epithelial cells in the mammary gland are shown in Table II, together with their known specificities. Figure 2 demonstrates the appearance of basal and luminal cells when stained separately or together by different keratin monoclonal antibodies. The luminal cell type has keratin determinants in common with simple epithelia elsewhere in the body, which are recognized by several antibodies that are monospecific for keratins 18 or 8 (Debus et al., 1982; Lane and Klymkowsky, 1982; Ramaekers et al., 1983a; Taylor-Papadimitriou et al., 1983). These monospecific antibodies to keratins 8 and 18 do not stain basal cells. Monospecific antibodies to keratin 7 also appear to stain specifically luminal cells (Fig. 3; F.C.S. Ramaekers, unpublished data) but, like antibodies to keratin 19, they can also show very weak staining of some basal cells in the large ducts (our observations). As discussed in Section 2.2, lack of basal cell staining does not necessarily exclude the possibility that these keratins are expressed in the basal cells. However, in the case of keratin 18, several antibodies recognizing different epitopes on the same protein (see Lane, 1982, for LE61 and LE65 anti-18) have shown a similar staining pattern, suggesting that these keratins are indeed absent from the myoepithelial cells and not merely masked.

Luminal cells are also recognized by monoclonal antibodies specific for keratin 19 (Bartek et al., 1985a), although expression of this keratin can be variable in the smaller ducts and terminal ductal lobular units (Bartek et al., 1985a; see also Figure 4B). Until recently, it was thought that basal cells throughout the gland were not stained by antibodies specific for keratin 19. Recently, however, we have observed that some basal cells in large ducts seen in nipple sections can show a weak positive reaction with these antibodies (Fig. 4A). Some pleurispecific monoclonal antibodies such as KA-4 also stain luminal cells without staining basal cells (Nagle et al., 1985, 1986). The antibody KA-4 sees keratins 14, 15, 16, and 19 on immunoblots, which suggests that its target in the luminal mammary gland cells is probably keratin 19, but staining by this sort of antibody is interpretable only in conjunction with biochemical data.

Antibodies have been developed that stain myoepithelial and not secretory mammary cells, but these are less well characterized than the monospecific antibodies described above. Nagle et al. (1986) describe an antibody, KA-1, that sees myoepithelial and not luminal cells in the large ducts and terminal lobular units but reacts with both cell types in the terminal ducts. They believe the antibody sees a determinant on keratins 4, 5, and 6 when these type II keratins are complexed (as heteropolymers in filament formation) with appropriate type I keratins (Nagle et al., 1986). By deduction from the biochemical analysis of Moll et al. (1982a), they conclude that KA-1 sees only keratin 5 in the mammary gland. Dairkee et al. (1985) described another monoclonal antibody,

Table II. Monoclonal Antibodies to Keratins That Recognize Human Mammary Gland Epithelia

Monospecific antibodies[a]		Target		Staining of cells[b]						Origin of data[c]
				Luminal cells			Basal cells			
mAb	Reference to mAb	Keratin	Tissue	LD	SD	L	LD	SD	L	
LE61	Lane (1982)	18	All simple	+	+	+	–	–	–	A
LE65	Lane (1982)	18	epithelia	+	+	+	–	–	–	A
CK1	Debus et al. (1982)	18	↓	+	ND	ND	–	ND	ND	S
CK2	Debus et al. (1982)	18	↓	+	ND	ND	–	ND	ND	S
CK3	Debus et al. (1982)	18	↓	+	ND	ND	–	ND	ND	S
CK4	Debus et al. (1982)	18	↓	+	ND	ND	–	ND	ND	S
RGE53	Ramaekers et al. (1983a)	18	↓	+	ND	ND	–	ND	ND	S,A
LE41	Lane (1982)	8	All simple	+	+	+	–	–	–	A
TROMA-1	Brulet et al. (1980)	8	epithelia	+	+	+	–	–	–	A
K7	Osborn et al. (1985)	7	Some simple epithelia	+	ND	ND	(+)	ND	ND	A
RCK105	Ramaekers (unpublished data)	7	Some simple epithelia	+	ND	ND	(+)	ND	ND	S,A
LP2K	Lane et al. (1985)	19	Some simple	+	+/–	+/–	(+)	–	–	A
BA16	Bartek et al. (1985a)	19	and some	+	+/–	+/–	(+)	–	–	A
BA17	Bartek et al. (1985a)	19	stratified	+	+/–	+/–	(+)	–	–	A
A53-B/A2	Karsten et al. (1985)	19	epithelia	+	+/–	+/–	(+)	–	–	A
312C8-1	Dairkee et al. (1986)	14	Basal cells	(+)	ND	ND	+	ND	ND	S

Pleurispecific antibodies			Staining of cells						
			Luminal cells			Basal cells			Origin of
mAb	Reference to mAb	Keratin target	LD	SD	L	LD	SD	L	data
CAM5.2	Makin et al. (1984)	7,8,(19?)	+	+	+	(+)	–	–	A
LP34	Taylor-Papadimitriou et al. (1983)	4,5,6,10,(14),(13),18	+	+	+	+	+	+	A
AE1	Woodcock-Mitchell et al. (1982)	10,14,15,16,19	+	ND	ND	+	ND	ND	A
AE3	Sun et al. (1985)	1,2,3,4,5,6,7,8	+	ND	ND	+	ND	ND	A
Kg8.13	Gigi et al. (1982)	1,5,6,7,8,10,11,18	+	ND	ND	+	ND	ND	S
LP1K	Lane et al. (1985)	1,2,4,5,6,8	+	ND	ND	+	ND	ND	A
KA1	Nagle et al. (1985)	4,5,6 in heteropolymers	–	+/–	–	+	+	+	S
KA4	Nagle et al. (1985)	14,15,16,19	+	+	+	–	–	–	S

[a]Monospecific antibodies to keratin 10 (suprabasal in skin) are not included because all mammary gland epithelial are negative.
[b]LD, large ducts; SD, small ducts; L, lobules; ND, not done; +, clearly positive staining in all cells; (+), very weak staining in most cells; +/–, some cells clearly positive, others unstained; –, no staining observed significantly above background.
[c]Origins of data are either S = source reference to antibody or A = data obtained/confirmed in authors' laboratories. In the latter case, staining reactions were assayed by two-stage immunoperoxidase staining of unfixed frozen sections.

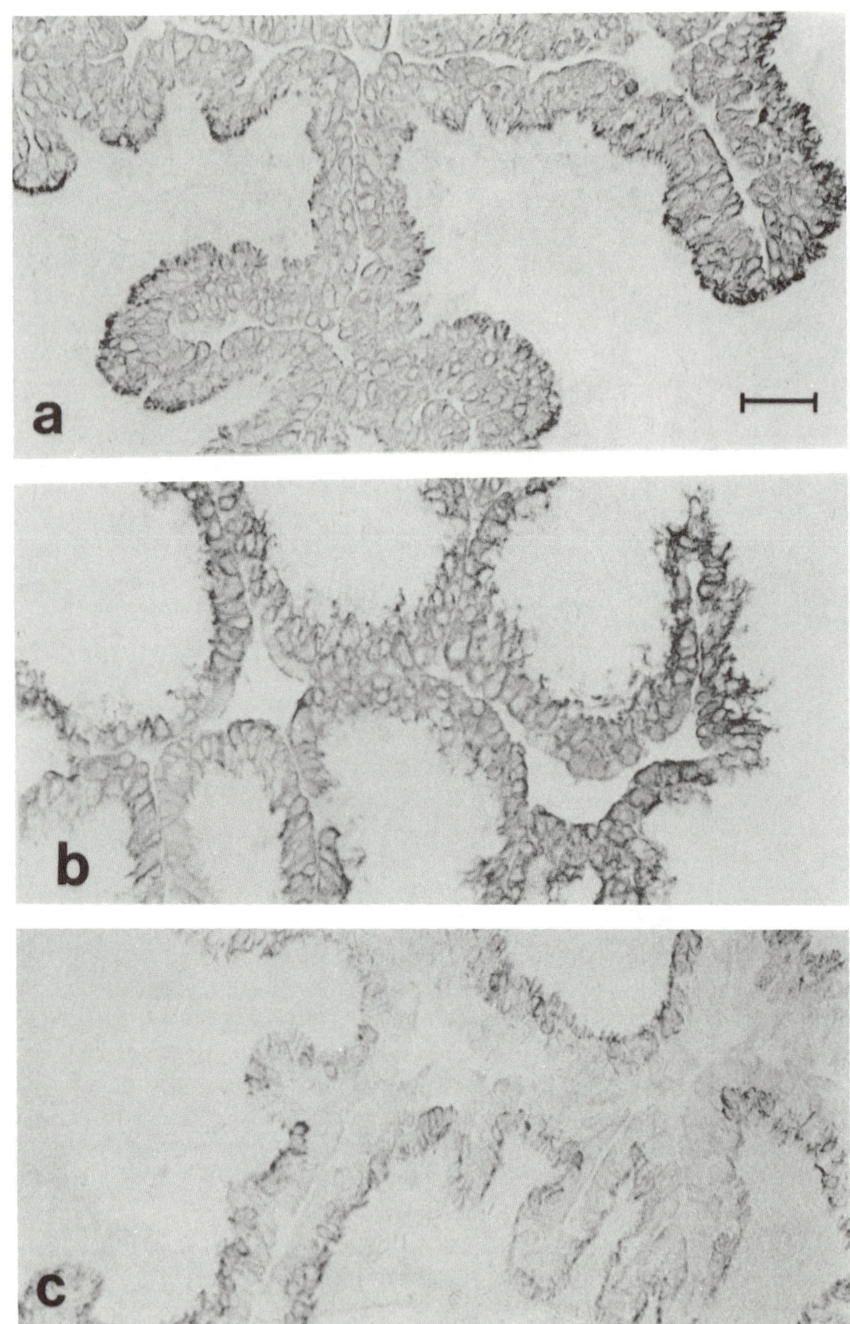
a
b
c

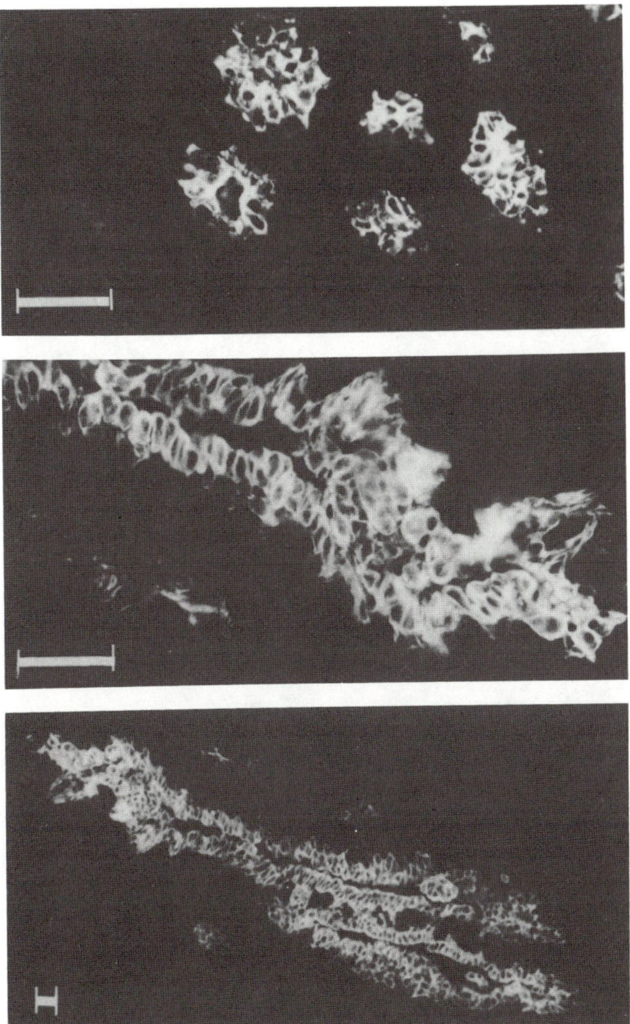

Figure 3. Sections of human mammary gland stained by indirect immunofluorescence with antibody RCK105, specific for human keratin 7. Bar = 25 μm. Courtesy of Dr. F.C.S. Ramaekers.

Figure 2. Selective staining of human mammary gland duct cells. Frozen sections were stained with culture supernatants containing monoclonal antibodies referred to in Table II and visualized by immunoperoxidase. (a) LP1K, staining both basal and luminal cell populations. (b) LE61 (to keratin 18) staining only luminal cells: note the thin foot processes by which the luminal cells keep in contact with the basal laminae. (c) LH8, staining basal cells: note the difference in morphology between the cells stained in (b) and (c). Bar = 25 μm.

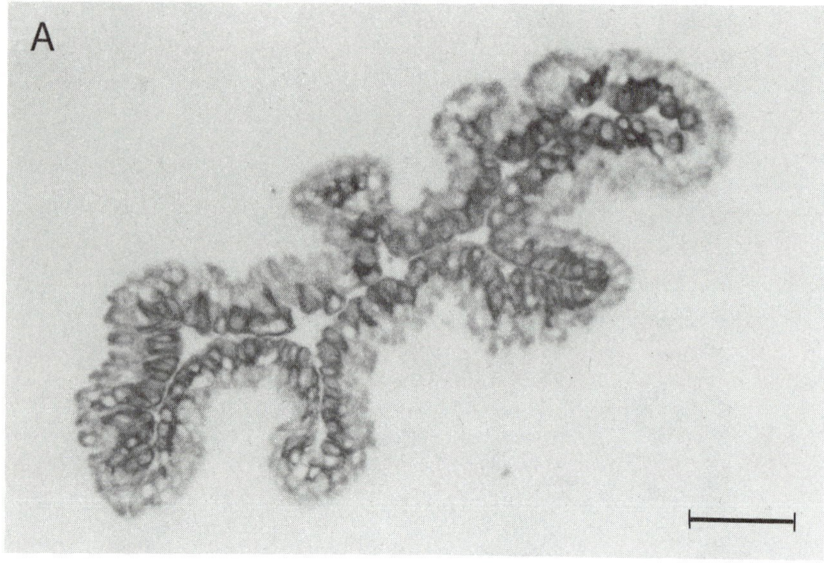

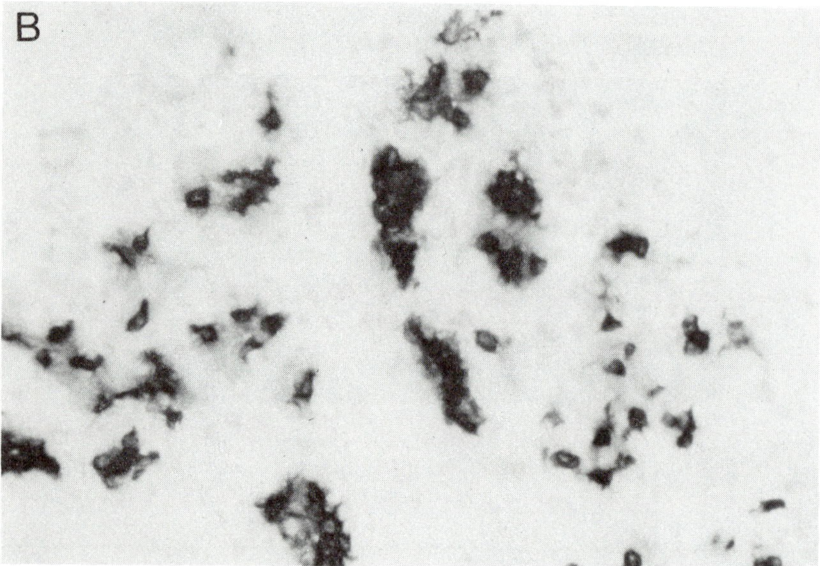

Figure 4. Immunoperoxidase staining of a section of normal human mammary gland by antibody LP2K (specific for keratin 19). (A) A large duct showing homogeneously strong staining of luminal cells and very weak staining of basal cells, and (B) a terminal lobular unit showing heterogeneity of staining (strongly positive or negative) of luminal cells. Bar = 25 μm.

312C8-1, reacting specifically with basal cells in the mammary gland which they attribute to a 51-kDa keratin isolated from a mammary carcinoma. This is presumably keratin 14, usually calculated as 50 kDa in molecular weight. However, some staining of luminal cells, particularly in large ducts, can also be observed (J. Bartek, personal communication).

In addition to the above antibodies, there is another group of antibodies that stain basal but not luminal cells in the mammary gland but which have not been characterized biochemically because they have not yet been persuaded to recognize denatured antigens in immunoblotting analyses. These include LH8, which was raised against a gel band containing keratin 14 (I.M. Leigh et al., unpublished data) and stains basal keratinocytes in skin, and PAb421 and PAb601, which were raised as antibodies to p53 nuclear protein and SV40 T antigen, respectively, but were found to bind to keratin filaments in basal epidermal keratinocytes (Leigh et al., 1985). In practice, such antibodies are very often not followed up because their reactivity is difficult to interpret, but it is probable that their specificity for basal cells in such a wide variety of locations is biologically significant. There are other monoclonal antibodies that are not against keratin filaments but that show this pattern of tissue reactivity, that is, specificity for basal cells whether in epidermis, mammary gland, or other tissues, such as the 4F2 (Patterson et al., 1984) and 23.10 (Gusterson et al., 1985) antibodies to cell surface glycoproteins. Nagle's KA-1 antikeratin monoclonal (Nagle et al., 1986) also stains epidermal basal cells, as does Dairkee's 312C8-1 antibody (J. Bartek, personal communication). These similarities between the basal epidermal keratinocytes and the basal cells lining the ducts and terminal ductal lobular units of the mammary gland could be related to the epidermal origin of the latter.

4.3. Subpopulations of Human Luminal Cells Detected by Keratin Differences

Direct experiments with human tissue for defining cell phenotypes at different stages of embryonic development or postnatally through puberty are difficult if not impossible to perform, so that it is hard to see how the absolute identification of stem cells and cell lineages can be achieved. However, some finer definition of cell phenotypes can be made using immunological markers, which identify subsets of the two major epithelial cell types seen in the adult gland, and there does appear to be a subpopulation of luminal cells in the small ducts which may express a dual keratin phenotype, superimposing the basal and luminal pattern. Clearly, one can postulate that such a cell type could give rise to both myoepithelial and secretory cells and thus may represent a stem cell.

Subsets of luminal epithelial cells have been identified using a series of antibodies reacting specifically with keratin 19 (Bartek et al., 1985a, 1986b). The antibodies BA16 and BA17, first reported by Bartek et al. as reacting specifically with keratin 19, were found to stain all luminal cells in the big ducts and most of the luminal cells in the terminal ductal lobular units and smaller ducts. However, a subset of unstained luminal cells was identified and these unstained cells were found predominantly in the smaller ducts and in the lobules of the terminal ductal lobular units themselves. The same cells expressed keratin 18 and in that respect are similar to other luminal cells. The spatial distribution in the gland of the luminal cells unreactive with BA16 and BA17 (unstained, possibly keratin 19−ve cells) was that predicted for a cell type with the proliferative potential to give rise to the new growth seen at pregnancy. The authors have suggested that, in view of the fact that this cell type also has a high growth potential in vitro and appears to be transformed readily by SV40 virus (Chang et al., 1982; Caron de Fromental et al., 1985; Chang, 1985, 1986; Bartek et al., 1986a; and Section 6.2.1), it may represent a cell phenotype in the secretory lineage (18+19−) with more proliferative potential than the more differentiated 18+19+ cell.

Another example of a subset of small duct luminal epithelial cells showing traces of a basal cell-like phenotype is that distinguished by staining with the antibody KA-1 (Nagle et al., 1986). Although this antibody is pleurispecific (see Table 2), keratin 5 is the only keratin of its identified targets which has been detected biochemically in the mammary gland. It was therefore assumed that KA-1 positive cells in the mammary gland contain keratin 5. KA-1 generally stains myoepithelial cells in the large ducts and in the lobules, but in the small ducts some luminal cells are stained as well. In other situations, such as epidermis, keratin 5 (56 kDa) has been described as characteristic of basal cells (Fuchs and Green, 1980).

It would be of interest to stain serial sections with the KA-1 antibody and the antibodies BA16 and BA17 to keratin 19 to see whether the expression of the KA-1 specific epitope in the mammary gland is seen only in cells that are negative for the BA16/BA17 epitopes, another feature of basal cells in this tissue. It is also important now to look closely at this small duct region with all the other keratin antibodies to see if any others show heterogeneous staining, since much of the staining and the biochemical analysis has only been done on large ducts. Preliminary studies on a few samples of normal breast show that the other two antibodies monospecific for keratin 19, that is, LP2K (Lane et al., 1985) and A53-B/A2 (Karsten et al., 1985), show a similar pattern of reaction to BA16 and BA17 (Bartek et al., 1986b; Bartek and Lane, unpublished data and Fig. 4B).

While it is clearly important to develop other monoclonal antibodies that react specifically with single keratins, the limited data available indicate that there appear to be cell types present in the luminal layer of the small or terminal ducts that in their profile of cytokeratin expression show some features in common with both the luminal and basal cells in the other part of the gland.

It might be expected that the phenotype of the cells of both epithelial lineages would differentiate as the duct function changes from mainly structural in the large ducts to predominantly contractile or secretory in the terminal units. Certainly, some of the basal cells in the large ducts can show a weak reaction with antibodies to keratin 19 and

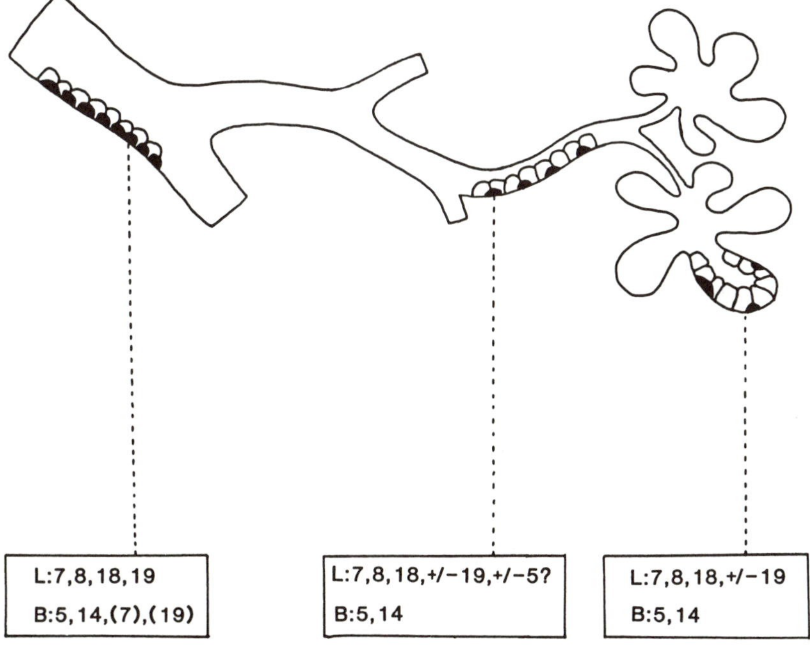

Figure 5. Keratin expression in basal and luminal cells in the human mammary gland predicted from immunohistochemical staining. Biochemical analysis of extracts of large ducts also indicates the presence of keratins 15 and 17, but no specific antibodies are available with which to localize these keratins. The +/− indicates that the keratin appears to be expressed in some but not all cells of this class, in this particular location in the gland. Parentheses indicate that very low levels of the keratin are detected. L = luminal cells, B = basal cells.

keratin 7, which react only with luminal cells in other parts of the gland (Fig. 4A). A summary of keratins expressed by basal and luminal cells in different parts of the gland as predicted from immunohistochemical staining is shown diagrammatically in Fig. 5.

An examination of the cells in the lactating gland might be expected to show up any differences in keratin expression that occur in the fully functioning basal or luminal cell. We have found that the human secretory cells stain clearly with antibodies to keratins 18 and 19; those against keratins 7 and 8 have to our knowledge not been tested. As yet, differences in the myoepithelial cells in the lactating mammary gland have not been identified using monoclonal antibodies.

4.4. Studies on Rodent Mammary Epithelia

Studies by Asch and Asch (1985a) have identified at least five keratins in mouse mammary gland. These were characterized according to the murine keratin catalog defined by Schiller et al. (1982), as keratins 8, 11, 14, 20, and 22, which are probably homologs of human keratins 5 and 8, possibly 14, 18, and 19 respectively. These investigators did not find any gross differences in keratin expression during normal development by biochemical analysis.

While the two basic cell types in the rodent mammary gland are the same as in the human gland, their evolution and differentiated keratin phenotype may or may not be the same since there are distinct differences in the physiology and structure of the gland between the two species. The question of how similar the cell lineages are in the human and the rat or mouse is a crucial one, since it is important to know which studies on carcinogenesis in the rodent are indeed relevant to the study of human breast cancer. As in the human, there does again appear to be an epithelial subpopulation with dual phenotype expression, although in rodents there is some evidence that this is basal and not luminal (Allen et al., 1984; Dulbecco et al., 1986).

The basal or myoepithelial cells in the adult rodent gland can be stained preferentially by a number of immunological reagents primarily recognizing stratified squamous epithelial cells (keratinocytes). This has been shown in rodent mammary gland sections with two antisera raised against bovine epidermal keratins (Franke et al., 1980; Asch et al., 1981), and with a monoclonal antibody, LP34 (Table III; Taylor-Papadimitriou et al., 1983), which in the rodent recognizes stratified squamous epithelia but not simple epithelia. These observations again suggest that the keratin profile of the myoepithelial cell may share common features with cells in the epidermis. All these antibody preparations, however, also

Table III. Antibodies to Cytokeratins Used to Identify Epithelial Cell Types in the Adult Rodent Mammary Gland

Antibody	Antigen	Specificity	Reference
Guinea pig polyclonal	Human skin keratins	Preferentially stains myoepithelial cells in mouse	Asch et al. (1981)
mAb LP34	Human psoriatic skin	Stains only myoepithelial cells in rat and mouse mammary gland	Taylor-Papadimitriou et al. (1983)
mAb 1A10	Bovine muzzle keratin	Stains only myoepithelial cells in rat mammary gland (55 kDa)	Allen et al. (1984)
mAb 24B42	Bovine muzzle keratin	Stains luminal cells at various stages of development in rat mammary gland (50, 68 kDa)	Allen et al. (1984)
mAb LE61	PtK1 cell detergent-insoluble extract	Stains luminal cells in mouse and rat mammary gland (reacts with human keratin 18)	Lane (1982)

stain the luminal cells in the human mammary gland. In the case of LP34, this appears to be because it recognizes human keratin 18 of simple epithelia but it does not react with the rodent equivalent. (LP34, however, recognizes several of the keratins expressed by human keratinocytes including keratins 5, 10, and 13, and its staining of rodent and human epidermis looks the same.) Antibodies LE61 and LE65 reacting with human keratin 18, which selectively stain luminal cells in the human, show a similar pattern of reactivity in the rat and mouse (Lane, 1982; Lane and Klymkowsky, 1982). This extends to the distinct staining we have observed with LE61 of rat luminal alveolar cells (E.B. Lane and J. Taylor-Papadimitriou, unpublished data) which contradicts a report by Dulbecco et al. (1983) describing these cells as negative.

Two antibodies raised by Allen and colleagues (1984) against bovine muzzle keratins are also useful in distinguishing between basal and luminal epithelial cells in the rat and have been used to examine the relation between these two cell types and cells in the end buds and in the embryo. The keratin specificity of these antibodies was given as bovine VI (antibody 1A10) and bovine Ib and VII (antibody 24B42), which would be homologous to human keratin 10 and keratins 2 and 14, respectively. Unfortunately, the keratin specificity on rodent tissues was not determined biochemically, and the identity of their tissue targets in the rodent mammary gland cannot be deduced from the bovine specificity given since bovine VI, or human 10, are not expressed basally in the homologous species. In the study by Allen and co-workers, it was found that in the 17-day embryo, when the mammary gland is developing from the epidermis, all the cells in the newly developing ducts were positive for both the basal (1A10) and luminal (24B42) epithelial keratin markers, although at this stage of development the basal cells of the epidermis express only the keratin recognized by the basal marker 1A10. The appearance of the luminal-specific keratins therefore marks the differentiation of the epidermal epithelium to mammary epithelium.

In the experiments of Allen et al. (1984) the cells near the basement membrane in the ducts of the newborn rat began to show positive staining with a polyclonal antiserum to myosin while staining positively with both keratin monoclonal antibodies; in addition, the cells close to the lumen showed reduced staining for the keratins recognized by 1A10. At puberty (3 weeks) in the end buds and young ducts some basal cells could still be detected which stained with both the luminal- and basal-specific antibodies. Thus, although these cells are basal and not luminal, the rodent gland appears to possess a subpopulation of dual phenotype cells, like the human small ducts, which are candidates for the stem cells with the potential to give rise to both cell lineages in the adult. Similar cells are reported to be present even in pregnant and lactating glands. These authors also suggest that somewhat more differentiated myoepithelial cells can give rise to luminal cells. The analogy with the production of differentiated cells from the basal layer of epidermis and other stratified epithelia is an obvious one and the idea is attractive. However, as yet there is little definite detailed information related to where the two lineages diverge and at what stage the differentiation along one of these lineages becomes irreversible.

5. Keratin Expression in Mammary Tumors

5.1. Human Tumors

One of the most widely used applications of the analysis of keratin expression is in tumor diagnosis. The presence of cytokeratins defines a tumor as a carcinoma and the presence of specific cytokeratins can also help in the subclassification of carcinomas. It is also possible to ask questions about the phenotype of the cell from which a tumor originated, since the profile of cytokeratin expression appears to be largely qualitatively unaltered in those malignancies where the cell of origin is known (Moll et al., 1983; Ramaekers et al., 1983b). In the mammary gland, one can ask specifically whether the phenotype of the malignant cell resembles that of the luminal or basal cell, and most of the data indicate that no features of the basal cell are seen in cells from primary or secondary breast cancers. Thus, the malignant cells in the two common human breast cancers, infiltrating lobular and infiltrating ductal carcinomas, stain positively with antibodies reactive with keratins 18 and 19 (Taylor-Papadimitriou et al., 1983; Bartek et al., 1985b) but do not react with the myoepithelial-specific antibodies LH8 (J. Burchell, A. Lewis, and I.M. Leigh, unpublished data) or KA-1 (Nagle et al., 1986). Another monoclonal antibody to keratin which is reported to stain specifically myoepithelial cells in tissue sections (M12C8-1) stained strongly and homogeneously only 3 out of 60 carcinoma specimens (Dairkee et al., 1985). Moll and colleagues (1983) have reported the presence in some anaplastic breast carcinomas of most of the keratins found in the normal mammary gland ducts, and even others not normally associated with mammary gland such as keratin 6, 11, and 16, although most of the tumors examined expressed only 7, 8, 18, and 19. Biochemical analysis of tissue does not necessarily reflect the keratin expression of the individual cancer cells and contributions could conceivably come from adjacent or enveloped normal tissue. It is also important to establish that these tumors are indeed primary and of breast origin, possibly by using other markers. That the phenotype of the malignant cells is in fact like that of the luminal cell is also suggested by the fact that the cancer cells express other markers normally found on luminal mammary epithelial cells (but not basal cells) such as milk fat globule membrane components (Taylor-Papadimitriou et al., 1983); the cancer cells, however, do not express milk proteins such as casein (Burchell et al., 1985; Burchell, 1986). Using antimyosin and antikeratin antibodies as markers for myoepithelial cells, Gusterson and colleagues (1982) have also concluded that very few myoepithelial cells are present in most infiltrating breast cancers, although myofibroblasts may be found in the stromal component. One interesting outcome of characterization of tumor cells with cytokeratin antibodies has been the demonstration of a profile of simple epithelial keratin expression in the malignant cells of Paget's disease, which corresponds to the luminal phenotype of the mammary gland (Moll et al., 1985; Nagle et al., 1985; Chaudary et al., 1986) and thus supports a mammary origin of this neoplasm rather than an epidermal one.

There are several features related to keratin expression which distinguish benign from malignant breast tumors. Within the benign tumors, such as fibroadenomas and sclerosing adenosis, myoepithelial cells are present and the myoepithelial cells can be stained with the basal cell marker antibody LH8 (J. Burchell and J. Taylor-Papadimitriou, unpublished data). In addition, the luminal cells of benign tumors show heterogeneity of staining with antibodies monospecific for keratin 19 (Bartek et al., 1985b, 1986a) in contrast to the homogeneously positive staining pattern seen with malignant tumors. Since it is the same cells seen in benign tumors that do not stain with any of the four different keratin 19-specific antibodies listed in Table II, it is likely that these cells are not expressing the keratin. The benign tumors probably arise from the polyclonal growth of many cells going through a few division cycles each, which would give a heterogeneous tumor cell population reflecting the heterogeneity of the cell population of origin. Furthermore, as the keratin 19−ve cells appear to represent a higher proportion of the luminal cells in benign tumors than is seen in the normal breast, the 19−ve cells may have a higher proliferative potential than that of the 19+ve cells. Since a malignant tumor is thought to develop clonally from one altered cell over many generations, it becomes difficult to identify the normal phenotype of the original cell if its progeny have some differentiation potential. Some early in situ lesions do contain keratin 19−ve cells and the possibility remains that this cell type may have been the target cell, which retains the ability to differentiate to a keratin 19+ve cell. However, an unambiguous interpretation of the static situation seen using tissue sections is not feasible without the framework of the detailed expression of keratins both in the normal developing breast and in the developing tumor.

5.2. Rodent Tumors

Asch and Asch (1985b) have examined keratin expression in normal, hyperplastic, and neoplastic mouse mammary gland; two-dimensional gel analysis of the keratin profiles suggested that some keratins are present in the abnormal tissue that are not found in the normal gland. However, it is conceivable that the keratins expressed in some hyperplastic alveolar nodules and tumors are found in small subsets of mammary epithelial cells in the normal gland, and this would only be shown by in situ immunohistochemistry using monospecific antibodies. In the rat, recent studies have suggested that the myoepithelial lineage is represented only in nonmetastasizing mammary tumors and is not evident in metastasizing tumors (Dunnington et al., 1984).

6. Keratin Expression in Cultured Mammary Epithelial Cells

6.1. Normal Cells

6.1.1. Human Mammary Epithelium

The need for an experimental culture system is particularly obvious in the case of the human mammary gland since experimentation in vivo is difficult if not impossible. Moreover, to characterize the phenotype of the cultured cells, it is crucial to have markers that are retained when the tissue integrity of the gland is disrupted and the cells are placed in medium containing growth factors. Although intermediate filament expression can be modified by long-term culture, the cytokeratin profile can be a comparatively stable feature of epithelial cells and may be largely maintained at least in short-term culture.

The major sources of normal mammary epithelial cells are human milk (Buehring, 1972; Taylor-Papadimitriou et al., 1977) and reduction mammoplasty tissue (Hallowes et al., 1980). These cells can be grown in monolayer culture on plastic (Stampfer et al., 1980) or embedded in collagen gels (Foster et al., 1983; Taylor-Papadimitriou et al., 1984; Durban et al., 1985) using a modification of the technique developed by Emerman and Pitelka (1977) for studying differentiation in mouse mammary epithelium. As might be expected, all the cells that are shed into milk appear to be the luminal epithelial cell type since they express keratins 8 and 18 (react positively with antibodies LE61, LE65, and LE41) (Chang and Taylor-Papadimitriou, 1983) and about 85% of colonies also express keratin 19 (react with antibodies BA16 and 17; Bartek et al., 1985a). Interestingly, the apparently keratin 19−ve colonies are large, supporting the idea that the 18+19− cells have a high proliferative potential.

The medium in which epithelial cells from milk are grown contains a cyclic AMP elevating agent that can be cholera toxin or an analog of cAMP (Taylor-Papadimitriou et al., 1980); such factors have been reported to induce an abortive squamous differentiation in normally secretory epithelial cells (Schaefer et al., 1980, 1983). In the studies of Schaefer and co-workers, the differentiation was characterized on morphological grounds but can now be defined using antibodies to keratins only expressed by suprabasal cells. The RKSE-60 antibody (Ramaekers et al., 1985) recognizes keratin 10 and positively stains some cells in senescing cultures of milk cells, but not in the earlier proliferating cultures (E. Durban and E.B. Lane, unpublished data). The milk epithelial cells do not grow well in monolayer culture on plastic in the absence of a cAMP elevating agent, but they do form proliferating structures in collagen gels. In these structures, even in the absence of cholera toxin, quite large areas of RKSE-60 +ve cells can be seen (Taylor-Papadimitriou et al., 1984); the cells expressing keratin 10 do not appear to express the simple epithelium keratins 18 and 19. These observations emphasize how important it is to characterize cell phenotype with markers directed to cellular components rather than to rely on morphology. They also show that commitment to secretory differentiation may not be totally inflexible, since cells in culture may be subverted to a different pathway.

The mammary organoids that are formed after collagenase digestion of reduction mammoplasty material and that form the starting material for tissue culture contain both basal and luminal cells. We have examined the keratin pattern in early cultures grown on plastic or in collagen gels in simple serum-containing media (Taylor-Papadimitriou et al., 1986). On plastic, two layers spread out from the organoid, and the upper layer shows a keratin profile (18+19+) characteristic of luminal epithelial cells as well as expressing the milk fat globule mucin—also expressed by this cell type. The lower layer, which one would expect to arise from the basal cells, is epithelial since the cells stain positively with LP34, but they are not stained with antibodies to keratins 18 and 19. However, the basal-specific antibody LH8 does not stain these cells either. Similarly, in collagen gels the basal cells quickly lose their positive reactivity with LH8, even though they maintain their normal tissue topography, and do not reexpress the specific antigen even when a new basement membrane is synthesized after 2–3 weeks in culture (Durban et al., 1985; Taylor-Papadimitriou et al., 1986). We therefore do not have a specific marker for the human basal cells in culture, beyond characterizing them as LP34+ and LE61−.

When cells from reduction mammoplasty tissue are cultured in more complex medium that may contain serum and medium conditioned by other cells (Stampfer et al., 1980) or pituitary extract (Hammond et al., 1984), the cells can be passaged for longer periods of time. In the medium developed by Stampfer, the cells senesce after approximately four passages (Stampfer and Bartley, 1985). In the serum-free medium developed by Hammond and colleagues, the cells can be subcultured for many more generations, but there is a selection for a small cuboidal cell type in the early passages (S.L. Hammond and R.G. Ham, personal communication). As yet, the keratin profiles of the cultured cells in the later passages have not been defined in detail. It is clearly important to examine the profile of keratin expression in these cells to see whether they could be stem cells with the ability to differentiate in a variety of ways.

6.1.2. Rodent Mammary Epithelium

A great deal of work has been done with mouse mammary epithelial cells from pregnant and lactating mice cultured in collagen gels, since in this system a partially differentiated phenotype can be induced (Emerman and Pitelka, 1977). Specific keratins are certainly present in cells cultured in this way (Hall and Bissell, 1986), some of which are recognized by antibodies AE1 and AE3 raised against human keratins (Woodcock-Mitchell et al., 1982). Selective staining of myo and secretory epithelial cells has not been reported in the collagen gel culture system. There is some evidence, however, that keratin determinants restricted in vivo to the myoepithelial cell lineage are retained in vitro in the rodent system. Thus, Asch and colleagues found that some cells were present in cultures from mouse mammary gland, which stained with the guinea pig antiserum found to react preferentially with myoepithelial cells in vivo (Asch et al., 1981). Furthermore, although Asch and Asch (1985a) found by two-dimensional gel analysis a relative increase in mouse keratin 11 (equivalent to human keratin 8, i.e., characteristic of luminal cells) in cells in primary culture, other keratins were detected that are usually associated with keratinocytes. Similarly, Warburton and colleagues (1985) have identified a cell type in cultures of virgin rat mammary gland which shows positive staining with the monoclonal antibody LP34 (staining only myoepithelial cells in the rat). These positively staining cells coexpressed vimentin (the intermediate filament protein of mesenchymal cells), which can be induced by tissue culture in many cell types. Cells showing markers characteristic of the secretory lineage, however, expressed only keratins, not vimentin.

The phenotype of the myoepithelial cell or basal cell may only be expressed fully when attached to a basement membrane and under an upper layer of luminal cells; when the tissue is disrupted, these membrane and cellular contacts are disrupted and it seems likely that changes in the intermediate filaments occur. As we have seen from Section 5, cells in the myoepithelial cell lineage do not seem to be represented in metastasizing tumors of either human or rat. However, a study of this lineage may be important because of the supportive role the basal cells appear to play in the growth and differentiation of cells in the secretory lineage.

6.2. Cultured Transformed Cells

6.2.1. Experimentally Transformed Cells

Although there is a considerable literature dealing with transformed mammary epithelial cell lines derived from the rat mammary gland, detailed characterization of the intermediate filaments in such cells has not been done. Cell lines have been obtained from the human mammary gland, by SV40 transformation of milk epithelial cells (Chang and Taylor-Papadimitriou, 1983; Chang, 1985,1986) and by chemical transformation of cells cultured from reduction mammoplasty material (Stampfer and Bartley, 1985). Both these sets of cell lines express keratins, but in the case of the milk derived fR cells, keratin 19 appears not to be expressed or only at very low levels (Chang, 1985; Bartek et al., 1986b). Since keratin 18 is expressed in the fR lines (LE61 +ve), the cells have a phenotype resembling the minor population of milk cell colonies referred to in Section 6.1.1, that is, the 15% of colonies that are large and 18+19− and that of the luminal cells in the smaller ducts that do not stain with antibodies directed to keratin 19. This cell type may be particularly sensitive to transformation by SV40, since the HBL100 cell line (Polonowski et al., 1976) shows a similar pattern of keratin expression to the fR lines (Bartek et al., 1986b). HBL100 was derived from normal milk cells but carries SV40 genetic information (Caron de Fromentel et al., 1985) and is thought to have arisen by transformation in vivo, probably via an SV40-carrying polio virus vaccine. However, it should be remembered that the profile of expression of keratins can be altered by SV40 transformation as is shown by the expression of keratin 18 (LE61 +ve) in SV40-transformed human keratinocytes (Taylor-Papadimitriou et al., 1982) and identification of the target cell by definition of the keratin profile of the transformant may not always be possible.

6.2.2. *Cells Cultured from Human Breast Tumors*

It has proved to be extremely difficult to culture identifiably malignant cells from primary human breast cancers, although cells from some benign tumors do proliferate in relatively simple medium (Stoker et al., 1976; Hallowes et al., 1977). Where cultures of epithelial cells from breast cancers have been obtained (Smith et al., 1986), the detailed profile of keratin expression has not been examined. There are, however, a number of cell lines that have been derived from metastatic cells found in serous effusions taken from breast cancer patients. All cell lines of this type that have been examined express keratins 8, 18, and 19 (E.B. Lane, unpublished data; Taylor-Papadimitriou et al., 1983; Quinlan et al., 1985; Bartek et al., 1986a) but some such as Cama 1, MDA 157, and T47D may express additional keratins. The two cell lines that were derived from Lasfargues from primary breast cancers—BT20 and BT474 (Lasfargues and Ozzello, 1958)—have also been shown to express keratin 19 (Bartek et al., 1985a). Biochemical analysis of BT20 extracts also showed that this cell line also expresses keratins 8 and 18 (E.B. Lane, unpublished data). In agreement with the analysis of breast cancer tissue and sections (see Sections 4 and 5), the data from cultured breast cancer cell lines indicate that the pattern of keratin expression in human breast cancer cells resembles that of the dominant luminal epithelial cell as seen in the normal gland.

7. Discussion

The wide spectrum of keratins identified in mammary gland ducts by two-dimensional gel electrophoresis (Moll et al., 1983) can readily be understood in the light of immunohistochemical data from tissue sections. The expression of keratins as deduced from histochemical and biochemical data together is summarized for the different cell types in the human mammary gland in Fig. 5. Antibodies that are monospecific for each of the keratins 8 and 18 all stain only the luminal cell type, indicating that these cells are "simple" epithelium in their keratin phenotype. The other two keratins often found in simple epithelium, that is, 7 and 19, are also found by immunohistochemical analysis predominantly in the luminal cells. Human myoepithelial cells, on the other hand, have a characteristic basal cell phenotype, which is shared by basal cells in epidermis and epidermal appendages.

Antibodies specific for basal keratinocytes in the epidermis stain basal cells in the mammary gland and in other eccrine epidermally derived glands probably because cells in these locations express keratins 5 and 14 in common. This may be interpreted as suggesting a common developmental pathway for all such basal cells, since at the time when these glands first start to develop in the embryo the basal epidermal cells already express their characteristic keratin phenotype. Data from the rodent system suggest that, in the early stages of development of the mammary gland, all cells in the ducts show a dual phenotype expressing keratins characteristic of the epidermal basal cell and of the adult luminal cell. The development of the mammary basal and luminal cells then occurs with the specific loss of one or other of the luminal-specific or basal-specific keratin determinants. This indicates that the myoepithelial lineage as well as the secretory lineage emerges, not directly from the epidermal cell, but via a mammary precursor stem cell, which according to Dulbecco and colleagues (1986) is also represented in the adult gland in the basal layer.

From the above discussion, it is clear that the mammary gland epithelium is neither a truly simple epithelium nor a stratified epithelium, but a "mixed" epithelium, containing both simple epithelial cells and cells that according to current dogma (Sun et al., 1984) belong to a keratinocyte-related lineage or phenotype. Interestingly, both cell types form contacts with the basement membrane, although these are more extensive for the basal cells. The similarity in keratin phenotype between the basal cells of the mammary gland and the basal cells of classical stratified squamous epithelia suggests that this phenotype is determined not by the ability of a cell to stratify, or even to leave the basal lamina, but by the ability of a cell to grow under another cell without a free surface. The actual "basal" (submerged) cell then is seen as a pivotal phenotype in epithelial evolution and the mixed epithelia of the mammary (and other) glands can then be viewed as intermediate in epithelial differentiation between simple epithelia and stratified squamous epithelia (see Fig. 1). This also requires another modification of Sun's hypothesis of keratin expression by differentiation-predicted pairs, in that keratins 5 and 14 should not be regarded as markers of keratinocytes or stratified squamous epithelial cells only, but rather as markers of the basal cell phenotype, that is, a cell type that grows in contact with the basal laminae but without a free surface.

Why a secretory gland should be composed of two epithelial cell types, or why a basal cell and a luminal cell should have such different keratin profiles, are questions for which we have no definitive answers but on which one can speculate a little. The accumulating structural and biochemical data on the different keratin polypeptides do suggest that the smaller keratins are (1) more soluble and (2) less likely to form such rigid structures in their compound filaments than the larger karatins. In that case, simple epithelial keratins such as 8 and 18 may be more appropriate for a secretory cell where a certain amount of cytoplasmic plasticity is required, while the stronger filament networks formed with keratins 5 and 14 are appropriate in basal cells to reinforce the structure of these thin epithelial ducts, which are not surrounded by muscle layers.

The proliferative relation between the two main cell types in the adult mammary gland is not yet clear. Candidate stem cells with a dual phenotype have been identified in the basal layer in the rodent and in the luminal layer in the human, but direct kinetic studies following the progeny of these cells have not been performed. In the human, the luminal phenotype can be shown at least to have proliferative potential, since this is the dominant phenotype found in primary cultures of mammary epithelium obtained from human milk (Bartek et al., 1985a) and in primary and metastatic breast cancers. In cultures of reduction mammoplasty tissue, proliferating cells are present which do not express simple epithelial keratins but they do not stain either with antibodies reactive with keratins found in myoepithelial cells in vivo. Thus, the basal phenotype as seen in the normal gland has not been identified positively in cultures of normal human mammary epithelium or in breast cancers, suggesting that the basal cell either has little proliferative potential or shows phenotypic alterations when removed from the basement membrane. The fact that mammary epithelial cells in culture and in cancers do not appear to express the keratin profile of the basal or myoepithelial cell at least indicates that the luminal cell phenotype is capable of extensive cell division. This, together with the fragmentary information on the possible location of a pleuripotent or stem cell population in the human mammary gland (probably in the small ducts), suggests that such cells are represented by a subfraction of the luminal cells.

It is perhaps important to point out that no conclusive evidence of truly anomalous keratin expression has yet been described. The evidence from biochemical and immunohistochemical findings on mammary epithelial cells, whether in situ in the gland, in tumors, or in tissue culture, all tends to support the constancy and predictability of expression of keratin proteins by epithelial cells. As in other systems, when the pattern of keratin expression in a cell line or in a tumor appears at first sight to be different from that of its tissue of origin, closer inspection has either revealed a subset of epithelial cells within the tissue that does show the pattern of expression in question, or else it transpires that the tumor or cell line probably originated elsewhere. A number of monospecific monoclonal antibodies are still needed, as markers for the remaining keratins that are still only recognizable by biochemical analysis, so that fine cellular anatomical detail of each tissue can be defined fully.

So far, the use of monoclonal antibodies to intermediate filaments has mostly confirmed conventional histological descriptions of normal tissues. What is now appearing, as an increasingly large range of antibodies with finer specificities are being used, is a further dimension in resolution for histology, in a description of local heterogeneity at the single-cell level. This application of monoclonal antibodies to modern histology is very important, since it is these subtle differences from cell to cell within the tissue that are critical to tissue differentiation and homeostasis. We will not understand in vivo tumorigenesis until we understand how two adjacent cells can follow two separate pathways toward differentiation and function, and why one cell is then more susceptible than the other to carcinogenic subversion.

ACKNOWLEDGMENTS: The authors would like to thank Dr. Jiri Bartek for useful discussions and some of the photographs, Dr. F. Ramaekers for providing the photographs for Fig. 3, and Liz Eaton for preparation and typing of the manuscript.

References

Allen, R., Dulbecco, R., Syka, P., Bowman, M., and Armstrong, B., 1984, Developmental regulation of cytokeratins in cells of the rat mammary gland studied with monoclonal antibodies, *Proc. Natl. Acad. Sci. USA* **81:**1203–1207.

Asch, B.B., Burstein, N.A., Vidrich, A., and Sun, T.-T., 1981, Identification of mouse mammary epithelial cells by immunofluorescence with rabbit and guinea pig anti-keratin antisera, *Proc. Natl. Acad. Sci. USA* **78:**5643–5647.

Asch, H.L., and Asch, B.B., 1985a, Expression of keratins and other cytoskeletal proteins in mouse mammary epithelium during the normal developmental cycle and primary culture, *Dev. Biol.* **107:**470–482.

Asch, H.L., and Asch, B.B., 1985b, Heterogeneity of keratin expression in mouse mammary hyperplastic alveolar nodules and adenocarcinomas, *Cancer Res.* **45:**2760–2768.

Bartek, J., Durban, E.M., Hallowes, R.C., and Taylor-Papadimitriou, J., 1985a, a subclass of luminal epithelial cells in the human mammary gland, defined by antibodies to cytokeratins, *J. Cell Sci.* **75:**17–33.

Bartek, J., Taylor-Papadimitriou, J., Miller, N., and Millis, R., 1985b, Patterns of expression of keratin 19 as detected with monoclonal antibodies in human breast tissues and tumours, *Int. J. Cancer* **36:**299–306.

Bartek, J., Bartkova, J., Schneider, J., Taylor-Papadimitriou, J., Kovarik, J., and Rejthar, A., 1986a, Expression of monoclonal antibody-defined epitopes of keratin 19 in human tumours and cultured cells, *Eur. J. Cancer Clin. Oncol.* **32:**1441–1452.

Bartek, J., Bartkova, J., Taylor-Papadimitriou, J., Rejthar, A., Kovarik, J., Lukas, Z., and Vojtesek, B., 1986b, Differential expression of keratin 19 in normal human epithelial tissues revealed by monospecific monoclonal antibodies, *Histochem. J.* **18:**565–575.

Brulet, P., Babinet, C., Kemler, R., and Jacob, F., 1980, Monoclonal antibodies against trophectoderm specific markers during mouse blastocyst formation, *Proc. Natl. Acad. Sci. USA* **77:**4113–4117.

Buehring, G.C., 1972, Culture of human mammary epithelial cells: Keeping abreast of a new method, *J. Natl. Cancer Inst.* **49:**1433–1434.

Burchell, J., 1986, Use of monoclonal antibodies in the study of differentiation and malignancy of the human mammary gland, PhD Thesis, CNAA.

Burchell, J., Bartek, J., and Taylor-Papadimitriou, J., 1985, Production and characterization of monoclonal antibodies to human casein. A monoclonal antibody that cross-reacts with casein and alpha-lactalbumin, *Hybridoma* **4:**341–350.

Caron de Fromentel, C., Nardeux, P.C., Soussi, T., Lavialle, C., Estrade, S., Carloni, G., Chandrasekaran, K., and Cassingena, R., 1985, Epithelial HBL-100 cell line derived from milk of an apparently healthy woman harbours SV40 genetic information, *Exp. Cell Res.* **160:**83–94.

Chang, S.E., 1985, In vitro transformation of human breast epithelial cells, in: *Breast Cancer: Origins, Detection and Treatment* (M.A. Rich, J.C. Hager, and J. Taylor-Papadimitriou, eds.), Martinus Nijhoff Publishing, Boston, pp. 205–226.

Chang, S.E., 1986, In vitro transformation of human epithelial cells, *Biochim. Biophys. Acta* **823:**161–194.

Chang, S.E., Keen, J., Lane, E.B., and Taylor-Papadimitriou, J., 1982, Establishment and characterization of SV40-transformed human breast epithelial cell lines, *Cancer Res.* **42:**2040–2053.

Chang, S.E., and Taylor-Papadimitriou, J., 1983, Modulation of phenotype in cultures of human milk epithelial cells and its relation to the expression of a membrane antigen, *Cell Differ.* **12:**143–154.

Chaudary, M.A., Millis, R.R., Lane, E.B., and Miller, N.A., 1986, Paget's disease of the nipple: A ten year review including clinical, pathological and immunohistochemical findings, *Breast Cancer Res. Treatment* **8:**139–147.

Dale, B.A., Holbrook, K.A., Kimball, J.R., Hoff, M., and Sun, T.-T., 1985, Expression of epidermal keratins and filaggrin during human fetal skin development, *J. Cell Biol.* **101:**1257–1269.

Dairkee, S.H., Blayney, C., Smith, H.S., and A.J. Hackett, 1985, Monoclonal antibody that defines human myoepithelium, *Proc. Natl. Acad. Sci. USA* **82:**7409–7413.

Debus, E., Weber, K., and Osborn, M., 1982, Monoclonal cytokeratin antibodies that distinguish simple from stratified squamous epithelial: Characterization of human tissues, *EMBO J.* **1:**1641–1647.

Dulbecco, R., Allen, W.R., Bologna, M., and M. Bowman, 1986, Marker evolution during the development of the rat mammary gland: Stem cells identified by markers and the role of myoepithelial cells, *Cancer Res.* **46:**2449–2456.

Dunnington, D.J., Kim, U., Hughes, C.M., Monaghan, P., Ormerod, E.J., and Rudland, P.S., 1984, Loss of myoepithelial cell characteristics in metastasizing rat mammary tumours relative to their nonmetastasizing counterparts, *J. Natl. Cancer Inst.* **72:**455–466.

Durban, E.M., Butel, J.S., Bartek, J., and Taylor-Papadimitriou, J., 1985, The importance of matrix interactions and tissue topography for the growth and differentiation of mammary epithelial cells in vitro, in: *Breast Cancer: Origins, Detection and Treatment* (M.A. Rich, J.C. Hager, and J. Taylor-Papadimitriou, eds.), Martinus Nijhoff Publishing, Boston, pp. 13–30.

Emerman, J.T., and Pitelka, D.R., 1977, Maintenance and induction of morphological differentiation in dissociated mammary epithelium on floating collagen membranes, *In Vitro* **13:**316–328.

Foster, C.S., Smith, C.A., Dinsdale, E.A., Monaghan, O., and Neville, A.M., 1983, Human mammary gland morphogenesis *in vitro*—the growth and differentiation of normal breast epithelium in collagen gel cultures defined by electron microscopy, monoclonal antibodies and autoradiographs, *Dev. Biol.* **96:**197–216.

Franke, W.W., Schmid, E., Freudenstein, C., Appelhans, B., Osborn, M., Weber, K., and Keenan, T.W., 1980, Intermediate-sized filaments of the prekeratin type in myoepithelial cells, *J. Cell Biol.* **84:**633–654.

Fuchs, E., and H. Green, 1980, Changes in keratin gene expression during terminal differentiation of the keratinocyte, *Cell* **19:**1033–1042.

Gigi, O., Geiger, B., Eshhar, Z., Moll, R., Schmid, E., Winter, S., Schiller, D.L., and Franke, W.W., 1982, Detection of a cytokeratin determinant common to diverse epithelial cells by a broadly cross-reacting monoclonal antibody, *EMBO J.* **1:**1429–1437.

Godsave, S.F., Wylie, C.C., Lane, E.B., and Anderton, B.H., 1984, Intermediate filaments in the *Xenopus* oocyte: The appearance and distribution of keratin-containing filaments, *J. Embryol. Exp. Morphol.* **83:**157–167.

Gusterson, B.A., Warburton, M.J., Mitchell, D., Ellison, M., Neville, A.M., and Rudland, P.S., 1982, Distribution of myoepithelial cells and basement membrane proteins in the normal breast and in benign and malignant breast diseases, *Cancer Res.* **42:**4763–4770.

Gusterson, B.A., McIlhinney, R.A.J., Patel, S., Knight, J., Monaghan, P., and Ormerod, M., 1985, The biochemical and immunocytochemical characterisation of an antigen on the membrane of basal cells of the epidermis, *Differentiation* **30:**102–110.

Hall, H.G., and Bissell, M.J., 1986, Characterization of the intermediate filament proteins of murine mammary gland epithelial cells, *Exp. Cell Res.* **162:**379–389.

Hallowes, R.C., Millis, R., Pigott, D., Shearer, M., Stoker, M.E.P., and Taylor-Papadimitriou, J., 1977, Results of a pilot study of cultures of human lacteal secretions and benign and malignant breast tumours, *Clin. Oncol.* **3:**81–90.

Hallowes, R.C., Bone, E.J., and Jones, W., 1980, A new dimension in the culture of human breast, in: *Tissue Culture in Medical Research,* Vol. 2 (R.J. Richards and K.T. Rajan, eds.), Pergamon Press, Oxford, pp. 215–245.

Hammond, S.L., Ham, R.G., and Stampfer, M.R., 1984, Serum-free growth of human mammary epithelial cells: Rapid clonal growth in defined medium and extended serial passage with pituitary extract, *Proc. Natl. Acad. Sci. USA* **81:**5435–5439.

Hanukoglu, I., and Fuchs, E., 1982, The cDNA sequence of a human epidermal keratin: Divergence of sequence but conservation of structure among intermediate filament proteins, *Cell* **31:**243–252.

Hanukoglu, I., and E. Fuchs, 1983, The cDNA sequence of a type II cytoskeletal keratin reveals constant and variable structural domains among keratins, *Cell* **33:**915–924.

Hogg, N.A.S., Harrison, C.J., and Tickle, C., 1983, Lumen formation in the developing mouse mammary gland, *J. Embryol. Exp. Morphol.* **73:**39–57.

Holbrook, K.A., 1979, Human epidermal embryogenesis, *Int. J. Dermatol.* **18:**329–356.

Jackson, B.W., Grund, C., Schmid, E., Burki, K., Franke, W.W., and Illmensee, K., 1980, Formation of cytoskeletal elements during mouse embryogenesis, *Differentiation* **17:**161–179.

Jackson, B.W., Grund, C., Winter, S., Franke, W.W., and Illmensee, K., 1981, Formation of cytoskeletal elements during mouse embryogenesis. II. Epithelial differentiation and intermediate-sized filaments in early post-implantation embryos, *Differentiation* **20:**203–216.

Johnson, L.D., Idler, W.W., Zhou, X-M., Roop, D.R., and Steinert, P.M., 1985, Structure of a gene for the human epidermal 67-kDa keratin, *Proc. Natl. Acad. Sci. USA* **82:**1896–1900.

Karsten, U., Papsdorf, G., Roloff, G., Stolley, P., Abel, H., Walther, I., and Weiss, H., 1985, Monoclonal anti-cytokeratin antibody from a hybridoma clone generated by electrofusion, *Eur. J. Cancer Clin. Oncol.* **21:**733–740.

Lane, E.B., 1982, Monoclonal antibodies provide specific intramolecular markers for the study of epithelial tonofilament organization, *J. Cell Biol.* **92:**665–673.

Lane, E.B., and Klymkowsky, M.W., 1982, Epithelial tonofilaments: Investigating their form and function using monoclonal antibodies, *Cold Spring Harbor Symp. Quant. Biol.* **46:**387–402.

Lane, E.B., Bartek, J., Purkis, P.E., and I.M. Leigh, 1985, Keratin antigens in differentiating skin, in: *Intermediate Filaments,* Vol. 455 (E. Wang, D. Fischman, R.H.K. Liem, and T.-T. Sun, eds.), New York Academy of Science, New York, pp. 241–258.

Lasfargues, E.Y., and Ozzello, L., 1958, Cultivation of human breast carcinomas, *J. Natl. Cancer Inst.* **21:**1131–1147.

Lazarides, E., 1980, Intermediate filaments as mechanical integrators of cellular space, *Nature (London)* **283:**249–256.

Lehtonen, E., Lehto, V.-P., Vartio, T., Badley, R.A., and Virtanen, I., 1983, Expression of cytokeratin polypeptides in mouse oocytes and preimplantation embryos, *Dev. Biol.* **100:**158–165.

Leigh, I.M., Pulford, K.A., Ramaekers, F.C.S., and Lane, E.B., 1985, Psoriasis: Maintenance of an intact monolayer basal cell differentiation compartment in spite of hyperproliferation, *Br. J. Dermatol.* **113:**53–64.

Makin, C.A., Bobrow, L.G., and Bodmer, W.F., 1984, Monoclonal antibody to cytokeratin for use in routine histopathology, *J. Clin. Pathol.* **37:**975–983.

Moll, R., Franke, W.W., Schiller, D.L., Geiger, B., and Krepler, R., 1982a, The catalog of human cytokeratins: Patterns of expression in normal epithelia, tumors and cultured cells, *Cell* **31:**11–24.

Moll, R., Moll, I., and Wiest, W., 1982b, Changes in the pattern of cytokeratin polypeptides in epidermis and hair follicles during skin development in human fetuses, *Differentiation* **23:**170–178.

Moll, R., Krepler, R., and Franke, W.W., 1983, Complex cytokeratin polypeptide patterns observed in certain human carcinomas, *Differentiation* **23:**256–269.

Moll, I., and Moll, R., 1985, Cells of extra-mammary Paget's disease express cytokeratins different from those of epidermal cells, *J. Invest. Dermatol.* **84:**3–8.

Moore, K.L., 1982, *The Developing Human,* 3rd ed., W.B. Saunders, Philadelphia.

Nagle, R.B., Lucas, D.O., McDaniel, K.M., Clark, V.A., and Schmalzel, G.M., 1985, New evidence linking mammary and extramammary Paget cells to a common cell phenotype, *Am. J. Clin. Pathol.* **83:**431–438.

Nagle, R.B., Boecker, W., Davis, J.R., Heid, H.W., Kaufmann, M., Lucas, D.O., and Jarasch, E.-D., 1986, Characterisation of breast carcinomas by two monoclonal antibodies distinguishing myoepithelial from luminal epithelial cells, *J. Histochem. Cytochem.* **34:**869–881.

Nelson, W.G., Battifora, H., Santana, H., and Sun, T.-T., 1984, Specific keratins as molecular markers for neoplasms with a stratified epithelial origin, *Cancer Res.* **44:**1600–1603.

Osborn, M., Altmannsberger, M., Debus, E., and Weber, K., 1985, Differentiation of the major human tumour groups using conventional and monoclonal antibodies specific for individual intermediate filament proteins, *Ann. N.Y. Acad. Sci.* **455:**649–668.

Oshima, R.G., Howe, W.E., Klier, F.G., Adamson, E.D., and Shevinsky, L.H., 1983, Intermediate filament protein synthesis in preimplantation murine embryos, *Dev. Biol.* **99:**447–455.

Patterson, J.A.K., Eisinger, M., Haynes, B.F., Berger, C.L., and Edelson, R.L., 1984, Monoclonal antibody 4F2 reactive with basal layer keratinocytes: Studies in the normal and a hyperproliferative state, *J. Invest. Dermatol.* **83:**210–213.

Peters, R.A., 1956, Hormones and the cytoskeleton, *Nature* **177:**426.

Pitelka, D.R., Hamamoto, S.T., Duafala, J.G., and Nemanic, M.K., 1973, Cell contacts in the mouse mammary gland, *J. Cell Biol.* **56:**797–818.

Polonowski, F.P., Gaffney, E.V., and Burke, R.E., 1976, HBL-100, a cell line established from human breast milk, *In Vitro* **12:**328 (abstract).

Quinlan, R., Schiller, D.L., Hatzfeld, M., Achstaetter, T., Moll, R., Jorcano, J., Magin, T.M., and Franke, W.W., 1985, Patterns of expression and organization of cytokeratin intermediate filaments, in: *Intermediate Filaments,* Vol. 455 (E. Wang, D. Fischman, R.H.K. Liem, and T.-T. Sun, eds.), New York Academy of Science, New York, pp. 282–306.

Ramaekers, F.C.S., Huysmans, A., Moesker, O., Kant, A., Jap, P., Herman, C., and Vooijs, P., 1983a, Monoclonal antibody to keratin filaments, specific for glandular epithelia and their tumors, *Lab. Invest.* **49:**353–361.

Ramaekers, F.C.S., Puts, J.J.G., Moesker, O., Kant, A., Huysmans, A., Haag, D., Jap, P.H.K., Herman, C.J., and Vooijs, G.P., 1983b, Antibodies to intermediate filament proteins in the immunohistochemical identification of human tumours: An overview, *Histochem. J.* **15:**691–713.

Ramaekers, F.C.S., Moesker, O., Huysmans, A., Schaart, G., Westerhof, G., Wagenaar, S.S., Herman, C.J., and Vooijs, G.P., 1985, Intermediate filament proteins in the study of tumor heterogeneity: An in-depth study of tumors of the urinary and respiratory tracts, *Ann. N.Y. Acad. Sci.* **455:**614–634.

Raychaudury, A., Marchuk, D., Lindhurst, M., and Fuchs, E., 1986, Three tightly-linked genes encoding human type I keratins: Conservation of sequence in the 5′-untranslated leader and 5′-upstream regions of coexpressed keratin genes, *Mol. Cell. Biol.* **6:**539–548.

Schaefer, F.V., Custer, R. P., and Sorof, S., 1980, Induction of abnormal development and differentiation in cultured mammary glands by cyclic adenine nucleotide and prostaglandins, *Nature* **286:**807–810.

Schaefer, F.V., Custer, R.P., and Sorof, S., 1983, Squamous metaplasia in human breast culture: Induction by cyclic adenine nucleotide and prostaglandins and influence of menstrual cycle, *Cancer Res.* **43:**279–286.

Schiller, D.L., Franke, W.W., and Geiger, B., 1982, A subfamily of relatively large and basic cytokeratin polypeptides as defined by peptide mapping is represented by one or several polypeptides in epithelial cells, *EMBO J.* **1:**761–769.

Smith, H.S., Wolman, S.R., Auer, G., and Hackett, A.J., 1986, Cell culture studies: A perspective on malignant progression of human breast cancer, in: *Breast Cancer: Origins, Detection and Treatment* (M.A. Rich, J.C. Hager, and J. Taylor-Papadimitriou, eds.), Martinus Nijhoff Publishing, Boston, pp. 75–89.

Stampfer, M., and Bartley, J.C., 1985, Long term growth of normal human mammary epithelial cells and establishment of partially transformed cell lines, in: *Growth and Differentiation of Cells in Defined Environment* (H. Murakami, I. Yamane, D.W. Barnes, J.P. Mather, I. Hayashi, and G.H. Sato, eds.), Springer-Verlag, New York, pp. 51–56.

Stampfer, M., Hallowes, R.C., and Hackett, A.J., 1980, Growth of normal human mammary cells in culture, *In Vitro* **16:**415–425.

Steinert, P.M., and Parry, D.A.D., 1985, Intermediate filaments: Conformity and diversity of expression and structure, *Ann. Rev. Cell Biol.* **1:**41–65.

Stoker, M.W.P., Pigott, D., and Taylor-Papadimitriou, J., 1976, Response to epidermal growth factors of cultured human mammary epithelial cells from benign tumours, *Nature* **264:**764–767.

Sun, T.-T., Eichner, R., Schermer, A., Cooper, D., Nelson, W.G., and Weiss, R.A., 1984, Classification, expression and possible mechanisms of evolution of mammalian epithelial keratins: A unifying model, in: *Cancer Cells 1/The Transformed Phenotype* (A.J. Levine, G.F. Vande Woude, W.C. Topp, and J.D. Watson, eds.), Cold Spring Harbor Laboratory, Cold Spring Harbor, NY.

Sun, T.-T., Tseng, S.C.G., Huang, A.J.-W., Cooper, D., Schermer, A., Lynch, M.H., Weiss, R., and Eichner, R., 1985, Monoclonal antibody studies of mammalian epithelial keratins: A review, *Ann. N.Y. Acad. Sci.* **455:**307–329.

Tannenbaum, M., Weiss, M., and Marx, A.J., 1979, Ultrastructure of the human mammary ductule, *Cancer* **23:**958–978.

Taylor-Papadimitriou, J., Shearer, M., and Tilly, R., 1977, Some properties of cells cultured from early lactation human milk, *J. Natl. Cancer Inst.* **58:**1563–1571.

Taylor-Papadimitriou, J., Purkis, P., and Fentiman, I.S., 1980, Cholera toxin and analogues of cyclic AMP stimulate the growth of cultured human mammary epithelial cells, *J. Cell. Physiol.* **102:**317–321.

Taylor-Papadimitriou, J., Purkis, P., Lane, E.B., McKay, I.A., and Chang, S.E., 1982, Effects of SV40 transformation on the cytoskeleton and behavioural properties of human keratinocytes, *Cell Diff.* **11:**169–180.

Taylor-Papadimitriou, J., Lane, E.B., and Chang, S.E., 1983, Cell lineages and interactions in neoplastic expression in the human breast, in: *Understanding Breast Cancer* (M.A. Rich, J.C. Hager, and P. Furmanski, eds.), Marcel Dekker, New York.

Taylor-Papadimitriou, J., Bartek, J., Durban, E., Burchell, J., Hallowes, R.C., Lane, E.B., and Millis, R., 1984, Monoclonal antibodies in the study of cell lineage, differentiation and malignancy in the human breast, in: *Monoclonal Antibodies and Breast Cancer* (R.L. Ceriani, ed.), Martinus Nijhoff Publishing, Boston, pp. 60–79.

Taylor-Papadimitriou, J., Burchell, J., Chang, S., Bartek, J., Gendler, S., and Durban, E.M., 1986, Use of monoclonal antibodies to define the phenotype of cells cultured from the human mammary gland, Proceedings of the Third International Cell Culture Congress, Sendai, Japan.

van Muijen, G.N.P., Ruitter, D.J., Franke, W.W., Achtstaetter, T., Haasnoot, W.H.B., Ponec, M., and Warnaar, S.O., 1986, Cell type heterogeneity of cytokeratin expression in complex epithelia and carcinomas as demonstrated by monoclonal antibodies specific for cytokeratins nos. 4 and 13, *Exp. Cell Res.* **162:**97–113.

Warburton, M.J., Ferns, S.A., Hughes, C.M., and Rudland, P.S., 1985, Characterization of rat mammary cell types in primary culture: Lectins and antisera to basement membrane and intermediate filament proteins as indicators of cellular heterogeneity, *J. Cell Sci.* **79:**287–304.

Weiss, R.A., Eichner, R., and Sun, T.-T., 1984, Monoclonal antibody analysis of keratin expression in epidermal disease: A 48- and 56-kdalton keratin as molecular markers for hyperproliferative keratinocytes, *J. Cell Biol.* **98:**1397–1406.

Woodcock-Mitchell, J., Eichner, R., Nelson, W.G., and Sun, T.T., 1982, Immunolocalization of keratin polypeptides in human epidermis using monoclonal antibodies, *J. Cell Biol.* **95:**580–588.

7

Proteins of the Milk-Fat-Globule Membrane as Markers of Mammary Epithelial Cells and Apical Plasma Membrane

I. H. Mather

1. Introduction

Currently, there is widespread interest in the identification of specific markers of mammary epithelial cells. This interest stems from attempts to delineate stages in the differentiation of mammary cells during development and to identify carcinoma-associated markers in neoplastic breast tissue. Markers are also needed for epithelial cells in primary and long-term mammary cultures in vitro. Within these concerns lie questions, for instance, about the identity of stem cells in mammary tissue, the expression of stage-specific developmental antigens, and the possible existence of tumor-specific markers. In addition, cell markers may often be used to delineate specific structures or domains of epithelial cells such as the apical or basal/lateral surfaces or specific intracellular compartments.

Despite their obvious importance, very few biochemical markers of mammary epithelial cells have been characterized (for a discussion of morphological markers see Pitelka, 1980). This is partly because the cellular heterogeneity of mammary tissue complicates the isolation of

I. H. Mather • Department of Animal Sciences, University of Maryland, College Park, Maryland 20742.

specific epithelial molecules that may be expressed in limited amounts, especially during early stages of development. For this reason, there has been recent interest in the use of the milk-fat-globule membrane (MFGM) as a potential source of epithelial antigens. MFGM is derived from epithelial cell membranes during the synthesis and secretion of milk triacylglycerols. Fat droplets in milk are coated with a layer of proteins and lipids of epithelial origin, which can easily be isolated from the fat fraction of milk. Several MFGM proteins have been purified and characterized and specific antibodies to them have been used to identify mammary epithelial cells, mammary carcinomas, and other cell types in a variety of circumstances. In addition, the secretion of fat droplets from the apical pole of the cell raises the possibility of obtaining antigens from MFGM that are highly concentrated or specific to the apical plasma membrane. Such apical markers have potential for studies on the biogenesis and maintenance of cell polarity during development.

The purpose of this chapter is to review our current knowledge of the proteins of MFGM and the advantages and pitfalls of using these antigens as specific cell and plasma membrane markers. For other reviews of the structure, function, and composition of MFGM, see Brunner (1969), Patton (1973), Anderson and Cawston (1975), Patton and Keenan (1975), and McPherson and Kitchen (1983).

2. Derivation of MFGM

2.1. Cellular Origin, Formation, and Secretion of MFGM

Evidence for the epithelial origin of MFGM comes from a large number of morphological studies at the resolution of the light and electron microscope (e.g., Jeffers, 1935; Bargmann and Knoop, 1959; Stein and Stein, 1967; Saacke and Heald, 1974). Furthermore, fat droplets only appear to be secreted from epithelial cells lining alveoli and intralobular ducts (e.g., see Saacke and Heald, 1974; Pitelka, 1980). Myoepithelial cells do not secrete fat, and although some epithelial cells in interlobular ducts may secrete casein* (Pitelka, 1980), there is little con-

*Evidence for this comes from the morphological identification of membrane-bounded vesicles containing casein micelles in ductal epithelial cells. It is assumed that these vesicles contain presecretory material that is subsequently released by exocytosis from the apical surface of these cells. However, it is equally possible that casein is taken up into ductal cells from the luminae by endocytosis.

vincing evidence that these cells synthesize and secrete membrane-coated lipid droplets.

In the past, the principal site of formation of MFGM was assumed to be the apical plasma membrane. However, it has become increasingly apparent that elements of MFGM may be derived directly from intracellular membranes including the rough endoplasmic reticulum, Golgi-derived secretory vesicles, as well as the cytoplasm. It is therefore worth considering the derivation of MFGM in some detail since the cellular origin and nature of the membrane proteins have a direct bearing on their potential usefulness as mammary cell markers and especially as markers of the apical plasma membrane.

The formation of MFGM requires the continued synthesis and export of triacylglycerols in the form of discrete droplets as well as the biogenesis of cellular membranes. Triacylglycerols are synthesized in the endoplasmic reticulum (for reviews see Bauman and Davis, 1974; Patton and Jensen, 1975; Moore and Christie, 1979; Mather and Keenan, 1983) and appear to accumulate in small droplets, less than 0.5 μm in diameter, on the cytoplasmic surface of the membrane cisternae. Following release from the endoplasmic reticulum, these droplets become the immediate cytoplasmic precursors of larger lipid droplets in basal and apical regions of the cell (Dylewski et al., 1984; Deeney et al., 1985; Keenan and Dylewski, 1985). These precursor lipid droplets, recently termed *lipovesicles* or *microlipid droplets* (Dylewski et al., 1984; Keenan and Dylewski, 1985), fuse with the outer surface of larger globules and contribute directly to the bulk lipid. Fat droplets increase in size most dramatically in the apical cytoplasm and especially during the process of secretion (Stemberger and Patton, 1981; Stemberger et al., 1984), although droplet growth occurs to some extent in all regions of the cytoplasm.

At all developmental stages, lipovesicles and intracellular lipid droplets are coated with an amorphous layer of material that stains darker than the bulk lipid (Saacke and Heald, 1974; Dylewski et al., 1984). This material occasionally has the apparent morphology of a "half membrane" (Patton and Keenan, 1975) or a tripartite lamellar structure (Dylewski et al., 1984) and appears to consist of phospholipids, sterols, cerebrosides, gangliosides, and proteins (Patton and Fowkes, 1967; Hood and Patton, 1973; Dylewski et al., 1984; Deeney et al., 1985). Many of the proteins may originate from the rough endoplasmic reticulum during the formation of lipovesicles, since electrophoretic analysis of the protein composition of isolated fractions of lipovesicles and rough endoplasmic reticulum show many similarities (Dylewski et al., 1984; Deeney et al., 1985). Rabbit antibodies to proteins of bovine cytoplasmic lipid droplets recognize two polypeptides with M_r values of approximately 44,000, which are also present in the rough endoplasmic reticulum, lipovesicles, and secreted MFGM (Deeney et al., 1985). At least one other protein, butyrophilin, has been identified in all these locations, although this protein is mainly concentrated in the apical plasma membrane and MFGM (discussed in Section 3.6). Surface proteins of intracellular lipid droplets may also originate from other membranes including the Golgi complex and secretory vesicles or be adsorbed from the cytoplasm, although there is no direct evidence for this.

Phospholipids, sterols, cerebrosides, and gangliosides may also be derived directly from the rough endoplasmic reticulum, during the formation of lipovesicles (Hood and Patton, 1973; Dylewski et al., 1984). Additionally, intracellular fat droplets may acquire lipids by post-synthetic association with membranes of the rough endoplasmic reticulum and the Golgi complex (Peixoto de Menezes and Pinto da Silva, 1979).

Following formation within the cell, lipid droplets coated with the amorphous layer discussed above are secreted with an additional outer bilayer membrane composed of proteins and lipids. There is general agreement that this membrane is at least partly derived from the apical surface and that fat droplets are coated with apical plasma membrane as they are discharged from the cell (Bargmann and Knoop, 1959; Bargmann et al., 1961; Kurosumi et al., 1968; Saacke and Heald, 1974; Peixoto de Menezes and Pinto da Silva, 1978; Franke et al., 1981). Secretory vesicle membrane may also contribute to the outer surface of secreted fat globules (Wooding, 1971a, 1973, 1977). In morphological studies using lactating mammary tissue from guinea pig, goat, and cow, Wooding observed frequent interactions between secretory vesicles and cytoplasmic lipid droplets. Progressive fusion of adjacent vesicles on the surface of fat droplets led to the formation of intracytoplasmic vacuoles containing fat droplets coated with vesicle membrane. Fat droplets were then released from the cell by exocytosis, following fusion of these vesicles with the apical plasma membrane. The concomitant interaction of individual fat droplets with the apical plasma membrane and secretory vesicles may lead to the formation of MFGM from both sources (for diagrams see Morré, 1977; Wooding, 1977; Mather and Keenan, 1983). Other investigators have also observed associations between secretory vesicles and cytoplasmic lipid droplets by both transmission electron microscopy (Morré, 1977; Franke and Keenan, 1979; Stemberger et al., 1984) and freeze-fracture techniques (Peixoto de Menezes and Pinto da Silva, 1978). Unfortunately, morphological studies alone cannot provide information on the extent that either the apical plasma membrane or secretory vesicle membrane contributes to the outer bilayer of MFGM, because the *rate* of formation of membrane from either source cannot be estimated. In addition, there are problems in preparing lipid-rich tissue for electron microscopy. The possibility that secretory vesicles are attracted to the surface of lipid droplets in the cytoplasm during the fixation process has never been adequately considered.

Biochemical data supporting both secretory mechanisms have been reported. Most of this evidence relies on the identification of enzymes in MFGM characteristic of either plasma membranes or the Golgi complex (Martel-Pradal and Got, 1972; Martel et al., 1973; Keenan et al., 1974; Powell et al., 1977). For instance, bovine MFGM is highly enriched in 5′-nucleotidase compared with total homogenates of mammary tissue (Keenan et al., 1979). This enzyme is widely regarded as a marker for the plasma membrane, although in at least some cells it is also present in endomembranes (e.g., see Widnell, 1972). On the other hand, galactosyl transferase is also present in human and bovine MFGM (Martel-Pradal and Got, 1972; Martel et al., 1973; Powell et al., 1977). Despite the recent demonstration of this enzyme on the surfaces of enterocytes and cultured cell lines (Roth et al., 1985; Shaper et al., 1985), galactosyl transferase appears to be largely restricted to the Golgi complex in mammary tissue (Moore et al., 1985). This is consistent with at least some contribution to MFGM from Golgi membranes.

Evaluation of the enzyme content of MFGM, however, is complicated by the presence of cytoplasmic inclusions, containing recognizable intracellular organelles, trapped between the outer membrane and the surface of the lipid droplets (Kurosumi et al., 1968; Wooding et al., 1970; Saacke and Heald, 1974). This material contributes directly to the membrane prepared from isolated milk-fat globules. There is much species variation in the extent of this problem. The amount of cytoplasmic material associated with milk-fat droplets in guinea pig, goat, and cow is low (Wooding et al., 1970; Janssen and Walstra, 1982); MFGM from rat and rabbit appears to be contaminated more heavily (Jarasch et al., 1977; Janssen and Walstra, 1982). Also, there is always the possibility that enzymes within endomembranes are added directly to the amorphous layer of material present on the surface of lipovesicles and intracytoplasmic droplets, which then become incorporated into MFGM at the apical surface.

Evidence that the outer bilayer of MFGM is at least partly derived from the apical plasma membrane comes from recent histological studies using antibodies to specific proteins. Both mucin-like glycoproteins of high M_r and butyrophilin appear to be concentrated in apical membranes in several species and both proteins are present in much lower concentrations in intracellular membranes including the Golgi complex (Franke et al., 1981; Johnson and Mather, 1985; Petersen and Van Deurs, 1986).

As fat droplets in the cytoplasm come into contact with either the apical plasma membrane or secretory vesicle membrane, a uniform dense layer of material is formed between the outer membrane bilayer and the surface of the lipid globules (Wooding, 1971a, 1973). This dense material is present in secreted fat globules and can be seen as a layer or coat, 10–50 μm in thickness on one side of isolated membrane (Fig. 1a; Keenan et al., 1971; Jarasch et al., 1977; Freudenstein et al., 1979). This coat is partly composed of protein, since it resists extraction with lipophilic solvents (Wooding and Kemp, 1975a,b), and is degraded by proteinases (Wooding and Kemp, 1975b; Greenwalt and Mather, 1985). Evidence (discussed in Sections 3.4 and 3.6) indicates that this coat is derived both from proteins in the cytoplasm and from the outer membrane bilayer.

Immediately after secretion, the MFGM is composed of at least four layers of material (Fig. 1b). These are, successively from the triacylglycerol core, (1) the amorphous layer of material derived from lipovesicles, (2) the protein coat, (3) the lipid bilayer, and (4) the glycocalyx, a complex of glycosaminoglycans and oligosaccharide chains, the latter in most instances covalently bound to integral membrane glycoproteins.

As the secreted fat globules accumulate in the alveolar luminae, membrane may be lost from the surface by a process of vesiculation and shedding (Wooding, 1971b). The fragmented MFGM contributes to a pool of membranes in skim milk which is also derived from several other sources (see Mather and Keenan, 1983, for discussion). Estimates for the extent of this loss vary widely and are undoubtedly affected by procedures used for the preparation of specimens for electron microscopy

---

Figure 1. Morphology and structure of MFGM. (a) MFGM isolated from bovine milk was fixed in glutaraldehyde, postfixed in OsO_4, and examined by transmission electron microscopy. The lipid bilayer and protein coat are indicated by small open arrowheads and large closed arrowheads, respectively. Bar = 100 nm. Micrograph courtesy of D.E. Greenwalt. (b) Diagram of the four layers of MFGM discussed in the text. In order from the triacylglycerol core these layers are: layer 1, the thin membrane possibly derived from intracellular lipovesicles; layer 2, the protein coat; layer 3, the lipid bilayer primarily derived from the apical plasma membrane and possibly secretory vesicle membrane; and layer 4, the glycocalyx. The possible location of major proteins of bovine MFGM is given in the right of the figure (see text). These positions are not intended to be mutually exclusive. As indicated by dashed lines, butyrophilin may be embedded in the lipid bilayer (see also Fig. 6d), and the high M_r mucins may be transmembrane proteins. The glycosylated domain of PAS-IV may contribute to the glycocalyx.

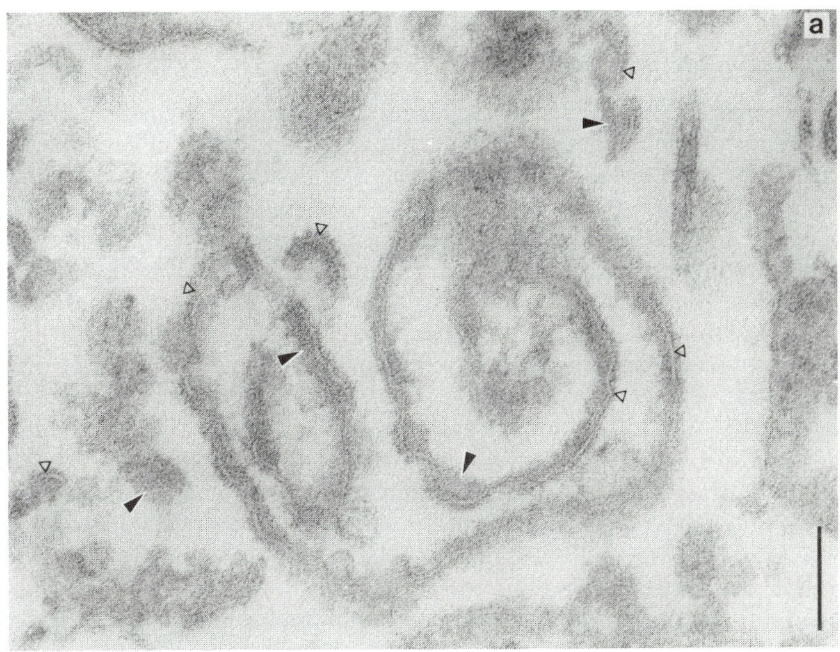
a

b

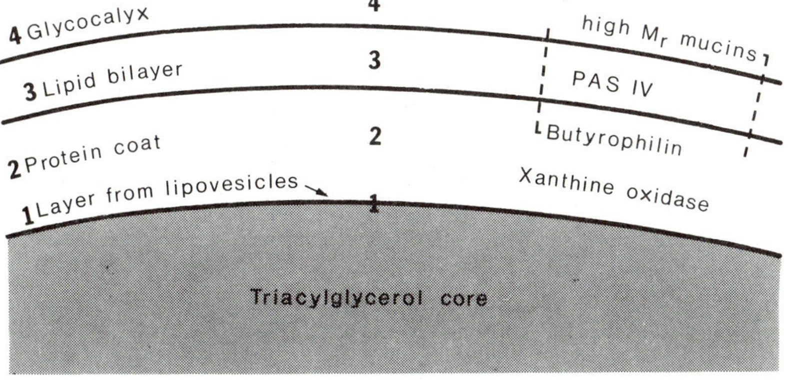
4
4 Glycocalyx
high M_r mucins
3
3 Lipid bilayer
PAS IV
2
Butyrophilin
2 Protein coat
Xanthine oxidase
1 Layer from lipovesicles
1
Triacylglycerol core

(e.g., compare the electron micrographs of Wooding, 1971b, with those of Horisberger et al., 1977, and Freudenstein et al., 1979).

2.2. Methods for Isolating MFGM

Preparation of MFGM is a relatively simple procedure that involves the removal of fat globules from milk and the release of membrane material from the surface of the droplets by physical or chemical means. Fat globules are usually separated from skim milk by centrifugation at relatively low *g* forces. In some cases, for example, bovine milk, the fat globules will separate under unit gravity in a relatively short time. This is because certain factors, including IgM, aggregate the fat globules into clusters which then rise to the surface at a faster rate than predicted from the size distribution of the individual droplets (Euber and Brunner, 1984). If low *g* forces are used, physical damage to the fat globules and MFGM should be minimal. However, approximately 75% of the fat globules of bovine milk are under 1 μm in diameter (Walstra, 1969). Although these droplets contribute only a few percent to the triacylglycerol content of milk, they account for a disproportionate amount of the total MFGM, because the surface to volume ratio is higher for smaller globules. Centrifugal forces up to 10,000*g* may therefore be necessary to ensure maximum yield of membrane, even in milk containing clustering factors.

Fat globules directly isolated from milk are contaminated with casein micelles and other secretory proteins. These are usually removed by several wash cycles while the membrane is still associated with the fat. Removal of caseins appears to be facilitated by the inclusion of salt in the washing medium (Basch et al., 1985). Unfortunately, membrane may be lost from the surface of the globules during this procedure, presumably because of mechanical erosion during the resuspension and centrifugation steps (Swope and Brunner, 1968; Anderson and Brooker, 1975). This can be a major problem with small samples of milk from, for example, laboratory rodents. To circumvent this, fat globules may be recovered in good yield from a single-step sucrose gradient following centrifugation at 1500*g* (Patton and Huston, 1986). Alternatively, membrane may be released directly from unwashed fat globules and recovered free of secretory protein either by density-gradient centrifugation (McPherson et al., 1984) or by washing the contaminated membranes with 0.1*M* citrate buffer (Johnson et al., 1985). In this latter method, citrate apparently destabilizes casein micelles so that they remain in the supernatant after centrifugation of the membrane and can be easily removed. Relative amounts of the major MFGM proteins from six different species are unaffected by this treatment (I.H. Mather and P.J. Madara, unpublished data).

Membrane may be released from fat globules (washed or unwashed) by either physical or chemical means. For large samples, the lipid droplets are usually suspended in buffer, cooled to less than 10°C, and subjected to mechanical agitation in, for example, a Waring blender or tissue homogenizer. During destabilization, the membrane is released into the aqueous phase and the fat aggregates into a granular mass. For small samples, the membrane is often released by subjecting the fat to several cycles of freezing and thawing. Membrane can be recovered either by centrifugation at approximately 100,000*g* (e.g., Mather and Keenan, 1975) or by precipitation with ammonium sulfate (Kitchen, 1974). Alternatively, membrane can be prepared from fat globules by the addition of detergents. If nonionic detergent (Triton X-100) is used in low concentrations, the MFGM can be recovered by centrifugation without the loss of major membrane-associated proteins (Patton, 1982).

Attempts have been made to purify MFGM by density-gradient centrifugation. This is of particular interest because the MFGM of some species, for example, rat and rabbit, may be contaminated with membranes derived from the cytoplasmic inclusions associated with some fat globules (Janssen and Walstra, 1982). Unfortunately, MFGM varies widely in buoyant density and as a consequence vesicles and sheets of membrane spread throughout sucrose gradients with densities ranging from under 1.05 to over 1.20 g/cm^3 (Kobylka and Carraway, 1972; Keenan et al., 1977; Kitchen, 1977; Mather et al., 1977). Gradient fractions contain variable quantities of lipid, but the same major MFGM proteins (however, see Kitchen, 1977). In one study, morphologically identifiable cytoplasmic membranes were recognized together with the cytoplasmic protein, actin, in a fraction of high density (Keenan et al., 1977). It may therefore be possible to remove some contaminating membranes, although this is rarely done, especially in species such as cow, in which cytoplasmic inclusions contribute very little material to MFGM.

There is good agreement among investigators on the identity of the major membrane-associated proteins, despite the large number of different methods used for preparing MFGM. In a recent comparison of six of the most widely used procedures, Basch et al. (1985) found only minor differences in the profile of bovine MFGM proteins detected by sodium dodecyl sulfate (SDS)–polyacrylamide gel electrophoresis (SDS-PAGE). The most variable factors were the relative amount of each protein in the fractions and the quantity of residual casein.

2.3. Nature of MFGM and Constituent Proteins

Isolated MFGM appears as flattened sheets, whorls, and vesicles of membrane (Keenan et al., 1970, 1971; Wooding and Kemp, 1975a,b). In favorable sections, the 10-nm-thick membrane bilayer is evident (small open arrowheads, Fig. 1a) and the protein coat appears as dense, fuzzy material of variable thickness (10–50 nm) on the "inner" face of the bilayer (large closed arrowheads, Fig. 1a). It is uncertain how much of the amorphous layer present on intracytoplasmic lipid droplets (Dylewski et al., 1984) is carried over into isolated MFGM (layer 1, Fig. 1b). While this layer can be distinguished on the surface of secreted globules under favorable conditions, it has never been seen in isolated MFGM by transmission electron microscopy. Furthermore, although several common proteins have been identified, most of the proteins of lipovesicles and intracytoplasmic lipid droplets are different from those of MFGM (Dylewski et al., 1984; Deeney et al., 1985). Presumably, the quantity of this layer in MFGM will depend on the sheer forces used to disrupt globules and the relative stability of the membrane layers. Certainly, shedding of MFGM into skim milk in the alveolar lumen appears to leave most of the amorphous material behind on the surface of the droplets (secondary membrane of Wooding, 1971b).

The physical disruption of fat globules releases a substantial amount of the globule-associated protein into the aqueous phase (Mather and Keenan, 1975; Mather et al., 1977). This raises questions on the nature of MFGM proteins, on whether they are associated with the lipid bilayer or the peripheral protein coat and glycocalyx. MFGM proteins have been classified as "integral" or "peripheral," using criteria developed for other biological membranes, such as the resistance of specific proteins to extraction with solutions containing 0.1 *M* Na_2CO_3 or high concentrations of salt (e.g., Johnson et al., 1985). However, the formation of MFGM almost certainly involves structural changes in the organization of the apical surface (Keenan et al., 1970; Peixoto de Menezes and Pinto da Silva, 1978; Freudenstein et al., 1979) and evidence is presented in Section 3.6 that the protein coat is derived, in part, from integral proteins of the lipid bilayer. The use of the terms integral and peripheral may introduce unnecessary confusion on the nature and properties of MFGM proteins. Certainly, it cannot be assumed that coat-associated MFGM proteins are necessarily peripheral components of the apical plasma membrane, or that integral proteins of the apical surface remain as integral components of the MFGM during and after secretion. These issues are discussed on an individual protein basis in succeeding sections.

3. Identity and Tissue Distribution of Major MFGM Proteins

3.1. Introduction

MFGM proteins are usually identified and classified according to their mobilities during separation by SDS-PAGE. Since separation is primarily based on differences in molecular size, estimates may be obtained for the apparent M_r values of individual proteins (Weber and Osborn, 1969). In the absence of further information, the individual bands of protein are usually assigned arabic or roman numerals in consecutive order starting with the protein of lowest mobility and consequently highest apparent M_r. Some investigators have only assigned numbers to the major proteins identified after staining with a dye, usually Coomassie Blue. Others have attempted to number all proteins. In addition, glycoproteins have often been identified by their ability to react with the periodic acid–Schiff (PAS) reagent and have been assigned separate numbers. The result, especially when attempts are made to compare the MFGMs of different species, can be unnecessarily confusing. For the sake of clarity, the Milk Protein Nomenclature Committee of the American Dairy Science Association recently suggested a scheme for classifying individual MFGM proteins, regardless of species (Eigel et al., 1984). This system is compared together with the classification systems used for bovine MFGM proteins by several investigators in Table I.

At least seven major bands of protein can be identified in bovine MFGM after separation by SDS-PAGE (Fig. 2a, Table I). Two components (PAS-I and PAS-III) contain large amounts of carbohydrate and stain strongly with the PAS reagent, but not with Coomassie Blue (compare lanes 1 and 2, Fig. 2a). Other proteins include the redox enzyme xanthine oxidase and the glycoprotein butyrophilin. Separation, by two-dimensional electrophoresis, combining SDS-PAGE with isoelectric focusing, has generally shown that the major protein bands are resolved into several related isoelectric variants (Table II). Most of the major bands are therefore not composed of many dissimilar proteins with coincident M_r values, although the rather insensitive Coomassie Blue stain has usually been employed to stain the separated proteins.

When the ultrasensitive silver reagent (Merril et al., 1981) is used to detect protein after one-dimensional SDS-PAGE, many minor bands of protein can be identified. Although these proteins may be authentic components of MFGM, some are undoubtedly the products of limited proteolytic breakdown of more abundant proteins. MFGM has been

Table I. Nomenclature for Bovine MFGM Proteins

Protein identified in Fig. 2a	Kobylka and Carraway (1972)	Anderson et al. (1974)	Mather and Keenan (1975)	Mather et al. (1980)	Eigel et al. (1984)[a]
PAS-I	2	A	I	I	MFGM-A_{10}-180, P
Xanthine oxidase	II	I	3	2	MFGM-A_{10}-155, C
PAS-III	4 (?)	C (?)	II	II or III ?	MFGM-A_{10}-100, P
PAS-IV	IV	III (?)	11	3/IV	MFGM-B_{10}-76, C, P
Butyrophilin	V	IV	12	4/V	MFGM-B_{10}-67, C, P
Band 15	VI	V	15	5/VI	MFGM-B_{10}-49.5, C, P
Band 16	VI	V	16	7/VII	MFGM-B_{10}-46, C, P

[a]In this notation, the gel is divided into four zones, A, B, C, and D (see Fig. 2). Zone A lies between the top of the separating gel and 94 kDa (the position of phosphorylase b protein standard); zone B lies between 94 and 43 kDa (the position of ovalbumin protein standard); zone C lies between 43 and 15 kDa (the position of α-lactalbumin protein standard); and zone D lies between 15 kDa and the position of the tracking dye. Most bovine MFGM proteins separate within zones A and B (see Fig. 2a). The figures denote the % (w/v) of polyacrylamide used, indicated as a subscript to the zone letter, and the apparent M_r when compared with a set of standards, separated in the same % (w/v) of polyacrylamide. Letters C and P are added to indicate whether the protein stains with Coomassie Blue and/or the PAS reagent, respectively. The values in column 6 in the table are derived from Fig. I of Mather et al. (1980). As an example, PAS-I (first protein on the list) separates in zone A in 10% (w/v) polyacrylamide with an apparent M_r of 180 kDa and stains with the PAS reagent but not Coomassie Blue. The Milk Protein Nomenclature Committee recommends that this nomenclature be cited at least once in the text, irrespective of the name given to each protein by individual investigators.

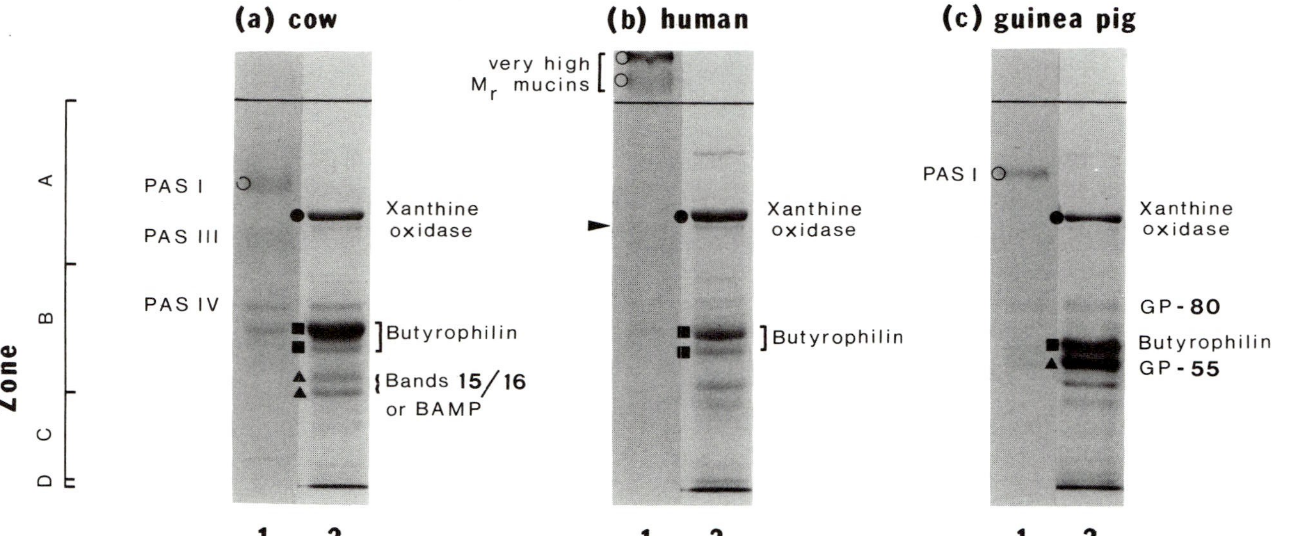

Figure 2. Comparison of bovine, human, and guinea pig MFGM by SDS-PAGE. Samples of MFGM from (a) bovine, (b) human, and (c) guinea pig milk were separated in stacking and separating gels containing, respectively, 4% (w/v) and 6% (w/v) polyacrylamide. A line in the figure separates the division between these two gels. Proteins were either stained with the PAS reagent (lanes 1) or Coomassie Blue (lanes 2). Glycoproteins and proteins are identified by names on either the right or left side of each panel. The four zones discussed in the legend to Table I are indicated to the left of the entire figure. Proteins with similar peptide maps or immunological properties are indicated by similar symbols: (○), high M_r mucin-like proteins; (●), xanthine oxidase; (■), butyrophilin; and (▲), bands 15/16 and GP-55. The major band of butyrophilin and a putative degradation product of butyrophilin are also indicated by square brackets to the right of panels (a) and (b). A similar "degradation" product is also present in guinea pig MFGM but is not resolved in 6% (w/v) polyacrylamide gels (see Johnson et al., 1985). For M_r values and isoelectric points of the major proteins see Table II.

Table II. Apparent M_r Values and Isoelectric Points for Major Bovine, Human, and Guinea Pig MFGM Proteins

Protein identified in Fig. 2	Cow		Human		Guinea pig	
	M_r ($\times 10^{-3}$)	Isoelectric points[a]	M_r ($\times 10^{-3}$)	Isoelectric points[a]	M_r ($\times 10^{-3}$)	Isoelectric points[a]
PAS-I/very high M_r mucins	180[c]	3.5–4.7[c]	N.D.[b]	N.D.	≥ 200[d]	≤ 4.0[d]
Xanthine oxidase	155[c,e]	6.9–7.6 (5–7)[f] 7.0–7.5 (3–4)[c,e,g,h]	155[h,i]	N.D.	155[d]	6.7–7.0 (≥3)[d]
PAS-IV	76[j]	7.8–8.5 (4)[j]	N.D.	N.D.	80[d]	6.9–7.3 (4)[d]
Butyrophilin	67[c,k]	5.55(1)[l] 5.2–5.3 (4)[k,m]	66[m]	5.4–5.6 (4)[m]	65[m] 63[d]	6.2–6.5 (4)[m] 5.7–6.15 (4)[d]
GP-55	—	—	—	—	55[d]	6.8–7.8 (4)[d]

[a]Isoelectric points quoted are the pH limits for the most acidic and most basic variants; figures in parentheses are the number of variants detected. Values in references c, f, and l were determined by flat-bed electrofocusing; all other isoelectric points were determined by two-dimensional polyacrylamide gel electrophoresis. [b]N.D., not determined. [c]Mather et al. (1980). [d]Johnson et al. (1985). [e]Jarasch et al. (1981). [f]Sullivan et al. (1982). [g]Bruder et al. (1982). [h]Bruder et al. (1983). [i]Heid (1983). [j]Greenwalt and Mather (1985). [k]Franke et al. (1981). [l]Mather (1978). [m]Heid et al. (1983).

shown to contain plasmin, which will degrade membrane proteins under certain conditions (Hofmann et al., 1979). Several of the major milk proteins are also subject to partial proteolysis during or after secretion (Eigel et al., 1979).

Comparison of the MFGM proteins of different species reveals both interesting similarities and differences. In all the dozen or more species that we and others have examined, the MFGM is composed of a simple pattern of major proteins. Subsequent sections will review our current knowledge of MFGM proteins with respect to chemical composition, immunological properties, and tissue distribution and where possible species comparisons will be made. The proteins of bovine MFGM are compared with those of the human and guinea pig membrane in Fig. 2 and Table II.

3.2. Glycoproteins of High M_r

The MFGMs of all species examined, including cow, goat, sheep, horse, guinea pig, rat, mouse, and human, contain at least one glycoprotein with an apparent M_r of over 100,000 (e.g., see Kobylka and Carraway, 1972; Huggins et al., 1980; Shimizu and Yamauchi, 1982; Johnson et al., 1985; data on goat, sheep, horse, and mouse from unpublished results of P.J. Madara and I.H. Mather). These glycoproteins characteristically stain very strongly with the PAS reagent, but poorly if at all with Coomassie Blue. The general lack of reactivity with protein dyes is probably because of the high content of carbohydrate, which in most well-characterized preparations is at least 50%, on a weight basis. These PAS-positive bands appear diffuse and often separate into several components with similar mobilities—which is frequently an indication of microheterogeneity in the composition of the oligosaccharide chains.

In rodents and ungulates, the glycoproteins separate on 10% (w/v) SDS–polyacrylamide gels with apparent M_r values* between 150,000 and 250,000 (e.g., cow and guinea pig; Mather and Keenan, 1975; Johnson et al., 1985; Fig. 2a,c). By contrast, the major glycoproteins of human MFGM barely penetrate into the stacking gel (3–4%, w/v polyacrylamide) and may therefore have M_r values in excess of 500,000 (Shimizu and Yamauchi, 1982; Fig. 2b). Glycoproteins of similarly high

*These estimates are unreliable because glycoproteins containing large quantities of carbohydrate migrate anomalously during SDS–PAGE (Segrest and Jackson, 1972). Comparisons with unglycosylated protein standards are valid only if determinations are made separately in gels containing different concentrations of polyacrylamide. At high concentrations of polyacrylamide, differences in mobility due to carbohydrate are minimized and the glycoproteins approach "ideal" behavior.

M_r have also been identified in monkey milk (cited in Shimizu et al., 1986), suggesting that these proteins may be a characteristic of primates.

Glycoproteins of high M_r that contain large quantities of carbohydrate have been purified from bovine, human, and guinea pig MFGM. The major bovine glycoprotein (PAS-I of Fig. 2a) has been purified to over 90% homogeneity using SDS-PAGE as a criterion of purity (*glycoprotein A*, Cawston et al., 1976; *glycoprotein 2*, Snow et al., 1977). Glycoprotein 2 contained large quantities of carbohydrate (~50% by weight) and sugars characteristic of both O- and N-linked oligosaccharide chains. Apparent M_r values of 70,000–100,000 and 148,000 were determined for glycoproteins 2 and A, respectively (Anderson et al., 1974; Cawston et al., 1976; Snow et al., 1977). Whether these differences are a reflection of the different methods used for estimating M_r or reflect actual differences in the composition of the isolates is unclear. Amino acid analyses for these two preparations were significantly different. This raises questions on the identity of either purified glycoprotein. The band of protein identified as PAS-I in Fig. 2a often appears as multiple components of nearly coincident mobility. Although this heterogeneity is usually ascribed to differences in sugar composition, PAS-I may also consist of more than one peptide chain. It is therefore possible that glycoproteins A and 2 were heterogeneous and contained differing quantities of glycoproteins with approximately similar M_r values. Alternatively, or in addition, the preparations may have been partially hydrolyzed by membrane-associated proteinases during isolation.

To my knowledge, the distribution of bovine PAS-I in cells and tissues has not been determined. This is clearly a glycoprotein that deserves further study.

The glycoproteins of very high M_r in human MFGM were first purified by Shimizu and Yamauchi (1982) and given the name PAS-O because they remain at the origin after SDS-PAGE (Fig. 2b). Apparently similar glycoproteins have now been isolated from human milk by other investigators (Ormerod et al., 1983; Sekine et al., 1985). The high levels of carbohydrate in these preparations and the profile of sugars detected (fucose, galactose, *N*-acetyl glucosamine, *N*-acetyl galactosamine, and sialic acid) are characteristic of mucin-like glycoproteins with oligosaccharide chains primarily bound to the peptide through O linkages to serine and threonine. These two amino acids account for over 20 mol % of the total in the PAS-O preparations of Shimizu and Yamauchi. Biochemical and immunological characterization of PAS-O has been complicated by the glycoprotein's polydisperse character and very high M_r. Of immediate concern is the possibility that the heterogeneity observed is due not only to differences in the number and composition of oligosaccharide chains, but also to the presence of more than one polypeptide. Recently, Shimizu et al. (1986) have shown that the original material identified at the top of polyacrylamide gels can be resolved into at least two components, one with a similar composition to PAS-O and a second component of even higher apparent M_r which has a significantly different amino acid composition. Unlike PAS-O, this second component binds to soybean agglutinin (*Glycine max*) and lacks epitopes, defined by several monoclonal antibodies, that are expressed on PAS-O. Shimizu et al. (1986) have called this second component HM glycoprotein-A (high M_r glycoprotein A) and renamed PAS-O, HM glycoprotein C. HM glycoprotein A contains higher amounts of carbohydrate than PAS-O, although the same sugars are present in approximately the same proportions (see also Fischer et al., 1984).

Both HM glycoproteins A and C also occur in a soluble form in skim milk (Shimizu et al., 1986) together with a third component, HM glycoprotein B, which may be a dimeric form of HM glycoprotein C. Mucin-like glycoprotein has also been isolated from skim milk by Ormerod et al. (1983). The purified preparation termed *epithelial membrane antigen* was markedly heterodisperse with estimated apparent M_r values ranging from 50,000 to 10^6. This preparation may have been partially degraded by proteinases, either in milk or during isolation, and additionally may have contained contaminating proteins. Shimizu et al. (1986) suggested that epithelial membrane antigen may consist of variable mixtures of HM glycoproteins A, B, and C, but the presence of material of comparatively low M_r (Ormerod et al., 1983) suggests the presence of additional polypeptides.

A glycoprotein of high M_r, PAS-I (Fig. 2c), has also recently been purified from guinea pig MFGM (V.G. Johnson, D.E. Greenwalt, and I.H. Mather, unpublished data). Serine and threonine account for approximately 30 mol % of the total amino acids and like the human and bovine glycoproteins, carbohydrate is a major component (at least 30–35% w/w). Preliminary sugar analysis has indicated the presence of galactose, mannose, *N*-acetyl glucosamine, *N*-acetyl galactosamine, and sialic acid, sugars characteristic of both O- and N-linked oligosaccharide chains. Monoclonal antibodies prepared against guinea pig PAS-I (Johnson and Mather, 1985) cross-react with both the human glycoprotein of high M_r (Greenwalt et al., 1985a) and weakly with bovine PAS-I (Johnson and Mather, 1985). At least some epitopes are therefore common to the high M_r glycoproteins of widely different species.

These mucin-like glycoproteins have excited much recent interest because they appear to be differentiation antigens that are highly concentrated in the apical membranes of secretory epithelial cells during

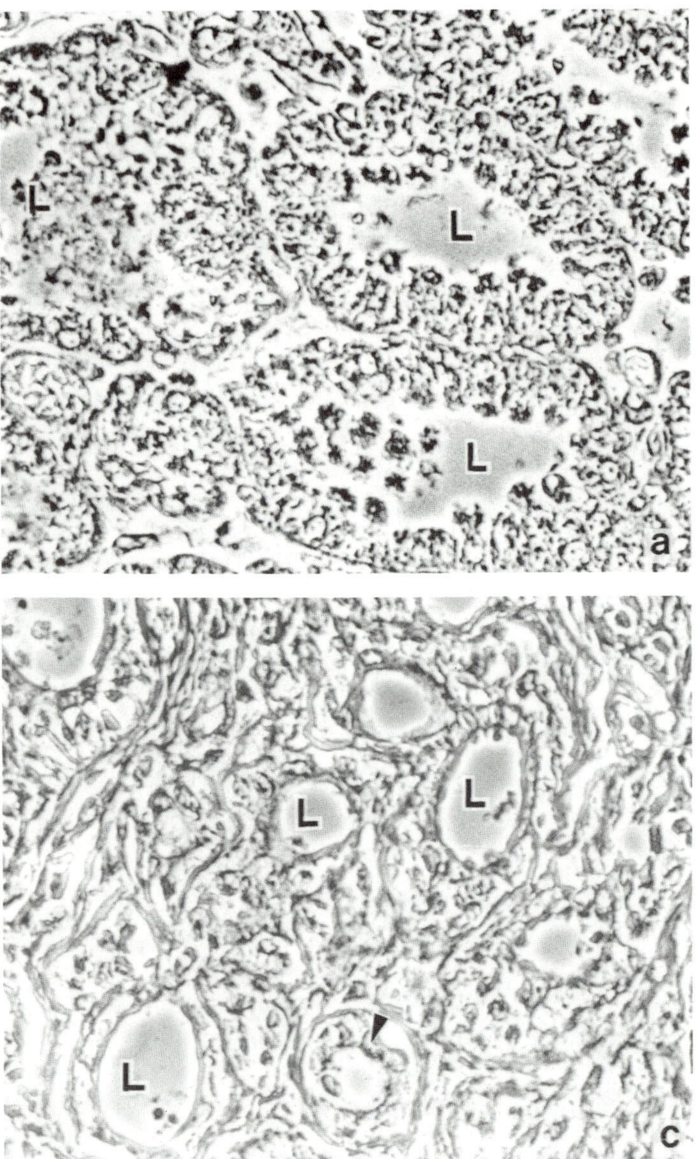

Figure 3. Distribution of the D-274 epitope in (a,b) lactating guinea pig mammary tissue and (c,d) infiltrating duct carcinoma of the human breast. Tissue samples were fixed in methacorn (Warburton et al., 1982) and embedded in paraffin. Dewaxed sections were sequentially incubated with monoclonal antibody D-274, biotinylated horse anti-(mouse IgG), and avidin-fluorescein. (a,b) In lactating guinea pig mammary tissue, apical surfaces of alveolar epithelial cells are intensely fluorescent. Basal regions of secretory cells, myoepithelial cells, and mesenchymal cells are without reaction. (c,d) Specimen of infiltrating duct carcinoma, showing pronounced apical staining of ducts and alveolar-like structures in the section. One duct remains unstained (arrowhead). (a,c) Phase contrast; (b,d) fluorescence; L, lumen. Bar = 50 μm. Micrographs courtesy of V.G. Johnson.

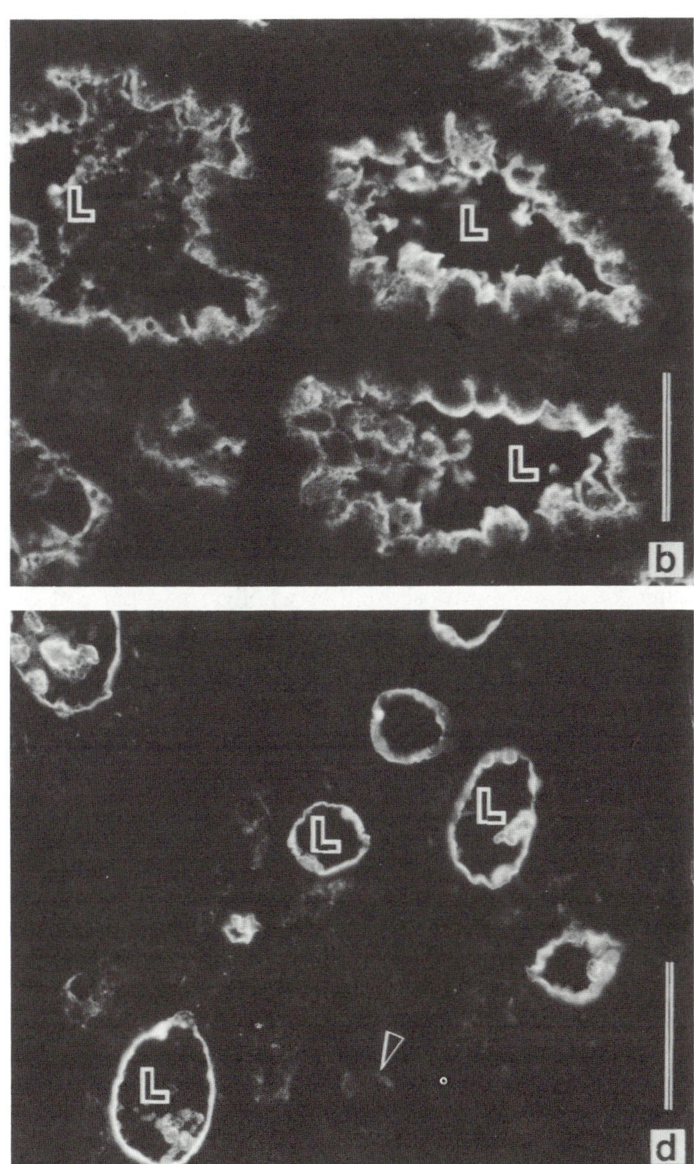

Figure 3. *(Continued)*

lactation (example for guinea pig PAS-I in Fig. 3a,b). No evidence has been obtained for the MFGM mucins in myoepithelial cells, capillary endothelial cells, fibroblasts, or other cells in mammary tissue. In addition, epitopes of the human mucin PAS-O, defined by several monoclonal antibodies, are expressed on the surface and in the cytoplasm and endomembranes of many breast carcinomas. This has raised the possibility of using such antibodies as "tumor markers" in a variety of clinical situations.

Much of this work stems from initial attempts to prepare monoclonal antibodies to human MFGM proteins (Taylor-Papadimitriou et al., 1981; Foster et al., 1982b). Because the MFGM mucins are especially immunogenic in the mouse, a large number of the initial hybrids obtained were found to secrete antibody to these proteins. At least a dozen well-characterized antibodies to the human MFGM mucins have now been described (Taylor-Papadimitriou et al., 1981; Foster et al., 1982b; Ceriani et al., 1983; Ellis et al., 1984; Hilkens et al., 1984; Kufe et al., 1984; Cordell et al., 1985; summarized in Table III), and an antibody prepared against guinea pig MFGM has been used to locate a mucin-associated epitope in human tissues (Greenwalt et al., 1985a).

Many of the epitopes recognized by the characterized antibodies have turned out to be composed either wholly, or in part, of carbohydrate (Table III; Burchell et al., 1983; Gooi et al., 1983; McIlhinney et al., 1985). None of these antibodies has been unambiguously shown to recognize an epitope associated with the peptide chain of any of the MFGM mucins. This is unfortunate because it cannot be assumed that changes observed in the expression of specific carbohydrate epitopes in tissues are due to changes in the levels of the mucin-like glycoproteins per se. Where possible, histochemical studies should be augmented by immunoblotting and peptide mapping techniques to identify the immunoreactive glycoproteins (e.g., see Burchell et al., 1983; Turnbull et al., 1986).

Epitopes recognized by many of the well-characterized antibodies to the high M_r glycoproteins (e.g., HMFG1, HMFG2, LICR LON M8, D-274) are maximally expressed in lactating mammary tissue (e.g., see Fig. 3a,b). Luminal borders of epithelial cells in alveoli and terminal ducts are heavily decorated with antibody. In mammary tissue from virgin guinea pigs, the epitopes recognized by D-16, -40, -256, -274, and -345 (Johnson and Mather, 1985; Table III) are virtually undetectable and in midpregnancy only limited staining of apical surfaces and secretory material in the luminae of alveoli in differentiated areas is observed. Likewise, in resting human breast tissue, mucin-related epitopes are expressed at lower levels than during lactation (e.g., see Arklie et al., 1981; Foster et al., 1982b).

At the resolution of the electron microscope, mucin-associated epitopes defined by monoclonal antibodies 115D8 (Hilkens et al., 1984) and E29 (Cordell et al., 1985) were detected primarily on the glycocalyx of apical membranes in human mammary epithelial cells (Petersen and Van Deurs, 1986). Membranes of the rough endoplasmic reticulum and the Golgi complex also bound either antibody, although the staining intensity was much reduced compared with the luminal surfaces.

None of the epitopes defined by the monoclonal antibodies is specific to the mammary gland, since in every study, reaction with other tissues has been observed. HMFG1, for example, cross-reacts with epithelial cells in bile ducts, pancreatic acinar cells, sebaceous glands, sweat gland, kidney, epididymus, uterus, and the alveoli and bronchioles of the lung (Arklie et al., 1981). HMFG2 showed a similar but not identical pattern and the LICR LON M8 and D-274 epitopes were also detected in a number of tissues other than the mammary gland (Foster et al., 1982b; Greenwalt et al., 1985a). In most tissues, staining was restricted to the exposed luminal borders of epithelia. The 115D8 epitope was detected in over 80% of all epithelia examined (Zotter et al., 1985). However, in the absence of additional biochemical data, the nature of the molecules expressing the specified epitopes in tissues other than mammary gland remains unknown (see Taylor-Papadimitriou et al., 1985, for discussion). Well-characterized antibodies to the peptide chain(s) of the MFGM mucins could be used to determine if there is indeed an apically expressed epithelial mucin, with similar characteristics in different tissues. Claims for such an "epithelial membrane antigen" (Heyderman et al., 1979; Sloane and Ormerod, 1981; Ormerod et al., 1983, 1985) are based on the use of polyclonal antibodies of doubtful specificity.

The identification of epitopes largely restricted to epithelial cells raises the possibility of using such determinants as cell markers in a number of pathological conditions. Although transformation to the malignant state is accompanied by a loss of epithelial characteristics, some properties of the differentiated phenotype may persist, including cell junctions and secretory product (Jamieson et al., 1981), cytokeratins (discussed in Chapter 6 of this volume), and cell surface antigens. Epitopes recognized by HMFG1 and 2, the LICR LON series, the 115D8 series, NCRC-11, E29, and so on are variably expressed in many carcinomas (Arklie et al., 1981; Epenetos et al., 1982; Foster et al., 1982a; Ellis et al., 1984; Hilkens et al., 1984; Kufe et al., 1984; Cordell et al., 1985; Greenwalt et al., 1985a; Lundy et al., 1985; Price et al., 1985; Zotter et al., 1985; Turnbull et al., 1986). In relatively benign conditions such as breast fibrocystic disease, the specified epitopes are associated with apical membranes and secreted luminal material. Such polarized expression persists in some malignant tumors (e.g., Fig. 3c,d) but it is less

Table III. Monoclonal Antibodies to Human MFGM Mucins

Antibody	Isotype	Immunogen	Protein specificity	Epitope
HMFG1[a,b,p]	IgG_1	Human MFGM	High M_r glycoprotein	Carbohydrate sequence possibly containing GlcNAc, Gal, GalNAc?
HMFG2[a,b,q]	IgG_1	Human MFGM boosted with milk epithelial cells	High M_r glycoprotein possibly different from HMFG1	Carbohydrate sequence possibly containing GlcNAc, Gal, GalNAc?, NANA?
LICR LON M8 [c,d]	IgG	Human MFGM	High M_r glycoprotein	Peptide/carbohydrate sequence
LICR LON M18[c,d,e]	IgM	Human MFGM	High M_r glycoprotein, many other proteins	Galβ1→4GlcNAcβ1→
BLMRL-HMFG-Mc5[f]	IgG_1	Human MFGM	High M_r glycoprotein	Not known
115D8[g]	IgG_{2b}	Human MFGM	High M_r glycoprotein	Not known

DF3[h,i]	IgG_1	Human breast carcinoma	High M_r glycoprotein	Peptide/carbohydrate sequence, possibly including GlcNAc and/or NANA
NCRC-11[j,k]	IgM	Human breast carcinoma	Glycoprotein > 400 kDa	Probably carbohydrate
E29[l,m]	Not reported	Human "epithelial membrane antigen"	High M_r glycoproteins 265–400 kDa	Not known
D-16[n]	IgG_1	Guinea pig MFGM	PAS-I in guinea pig and cow, high M_r mucins in human	Not known
D-40, D-256[n,o] D-274, D-345	IgM	Guinea pig MFGM	PAS-I in guinea pig and cow, high M_r mucins in human	Not known

[a]Taylor-Papadimitriou et al. (1981). [b]Burchell et al. (1983). [c]Foster et al. (1982b). [d]McIlhinney et al. (1985). [e]Gooi et al. (1983). [f]Ceriani et al. (1983). [g]Hilkens et al. (1984). [h]Kufe et al. (1984). [i]Sekine et al. (1985). [j]Ellis et al. (1984). [k]Price et al. (1985). [l]Cordell et al. (1985). [m]Heyderman et al. (1985). [n]Johnson and Mather (1985). [o]Greenwalt et al. (1985a). [p]Originally referred to as 1.10.F3. [q]Originally referred to as 3.14.A3.

common, and the epitopes are increasingly detected on intracellular membranes (Petersen and Van Deurs, 1986) and possibly the cytoplasm. Expression is markedly heterogeneous, both in benign and malignant conditions, and both well-stained and entirely negative ducts and alveoli are frequently recognized in adjacent areas of tissue (arrowheads, Fig. 3c,d; for discussion of heterogeneity in epithelial and tumor cells see Edwards, 1985).

In tumor cells, the intracellular location of epitopes normally expressed on apical membranes suggests the disordered processing and/or misdirection of the mucin-like glycoproteins. In support of this concept, some epitopes, for example, HMFG1 and HMFG2, can be detected on components of lower M_r than the terminally processed MFGM mucins in mammary tumors and cell lines (Burchell et al., 1983; Turnbull et al., 1986). These components may be intracellular forms of the high M_r mucins, containing partially completed oligosaccharide chains. If the epitope is contained within these oligosaccharides then not only will intracellular forms of variable size be detected, but also the antibody may bind in increased amounts because the epitope is more accessible. This may explain why some carcinomas apparently express increased amounts of carbohydrate epitopes that are either absent or detected at low levels in the parent epithelia. On the other hand, some epitopes are masked on tumors because of the incorporation of additional sugars. The sugar sequence, Galβ1→4GlcNAcβ1→, is almost entirely cryptic on carcinoma cells because of excess sialylation. Removal of sialic acid with neuraminidase allows binding of antibody to the exposed epitope and reveals expression of this determinant in a heterogeneous fashion throughout the tumors (Foster and Neville, 1984).

Future progress in this area should be rapid given the clinical interest in the human proteins. We need to know more about the chemical nature of the mucins associated with both MFGM and tumor cells, on how many peptide chains are synthesized, and whether these polypeptides are common to epithelia in tissues other than the mammary gland. In addition, further characterization of the MFGM mucins of other species, including ruminants and rodents, should provide interesting comparative data and allow study of the possible function of this group of molecules in terminally differentiated tissues.

3.3. PAS-III

A second glycoprotein, PAS-III (Fig. 2a), which also stains with the PAS reagent but not with Coomassie Blue, is present in the MFGMs of cow, goat, and sheep. In 10% (w/v) polyacrylamide gels, the apparent M_r

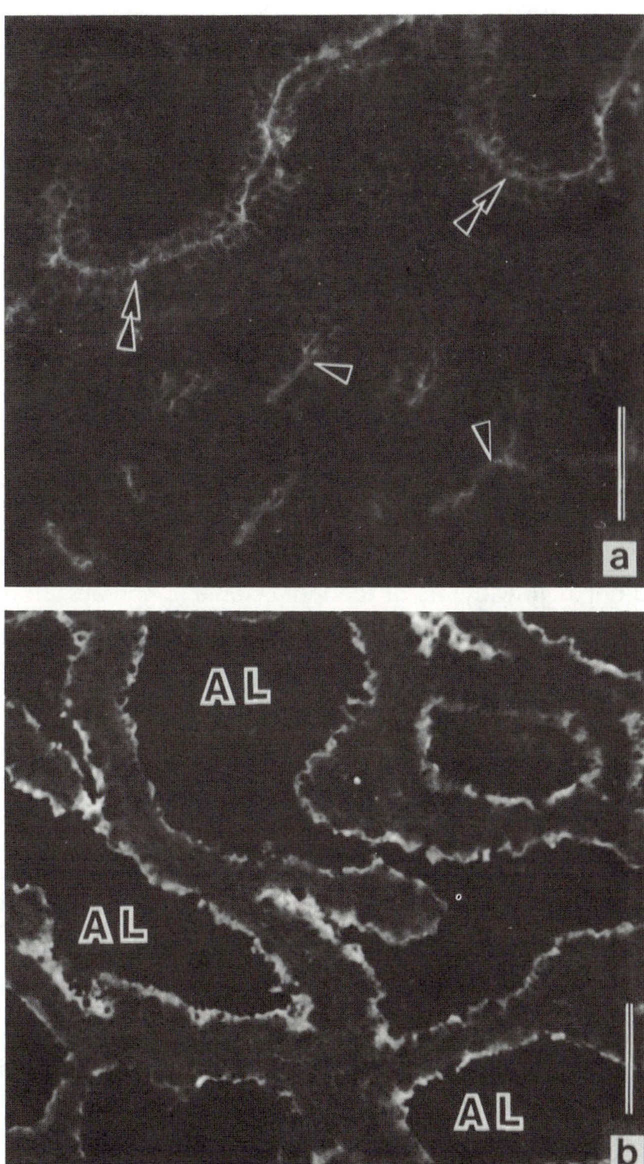

Figure 4. Localization of PAS-III in bovine mammary tissue by immunofluorescence microscopy. Distribution of PAS-III in frozen, acetone-fixed mammary tissue from (a) an 18-month-old heifer and (b) a lactating cow, determined by sequential incubation with monoclonal antibodies A-143 in (a) and A-57 in (b) followed by fluorescein-conjugated rabbit anti-(mouse IgG). (a) Before lactation PAS-III is associated with ducts seen in cross-section (single arrowheads) and longitudinal section (double arrowheads) and there is little staining of mesenchymal cells. (b) During lactation apical surfaces of alveolar epithelial cells are brightly decorated with antibody. AL, alveolar lumen. Bar = 50 μm.

of the bovine protein ranges from 95,000 to over 100,000. Immunoblotting with specific rabbit antibodies indicates that the proteins of caprine and bovine MFGM are immunologically similar and have similar apparent M_r values (P.J. Madara and I.H. Mather, unpublished data). We have been unable to detect PAS-III-like proteins with these antibodies in the MFGMs of horse, human, or guinea pig. Neither the polyclonal antibody nor four monoclonal antibodies to PAS-III showed cross-reactivity with bovine PAS-I, indicating that these two glycoproteins are probably unrelated.

Like the high M_r glycoproteins discussed in Section 3.2, PAS-III is highly concentrated in the apical pole of alveolar secretory cells during lactation (Fig. 4b). At the resolution of the light microscope, there is little evidence for the presence of PAS-III epitopes recognized by monoclonal antibodies A-42, -57, -127, and -143 in basal regions of epithelial cells (example for A-57 in Fig. 4b). Other cells in lactating mammary tissue including capillary endothelial cells, myoepithelial cells, and stromal elements did not stain with any of the monoclonal antibodies. In one sample of mammary tissue from a virgin cow (18-month-old heifer), PAS-III-associated epitopes were detected in epithelial cells lining ducts (Fig. 4a). Although these ductal structures were barely visible in the phase contrast image, the apical surfaces were easily recognizable after decoration with fluorescently labeled antibody. In addition, staining appeared to be specific to epithelial cells. PAS-III-associated epitopes are therefore expressed in relatively undifferentiated mammary tissue and may be used to identify epithelial cells in prelactating ruminant glands.

3.4. Xanthine Oxidase (E.C. 1.2.3.2)

Detection of xanthine oxidase in milk dates from the early days of biological chemistry (Morgan et al., 1923, and references cited therein). The enzyme was first extensively purified from milk by Ball in 1939 and since that time has been purified to homogeneity, crystallized, and widely characterized with respect to substrate specificity and mechanism of enzyme action (reviewed by Bray, 1975; Coughlan, 1980; Hille and Massey, 1985). Xanthine oxidase consists of two monomers with M_r values of approximately 150,000 (Waud et al., 1975) and contains iron–sulfur groups, molybdenum, FAD, and a pterin cofactor. In fat globules, xanthine oxidase is present in both a soluble and a membrane-bound form and approximately 50% of the enzyme is released into the aqueous phase when fat droplets are disrupted to isolate MFGM (Briley and Eisenthal, 1974; Mather et al., 1977; Bruder et al., 1982). At least a fraction of the enzyme in the aqueous phase is truly soluble since it is retained in Sephadex G-200 during gel filtration (Briley and Eisenthal, 1974). Of the enzyme associated with MFGM, 60–80% of the activity can be released by washing membrane fractions with 1.5 *M* KCl and 1% (v/v) Triton X-100 (Bruder et al., 1982). The residual enzyme appears to be tightly membrane bound.

In unwashed bovine MFGM, xanthine oxidase accounts for approximately 13% of the total membrane-associated protein (band 2 of Mather et al., 1980) and after SDS-PAGE it can be identified as a major Coomassie-Blue-positive band of apparent M_r 155,000 (Fig. 2a; Waud et al., 1975; Mangino and Brunner, 1977; Mather et al., 1977). The enzyme does not appear to react with the PAS reagent, indicating that carbohydrate is either absent or present in very low quantities (compare lanes 1 and 2, Fig. 2a). Isoelectric points for the bovine enzyme range from 6.9 to 7.5 (Table II) and anywhere from three to seven isoelectric variants have been detected after analytical or preparative electrofocusing (Jarasch et al., 1981; Bruder et al., 1982; Sullivan et al., 1982).

A similar Coomassie-Blue-positive/PAS-negative protein has been identified in the MFGMs of at least 10 other species after SDS-PAGE (Fig. 2; see also, for human MFGM, Freudenstein et al., 1979; for rat, Huggins et al., 1980; for goat, sheep, and pig, Heid et al., 1983; and for guinea pig, Johnson et al., 1985). By the use of peptide mapping techniques and immunological methods, this protein has been identified as xanthine oxidase in human (Bruder et al., 1983; Heid, 1983) and guinea pig MFGM (Johnson et al., 1985). Furthermore, the similarities in M_r and the isoelectric variants point to the identity of these proteins (Table II). However, in no case other than bovine MFGM has a direct correlation been made between xanthine oxidase activity and the 155,000 M_r protein.

Imam et al. (1982) have described the purification of a glycoprotein, EMGP-155, from human MFGM with an M_r of 155,000. The methods used for isolation included the extraction of human MFGM with 1.5 *M* $MgCl_2$ solutions and the removal of concanavalin-A-binding proteins by lectin-affinity chromatography. In our hands with bovine MFGM, these procedures produce fractions that are highly enriched in xanthine oxidase, and the M_r reported by Imam et al. (1982) tends to agree with this. It is puzzling therefore that the isolated protein was reported to stain strongly with the PAS reagent and contain 21% carbohydrate by weight. A glycoprotein of apparent M_r 140,000 in human MFGM can be resolved from xanthine oxidase by SDS-PAGE (arrowhead, Fig. 2b). It is possible therefore that this was the EMGP-155 glycoprotein isolated. However, in the absence of other data (peptide maps and separation by two-dimensional gel electrophoresis) it is difficult to determine whether this preparation was truly homogeneous or contaminated with xanthine oxidase. The rather insensitive method of immunodiffusion in agarose gels was used as a criterion of purity.

The distribution of xanthine oxidase in cells and tissues has been determined by a combination of immunocytochemistry at the resolution of the light and the electron microscope, and by immunoassays using monospecific polyclonal and monoclonal antibodies (Jarasch et al., 1981; Bruder et al., 1982, 1983). Enzyme was detected in most tissues examined including mammary gland, liver, small intestine, heart, lung, and thymus. In the mammary gland, xanthine oxidase was highly concentrated in the apical cytoplasm of alveolar–epithelial cells during lactation, as might be expected in view of the apical derivation of MFGM. However, the enzyme was also detected throughout the cytoplasm including basal regions of secretory cells and additionally was localized in capillary endothelial cells (Jarasch et al., 1981). The enzyme was absent from the capillary cells of large blood vessels and other mesenchymal cells and myoepithelial cells. In tissues other than mammary gland, xanthine oxidase was concentrated primarily in capillary endothelial cells. Endothelial cells containing the enzyme included those lining the sinusoids of liver, the capillaries of myocardium, and the capillaries of the lamina propria and the lamina muscularis of the small and large intestine. Xanthine oxidase was also detected in thymus, white adipose tissue, and lung. Enzyme was distributed throughout the cytoplasm of endothelial cells in all locations examined and epithelial cells appeared to be without reaction.

These results were surprising because it had always been assumed that the bulk of xanthine oxidase in tissues was present in parenchymal cells. As it turns out, it is only in the secretory cells of mammary tissue during lactation that xanthine oxidase is expressed in epithelial cells in large amounts (Bruder et al., 1983; Ringo and Rocha, 1983). The large concentration of xanthine oxidase in secreted fat globules and isolated MFGM, compared with levels in mammary cells (Mather et al., 1982; Bruder et al., 1983), implies that the enzyme is selectively concentrated in the MFGM during secretion. Limited evidence suggests that xanthine oxidase is concentrated in the protein coat structure of MFGM (Fig. 1a,b). The enzyme is inaccessible to lactoperoxidase-catalyzed iodination reactions in intact washed fat globules (Mather and Keenan, 1975; component 3 of this reference is xanthine oxidase; Patton and Hubert, 1983) and is also inaccessible to specific antibodies, unless the fat globules are disrupted to expose enzyme (Nielsen and Bjerrum, 1977), suggesting an "internal" location. The release of xanthine oxidase into the aqueous phase following disruption of washed fat globules, and the "peripheral" nature of the enzyme in isolated MFGM, also implies that the enzyme is located on the internal "cytoplasmic" face of MFGM in association with the protein coat.

It is reasonable to assume that the accumulation of xanthine oxidase in the protein coat of MFGM is in some way related to a specific function of the enzyme in fat secretion (see Jarasch et al., 1981, for discussion). However, what this function might be is not obvious; neither is the restricted location of the enzyme in capillary endothelial cells in diverse tissues easy to reconcile with the enzyme's biochemical properties.

Despite its secretion from the apical pole of mammary cells, xanthine oxidase is suitable as a marker neither for epithelial cells nor for the apical plasma membrane. However, the enzyme should have great utility as a marker of capillary endothelial cells in many tissues. In addition, the elevated levels of xanthine oxidase activity seen toward the end of pregnancy and during lactation in mammary epithelial cells (Bruder et al., 1983; Ringo and Rocha, 1983) may be used as a biochemical marker of cellular differentiation.

3.5. PAS-IV

PAS-IV (Fig. 2a) is a relatively basic glycoprotein of apparent M_r 76,000 (Table II) which was recently isolated from bovine MFGM (Greenwalt and Mather, 1985). Immunologically similar proteins, with approximately the same M_r values, have also been identified in human and guinea pig MFGM (GP-80 in guinea pig membranes, Fig. 2c). By several criteria, PAS-IV was determined to be an "integral" protein of the MFGM (Fig. 1b). The glycoprotein was resistant to degradation by proteinases in unfractionated membrane but was rapidly degraded when solubilized by detergents, indicating a close association with the membrane bilayer. PAS-IV was recovered from the detergent phase of Triton X-114 solutions at room temperature, which is a property of integral membrane proteins with amphiphilic properties (Bordier, 1981), and amino acid analysis revealed a high proportion of amino acids with nonpolar residues.

By the use of immunofluorescence techniques, the distribution of PAS-IV was determined in a number of tissues including the mammary gland. The glycoprotein was detected in high concentrations on the apical surfaces of secretory epithelial cells in lactating mammary tissue and in apparently lower amounts on lateral and basal plasma membranes (Fig. 5a). Additional staining of basal cells underlying the epithelial pavement was also observed (single arrowheads, Fig. 5a). These cells were identified as capillary endothelial cells by comparing the dis-

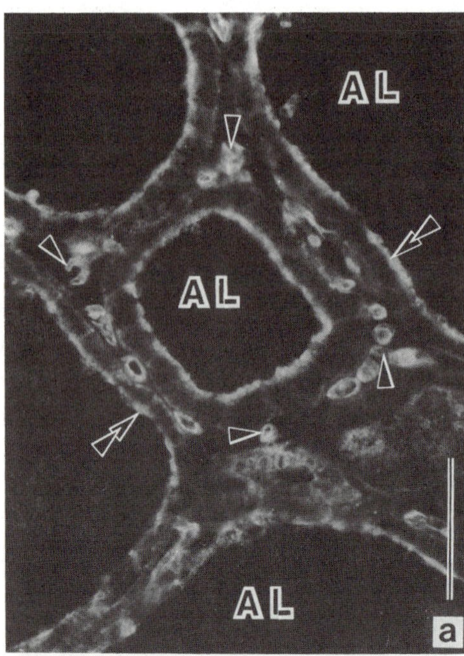

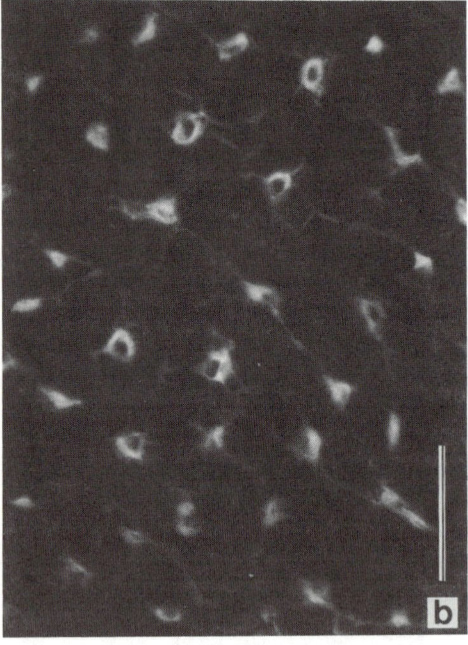

Figure 5. Localization of bovine PAS-IV in (a) mammary gland and (b) heart, determined by immunofluorescence microscopy. (a) Distribution of PAS-IV in methacorn-fixed paraffin-embedded lactating bovine mammary tissue, determined by sequential incubations with affinity-purified rabbit antibodies, biotinylated goat anti-(rabbit IgG), and avidin-fluorescein. Capillary endothelial cells (single arrowheads) and apical membranes of secretory epithelial cells (double arrowheads) are brightly stained. AL, alveolar lumen. Bar = 50 μm. (b) Distribution of PAS-IV in frozen, acetone-fixed bovine heart, determined by sequential incubations with monoclonal antibody E-1, biotinylated horse anti-(mouse IgG), and avidin-fluorescein. Capillary cells throughout the myocardium are brightly fluorescent. Bar = 50 μm. Full experimental details are in Greenwalt and Mather (1985) and Greenwalt et al. (1985b). Micrographs courtesy of D.E. Greenwalt.

tribution of PAS-IV with factor VIII antigen, a widely used marker for endothelia. In other tissues, PAS-IV appeared to be almost exclusively located in capillaries (example for heart in Fig. 5b). In one exception, the apical surfaces of the epithelial cells of lung bronchioles were intensely stained and the endothelium was without reaction. Immunoblotting and peptide mapping techniques confirmed that the immunoreactive proteins in MFGM, heart, and lung were very similar (Greenwalt et al., 1985b).

Unlike xanthine oxidase and factor VIII antigen, PAS-IV is firmly bound to membranes. This makes the glycoprotein an ideal marker for identifying endothelial cells, especially in heterogeneous populations of dispersed cells obtained for biochemical studies from solid tissues. Whether PAS-IV is expressed in long-term cultures of endothelial cells is uncertain. Preliminary tests with endothelial cell cultures indicated that unfortunately it probably is not (I.H. Mather and P.M. Gullino, unpublished data).

3.6. Butyrophilin

The major Coomassie-Blue-positive protein of bovine MFGM is an acidic glycoprotein of M_r 67,000 comprised of four variants, with isoelectric points from pH 5.2 to 5.3 (Fig. 2a, lane 2; Table II). This glycoprotein, originally assigned the numbers band V (Kobylka and Carraway, 1972) or component 12 (Mather and Keenan, 1975), was given the name butyrophilin* by Franke et al. (1981) to describe its pronounced hydrophobic properties. Repeated extraction of MFGM with solutions containing nonionic detergents or high concentrations of salt leads to enrichment of this protein in the insoluble residue, at the expense of more "peripheral" components of the membrane (Mather et al., 1977; Freudenstein et al., 1979). Similarly, insoluble proteins with M_r values in the range 63,000–68,000 and with relatively acidic isoelectric points have been identified in the MFGMs of several other species, for example, human, sheep, goat, and pig (Heid et al., 1983). The two-dimensional maps of the four bovine variants are virtually identical and they show many similarities to variants of the human protein (Heid, 1983; Heid et al., 1983). Immunological similarities between the proteins of bovine, caprine, and ovine MFGM have also been reported (Freudenstein et al., 1979; Franke et al., 1981). In addition, the MFGMs of rat and guinea pig contain proteins of approximately similar M_r, but

*Meaning "associated with milk fat" or "having affinity to milk fat." From the Greek *butyros*, for butter, and *philos*, having affinity for.

with rather more basic isoelectric points. Despite these differences, the peptide maps of the bovine and guinea pig proteins are similar, but not identical (Heid et al., 1983; Johnson et al., 1985), and the monoclonal antibody D-120 which binds to the guinea pig protein cross-reacts with bovine butyrophilin (Johnson and Mather, 1985). For these reasons, Heid et al. (1983) suggested that the name butyrophilin be extended to the proteins of all these species.

Because butyrophilin has been identified from electrophoretic profiles and has no known enzyme function, it is important to establish that the protein is unrelated to other MFGM proteins within the same species. Evidence for at least one presumptive proteolytic fragment of butyrophilin, of slightly lower M_r, in the MFGMs of several species (e.g., see Fig. 2 and legend) and possible aggregates of butyrophilin have been reported (Heid et al., 1983; Basch et al., 1985). However, in most cases, the other major proteins of bovine MFGM are distinctly different from butyrophilin, at least using peptide mapping and immunological comparisons as criteria (Franke et al., 1981; Heid, 1983).

Bovine butyrophilin has been purified and characterized (Freudenstein et al., 1979; Franke et al., 1981; Keenan et al., 1982). The protein contains glutamate (or glutamine), aspartate (or asparagine), threonine, valine, leucine, and glycine as principal amino acids (Freudenstein et al., 1979) and 1–2 moles of tightly bound (possibly covalently linked) fatty acid per mole of protein (Keenan et al., 1982). It is not immediately obvious from the amino acid composition why butyrophilin has such hydrophobic properties. Possibly, the protein contains a limited transmembrane sequence of amino acids containing nonpolar residues that are associated with the lipid bilayer. Alternatively, the presence of tightly bound fatty acids may confer hydrophobic characteristics to the protein.

Two analyses for the carbohydrate content of bovine butyrophilin indicated the presence of glucosamine (probably *N*-acetyl glucosamine), mannose, glucose, galactose, and fucose (Freudenstein et al., 1979; Heid et al., 1983). Galactosamine and sialic acid were also detected in one preparation (Freudenstein et al., 1979), although this was not confirmed in a later study from the same group (Heid et al., 1983). Treatment of butyrophilin with neuraminidase had no effect on the isoelectric points of the variants, also indicating that sialic acid is probably absent, and analysis of human butyrophilin revealed a similar sugar composition (Heid et al., 1983).

Imam et al. (1981) also purified a protein from human MFGM, EMGP-70, with a similar apparent M_r (70,000) to butyrophilin. However, the identity of this protein remains uncertain. An almost quantitative yield of soluble protein was obtained by extracting washed human cream with solutions containing 1.5 *M* $MgCl_2$. These are conditions previously shown to extract *loosely associated proteins* from bovine MFGM, leaving butyrophilin (or band 12) in the insoluble fraction (Mather and Keenan, 1975). Comparisons of the amino acid and sugar compositions also showed differences (Freudenstein et al., 1979; Imam et al., 1981; Heid et al., 1983), and the reported isoelectric points (pH 6.0–6.4, Imam et al., 1984) were more basic than those reported by Heid et al. (1983) for human butyrophilin. It is unfortunate that these preparations have not been compared directly by peptide mapping and immunological techniques.

By the use of immunofluorescence and electron microscopy, the distribution of bovine butyrophilin was determined in lactating mammary tissue (Franke et al., 1981). The apical surfaces of alveolar epithelial cells were brightly decorated with fluorescently labeled antibody and at the resolution of the electron microscope, antigen appeared concentrated in the protein coat of budding lipid droplets, and on the apical plasma membrane. No evidence of butyrophilin in the basal cytoplasm of secretory epithelial cells, myoepithelial cells, or mesenchymal cells was observed. Butyrophilin appears specific to lactating mammary tissue, since the antigen was not detected in the glands of 6-month-old or 18-month-old virgin cows, or in bovine liver, intestine, heart, thymus, brain, or white adipose tissue.

We have found a similar distribution for butyrophilin in guinea pig mammary tissue using four monoclonal antibodies, D-120, -263, -271, and -387 (Johnson and Mather, 1985), and affinity-purified rabbit antibodies (Fig. 6). The accumulation of butyrophilin in the apical surface (Fig. 6a), especially in areas associated with budding lipid droplets (Fig. 6b,c), may be seen to advantage by the use of colloidal gold–protein A conjugates and electron microscopy. In isolated MFGM (Fig. 6d,e), butyrophilin appears to be associated both with the lipid bilayer (small open arrowheads) and the protein coat (single closed arrowheads), although some areas of the coat appear unreactive with antibody (double arrowheads).

The presence of butyrophilin in a protein coat contiguous with the cytoplasm is at variance with the general observation that the carbohydrate moieties of glycoproteins are associated with the external surfaces of plasma membranes (Hirano et al., 1972). To explain this, Freudenstein et al. (1979) suggested that butyrophilin is either added directly to the apical membrane from *nonmembranous cytoplasmic components* (an unconventional viewpoint) or is derived from the apical plasma membrane, following the rearrangement of integral membrane proteins during the budding of lipid droplets. This latter view is in agreement with freeze-

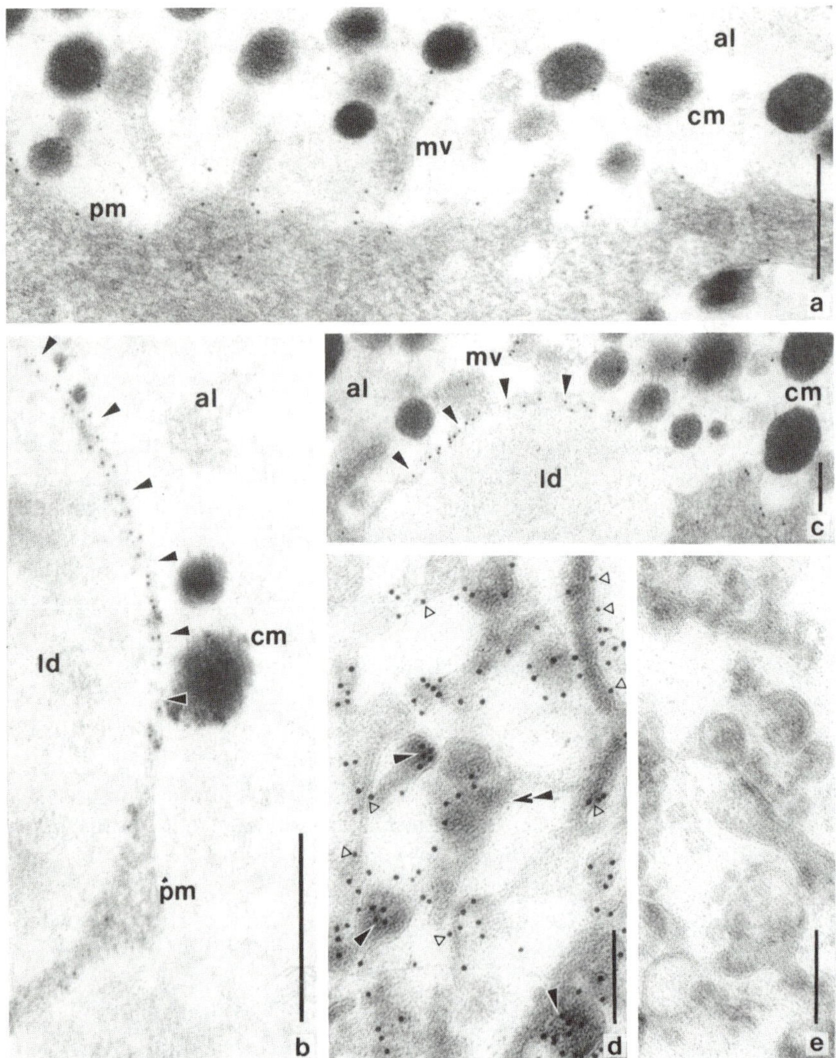

Figure 6. Localization of guinea pig butyrophilin in lactating mammary gland and MFGM by electron microscopy. Lactating guinea pig mammary tissue and isolated MFGM were fixed in glutaraldehyde and embedded in Lowicryl. Sections of tissue were sequentially incubated with affinity-purified rabbit antibody to butyrophilin and protein A–colloidal gold (10nm). (a) Butyrophilin is present in the apical surface of secretory cells, including microvilli, and is especially concentrated (b,c) in areas where the apical surface is most closely associated with budding lipid droplets (arrowheads). (d) In isolated MFGM, butyrophilin appears to be associated both with the lipid bilayer (small open arrowheads) and the protein coat (single closed arrowheads), although some areas of the protein coat are unlabeled (double arrowheads). (e) Specimens successively treated with fractionated serum from unimmunized rabbits and protein A–colloidal gold remain unlabeled. al, Alveolar lumen; cm, casein micelle; ld, lipid droplet; mv, microvillus; pm, plasma membrane. Bars = 0.5 μm in (a) and (b) and 0.2 μm in (c), (d), and (e).

fracture studies, which have shown that the characteristic intramembranous particles associated with fractured surfaces of apical plasma membrane are absent in areas of membrane that are in direct contact with budding lipid droplets (Peixotes de Menezes and Pinto da Silva, 1978; Zerban and Franke, 1978). These particles may be cleared from the bilayer surrounding lipid droplets by exclusion in the lateral plane of the membrane, in which case they would be expelled entirely from MFGM (which is clearly not possible in the case of butyrophilin). Alternatively, they may be "extracted" in a longitudinal direction toward the closely apposed hydrophobic lipid droplets and become an integral component of the coat (Fig. 7a). The apparent increase in the amount of butyrophilin surrounding fat droplets compared with the apical plasma membrane (compare Fig. 6a with b and c) may therefore be a consequence of the increased accessibility of antibody to epitopes of butyrophilin in the protein coat. Another possibility is that butyrophilin is "recruited" or "capped" by fat droplets during the budding process (Fig. 7b) and then incorporated into the protein coat. Either or both phenomena may be a cause or an effect of lipid droplet secretion.

Apart from butyrophilin, rearrangement of many of the other components of the apical surface may occur during the secretion of lipid

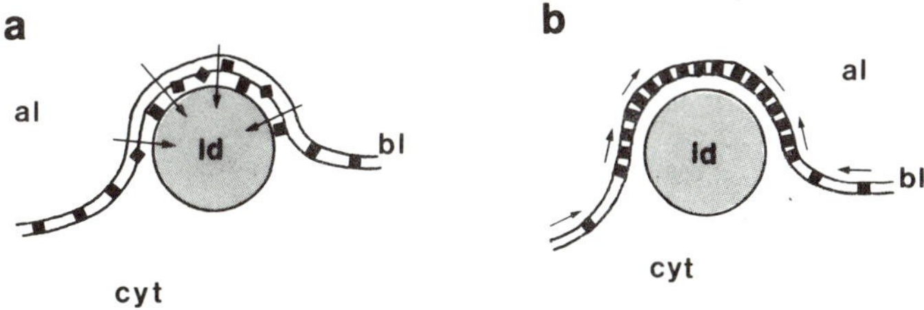

Figure 7. Possible schemes to explain the distribution of butyrophilin and the formation of the protein coat of MFGM during the budding of milk-fat droplets from the apical plasma membrane. Membrane proteins in the figure are indicated by squares (■). (a) In areas of membrane that are not associated with intracellular lipid droplets, the proteins are true integral components of the bilayer. Following or during apposition of fat droplets with the apical surface, a local rearrangement of membrane constituents occurs and membrane proteins are either partially or completely "extracted" (arrows) from the bilayer and become components of the protein coat. The increased labeling of the apical surface in areas in contact with budding lipid droplets (Fig. 6b,c) is seen to be a consequence of the increased accessibility of antibody to exposed epitopes. Not shown is the possibility that xanthine oxidase from the cytoplasm becomes associated with the protein coat during this process, see text. (b) As the fat droplets approach the apical membrane, butyrophilin and other membrane proteins may accumulate around the droplets by lateral movement (arrows) within the plane of the bilayer ("capping"). The possibilities in (a) and (b) are not mutually exclusive. Either phenomenon could be a cause or a result of lipid droplet secretion. al, Alveolar lumen; bl, bilayer; cyt, cytoplasm; ld, lipid droplet.

droplets. Deeney et al. (1985) effectively stripped off the bilayer membrane from fat droplets by controlled homogenization and obtained a fraction of bovine lipid globules that were still partially covered with elements of the protein coat. Analysis of these fractions showed marked enrichment in many of the major MFGM proteins, including butyrophilin.

This discussion is important to those interested in MFGM proteins as membrane markers, because the presence of a protein coat, which was presumed to be derived predominantly from the cytoplasm (Wooding, 1971a), cast considerable doubt in the minds of many investigators on the identity of MFGM proteins as integral components of the membrane bilayer. With the exception of xanthine oxidase, such concern may be misfounded because many of the membrane proteins, including butyrophilin, are firmly bound to intracellular membranes (Mather et al., 1984; P.J. Madara and I.H. Mather, unpublished data) and are probably only incorporated into the protein coat of MFGM during secretion of lipid droplets from the cell.

Butyrophilin is a marker of differentiation in mammary cells, since it is expressed at high levels during lactation but not during pregnancy (Franke et al., 1981; Heid et al., 1983). This raises the possibility of using butyrophilin as a marker of differentiation in human breast tumors, in an analogous manner to the work with the high M_r mucins of MFGM. However, I know of no such studies. Imam and co-workers (Imam and Tökés, 1981; Imam et al., 1984) have described the distribution of the EMGP-70 glycoprotein in normal mammary cells and malignant breast tumors. EMGP-70 was localized on the apical surfaces of mammary cells in resting and lactating breast tissue and in benign lesions. In tumor cells, the glycoprotein was heterogeneously distributed on cell membranes and in intracellular locations, in an analogous fashion to the PAS-O epitopes discussed in Section 3.2. However, the localization of EMGP-70 in nonlactating cells and the discrepancies in the composition of this glycoprotein, when compared with butyrophilin, raise considerable doubt as to its identity.

3.7. Glycoprotein B, Bovine-Associated Mucoprotein (BAMP), and GP-55

A number of fractions have been prepared from bovine MFGM enriched in glycoproteins with estimated M_r values from 43,000 to 55,000 (Butler and Oskvig, 1974; Mather and Keenan, 1975; Basch et al., 1976; Keenan et al., 1977; Butler et al., 1980; Pringnitz et al., 1985). Many of these preparations consist of two components with closely spaced M_r values, which share some identical immunological properties

(Mather et al., 1980) and tryptic peptides (Johnson et al., 1985). Because of these similarities, it has proved difficult to separate the individual glycoproteins by a number of chromatographic techniques. These glycoproteins, termed bands 15/16 (Fig. 2a; Mather and Keenan, 1975), are released into the soluble phase on treatment of washed fat globules with 1.5 *M* $MgCl_2$ solutions. Studies with lactoperoxidase and ^{125}I showed that bands 15/16 are readily iodinated in intact fat globules, suggesting that they are present on the globule surface (Mather and Keenan, 1975).

Whether such surface-associated components are present on the MFGMs of other species remains to be established. Human MFGM contains variable quantities of peptides with similar apparent M_r values (Fig. 2b), and the most prominent Coomassie-Blue-positive component of guinea pig MFGM, GP-55, is a glycoprotein of M_r 55,000 (Fig. 2c), which may have some similarities to bands 15/16 (Johnson et al., 1985).

Basch et al. (1976) purified a glycoprotein with an apparent M_r of 49,500 from bovine MFGM, termed glycoprotein B, which appears to be related, if not identical, to bands 15/16 (Basch et al., 1985). Glycoprotein B contained 14.3% (w/v) carbohydrate including mannose, galactose, glucose, glucosamine, galactosamine, and *N*-acetyl neuraminic acid, suggesting the presence of both N- and O-linked oligosaccharides. The amino acid composition was similar to a glycoprotein doublet purified by Keenan et al. (1977), with estimated M_r values of 48,000 and 50,000, suggesting that these preparations were enriched in the same polypeptides.

In separate studies, Butler and colleagues described the preparation of rabbit antisera to so-called, bovine-associated mucoprotein (BAMP). This glycoprotein complex was originally isolated by Jackson et al. (1962), by extracting $(NH_4)_2SO_4$-precipitated bovine MFGM with organic solvents and releasing a soluble complex from the defatted residue with distilled water. By the criteria of the times, the preparation was reasonably pure, although at least two contaminating whey proteins were identified by immunological techniques (Coulson and Jackson, 1962). More recent studies have shown the preparation to be markedly heterogeneous, but nevertheless a considerable enrichment of bands 15/16 is present and these can be purified as a complex (Pringnitz et al., 1985). Antibody to the original preparation of Jackson et al. (1962) was used to determine the tissue distribution of BAMP (Butler and Oskvig, 1974; Butler et al., 1980). Staining of all surfaces of bovine mammary epithelial cells, especially the apical surfaces, was detected by the use of immunofluorescence techniques. Fluorescence was also detected on the surfaces of salivary gland, in bronchoalveolar secretions, and many other adult and some fetal bovine tissues. Most interestingly, *human* tumors (e.g., breast carcinomas, optic melanoma, retinal blastoma, thyroid carcinoma) and some fetal epithelial cells were strongly positive even though antigen was not detected in disease-free human tissues. Precipitating antibodies to BAMP were isolated from the sera of patients with cancer and some conditions caused by autoimmune phenomena (e.g., systemic lupus erythematosis). These data were interpreted as evidence that bovine BAMP is immunologically related to a human carcinoembryonic antigen (incidentally distinct from the widely characterized carcinoembryonic antigen, and α-fetoprotein). In pathological conditions, this fetal antigen appears to be expressed on cell surfaces and leads to the generation of autoantibodies. With the advent of more sensitive methods for determining the specificity of antisera, it will be interesting to determine if indeed there is one BAMP-related human antigen or whether the rabbit antisera contained antibodies to epitopes expressed on several, otherwise unrelated, molecules.

The tissue distribution of glycoprotein GP-55 of guinea pig MFGM (Fig. 2c), which may be related to bands 15/16 (Johnson et al., 1985), has been little studied. Epitopes recognized by monoclonal antibodies D-3, -101, -110, and -248 appear concentrated in the apical pole of mammary epithelial cells during lactation but are absent from tissue taken even in late pregnancy (Johnson and Mather, 1985). This glycoprotein may therefore be yet another example of a differentiation-specific antigen of MFGM and mammary cells. However, the suitability of this glycoprotein as a cell marker may be compromised by the occurrence of both soluble and membrane-bound forms in both cells and milk (Mather et al., 1984), properties also shared by bovine bands 15/16 (BAMP) (Pringnitz et al., 1985).

3.8. Comment on Antibody Specificity

In the quest for specific epithelial or mammary markers, several investigators have used unfractionated MFGM as a source of immunogen for preparing polyclonal antibodies (usually in rabbits). These antisera were then made "specific" by absorption protocols against dissimilar antigens (Ceriani et al., 1977; Heyderman et al., 1979; Sasaki et al., 1981) or used without further treatment (Warburton et al., 1982). By the use of such techniques, claims were made for the preparation of antibodies specific for mammary cells (Ceriani et al., 1977, 1982; Sasaki et al., 1981), or epithelial cells (Heyderman et al., 1979; Ormerod et al., 1983). However, in no case has convincing data on the biochemical specificity of these antibodies been published. Major problems include identifying which "dissimilar" antigens to use for the absorption protocols and how to remove antibodies to carbohydrate epitopes that are widely distributed in nature. Since carbohydrates are especially immunogenic (e.g., see Alexander and Elder, 1984), a high proportion of the antibodies in polyclonal antisera may recognize oligosaccharide determinants. In addition, it is obvious from previous sections that several MFGM proteins are widely distributed in tissues other than the mammary gland and are expressed in mesenchymal cells as well as cells of ectodermal origin (xanthine oxidase and PAS-IV). It is therefore difficult to see how antibodies to unfractionated MFGM, which contains a multitude of different epitopes, can be made sufficiently specific to be of practical use. With the advent of highly sensitive immunoblotting and peptide mapping techniques, it should be possible to test these antisera against a panel of membrane and tissue fractions and to determine their specificities with some confidence.

4. Conclusions

Specific MFGM proteins are potentially useful as markers of mammary tissue, mammary epithelial cells, and the apical surface of these cells. In addition, some proteins are specific to lactating mammary tissue and may therefore be useful as differentiation markers. Other proteins are expressed in cells other than mammary epithelial cells, most notably endothelial cells of capillaries in many tissues. In this concluding section, some points about these proteins are worth emphasizing:

1. With the exception of xanthine oxidase, MFGM proteins have been identified as bands of denatured protein by SDS-PAGE. It therefore behooves the investigator to establish that proteins purified from MFGM are biochemically unrelated, for example, as proteolytic fragments of the same protein, and that the proteins have not been previously characterized from other sources. The major MFGM mucins, PAS-IV, butyrophilin, and bands 15/16 appear to be biochemically unrelated to each other and to xanthine oxidase. Whether these proteins have been independently identified and previously characterized from tissues other than the mammary gland is more difficult to establish. Certainly, butyrophilin appears unique to mammary tissue and is unlike other well-characterized mammary proteins, and PAS-IV and bands 15/16 or BAMP are different from other potentially similar proteins (Butler et al., 1980; Greenwalt and Mather, 1985).

2. The derivation of MFGM from *terminally differentiated cells* places some significant limitations on the kind of protein marker that can be isolated. The high M_r mucins, xanthine oxidase, PAS-III, PAS-IV, butyrophilin, and GP-55 are all maximally expressed during lactation and are absent or present at much lower concentrations in the epithelial cells of glands from virgin or pregnant animals. Expression of these antigens correlates to varying degrees with the extent of mammary differentiation. Most MFGM antigens will therefore be either differentiation specific or expressed at several stages of mammary development including lactation. Theoretically, it should be possible to isolate antigens from colostral membranes, which may be specific to mammary cells during pregnancy. However, the chances of identifying such *stage-specific* antigens in colostral fat-globule membrane are remote because copious fat synthesis and secretion only occur in terminally differentiated cells (e.g., see Chatterton et al., 1975). In addition, the *prepartum* removal of colostrum rapidly changes the composition and nature of the secretion to that of "normal" milk (Linzell and Peaker, 1974), including components of the MFGM (D.S. Armstrong and I.H. Mather, unpublished data), which further reduces the chance of identifying pregnancy-specific proteins.

There is also no possibility of identifying a marker specific to mammary tumors. The most that can be hoped for is a protein, like the high M_r mucins, that carries epitopes which are still expressed in malignant cells. Potentially promising approaches for the identification of "malignant cell markers" include the production of antibody-secreting hybrids by fusion of myeloma cells with lymphocytes from breast cancer patients (Schlom et al., 1980) and the use of membranes from metastatic tumor cells as a source of antigens for the preparation of specific antibodies (Nuti et al., 1982).

3. The only mammary-specific MFGM protein characterized to date appears to be butyrophilin. Other proteins including xanthine oxidase and PAS-IV and possibly bands 15/16 or BAMP are widely distributed in other organs. MFGM also contains histocompatability antigens (Wiman et al., 1979; Newman et al., 1980) and many enzymes such as 5′-nucleotidase, phosphodiesterase, and alkaline phosphatase (reviewed by Anderson and Cawston, 1975; Patton and Keenan, 1975; McPherson and Kitchen, 1983) that are common to many cells and tissues. The specific expression of butyrophilin in lactating mammary gland and its association with budding lipid droplets imply that this protein may function in the process of lipid secretion, although all the evidence for this is circumstantial. Butyrophilin deserves further study, not only in relation

to possible function but also as a potential mammary-specific marker that could be used to identify human breast carcinoma cells.

4. Several MFGM proteins appear specific to epithelial cells. These include the high M_r mucins, butyrophilin, and bands 15/16 or BAMP. Since butyrophilin and the mucins are expressed in mammary cells in culture (Lee et al., 1984; Edwards et al., 1984), these proteins may be useful for identifying epithelial cells in heterogeneous populations in vitro (e.g., as in organ culture or cultures on floating collagen gels).

5. MFGM may be derived from elements of the rough endoplasmic reticulum, secretory vesicle membranes, and the cytoplasm, as well as the apical plasma membrane. The use of MFGM proteins as apical markers should therefore be circumscribed by a rigorous demonstration that individual proteins are concentrated in the apical surface and are largely absent from intracellular membranes and the cytoplasm. Localization of MFGM antigens at the resolution of the electron microscope is essential for this purpose. Using this criterion, butyrophilin (Franke et al., 1981; Fig. 6) and the high M_r mucins (Petersen and Van Deurs, 1986) are the only major MFGM proteins that appear to be associated predominantly with apical plasma membranes. Xanthine oxidase is present in the cytoplasm of both mammary epithelial and endothelial cells and PAS-IV is associated with basal and lateral plasma membranes and endothelial cell surfaces. Judging from the immunofluorescence data, PAS-III (Fig. 4) may largely be concentrated in apical surfaces, although the distribution of this protein has not been studied at the resolution of the electron microscope.

MFGM proteins are a diverse group of molecules sharing one common characteristic—by accident of birth they are all derived from mammary epithelial cells. The ready availability of MFGM proteins provides the investigator with a unique source of epithelial proteins. We need to know more about the possible functions of these proteins in the mammary gland and other tissues, and details of the biosynthesis and processing of MFGM proteins and how their expression in mammary cells is regulated. With the advent of molecular cloning techniques, a detailed description of specific MFGM components will be possible which should remove some of the current uncertainties about the nature and identity of these proteins.

Acknowledgments: I thank Dr. Werner W. Franke and Frau Caecilia Kuhn of the German Cancer Research Center, Heidelberg, F.R.G., for introducing me to the technique of immunofluorescence microscopy which has played such an essential role in our recent work. Part of the preliminary data on PAS-III discussed in Section 3.3 and Fig. 4 were gathered while the author was on sabbatical leave in Dr. Franke's laboratory. My colleagues, Dr. Virginia G. Johnson and Dr. Dale E. Greenwalt, are gratefully acknowledged for permission to reproduce the photomicrographs in Figs. 1, 3, and 5 and I thank Ms. Patricia J. Madara for her unfailing technical assistance. I am also indebted to Ms. Margaret Kempf for all secretarial help. The work from my laboratory discussed in this chapter was funded in part by grants PCM 79-13403, PCM 82-03936, and DCB 85-13333 from the National Science Foundation. This paper is Scientific Article No. A-4514, Contribution No. 7507 of the Maryland Agricultural Experiment Station, Department of Animal Sciences.

References

Alexander, S., and Elder, J.H., 1984, Carbohydrate dramatically influences immune reactivity of antisera to viral glycoprotein antigens, *Science* **226:**1328–1330.

Anderson, M., and Brooker, B.E., 1975, Loss of material during the isolation of milk fat globule membrane, *J. Dairy Sci.* **58:**1442–1448.

Anderson, M., and Cawston, T.E., 1975, Reviews of the progress of dairy science. The milk-fat globule membrane, *J. Dairy Res.* **42:**459–483.

Anderson, M., Cawston, T., and Cheeseman, G.C., 1974, Molecular-weight estimates of milk-fat-globule–membrane protein–sodium dodecyl sulphate complexes by electrophoresis in gradient acrylamide gels, *Biochem. J.* **139:**653–660.

Arklie, J., Taylor-Papadimitriou, J., Bodmer, W., Egan, M., and Millis, R., 1981, Differentiation antigens expressed by epithelial cells in the lactating breast are also detectable in breast cancers, *Int. J. Cancer* **28:**23–29.

Ball, E.G., 1939, Xanthine oxidase: Purification and properties, *J. Biol. Chem.* **128:**51–67.

Bargmann, W., and Knoop, A., 1959, Über die Morphologie der Milchsekretion Licht- und Elektronenmikroskopische Studien an der Milchdrüse der Ratte, *Z. Zellforsch.* **49:**344–388.

Bargmann, W., Fleischhauer, K., and Knoop, A., 1961, Über die Morphologie der Milchsekretion. II Zugleich eine Kritik am Schema der Sekretionsmorphologie, *Z. Zellforsch.* **53:**545–568.

Basch, J.J., Farrell, H.M., and Greenberg, R., 1976, Identification of the milk fat globule membrane proteins I. Isolation and partial characterization of glycoprotein B, *Biochim. Biophys. Acta* **448:**589–598.

Basch, J.J., Greenberg, R., and Farrell, H.M., 1985, Identification of the milk fat globule membrane proteins. II. Isolation of major proteins from electrophoretic gels and comparison of their amino acid compositions, *Biochim. Biophys. Acta* **830:**127–135.

Bauman, D.E., and Davis, C.L., 1974, Biosynthesis of milk fat, in: *Lactation, A Comprehensive Treatise,* Vol. II (B.L. Larson and V.R. Smith, eds.), Academic Press, New York, pp. 31–75.

Bordier, C., 1981, Phase separation of integral membrane proteins in Triton X-114 solution, *J. Biol. Chem.* **256:**1604–1607.

Bray, R.C., 1975, Molybdenum iron–sulfur flavin hydroxylases and related enzymes, in: *The Enzymes,* Vol. XII (P.D. Boyer, ed.), 3rd ed., Academic Press, New York, pp. 299–419.

Briley, M.S., and Eisenthal, R., 1974, Association of xanthine oxidase with the bovine milk-fat-globule membrane. Catalytic properties of the free and membrane-bound enzyme, *Biochem. J.* **143:**149–157.

Bruder, G., Heid, H., Jarasch, E.-D., Keenan, T.W., and Mather, I.H., 1982, Characteristics of membrane-bound and soluble forms of xanthine oxidase from milk and endothelial cells of capillaries, *Biochim. Biophys. Acta* **701:**357–369.

Bruder, G., Heid, H.W., Jarasch, E.-D., and Mather, I.H., 1983, Immunological identification and determination of xanthine oxidase in cells and tissues, *Differentiation* **23:**218–225.

Brunner, J.R., 1969, Milk lipoproteins, in: *Structural and Functional Aspects of Lipoproteins in Living Systems* (E. Tria and A.M. Scanu, eds.), Academic Press, New York, pp. 545–578.

Burchell, J., Durbin, H., and Taylor-Papadimitriou, J., 1983, Complexity of expression of antigenic determinants, recognized by monoclonal antibodies HMFG-1 and HMFG-2, in normal and malignant human mammary epithelial cells, *J. Immunol.* **131:**508–513.

Butler, J.E., and Oskvig, R., 1974, Cancer, autoimmunity and IgA-deficiency related by a common antigen–antibody system, *Nature* **249:**830–832.

Butler, J.E., Pringnitz, D.J., Martens, C.L., and Crouch, N., 1980, Bovine-associated mucoprotein. I. Distribution among adult and fetal bovine tissues and body fluids, *Differentiation* **17:**31–40.

Cawston, T.E., Anderson, M., and Cheeseman, G.C., 1976, Isolation, preparation and the amino acid composition of 4 milk-fat globule membrane proteins solubilized by treatment with sodium dodecyl sulphate, *J. Dairy Res.* **43:**401–409.

Ceriani, R.L., Thompson, K., Peterson, J.A., and Abraham, S., 1977, Surface differentiation antigens of human mammary epithelial cells carried on the human milk fat globule, *Proc. Natl. Acad. Sci. USA* **74:**582–586.

Ceriani, R.L., Sasaki, M., Sussman, H., Wara, W.M., and Blank, E.W., 1982, Circulating human mammary epithelial antigens in breast cancer, *Proc. Natl. Acad. Sci. USA* **79:**5420–5424.

Ceriani, R.L., Peterson, J.A., Lee, J.Y., Moncada, R., and Blank, E.W., 1983, Characterization of cell surface antigens of human mammary epithelial cells with monoclonal antibodies prepared against human milk fat globule, *Somat. Cell Genet.* **9:**415–427.

Chatterton, R.T., Harris, J.A., and Wynn, R.M., 1975, Lactogenesis in the rat: An ultrastructural study of the initiation of the secretory process, *J. Reprod. Fertil.* **43:**479–484.

Cordell, J., Richardson, T.C., Pulford, K.A.F., Ghosh, A.K., Gatter, K.C., Heyderman, E., and Mason, D.Y., 1985, Production of monoclonal antibodies against human epithelial membrane antigen for use in diagnostic immunocytochemistry, *Br. J. Cancer* **52:**347–354.

Coughlan, M.P., 1980, Aldehyde oxidase, xanthine oxidase and xanthine dehydrogenase: Hydroxylases containing molybdenum, iron–sulphur and flavin, in: *Molybdenum and Molybdenum-Containing Enzymes* (M.P. Coughlan, ed.), Pergamon, Oxford, pp. 119–185.

Coulson, E.J., and Jackson, R.H., 1962, The mucoprotein of the fat/plasma interface of cow's milk. II. Immunochemical characterization, *Arch. Biochem. Biophys.* **97:**378–382.

Deeney, J.T., Valivullah, H.M., Dapper, C.H., Dylewski, D.P., and Keenan, T.W., 1985, Microlipid droplets in milk secreting mammary epithelial cells: evidence that they originate from endoplasmic reticulum and are precursors of milk lipid globules, *Eur. J. Cell Biol.* **38:**16–26.

Dylewski, D.P., Dapper, C.H., Valivullah, H.M., Deeney, J.T., and Keenan, T.W., 1984, Morphological and biochemical characterization of possible intracellular precursors of milk lipid globules, *Eur. J. Cell Biol.* **35:**99–111.

Edwards, P.A.W., 1985, Heterogeneous expression of cell-surface antigens in normal epithelia and their tumours, revealed by monoclonal antibodies, *Br. J. Cancer* **51:**149–160.

Edwards, P.A.W., Brooks, I.M., and Monaghan, P., 1984, Expression of epithelial antigens in primary cultures of normal breast analysed with monoclonal antibodies, *Differentiation* **25:**247–258.

Eigel, W.N., Hofmann, C.J., Chibber, B.A.K., Tomich, J.M., Keenan, T.W., and Mertz, E.T., 1979, Plasmin-mediated proteolysis of casein in bovine milk, *Proc. Natl. Acad. Sci. USA* **76:**2244–2248.

Eigel, W.N., Butler, J.E., Ernstrom, C.A., Farrell, H.M., Harwalkar, V.R., Jenness, R., and Whitney, R. Mcl., 1984, Nomenclature of proteins of cow's milk: Fifth revision, *J. Dairy Sci.* **67:**1599–1631.

Ellis, I.O., Robins, R.A., Elston, C.W., Blamey, R.W., Ferry, B., and Baldwin, R.W., 1984, A monoclonal antibody, NCRC-11, raised to human breast carcinoma. 1. Production and immunohistological characterization, *Histopathology* **8:**501–516.

Epenetos, A.A., Britton, K.E., Mather, S., Shepherd, J., Granowska, M., Taylor-Papadimitriou, J., Nimmon, C.C., Durbin, H., Hawkins, L.R., Malpas, J.S., and Bodmer, W.F., 1982, Targeting of iodine-123-labelled tumour-associated monoclonal antibodies to ovarian, breast, and gastrointestinal tumours, *Lancet* **2:**999–1004.

Euber, J.R., and Brunner, J.R., 1984, Reexamination of fat globule clustering and creaming in cow milk, *J. Dairy Sci.* **67:**2821–2832.

Fischer, J., Klein, P.-J., Farrar, G.H., Hanisch, F.-G., and Uhlenbruck, G., 1984, Isolation and chemical and immunochemical characterization of the peanut-lectin-binding glycoprotein from human milk-fat-globule membranes, *Biochem. J.* **224:**581–589.

Foster, C.S., and Neville, A.M., 1984, Monoclonal antibodies to the human mammary gland: (III) Monoclonal antibody LICR-LON-M18 identifies impaired expression and excess sialylation of the I (Ma) cell-surface antigen by primary breast carcinoma cells, *Hum. Pathol.* **15:**502–513.

Foster, C.S., Dinsdale, E.A., Edwards, P.A.W., and Neville, A.M., 1982a, Monoclonal antibodies to the human mammary gland: (II) Distribution of determinants in breast carcinomas, *Virchows Arch. [Pathol. Anat.]* **394:**295–305.

Foster, C.S., Edwards, P.A.W., Dinsdale, E.A., and Neville, A.M., 1982b, Monoclonal antibodies to the human mammary gland: (I) Distribution of determinants in non-neoplastic mammary and extra-mammary tissues, *Virchows Arch. [Pathol. Anat.]* **394:**279–293.

Franke, W.W., and Keenan, T.W., 1979, Interaction of secretory vesicle membrane coat structures with membrane free areas of forming milk lipid globules, *J. Dairy Sci.* **62:**1322–1325.

Franke, W.W., Heid, H.W., Grund, C., Winter, S., Freudenstein, C., Schmid, E., Jarasch, E.-D., and Keenan, T.W., 1981, Antibodies to the major insoluble milk fat globule membrane-associated protein: Specific location in apical regions of lactating epithelial cells, *J. Cell Biol.* **89:**485–494.

Freudenstein, C., Keenan, T.W., Eigel, W.N., Sasaki, M., Stadler, J., and Franke, W.W., 1979, Preparation and characterization of the inner coat material associated with fat globule membranes from bovine and human milk, *Exp. Cell Res.* **118:**277–294.

Gooi, H.C., Uemura, K., Edwards, P.A.W., Foster, C.S., Pickering, N., and Feizi, T., 1983, Two mouse hybridoma antibodies against human milk-fat globules recognise the I (Ma) antigenic determinant β-D-Galp-(1→4)-βD-GlcpNAc-(1→6), *Carbohydr. Res.* **120:**293–302.

Greenwalt, D.E., and Mather, I.H., 1985, Characterization of an apically derived epithelial membrane glycoprotein from bovine milk, which is expressed in capillary endothelia in diverse tissues, *J. Cell Biol.* **100:**397–408.

Greenwalt, D.E., Johnson, V.G., Kuhajda, F.P., Eggleston, J.C., and Mather, I.H., 1985a, Localization of a membrane glycoprotein in benign fibrocystic disease and infiltrating duct carcinomas of the human breast with the use of a monoclonal antibody to guinea pig milk fat globule membrane, *Am. J. Pathol.* **118:**351–359.

Greenwalt, D.E., Johnson, V.G., and Mather, I.H., 1985b, Specific antibodies to PAS IV, a glycoprotein of bovine milk-fat-globule membrane, bind to a similar protein in cardiac endothelial cells and epithelial cells of lung bronchioles, *Biochem. J.* **228:**233–240.

Heid, H.W., 1983, Biochemical and immunological characterization of the proteins of the milk fat globule membrane, PhD dissertation, University of Heidelberg.

Heid, H.W., Winter, S., Bruder, G., Keenan, T.W., and Jarasch, E.-D., 1983, Butyrophilin, an apical plasma membrane-associated glycoprotein characteristic of lactating mammary glands of diverse species, *Biochim. Biophys. Acta* **728:**228–238.

Heyderman, E., Steele, K., and Ormerod, M.G., 1979, A new antigen on the epithelial membrane: Its immunoperoxidase localisation in normal and neoplastic tissue, *J. Clin. Pathol.* **32:**35–39.

Heyderman, E., Strudley, I., Powell, G., Richardson, T.C., Cordell, J.L., and Mason, D.Y., 1985, A new monoclonal antibody to epithelial membrane antigen (EMA)-E29. A comparison of its immunocytochemical reactivity with polyclonal anti-EMA antibodies and with another monoclonal antibody, HMFG-2, *Br. J. Cancer* **52:**355–561.

Hilkens, J., Buijs, F., Hilgers, J., Hageman, Ph., Calafat, J., Sonnenberg, A., and van der Valk, M., 1984, Monoclonal antibodies against human milk-fat globule membranes detecting differentiation antigens of the mammary gland and its tumors, *Int. J. Cancer* **34:**197–206.

Hille, R., and Massey, V., 1985, Molybdenum-containing hydroxylases: Xanthine oxidase, aldehyde oxidase, and sulfite oxidase, in: *Molybdenum Enzymes* (T.G. Spiro, ed.), Wiley, New York, pp. 443–518.

Hirano, H., Parkhouse, B., Nicolson, G.L., Lennox, E.S., and Singer, S.J., 1972, Distribution of saccharide residues on membrane fragments from a myeloma-cell homogenate: Its implications for membrane biogenesis, *Proc. Natl. Acad. Sci. USA* **69:**2945–2949.

Hofmann, C.J., Keenan, T.W., and Eigel, W.N., 1979, Association of plasminogen with bovine milk fat globule membrane, *Int. J. Biochem.* **10:**909–917.

Hood, L.F., and Patton, S., 1973, Isolation and characterization of intracellular lipid droplets from bovine mammary tissue, *J. Dairy Sci.* **56:**858–863.

Horisberger, M., Rosset, J., and Vonlanthen, M., 1977, Location of glycoproteins on milk fat globule membrane by scanning and transmission electron microscopy, using lectin-labelled gold granules, *Exp. Cell Res.* **109:**361–369.

Huggins, J.W., Trenbeath, T.P., Chesnut, R.W., Carraway, C.A.C., and Carraway, K.L., 1980, Purification of plasma membranes of rat mammary gland. Comparisons of subfractions with rat milk fat globule membrane, *Exp. Cell Res.* **126:**279–288.

Imam, A., and Tökés, Z.A., 1981, Immunoperoxidase localization of a glycoprotein on plasma membrane of secretory epithelium from human breast, *J. Histochem. Cytochem.* **29:**581–584.

Imam, A., Laurence, D.J.R., and Neville, A.M., 1981, Isolation and characterization of a major glycoprotein from milk-fat-globule membrane of human breast milk, *Biochem. J.* **193:**47–54.

Imam, A., Laurence, D.J.R., and Neville, A.M., 1982, Isolation and characterization of two individual glycoprotein components from human milk-fat-globule membranes, *Biochem. J.* **207:**37–41.

Imam, A., Taylor, C.R., and Tökés, Z.A., 1984, Immunohistochemical study of the expression of human milk fat globule membrane glycoprotein 70, *Cancer Res.* **44:**2016–2022.

Jackson, R.H., Coulson, E.J., and Clark, W.R., 1962, The mucoprotein of the fat/plasma interface of cow's milk. I. Chemical and physical characterization, *Arch. Biochem. Biophys.* **97:**373–377.

Jamieson, J.D., Ingber, D.E., Muresan, V., Hull, B.E., Sarras, M.P., Maylié-Pfenninger, M.-F., and Iwanij, V., 1981, Cell surface properties of normal, differentiating, and neoplastic pancreatic acinar cells, *Cancer* **47:**1516–1525.

Janssen, M.M.T., and Walstra, P., 1982, Cytoplasmic remnants in milk of certain species, *Neth. Milk Dairy J.* **36:**365–368.

Jarasch, E.-D., Bruder, G., Keenan, T.W., and Franke, W.W., 1977, Redox constituents in milk fat globule membranes and rough endoplasmic reticulum from lactating mammary gland, *J. Cell Biol.* **73:**223–241.

Jarasch, E.-D., Grund, C., Bruder, G., Heid, H.W., Keenan, T.W., and Franke, W.W., 1981, Localization of xanthine oxidase in mammary-gland epithelium and capillary endothelium, *Cell* **25:**67–82.

Jeffers, K.R., 1935, Cytology of the mammary gland of the albino rat. I. Pregnancy, lactation and involution, *Am. J. Anat.* **56:**257–277.

Johnson, V.G., and Mather, I.H., 1985, Monoclonal antibodies prepared against PAS-I, butyrophilin, and GP-55 from guinea-pig milk-fat-globule membrane bind specifically to the apical pole of secretory-epithelial cells in lactating mammary tissue, *Exp. Cell Res.* **156:**144–158.

Johnson, V.G., Greenwalt, D.E., Heid, H.W., Mather, I.H., and Madara, P.J., 1985, Identification and characterization of the principal proteins of the fat-globule membrane from guinea-pig milk, *Eur. J. Biochem.* **151:**237–244.

Keenan, T.W., and Dylewski, D.P., 1985, Aspects of intracellular transit of serum and lipid phases of milk, *J. Dairy Sci.* **68:**1025–1040.

Keenan, T.W., Morré, D.J., Olson, D.E., Yunghans, W.N., and Patton, S., 1970, Biochemical and morphological comparison of plasma membrane and milk fat globule membrane from bovine mammary gland, *J. Cell Biol.* **44:**80–93.

Keenan, T.W., Olson, D.E., and Mollenhauer, H.H., 1971, Origin of the milk fat globule membrane, *J. Dairy Sci.* **54:**295–299.

Keenan, T.W., Morré, D.J., and Huang, C.M., 1974, Membranes of the mammary gland, in: *Lactation, A Comprehensive Treatise,* Vol. II (B.L. Larson and V.R. Smith, eds.), Academic Press, New York, pp. 191–233.

Keenan, T.W., Freudenstein, C., and Franke, W.W., 1977, Membranes of mammary gland. XIII. A lipoprotein complex derived from bovine milk fat globule membrane with some preparative characteristics resembling those of actin, *Cytobiologie* **14:**259–278.

Keenan, T.W., Sasaki, M., Eigel, W.N., Morré, D.J., Franke, W.W., Zulak, I.M., and Bushway, A.A., 1979, Characterization of a secretory vesicle-rich fraction from lactating bovine mammary gland, *Exp. Cell Res.* **124:**47–61.

Keenan, T.W., Heid, H.W., Stadler, J., Jarasch, E.-D., and Franke, W.W., 1982, Tight attachment of fatty acids to proteins associated with milk lipid globule membrane, *Eur. J. Cell Biol.* **26:**270–276.

Kitchen, B.J., 1974, A comparison of the properties of membranes isolated from bovine skim milk and cream, *Biochim. Biophys. Acta* **356:**257–269.

Kitchen, B.J., 1977, Fractionation and characterization of the membranes from bovine milk fat globules, *J. Dairy Res.* **44:**469–482.

Kobylka, D., and Carraway, K.L., 1972, Proteins and glycoproteins of the milk fat globule membrane, *Biochim. Biophys. Acta* **288:**282–295.

Kufe, D., Inghirami, G., Abe, M., Hayes, D., Justi-Wheeler, H., and Schlom, J., 1984, Differential reactivity of a novel monoclonal antibody (DF3) with human malignant versus benign breast tumors, *Hybridoma* **3:**223–232.

Kurosumi, K., Kobayashi, Y., and Baba, N., 1968, The fine structure of mammary glands of lactating rats, with special reference to the apocrine secretion, *Exp. Cell Res.* **50:**177–192.

Lee, E.Y.-H., Parry, G., and Bissell, M.J., 1984, Modulation of secreted proteins of mouse mammary epithelial cells by the collagenous substrata, *J. Cell Biol.* **98:**146–155.

Linzell, J.L., and Peaker, M., 1974, Changes in colostrum composition and in the permeability of the mammary epithelium at about the time of parturition in the goat, *J. Physiol.* **243:**129–151.

Lundy, J., Thor, A., Maenza, R., Schlom, J., Forouhar, F., Testa, M., and Kufe, D., 1985, Monoclonal antibody DF3 correlates with tumor differentiation and hormone receptor status in breast cancer patients, *Breast Cancer Res. Treat.* **5:**269–276.

Mangino, M.E., and Brunner, J.R., 1977, Isolation and partial characterization of xanthine oxidase associated with the milk fat globule membrane of cow's milk, *J. Dairy Sci.* **60:**841–850.

Martel, M.B., Dubois, P., and Got, R., 1973, Membranes des globules lipidiques du lait humain. Preparation, etude morphologique et composition chimique, *Biochim. Biophys. Acta* **311:**565–575.

Martel-Pradal, M.B., and Got, R., 1972, Presence d'enzymes marqueurs des membranes plasmiques, de l'appareil de Golgi et du reticulum endoplasmique dans les membranes des globules lipidiques de lait maternel, *FEBS Lett.* **21:**220–222.

Mather, I.H., 1978, Separation of the proteins of bovine milk-fat globule membrane by electrofocusing, *Biochim. Biophys. Acta* **514:**25–36.

Mather, I.H., and Keenan, T.W., 1975, Studies on the structure of milk fat globule membrane, *J. Membr. Biol.* **21:**65–85.

Mather, I.H., and Keenan, T.W., 1983, Function of endomembranes and the cell surface in the secretion of organic milk constituents, in: *Biochemistry of Lactation* (T.B. Mepham, ed.), Elsevier Science Publishers, Amsterdam, pp. 231–283.

Mather, I.H., Weber, K., and Keenan, T.W., 1977, Membranes of mammary gland. XII. Loosely associated proteins and compositional heterogeneity of bovine milk fat globule membrane, *J. Dairy Sci.* **60:**394–402.

Mather, I.H., Tamplin, C.B., and Irving, M.G., 1980, Separation of the proteins of bovine milk-fat-globule membrane by electrofocusing with retention of enzymatic and immunological activity, *Eur. J. Biochem.* **110:**327–336.

Mather, I.H., Sullivan, C.H., and Madara, P.J., 1982, Detection of xanthine oxidase and immunologically related proteins in fractions from bovine mammary tissue and milk after electrophoresis in polyacrylamide gels containing sodium dodecyl sulphate, *Biochem. J.* **202:**317–323.

Mather, I.H., Bruder, G., Jarasch, E.-D., Heid, H.W., and Johnson, V.G., 1984, Protein synthesis in lactating guinea-pig mammary tissue perfused in vitro. II. Biogenesis of milk-fat-globule membrane proteins, *Exp. Cell Res.* **151:**277–282.

McIlhinney, R.A.J., Patel, S., and Gore, M.E., 1985, Monoclonal antibodies recognizing epitopes carried on both glycolipids and glycoproteins of the human milk fat globule membrane, *Biochem. J.* **227:**155–162.

McPherson, A.V., and Kitchen, B.J., 1983, Reviews of the progress of dairy science: The bovine milk fat globule membrane—its formation, composition, structure and behaviour in milk and dairy products, *J. Dairy Res.* **50:**107–133.

McPherson, A.V., Dash, M.C., and Kitchen, B.J., 1984, Isolation of bovine milk fat globule membrane material from cream without prior removal of caseins and whey proteins, *J. Dairy Res.* **51:**113–121.

Merril, C.R., Dunau, M.L., and Goldman, D., 1981, A rapid sensitive silver stain for polypeptides in polyacrylamide gels, *Anal. Biochem.* **110:**201–207.

Moore, A., Boulton, A.P., Heid, H.W., Jarasch, E.-D., and Craig, R.K., 1985, Purification and tissue-specific expression of casein kinase from the lactating guinea-pig mammary gland, *Eur. J. Biochem.* **152:**729–737.

Moore, J.H., and Christie, W.W., 1979, Lipid metabolism in the mammary gland of ruminant animals, *Prog. Lipid Res.* **17:**347–395.

Morgan, E.J., Stewart, C.P., and Hopkins, F.G., 1923, On the anaerobic and aerobic oxidation of xanthin and hypoxanthin by tissues and by milk, *Proc. Soc. London Ser. B* **94:**109–131.

Morré, D.J., 1977, The Golgi apparatus and membrane biogenesis, in: *Cell Surface Reviews*, Vol. 4 (G. Poste and G.L. Nicolson, eds.), North-Holland, Amsterdam, pp. 1–83.

Newman, R.A., Ormerod, M.G., and Greaves, M.F., 1980, The presence of HLA-DR antigens on lactating human breast epithelium and milk fat globule membranes, *Clin. Exp. Immunol.* **41:**478–486.

Nielsen, C.S., and Bjerrum, O.J., 1977, Crossed immunoelectrophoresis of bovine milk fat globule membrane protein solubilized with non-ionic detergent, *Biochim. Biophys. Acta* **466:**496–509.

Nuti, M., Teramoto, Y.A., Mariani-Costantini, R., Horan Hand, P., Colcher, D., and Schlom, J., 1982, A monoclonal antibody (B72.3) defines patterns of distribution of a novel tumor-associated antigen in human mammary carcinoma cell populations, *Int. J. Cancer* **29:**539–545.

Ormerod, M.G., Steele, K., Westwood, J.H., and Mazzini, M.N., 1983, Epithelial membrane antigen: Partial purification, assay and properties, *Br. J. Cancer* **48:**533–541.

Ormerod, M.G., McIlhinney, J., Steele, K., and Shimizu, M., 1985, Glycoprotein PAS-O from the milk fat globule membrane carries antigenic determinants for epithelial membrane antigen, *Mol. Immunol.* **22:**265–269.

Patton, S., 1973, Origin of the milk fat globule, *J. Am. Oil Chem. Soc.* **50:**178–185.

Patton, S., 1982, Release of remnant plasma membrane from milk fat globules by Triton X-100, *Biochim. Biophys. Acta* **688:**727–734.

Patton, S., and Fowkes, F.M., 1967, The role of the plasma membrane in the secretion of milk fat, *J. Theoret. Biol.* **15:**274–281.

Patton, S., and Jensen, R.G., 1975, Lipid metabolism and membrane functions of the mammary gland, in: *Progress in the Chemistry of Fats and Other Lipids*, Vol. XIV, Part 4 (R.T. Holman, ed.), Pergamon Press, Oxford, pp. 163–277.

Patton, S., and Keenan, T.W., 1975, The milk fat globule membrane, *Biochim. Biophys. Acta* **415:**273–309.

Patton, S., and Hubert, J., 1983, Binding of Concanavalin A to milk fat globules and release of the lectin-membrane complex by Triton X-100, *J. Dairy Sci.* **66:**2312–2319.

Patton, S., and Huston, G.E., 1986, A method for isolation of milk fat globules, *Lipids* **21:**170–174.

Peixoto de Menezes, A., and Pinto da Silva, P., 1978, Freeze-fracture observations of the lactating rat mammary gland. Membrane events during milk fat secretion, *J. Cell Biol.* **76:**767–778.

Peixoto de Menezes, A., and Pinto da Silva, P., 1979, Fat droplet formation in rat lactating mammary gland and mammary carcinomas viewed by freeze-fracture, *Lab. Invest.* **40:**545–553.

Petersen, O.W., and Van Deurs, B., 1986, Characterization of epithelial membrane antigen expression in human mammary epithelium by ultrastructural immunoperoxidase cytochemistry, *J. Histochem. Cytochem.* **34:**801–809.

Pitelka, D.R., 1980, Evaluation of morphological markers of mammary epithelial cells, in: *Cell Biology of Breast Cancer* (C.M. McGrath, M.J. Brennan, and M.A. Rich, eds.), Academic Press, New York, pp. 3–15.

Powell, J.T., Järlfors, U., and Brew K., 1977, Enzymic characteristics of fat globule membranes from bovine colostrum and bovine milk, *J. Cell Biol.* **72:**617–627.

Price, M.R., Edwards, S., Owainati, A., Bullock, J.E., Ferry, B., Robins, R.A., and Baldwin, R.W., 1985, Multiple epitopes on a human breast-carcinoma-associated antigen, *Int. J. Cancer* **36:**567–574.

Pringnitz, D.J., Butler, J.E., and Guidry, A.J., 1985, *In vivo* proteolytic activity of the mammary gland. Contribution to the origin of secretory component, β_2-microglobulin and bovine-associated mucoprotein (BAMP) in cow's milk, *Vet. Immunol. Immunopathol.* **9:**143–160.

Ringo, D.L., and Rocha, V., 1983, Xanthine oxidase, an indicator of secretory differentiation in mammary cells, *Exp. Cell Res.* **147:**216–220.

Roth, J., Lentze, M.J., and Berger, E.G., 1985, Immunocytochemical demonstration of ecto-galactosyltransferase in absorptive intestinal cells, *J. Cell Biol.* **100:**118–125.

Saacke, R.G., and Heald, C.W., 1974, Cytological aspects of milk formation and secretion, in: *Lactation, A Comprehensive Treatise,* Vol. II (B.L. Larson and V.R. Smith, eds.), Academic Press, New York, pp. 147–189.

Sasaki, M., Peterson, J.A., and Ceriani, R.L., 1981, Quantitation of human mammary epithelial antigens in cells cultured from normal and cancerous breast tissues, *In Vitro* **17:**150–158.

Schlom, J., Wunderlich, D., and Teramoto, Y.A., 1980, Generation of human monoclonal antibodies reactive with human mammary carcinoma cells, *Proc. Natl. Acad. Sci. USA* **77:**6841–6845.

Segrest, J.P., and Jackson, R.L., 1972, Molecular weight determination of glycoproteins by polyacrylamide gel electrophoresis in sodium dodecyl sulphate, *Methods Enzymol.* **28:**54–63.

Sekine, H., Ohno, T., and Kufe, D.W., 1985, Purification and characterization of a high molecular weight glycoprotein detectable in human milk and breast carcinomas, *J. Immunol.* **135:**3610–3615.

Shaper, N.L., Mann, P.L., and Shaper, J.H., 1985, Cell surface galactosyltransferase: Immunochemical localization, *J. Cell. Biochem.* **28:**229–239.

Shimizu, M., and Yamauchi, K., 1982, Isolation and characterization of mucin-like glycoprotein in human milk fat globule membrane, *J. Biochem.* (*Tokyo*) **91:**515–524.

Shimizu, M., Yamauchi, K., Miyauchi, Y., Sakurai, T., Tokugawa, K., and McIlhinney,

R.A.J., 1986, High-M_r glycoprotein profiles in human milk serum and fat-globule membrane, *Biochem. J.* **233:**725–730.

Sloane, J.P., and Ormerod, M.G., 1981, Distribution of epithelial membrane antigen in normal and neoplastic tissues and its value in diagnostic tumor pathology, *Cancer* **47:**1786–1795.

Snow, L.D., Colton, D.G., and Carraway, K.L., 1977, Purification and properties of the major sialoglycoprotein of the milk fat globule membrane, *Arch. Biochem. Biophys.* **179:**690–697.

Stein, O., and Stein, Y., 1967, Lipid synthesis, intracellular transport, and secretion. II. Electron microscopic radioautographic study of the mouse lactating mammary gland, *J. Cell Biol.* **34:**251–263.

Stemberger, B.H., and Patton, S., 1981, Relationships of size, intracellular location, and time required for secretion of milk fat droplets, *J. Dairy Sci.* **64:**422–426.

Stemberger, B.H., Walsh, R.M., and Patton, S., 1984, Morphometric evaluation of lipid droplet associations with secretory vesicles, mitochondria and other components in the lactating cell, *Cell Tiss. Res.* **236:**471–475.

Sullivan, C.H., Mather, I.H., Greenwalt, D.E., and Madara, P.J., 1982, Purification of xanthine oxidase from the fat-globule membrane of bovine milk by electrofocusing. Determination of isoelectric points and preparation of specific antibodies to the enzyme, *Mol. Cell. Biochem.* **44:**13–22.

Swope, F.C., and Brunner, J.R., 1968, The fat globule membrane of cow's milk: A reassessment of isolation procedures and mineral composition, *Milchwissenschaft* **23:**470–473.

Taylor-Papadimitriou, J., Peterson, J.A., Arklie, J., Burchell, J., Ceriani, R.L., and Bodmer, W.F., 1981, Monoclonal antibodies to epithelium-specific components of the human milk fat globule membrane: Production and reaction with cells in culture, *Int. J. Cancer* **28:**17–21.

Taylor-Papadimitriou, J., Burchell, J., Moss, F., and Beverley, P., 1985, Monoclonal antibodies to epithelial membrane antigen and human milk fat globule mucin define epitopes expressed on other molecules, *Lancet* **1:**458.

Turnbull, J.E., Baildam, A.D., Barnes, D.M., and Howell, A., 1986, Molecular expression of epitopes recognized by monoclonal antibodies HMFG-1 and HMFG-2 in human breast cancers: Diversity, variability and relationship to prognostic factors, *Int. J. Cancer* **38:**89–96.

Walstra, P., 1969, Studies on milk fat dispersion. II. The globule-size distribution of cow's milk, *Neth. Milk Dairy J.* **23:**99–110.

Warburton, M.J., Mitchell, D., Ormerod, E.J., and Rudland, P., 1982, Distribution of myoepithelial cells and basement membrane proteins in the resting, pregnant, lactating, and involuting rat mammary gland, *J. Histochem. Cytochem.* **30:**667–676.

Waud, W.R., Brady, F.O., Wiley, R.D., and Rajagopalan, K.V., 1975, A new purification procedure for bovine milk xanthine oxidase: Effect of proteolysis on the subunit structure, *Arch. Biochem. Biophys.* **169:**695–701.

Weber, K., and Osborn, M., 1969, The reliability of molecular weight determinations by dodecyl sulfate–polyacrylamide gel electrophoresis, *J. Biol. Chem.* **244:**4406–4412.

Widnell, C.C., 1972, Cytochemical localization of 5′-nucleotidase in subcellular fractions isolated from rat liver. I. The origin of 5′-nucleotidase activity in microsomes, *J. Cell Biol.* **52:**542–558.

Wiman, K., Curman, B., Trägårdh, L., and Peterson, P.A., 1979, Demonstration of HLA-DR-like antigens on milk fat globule membranes, *Eur. J. Immunol.* **9:**190–195.

Wooding, F.B.P., 1971a, The mechanism of secretion of the milk fat globule, *J. Cell Sci.* **9:**805–821.

Wooding, F.B.P., 1971b, The structure of the milk fat globule membrane, *J. Ultrastruct. Res.* **37:**388–400.

Wooding, F.B.P., 1973, Formation of the milk fat globule membrane without participation of the plasmalemma, *J. Cell Sci.* **13:**221–235.

Wooding, F.B.P., 1977, Comparative mammary fine structure, in: *Comparative Aspects of Lactation* (M. Peaker, ed.), Academic Press, London, pp. 1–41.

Wooding, F.B.P., and Kemp, P., 1975a, Ultrastructure of the milk fat globule membrane with and without triglyceride, *Cell Tiss. Res.* **165:**113–127.

Wooding, F.B.P., and Kemp, P., 1975b, High-melting-point triglycerides and the milk-fat-globule membrane, *J. Dairy Res.* **42:**419–426.

Wooding, F.B.P., Peaker, M., and Linzell, J.L., 1970, Theories of milk secretion: Evidence from the electron microscopic examination of milk, *Nature* **226:**762–764.

Zerban, H., and Franke, W.W., 1978, Milk fat globule membranes devoid of intramembranous particles, *Cell Biol. Int. Rep.* **2:**87–98.

Zotter, S., Lossnitzer, A., Kunze, K.-D., Müller, M., Hilkens, J., Hilgers, J., and Hageman, P., 1985, Epithelial markers for paraffin-embedded human tissues. Immunohistochemistry with monoclonal antibodies against milk fat globule antigens, *Virchows Arch. [Pathol. Anat.]* **406:**237–251.

8

Receptor-Mediated Transepithelial Transport of Polymeric Immunoglobulins

Roberto Solari and Jean-Pierre Kraehenbuhl

1. Introduction

The transfer of acquired immunity from mother to offspring is essential to ensure survival of the newborn on leaving the sterile environment of the uterus. Since the fetus does not come into contact with microbial or dietary antigens, its immune system is not primed to respond to the challenges it will receive once exposed to the external environment. This passive immunization is largely due to the transmission of maternal IgG to the offspring either via the placenta (human and rabbit), via the intestinal absorption of colostrum (horse, swine, cow, and goat), or via a combination of these routes (rodents and dog). The permeability of the placenta to maternal IgG can be correlated, albeit not perfectly, with the number of membrane barriers separating the maternal and fetal circulations. Consequently, the newborn of most species are dependent, to varied extents, on antibodies derived from maternal mammary secretions. The spectrum of immunoglobulin classes present in the milk is a reflection of the defense requirements in each case. In those species where IgG is transferred totally in utero, IgA is the principal immu-

Roberto Solari • Department of Immunobiology, Glaxo Group Research Limited, Greenford, Middlesex UB6 OHE, United Kingdom. ***Jean-Pierre Kraehenbuhl*** • Swiss Institute for Experimental Cancer Research, Lausanne University, Lausanne, Switzerland.

noglobulin class in colostrum and milk. Where IgG is transferred postpartum via the intestinal absorption of colostrum, IgG is the predominant immunoglobulin class. After closure of the neonatal gut to colostral absorption, the milk immunoglobulin composition changes in the nonruminants (swine, horse) and IgA becomes the principal immunoglobulin. Ruminants, however, are deficient in both colostrum and milk IgA because this would impair the formation of the normal digestive flora required in the rumen. In addition to antibodies, maternal colostrum and milk contain a battery of antimicrobial agents such as lysozyme, complement, and lactoferrin and cells of the lymphoid and reticuloendothelial system. Although these components may play an ancillary role, the critical factor responsible for the immunological defense of the neonate appears to be the transfer of maternal immunoglobulin.

The maternal IgA antibodies found in milk are generally not absorbed by the intestine of the neonate, and their protective function acts at the level of the mucosal surface by mechanisms which are not yet fully understood. The apparent resistance of milk IgA to digestion within the intestine would facilitate its role in mucosal immunity (Brown et al., 1970; Porter, 1973; Underdown and Dorrington, 1974; Lindh, 1975). There is an accumulating body of evidence that associates IgA with the antibacterial and antiviral properties of human colostrum and milk (Hodes et al., 1964; Warren et al., 1964; Adinolfi et al., 1966; Akao et al., 1971; Hanson et al., 1979; Porter 1979; Ogra et al., 1983; Mestecky et al., 1984) and its role in the prevention of food allergies among children (Cruz and Hanson, 1983; Crago and Mestecky, 1984). It has also been implicated in the defense against transmissible gastroenteritis virus (TGE) and porcine rotavirus in newborn pigs (Saif and Bohl, 1979).

The IgA present in milk appears principally to be synthesized locally in the mammary gland by plasma cells in the lamina propria (Weisz-Carrington et al., 1977; Russell et al., 1982; Brandtzaeg, 1983), although serum-derived IgA may also be transported into the milk at certain stages of lactation (Sheldrake et al., 1984). In general, the proportion of serum-derived to locally produced IgA in the milk decreases through pregnancy and lactation. The appearance of specific IgA antibodies in milk has been shown to be elicited by the intestinal administration of the antigen to the mother (Goldblum et al., 1975; Roux et al., 1977; Weisz-Carrington et al., 1978; Hanson et al., 1979; Lamm et al., 1979; Montgomery et al., 1979; Ogra et al., 1983). This intestine–mammary gland–intestine axis which results in the neonate being passively immunized against enteric antigens experienced by the mother is part of a more wide-reaching network known as the common mucosal immune system.

2. The Common Mucosal Immune System

The significance of IgA in colostrum and milk is better appreciated when one considers the mucosal immune system as a whole. The mucosal surfaces of the body are constantly exposed to environmentally borne antigens and pathogens, and these tissues are the sites of an extensive immunological network responsible for their defense against infection. Within many mucosal tissues are found aggregated lymphoid nodules known generally as mucosal-associated lymphoid tissue, or MALT. The principal locations of such nodules are in the gut (GALT), for example, the Peyer's patches, or in the bronchi (BALT) (Bienenstock and Befus, 1980, 1983, 1984). These nodules of lymphoid tissue are overlaid with a specialized follicle-associated epithelium (FAE) which is made up of microfold or M cells. The transport of soluble proteins, nonadherent particles, and bacteria across M cells covering Peyer's patches and the mammalian appendix is well documented (Shimizu and Andrew, 1967; Bockman and Cooper, 1973; Owen and Jones, 1974; Leferre et al., 1978; Ducroc et al., 1983; Keljo and Hamilton, 1983; Owen et al., 1983). Recently, it has been shown that microorganisms that adhere to the apical membrane of M cells are rapidly transported from the luminal space into MALT (Wolf et al., 1981; Neutra et al., 1982; Bye et al., 1984). It would appear that the FAE is actively engaged in sampling the luminal content of the gut and bronchi and stimulating lymphocytes present in the MALT with antigens present in the external environment. When in vitro cultures of Peyer's patch cells respond to antigen, a substantial amount of the antibody produced is IgA. It is not clear whether this is due to the precommitment of MALT B cells to IgA secretion or whether MALT T cells produce helper factors that cause a class switch to IgA. Several studies have shown that Peyer's patch T cells can provide IgA-specific help in culture (Elson et al., 1979; Kiyonott et al., 1982; Kawanishi et al., 1983; Kawanishi and Strober, 1983; Campbell and Vose, 1985), whereas other studies show that IgA-precommitted B cells localize preferentially in the MALT (Tseng, 1982; Arny et al., 1984). Whichever mechanism proves to be correct, it is clear that the majority of MALT B cells express cell surface IgA, which can be shown to repopulate mucosal tissues with IgA producing cells when transferred into lethally irradiated recipients or congenic animals. Such repopulation studies with IgA precursor cells led to the concept of a common mucosal immune system in which B cells are driven to proliferate in MALT and subsequently repopulate the intestine, bronchus, breast, cervix, and lacrimal and salivary glands with IgA dimer secreting plasma cells

(Bienenstock and Befus, 1980, 1983) (Fig. 1). In order for these antibodies to protect mucosal surfaces from environmental antigens, they must cross the mucous or exocrine gland epithelium and be released into external secretions. However, they cannot simply diffuse through this epithelial barrier since the cells are sealed together by tight junctions

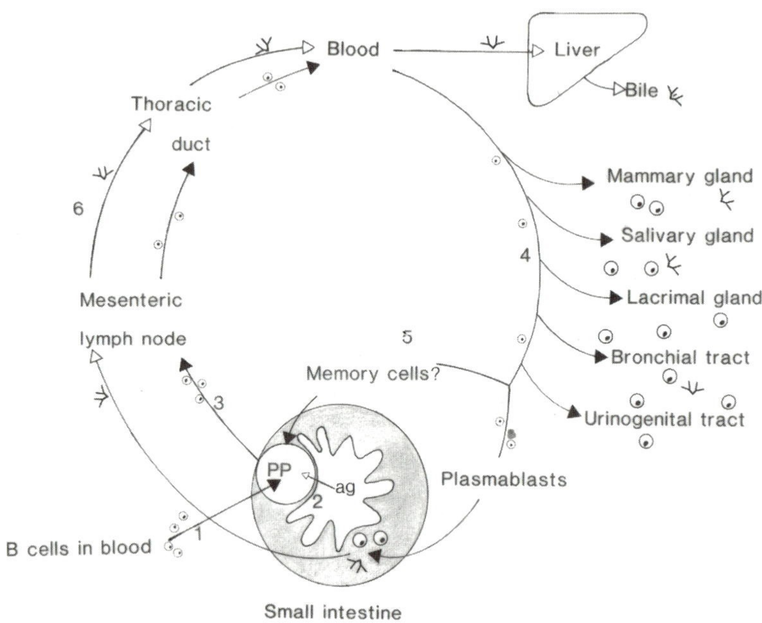

Figure 1. Schematic representation of the mucosal immune system. (1) Two mechanisms have been proposed to explain the origin of B cells in MALT. Immature circulating B cells may arrive in MALT either by chance or because they are precommitted to a mucosal distribution. MALT B cells may either be precommitted to IgA synthesis or may depend on T-helper cells to produce a switch to IgA synthesis (Phillips-Quagliata et al., 1983). (2) In the small intestine, environmental antigens traverse the follicle-associated epithelia (FAE) of the Peyer's patch and prime the underlying B cells. (3) B cells drain out of the Peyer's patch into the mesenteric lymph node (MLN) where proliferation and differentiation take place. The cells leaving the MLN are mainly plasmablasts and memory blasts. (4) Plasmablasts home to the lamina propria of exocrine and mucosal tissue where they eventually become trapped as their migratory ability decreases with maturation into polymeric IgA secreting plasma cells. Secreted IgA (-Y-) finds its way both to mucosal surfaces and into the blood stream. (5) Memory cells may home back to the GALT, and so help in further antigen-driven clonal expansion. (6) Polymeric IgA antibodies and pIgA antibody–antigen complexes (Peppard et al., 1982), which reach the circulation, are removed by the liver and secreted into bile (-▷). Drainage of the intestinal mucosa is the major source of blood pIgA, and it enters the bloodstream at the thoracic duct (Kleinman et al., 1982). After Montgomery et al. (1984).

at their apical poles. Consequently, the dimeric IgA antibodies must be transported through the epithelial cells by a specific mechanism.

3. Secretory IgA and Secretory Component

The study of the transepithelial transport of IgA dimer began with the observation that the most abundant immunoglobulin in external secretions is a modified form of dimeric IgA known as secretory IgA (sIgA) (Fig. 2). Analysis of this immunoglobulin reveals it to be a complex of two IgA monomers joined together by a 12-kDa glycoprotein known as the J-chain (Halpern and Koshland, 1970; Wilde and Koshland, 1973) and associated with an 80-kDa glycoprotein known as secretory component (SC) (Tomasi and Zigelbaum, 1963; Tomasi et al., 1965; South et al., 1966; Asofsky and Small, 1967; Cebra and Small, 1967; Tomasi and Grey, 1972). Whereas the J-chain containing IgA

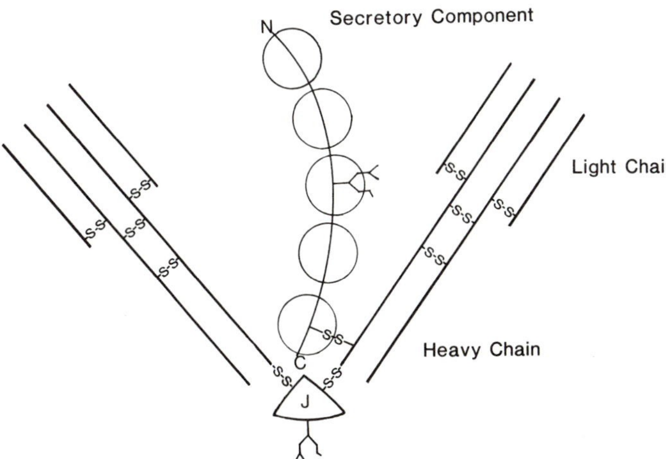

Figure 2. Schematic representation of the secretory IgA molecule (SIgA). Two IgA molecules, each comprising two light and two heavy chains, are cross-linked via a 12-kDa glycoprotein known as the joining or J-chain, to form an IgA dimer. The IgA dimer is bound to an 80-kDa glycoprotein known as secretory component (SC). SC represents the ectoplasmic domain of the polymeric Ig receptor. Binding of SC to the IgA dimer can be either via a disulfide bond, probably between domain 5 of SC and an α-chain, or by ionic interactions. Whereas most human SC is disulfide-bound to the α-chain of dimeric IgA (Tomasi and Grey, 1972), in the rabbit variable amounts are disulfide-bound (Grey et al., 1971) and covalent binding has been shown to depend on the IgA subclass (Knight et al., 1975). SC may protect the IgA dimer from proteolysis in external secretions (Brown et al., 1970; Porter, 1973; Underdown and Dorrington, 1974; Lindh, 1975).

dimer is synthesized and secreted by plasma cells present in the lamina propria of mucous or exocrine tissues, SC has been shown to be synthesized by the epithelial cells themselves and was consequently suspected of playing a role in IgA dimer transport. Immunocytochemical localization of SC in epithelial cells known to transport IgA dimer showed that SC was present intracellularly in the biosynthetic apparatus of the cell and also along the basolateral plasma membrane (Brandtzaeg, 1974; Brown et al., 1976; Huang et al., 1976; Crago et al., 1978; Kuhn and Kraehenbuhl, 1979b; Nagura et al., 1979; Socken et al., 1979). Cells bearing SC antigenic determinants were subsequently shown to bind IgA dimer specifically and with high affinity, and this binding could be competed for by SC and abolished by preincubation with anti-SC antibodies (Kuhn and Kraehenbuhl, 1979b). Furthermore, the transport of IgA dimer from blood to bile by the liver and the binding of IgA dimer to isolated hepatocytes in vitro were impaired by preincubation of the IgA dimer with SC (Fischer et al., 1979; Nagura et al., 1979).

Although this evidence suggested that SC was involved in the transcytosis of IgA dimer, it was unclear how a secretory protein could fulfill this role. The breakthrough came when SC mRNA purified from rabbit mammary glands was translated in a cell-free system in the presence of dog pancreas microsomal vesicles. The translation product was not soluble SC as found either free or bound to IgA dimer in secretions (SCs) but a transmembrane glycoprotein (SCm) which was 30 kDa larger than SCs. Comparison of SCm purified from rabbit mammary gland or liver membrane preparations and SCs purified from rabbit milk or bile reveals extensive structural homology when analyzed by peptide mapping (Kuhn and Kraehenbuhl, 1981). Peptide map analysis of the rat liver SCm and rat bile SCs confirms these findings (Fig. 3). The precursor–product relation between SCm and SCs was further demonstrated by biosynthetic labeling pulse-chase experiments in the rabbit mammary gland (Solari and Kraehenbuhl, 1984).

Several models have been proposed to explain how SCm mediates the transcytosis of IgA dimer (reviewed by Brandtzaeg, 1981); however, the common theme appears to be that SCm is cleaved while transporting IgA dimer from the basolateral to the apical plasma membrane of the epithelial cell, resulting in the release of SCs bound to IgA dimer into external secretions. This unique receptor-mediated transcytosis mechanism has led some workers to describe SCm as a *sacrificial receptor* (Kuhn and Kraehenbuhl, 1982). However, the observation that SCm is responsible for the transcytosis of polymeric IgA and also IgM has led to it being renamed the polymeric immunoglobulin receptor (pIgR), and we propose to use this nomenclature in future reference.

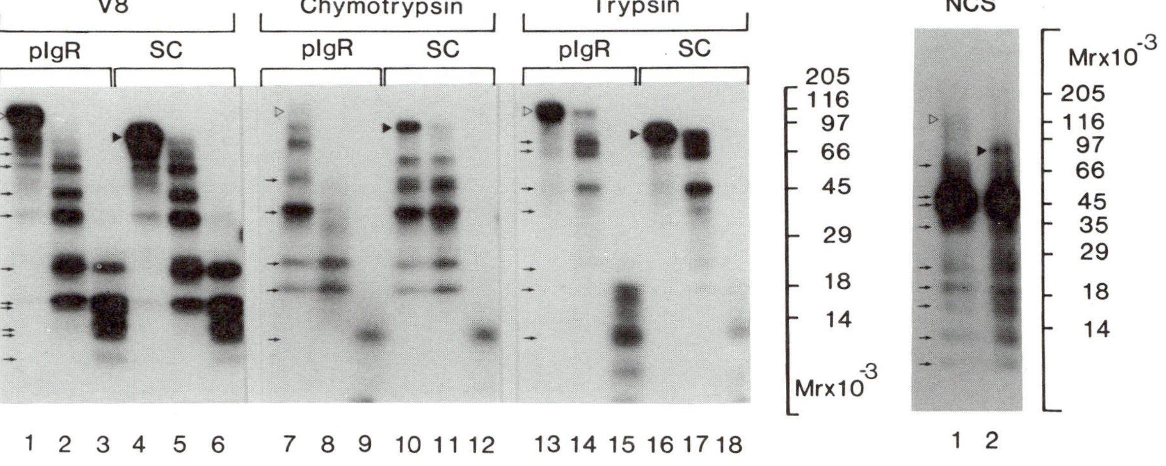

Figure 3. Peptide map analysis of the pIgR and SC. (A) The pIg receptor was immunoprecipitated from rat liver microsomes using the monoclonal 166 antibody (Mab 166) (Solari et al., 1985), run on an SDS-PAGE, and the receptor was excised from the stained gel. Whole rat bile was run on SDS-PAGE and the band corresponding to SCs was excised from the stained gel. Both proteins were iodinated in the gel slice (Elder et al., 1977; Speicher et al., 1982) and run on a second SDS-PAGE. The gel was cut into 2-mm slices, and each slice was counted. The gel slices containing the iodinated pIg receptor and SCs were incubated in 0.5% SDS, 0.1 *M* TRIS/HCl, pH 7.6, to elute the labeled proteins. The eluted pIg receptor and SCs were incubated at 37°C for 2 h with various proteases as follows: Lanes 1–6 digestion with V8 protease; lanes 1 and 4 = 50 ng; lanes 2 and 5 = 500 ng; lanes 3 and 6 = 5000 ng; lanes 7–12 digestion with chymotrypsin; lanes 7 and 10 = 0.5 μg; lanes 8 and 11 = 5 μg; lanes 9 and 12 = 25 μg; lanes 13–18 digestion with trypsin; lanes 13 and 16 = 0.5 μg; lanes 14 and 17 = 5 μg; lanes 15 and 18 = 25 μg. The Trypsin was added in 4 aliquots every 30 min. The reactions were terminated by boiling in sample buffer, followed by electrophoresis on an 8–20% SDS-PAGE. The dried gel was subsequently analyzed by autoradiography. The positions of the intact pIg receptor (△) and SCs (▲) are shown. Arrows indicate peptides common to both proteins. (B) The pIg receptor and SC were excised from a stained SDS-PAGE and iodinated. The iodinated gel slices were treated with *N*-chlorosuccinimide as previously described (Lischwe and Ochs, 1982) and run on an 8–25% SDS-PAGE. The positions of the pIg receptor (△) and SC (▲) are shown. Arrows indicate peptides common to both proteins.

4. Structure of the pIg Receptor

The primary structure of the pIg receptor (Fig. 4) has recently been deduced by cloning and sequencing the DNA complementary to the receptor's mRNA isolated from rabbit liver and lactating mammary gland (Mostov et al., 1984). The complete pIg receptor translation product consists of 773 amino acids, which can be divided into an 18-amino-acid N-terminal signal peptide, a 629-amino-acid extracellular sequence, a 23-amino-acid membrane-spanning segment, and a cytoplasmic tail of 103 amino acids. The extracellular sequence, which is responsible for binding to pIg, contains 18 cysteine residues, 10 of which could be grouped into regularly spaced pairs in which the members of each pair are separated by 60–70 amino acids. The sequences surrounding the pairs of cysteines have a high degree of internal homology, suggesting that the extracellular segment of the receptor has five repeating domains 100–115

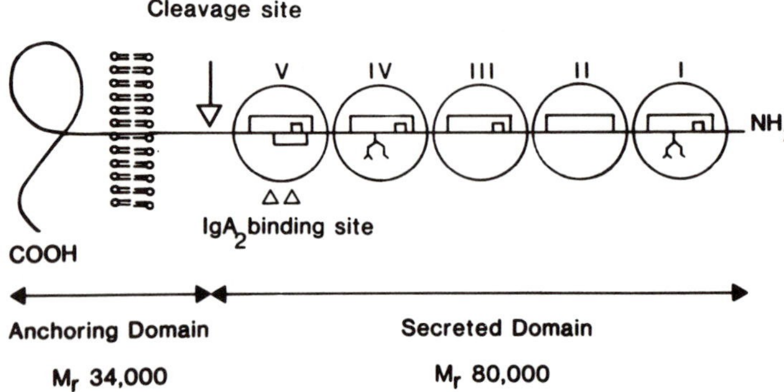

Figure 4. Structure of the pIg receptor. On the basis of cDNA sequence data for the receptor (Mostov et al., 1985) and amino acid sequencing of the secreted domain (Eiffert et al., 1984), we can draw this composite representation of the receptor. It is a transmembrane glycoprotein with a M_r of 110–120 kDa depending on species. In the human, there are seven N-linked oligosaccharide chains but only two in the rabbit. The receptor can be divided into the 35-kDa membrane anchoring sequence and the 80-kDa secreted sequence. The secreted sequence, or SCs, is made up of five mutually homologous immunoglobulin-like domains, about 104–114 residues long. All the domains contain a large disulfide bridge between cysteines spaced about 70 residues apart, and most domains also contain an additional small disulfide bridge between cysteins spaced about 7 residues apart. The fifth domain contains a further pair of cysteines which are thought to participate in covalent bonding with the pIg ligand. The 35-kDa membrane anchoring sequence has a 10-kDa extracellular portion and a 23-amino-acid membrane-spanning sequence made up of mainly hydrophobic residues. The cytoplasmic tail is 103 amino acids long and contains the receptor's phosphorylation site. The receptor may be phosphorylated in the Golgi complex. The exact site and mechanism of cleavage of SCs from its membrane anchoring domain have yet to be determined.

residues in length. These repeating units are similar in length and in the position of paired cysteine residues to immunoglobulin domains. Comparison of the pIg receptor's sequence with data banks shows extensive homology with numerous members of the immunoglobulin superfamily, and the best correspondence with immunoglobulin κ-chain variable region domains. The primary structure of the pIg receptor's extracellular domain has been confirmed by the amino acid sequencing of human SCs purified from colostrum (Eiffert et al., 1984). Sequence comparisons show that the amino acid chain can be divided into five successive and mutually homologous domains 104–114 residues in length. The internal homology is so marked that in many positions the same residues occur in all homologous regions. Sequencing of human SCs by protein chemistry techniques shows that the protein contains 20 cysteine residues, all of which are bound by disulfide bridges. In each domain, except for the second, disulfide bridges are found between cysteines about 70 residues apart (residues 24–101) and cysteines 7–10 residues apart (residues 42–52). In the fifth domain, two further cysteines are found in positions 28 and 70. This information reveals that each homologous domain (except for the second) is divided by two bridges into one large loop and one small loop. Dot matrix analysis of the rabbit sequence also suggested that there might be less constant repeating units within the larger 106–115 amino acid domains. In the fifth domain of the human sequence, there is an extra loop and binding of the receptor to the α-chain of IgA may occur via disulfide rearrangement of this bridge. In human SC, the two cysteines involved in the disulfide bonds with IgA dimer are surrounded by the sequences His-Phe-Pro-Cys-Lys-Tyr-Phe and Asn-Asp-His-Cys-Glu-Asp (Cunningham-Rundles and Lamm, 1975). The cysteines involved in the rabbit are not known, but the closest homologies to these sequences surround the cysteines in positions 464 and 481. This suggests that in the rabbit it is also the fifth domain of the receptor that becomes covalently linked to its ligand. Comparison of the extracellular domains of the rabbit pIg receptor and human SCs shows some 60% homology, and, by analogy, the small and large loop structure should also be present in the rabbit in domains 1,2, and 5.

Whereas the first five extracellular domains of the pIg receptor show structural homology with immunoglobulin domains, the sixth domain appears to be somewhat different. Although it also has sequence homology with the immunoglobulin domains, it has lost the second member of the conserved cysteine pair. Moreover, the C-terminus has been replaced by a hydrophobic membrane-spanning sequence that is homologous with an immunoglobulin κ-chain variable region sequence.

The common ancestry of molecules involved in recognition in the immune system is a most interesting observation. The immunoglobulins, histocompatibility antigens (Strominger et al., 1980), and the T-cell receptor (Hendrick et al., 1984a,b; Yanagi et al., 1984) all have the basic immunoglobulin domain, in addition to molecules such as Thy 1, which may be involved in cell–cell interactions and development (Williams and Gagnon, 1982). In the case of the pIg receptor, interaction of the immunoglobulin-like domains with the domains of its ligand is reminiscent of the binding of immunoglobulin chains to one another. Whether all classes of immunoglobulin receptor will be based on this common system is not yet known.

In most species so far examined, both the pIg receptor and SCs appear homogeneous with respect to size. However, in the rabbit there is considerable heterogeneity, and high and low molecular weight families can be identified that differ by at least 25 kDa. Furthermore, in some rabbits, each family can be resolved by SDS-PAGE into two polypeptides, whereas in other rabbits at least four polypeptides can be identified. This considerable heterogeneity in rabbits is the result of several processes. First, the intrafamily polymorphism was explained by the serological demonstration of two allotypes, t^{61} and t^{62}, which are allelic genes at an autosomal locus (Knight et al., 1975; Kuhn et al., 1983). Homozygotes expressed two polypeptides in each family, whereas heterozygotes expressed four. Second, the generation of high and low molecular weight families is the result of an intramolecular deletion in the secreted domain of the receptor, since both —COOH and —NH_2 termini of the high and low molecular weight families of SCs are identical (Kuhn et al., 1983). The low molecular weight family would appear to be generated by alternate splicing of mRNA's coding from the high molecular weight family (Deitcher et al., 1986). The biological significance of this polymorphism in the rabbit is not yet fully understood. Both high and low molecular weight families are functional in IgA dimer transport (Kuhn et al., 1983); however, it would appear that only the high molecular weight family is capable of forming a covalent liaison with IgA dimer (Solari et al., 1985). Analysis of this intramolecular deletion may consequently provide information pertinent to the liaison between ligand and receptor.

The sequence data also provides information relevant to the receptor's routing through the cell. First, one can determine that in the rabbit there are two potential sequences for N-linked glycosylation, whereas in human SCs there are seven. Second, and perhaps more interesting in terms of receptor traffic, there are 19 hydroxy amino acids on the cytoplasmic tail of the rabbit receptor that could be phosphorylated.

5. Transcellular Transport of Polymeric Ig

The first step in the transcytosis of pIg across mucosal or exocrine epithelial cells is the binding of the ligand to its receptor at the basolateral cell surface. The association constant for the interaction between the purified receptor and dimeric IgA has been calculated to be 1.2×10^8 M^{-1}, similar to that reported for the binding of SCs to IgA dimer (Kuhn and Kraehenbuhl, 1979a, 1981). However, this value is one order of magnitude higher than the dissociation constant for the interaction between IgA dimer and viable mammary cells or liver and mammary microsomes (Kuhn and Kraehenbuhl, 1979b). The difference could reflect the detergent solubilization required to purify the pIg receptor. The most intensively studied system of pIg transcytosis is the transport of IgA dimer from blood to bile by the rat hepatocyte. Several studies have demonstrated that IgA dimer, when injected into the systemic circulation of a rat or into the portal vein of an isolated perfused liver, is efficiently transported to the bile, reaching a maximum concentration 30–60 min after injection (Jackson et al., 1978; Orlans et al., 1978, 1983; Fisher et al., 1979; Mullock et al., 1980c; Renston et al., 1980; Lemaitre-Coelho et al., 1981; Delacroix et al., 1982; Schiff et al., 1984; Hoppe et al., 1985). Morphological analysis of the rat hepatocyte using immunocytochemistry and autoradiography suggests that the pIg receptor is distributed along the sinusoidal plasma membrane mainly in pits and small tubules (Birbeck et al., 1979; Renston et al., 1980; Takahashi et al., 1982; Geuze et al., 1984; Hoppe et al., 1985), which is in contrast to a more diffuse distribution along the basolateral plasma membrane of enterocytes (Brown et al., 1976; Nagura et al., 1979).

Both cell fractionation (Mullock et al., 1979, 1980a, 1983; Limet et al., 1982, 1985) and morphological techniques (Birbeck et al., 1979; Renston et al., 1980; Takahashi et al., 1982; Geuze et al., 1984; Hoppe et al., 1985) reveal that the IgA dimer is subsequently endocytosed into vesicles with diameters between 100 and 140 nm and rapidly transported to the canalicular plasma membrane. However, dimeric IgA is only one of the many proteins endocytosed by receptor-mediated processes at the hepatocyte sinusoidal plasma membrane. These various ligands can be either transported to bile, returned to the blood, or delivered to lysosomes where they are degraded. Clearly, the hepatocyte must be able to sort each ligand to its correct destination, but how and where this sorting occurs remain controversial. One possibility is that ligands destined for different compartments are sorted at the sinusoidal plasma membrane into specific endocytic vesicles (Schiff et al., 1984).

This possibility is supported by the observation that choloroquine and dansyl cadaverine inhibit the processing of asialo-orosomucoid by the isolated perfused liver while having no effect on IgA dimer transport from blood to bile, and that taurocholate inhibits IgA dimer transport but has no effect on asialo-orosomucoid (Underdown et al., 1983). However, it would appear equally possible that ligands are sorted to their various destinations within the cell. It has been demonstrated by density shift techniques that the same endosomal vesicles contained both IgA dimer, which is destined to be secreted into bile, and asialoglycoproteins, which are destined for the lysosome (Courtoy et al., 1984; Limet et al., 1985). Further evidence for the intracellular sorting of ligands makes use of the observation that certain subtypes of human IgA dimer can bind to the asialogylcoprotein receptor via O-linked sugars present in their hinge region (Stockert et al., 1982). Analysis of the uptake of human IgA by the rat liver demonstrates that its endocytosis from the blood is mediated by the asialoglycoprotein receptor rather than the pIg receptor. The human IgA avoids the usual fate of asialoglycoproteins, namely, degradation in the lysosome, by switching to the pIg receptor in a prelysosomal compartment and is eventually secreted into bile bound to SCs (Schiff et al., 1986). This would require both the asialoglycoprotein and pIg receptors to be present within the same endocytic vesicle.

Morphological data also provide conflicting evidence for the sorting of endocytosed ligands. Studies on IgA transport in the rat liver using electron microscopic autoradiography suggested that ligands destined for transcytosis or degradation were endocytosed into separate vesicles at the sinusoidal plasma membrane (Renston et al., 1980; Jones et al., 1982). However, evidence that different receptors and their ligands are endocytosed within the same vesicles comes from double-labeling immuno-electron microscopy on ultrathin cryosections of rat liver (Geuze et al., 1984). These techniques demonstrate the presence of the pIg receptor, the asialoglycoprotein receptor, and the mannose-6-phosphate receptor in Golgi, along the entire plasma membrane and within the same coated pits and vesicles. All three receptors were found in the compartment of uncoupling of receptors and ligand (CURL), where sorting of the different receptors to their various destinations appeared to take place. Although the mechanisms for the transcytosis of IgA dimer containing vesicles are not clearly understood, the process would appear to depend on microtubules since it can be inhibited by colchicine (Mullock et al., 1980c).

In addition to the need for sorting of the pIg receptor, the membrane anchoring domain must also be cleaved during transcellular transport to allow the exocytosis of sIgA from the apical plasma membrane. In enterocytes, cleavage may occur in transcytotic vesicles (Mostov and Blobel, 1982), whereas in the liver it would appear that this cleavage occurs at the final destination of the receptor, namely, the apical plasma membrane. The evidence for the latter is that SCs cannot be detected in any cellular fraction and that intact receptor can be demonstrated in plasma membrane preparations enriched in the canalicular domain (unpublished data). Moreover, IgA dimer can still be detected bound to the luminal surface of the canalicular plasma membrane (Geuze et al., 1984). Although we can speculate about the site of receptor cleavage, we still do not understand the mechanism. Comparison of the C-terminus of rabbit milk SCs, as determined by carboxypeptidase Y digestion with the primary stucture of the rabbit pIg receptor as determined by cloning and sequencing the cDNA, provides three possible cleavage sites (Mostov et al., 1984). However, all three of these sites would require cleavage between two acidic amino acids, and consequently if the cleavage is proteolytic it involves a mechanism not yet documented. However, analysis of the C-terminus of human SCs demonstrates heterogeneity of the amino acid sequence (Eiffert et al., 1984). Consequently, cleavage may occur either at a unique site followed by a variable amount of proteolytic digestion or at one of several suitable sites.

Recently, the cloned pIg receptor cDNA has been functionally expressed by its introduction into fibroblasts (Deitcher et al., 1986), and it was demonstrated that the fibroblasts could cleave the pIg receptor and secrete SC. Since fibroblasts do not normally express the pIg receptor, this suggests that if receptor cleavage is proteolytic, then the protease must be ubiquitous. Another possibility is that the receptor is autocatalytically cleaved as a result of a particular modification occurring at the apical plasma membrane. If the mechanism of receptor cleavage is unclear, then so too is the fate of the 34-kDa membrane anchor that must be generated upon release of the ectoplasmic domain of the receptor into external secretions. Recent studies making use of a monoclonal antibody directed against the cytoplasmic tail of the receptor have revealed the presence of the 34-kDa membrane anchoring domain of the receptor in microsomal fractions (unpublished data), in addition to a 32-kDa protein in the cytosol and 31- and 29-kDa proteins in the bile (Solari et al., 1986). The suggestion is that the 34-kDa membrane anchor undergoes a series of modifications that permit it to be eliminated from the canalicular membrane and released into the bile. Whether the membrane anchoring domain is eliminated into external secretions in all epithelial cells expressing the receptor is not known, and one suspects that the hepatocyte may prove to be unusual in this respect.

6. Receptor Biosynthesis

The transcytosis of pIg provides an interesting model for studying the sorting of endocytosed ligands. However, this is only half of the pIg receptor story, and to understand the receptor's complex routing one must also examine its biosynthesis. The routing of the pIg receptor is of particular interest because it is sorted to several cellular destinations in a specific sequence and so provides an interesting model to study protein sorting within the cell. Such investigations have been performed in the rabbit mammary gland (Solari and Kraehenbuhl, 1984), the rat liver (Sztul et al., 1983, 1985a,b), and an adenocarcinoma cell line derived from the colon (Mostov and Blobel, 1982). In cell-free translation experiments, it was first demonstrated that the pIg receptor was synthesized on the rough endoplasmic reticulum (RER) and cotranslationally core-glycosylated (Mostov et al., 1980). Subsequent pulse-chase studies in the rabbit mammary gland confirmed that the receptor is synthesized as a core-glycosylated glycoprotein that is sensitive to Endoglycosidase H (Endo H) digestion. Transport of the newly synthesized receptor from the RER to the Golgi complex was deduced by the acquisition of resistance to Endo H since resistance is due to the combined action of the enzymes GlcNAC transferase I and mannosidase II, both of which are located in median Golgi cisternae (Dunphy and Rothman, 1983; Goldberg and Kornfeld, 1983; Dunphy et al., 1985). These observations demonstrated a half-time of 30 min for the appearance of Endo H resistant forms of the receptor (Solari and Kraehenbuhl, 1984). Studies on the receptor's processing in the rat liver allow a combination of biosynthetic labeling and cellular fractionation. Such experiments demonstrate that the receptor is synthesized as a core-glycosylated glycoprotein in RER-enriched fractions and is terminally glycosylated in Golgi-enriched fractions with a half-time of about 30 min (Fig. 5). The unusual feature of these results is that the biosynthetically labeled receptor appears to reside in Golgi-enriched fractions for relatively long periods of time, even after the peak of SCs secretion into bile has passed (Sztul et al., 1985b). Separation of the Golgi into *heavy* and *light* fractions results in a relative enrichment of *early* and *late* components of the Golgi biosynthetic apparatus (Ehrenreich et al., 1973; Bergeron et al., 1978), and analysis of the flux of biosynthetically labeled receptor through these compartments is possible (Sztul et al., 1985b). The receptor is first detected in the heavy Golgi fraction and subsequently in the light fraction; however, some of the receptor in the heavy fraction still remains after all has been chased out of the light fraction. There are two possible interpretations of these results. First, the heavy Golgi fraction is contaminated with endocytic vesicles, which are transporting the receptor from the sinusoidal to the canalicular plasma membrane; second, there are two pools of receptor that turn over at different rates, one of which moves through the Golgi rapidly and one of which has a long residency time in the *earlier* Golgi cisternae.

Pulse-chase experiments in the lactating rabbit mammary gland have been performed followed by immunoprecipitation of the pIg receptor and SCs using a panel of antibodies directed against different domains of the molecule (Solari and Kraehenbuhl, 1984). Sequential immunoprecipitation of the receptor using the different antibodies in cascades revealed that the receptor existed as several pools and that these pools could be shown to have different turnover rates within the cell. The significance of having two or more pools of a receptor turning over at different rates is still unclear. What is clear, however, is that after processing of the receptor in the Golgi, its subsequent routing to the basolateral membrane, where pIg binding and endocytosis occurs, and the cleavage of the membrane anchoring domain and release from the apical plasma membrane of SCs, both free and covalently bound to pIg, take place very rapidly (Solari and Kraehenbuhl, 1984). Biosynthetically labeled SCs can be detected in milk as early as 30–60 min after synthesis of the receptor on the RER.

One of the most interesting aspects of the pIg receptor is its complex routing through the cell. For the pIg receptor to transport pIg vectorially in a basolateral–apical direction, the receptor must clearly be expressed at the cell's basolateral plasma membrane where it can encounter its ligand. The question is, however, does a mechanism exist that directs the receptor to this membrane domain after its maturation in the Golgi complex, or is the receptor randomly distributed to both apical and basolateral domains? Two lines of evidence so far suggest that there is a post-Golgi sorting mechanism. The first comes from studies on the rabbit mammary gland (Solari and Kraehenbuhl, 1984). In the rabbit, the receptor binds covalently to certain IgA dimer allotypes (Kuhn and Kraehenbuhl, 1979a), and consequently the appearance in milk of biosynthetically labeled SCs covalently bound to IgA dimer is evidence that the receptor was routed to the basolateral plasma membrane prior to

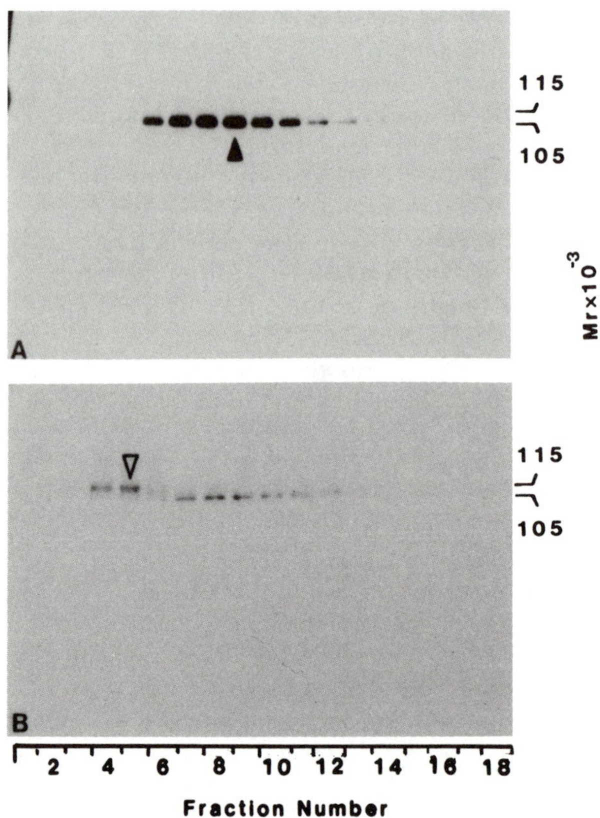

Figure 5. Biosynthesis of the pIg receptor in the rat liver. Livers were surgically removed from OFA rats and maintained in a recirculating perfusion system. The livers were pulsed by the injection of 500 μCi of ^{35}S cysteine into the perfusion medium which was allowed to circulate for 7 min prior to being washed out and the addition of excess cold cysteine. The pulsed livers were subsequently chased for various periods of time prior to their homogenization and fractionation. The microsomal pellets were separated by centrifugation on linear 1.11–1.25 g/ml sucrose density gradients as described previously (Solari et al., 1986). After equilibration, the gradients were fractionated into 18 × 2-ml aliquots (fraction 1 being the top and fraction 18 the bottom of the gradient). Each fraction was immunoprecipitated with the monoclonal antibody 166 and the adsorbed material was analyzed by SDS-PAGE and fluorography. Panel (A) shows the distribution of labeled pIg receptor after a zero chase. All the receptor is in the 105-kDa core-glycosylated form, and coequilibrates in the center of the gradient with rER marker enzyme activity (▲). Panel (B) shows the distribution of receptor after a 30-min chase. Approximately half of the labeled receptor has been converted to the 115-, 118-kDa terminally glycosylated form and now coequilibrates with Golgi marker enzyme activity (△). Panels (C) and (D) represent 60- and 120-min chase periods, respectively. At these time points, the 105-kDa receptor has been chased out of the RERcompartment and accumulates in the Golgi-enriched fractions as the 115-, 118-kDa terminally glycosylated form.

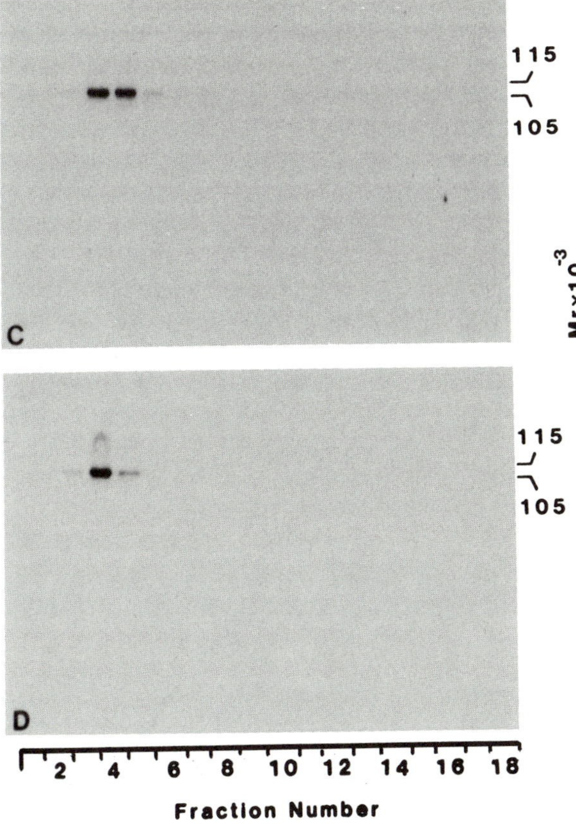

Figure 5. (Continued)

transcytosis to the apical cell surface. A panel of antibodies was raised that recognized only free SCs or both free SCs and SCs covalently bound to IgA dimer, and these antibodies were used to immunoprecipitate milk after biosynthetic labeling of rabbit mammary gland tissue. The results demonstrated that covalently linked and noncovalently linked SCs were secreted into the milk with identical kinetics, suggesting that probably all the receptor is sorted to the basolateral plasma membrane after leaving the Golgi. The second line of evidence comes from the expression of the receptor's cloned cDNA in polarized MDCK epithelial cells (Mostov and Deitcher, 1986). These studies indicate that 90% of the newly synthesized receptor that is ultimately cleaved and secreted into the apical medium as SCs goes first to the basolateral plasma membrane. Such

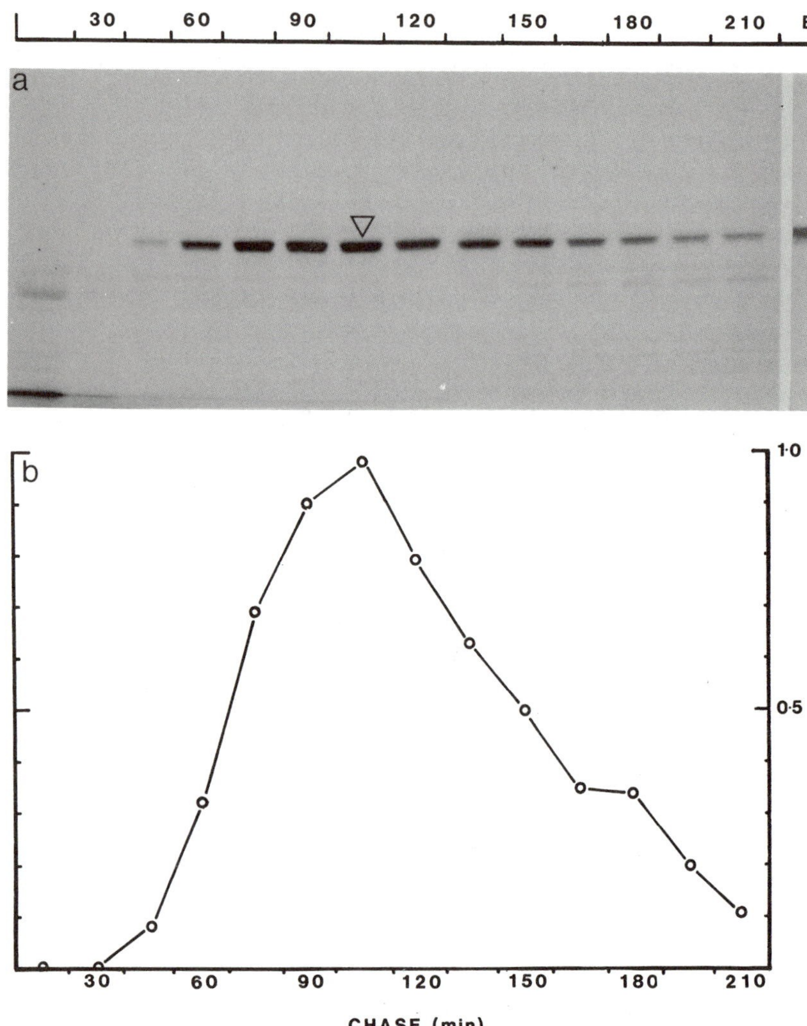

Figure 6. Secretion of SCs into bile. Rat livers were pulsed with 500 μCi of ^{35}S-cysteine by injection into the hepatic portal vein in situ (panel a). Bile was collected at 15-min intervals after injection via a canula placed in the bile duct. The 30-μl samples of bile collected at each time interval were analyzed by SDS-PAGE under reducing conditions followed by fluorography. The secreted ectoplasmic domain of the receptor, SCs, was the major biosynthetically labeled protein to be secreted into the bile. It was identified by Western blotting of a bile sample with a polyclonal antibody directed against the ectoplasmic domain of the receptor (panel a, lane B) and by peptide map analysis (see Fig. 3). Quantification of labeled SCs secretion into the bile was performed by scanning the fluorographic images from three separate experiments and the mean result is shown in panel (b). The peak of labeled SCs secretion into the bile occurs between 90 and 105 min postinjection (△).

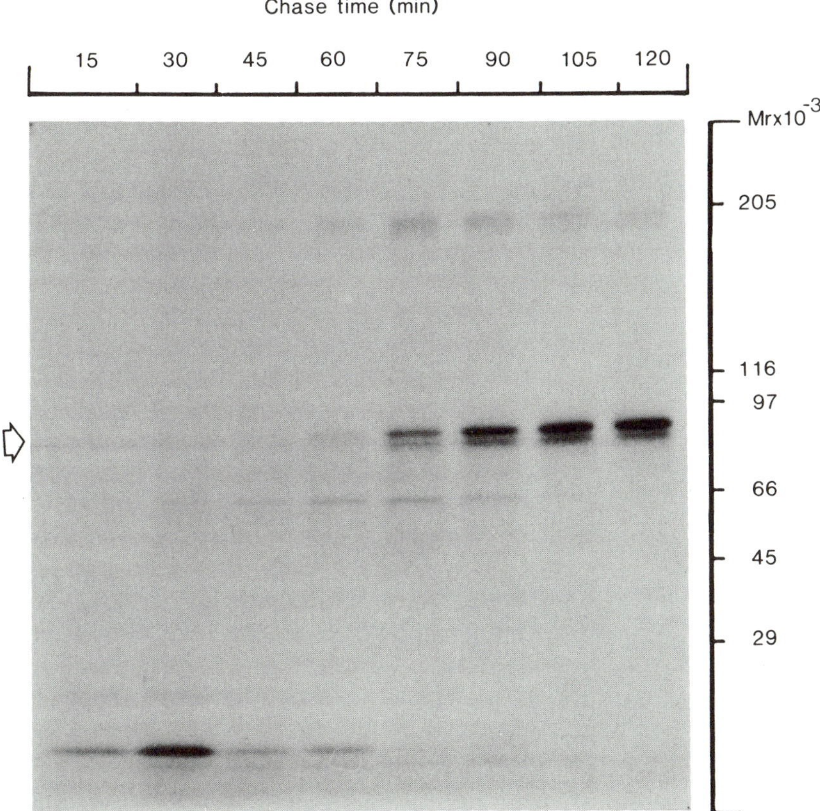

Figure 7. Secretion of SC into the bile in the absence of pIg. A rat liver was surgically removed and maintained at 37°C in an isolated recirculating apparatus as previously described (Dunn et al., 1983). After a 30-min equilibration period, during which time the medium was exchanged twice with fresh medium, a pulse of 0.5 mCi of ^{35}S-cysteine was added. Bile was collected at 15-min intervals over the next 2 h. The 10-μl aliquots of each bile sample were analyzed by SDS-PAGE and fluorography. SC is the major protein synthesized by the liver to be secreted into bile (△), and it is first detected after 45–60 min, which is similar to the in situ experiments (Fig. 6). Consequently, secretion of SC appears to continue even in the absence of pIg in the medium. The identification of this protein as SCs was performed by peptide map analysis (Fig. 3) and by Western blot analysis with antibodies raised against the pIg receptor.

post-Golgi sorting mechanisms may play a fundamental role in cellular organization, since studies on the expression of viral envelope proteins in polarized epithelial cell lines such as MDCK demonstrate that proteins destined for the apical or basolateral plasma membrane domains of the cell are sorted after processing in the Golgi complex (Rindler et al., 1984, 1985; Fuller et al., 1985).

It has been proposed that the pIg receptor is synthesized and routed through the cell and that SCs is secreted from the apical plasma membrane even in the absence of ligand. Evidence for this observation comes from the collection of bile from isolated perfused livers. In this situation, there is no ligand available at the sinusoidal plasma membrane yet SCs continues to be secreted into bile (Mullock et al., 1980b). We have performed biosynthetic labeling experiments in the isolated perfused liver using ^{35}S-cysteine. These studies indicate that even in the absence of ligand, the pIg receptor is synthesized on the RER and processed in the Golgi at what appears to be the normal rate (unpublished data). Moreover, SCs is secreted into the bile with similar kinetics to the in vivo situation (Figs. 6 and 7). The functional expression of the pIg receptor's cloned cDNA in fibroblasts and MDCK cells also confirms these observations (Deitcher et al., 1986; Mostov and Deitcher, 1986). The biosynthesis of the receptor and secretion of SCs into the medium were affected neither qualitatively nor quantitatively by the presence of dimeric IgA. Consequently, it would appear that the pIg receptor functions as a continuous self-destructing conveyor belt.

7. *Receptor Phosphorylation*

We have shown that the pIg receptor undergoes several modifications during its transcellular routing, such as glycosylation and cleavage of its membrane anchoring domain. It has recently been demonstrated by labeling the rabbit mammary gland (Fig. 8) and rat liver with ^{32}P-orthophosphate followed by cell fractionation and immunoprecipitation that the pIg receptor is phosphorylated. The fractionation studies in the rat liver demonstrate that it is only the terminally glycosylated form of the receptor that is phosphorylated, and this phosphorylated form can only be detected in fractions enriched in the Golgi complex (Solari and Kraehenbuhl, 1987). These Golgi fractions are not pure and are notably contaminated with endosomes; consequently, one cannot be sure of the exact site of phosphorylation. However, the possibility that the pIg receptor is phosphorylated in the Golgi is strengthened by findings that a cyclic-AMP-dependent protein kinase II is associated with this organelle (Nigg et al., 1985) and that a range of proteins can be phosphorylated in

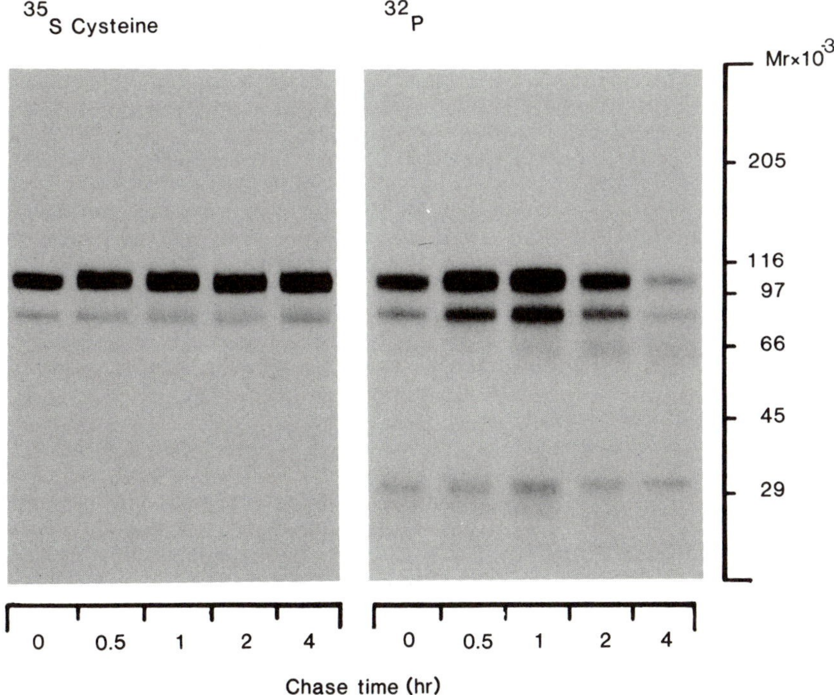

Figure 8. Phosphorylation of the pIg receptor in the rabbit mammary gland. Minilobules were dissected from a lactating rabbit mammary gland and pulsed with either ^{35}S-cystein or ^{32}P-orthophosphate as previously described (Solari and Kraehenbuhl, 1984). After the pulse, the minilobules were chased for various periods of time. A cell extract was made from each time point and was immunoprecipitated with the monoclonal 166 antibody (Solari et al., 1985), followed by analysis on SDS-PAGE and fluorography of autoradiography. The ^{35}S-cysteine labeling demonstrates the high and low M_r doublets typical of the heterogeneous rabbit pIg receptor. The ^{35}S-labeled receptor recognized by the Mab 166 has a slow turnover as previously described (Solari and Kraehenbuhl, 1984). Labeling with ^{32}P reveals that both upper and lower doublets of the receptor are phosphorylated. The phosphorylated receptor apparently has a more rapid turnover, although this could be the result of dephosphorylation by phosphatase action.

vitro by incubating highly purified rat liver Golgi fractions with γ-^{32}P-ATP by what appears to be an integral membrane kinase (Capasso et al., 1985).

The pIg receptor has potential sites for phosphorylation on both ectoplasmic and cytoplasmic facing sequences; however, it has been determined that the receptor in the rat liver is exclusively phosphorylated on its cytoplasmic tail (Solari and Kraehenbuhl, 1987). This was achieved by purification of Golgi cisternae after labeling of the liver with ^{32}P-orthophosphate, followed by digestion of the protruding cytoplasmic tail of the receptor with trypsin. Removal of the cytoplasmic tail results in a drop in M_r of 20 kDa and the loss of all the ^{32}P label.

There are 19 hydroxy amino acids on the cytoplasmic tail of the rabbit receptor which could be phosphorylated—11 serines, 6 threonines, and 2 tyrosines. From the sequencing of proteins phosphorylated by different protein kinases, the following consensus sequences have been proposed. All serine/threonine-protein kinases so far examined select serine or threonine when surrounded by positively charged amino acids (Hunter and Cooper, 1985). Canonical recognition sequences have been proposed for cAMP-dependent protein kinase (Lys-Arg-X-X-Ser-) and for Ca^{2+}/calmodulin-dependent protein kinase (Lys-Arg-X-Ser-X-Arg-) (Krebs and Beavo, 1979). Although none of these sequences is present on the cytoplasmic tail of the rabbit receptor, serine 725 is surrounded by the sequence -Lys-Arg-X-Ser, which has been shown to be a suitable substrate for cGMP- and cAMP-dependent kinase (Lincoln and Corbin, 1977) and Ser and Thr surrounded by positively charged amino acids are located at positions 664 and 698. In addition, the autophosphorylation sites of viral protein tyrosine kinases have the common feature of a basic amino acid 7 residues to the —NH_2 terminal side of the tyrosine and one or more acidic amino acids among the intervening sequence (Hunter and Cooper, 1985). Tyr 735 is surrounded by such a consensus sequence: Lys-Glu-Glu-Ala-As-Leu-Ala-Tyr- (Table I). Although recent studies have shown that the receptor is phosphorylated on serines (Larkin et al., 1986), this information suggests that the receptor may be phosphorylated at different sites during its intracellular processing. It has been suggested that the cytoplasmic tail of the receptor may contain the necessary information for correct sorting. If phosphorylation is important for the sorting of the receptor, then its complex intracellular routing may be controlled by a series of phosphorylation–dephosphorylation events on specific residues. Phosphorylation of the cytoplasmic tail in the Golgi complex may provide the correct signal for the receptor to be routed to the basolateral plasma membrane. On arrival at the basolateral membrane, the cytoplasmic tail might be dephosphorylated or phosphorylated at an alternate site, which would re-

Table I. Potential Phosphorylation Sites

Tyrosine (735)	Lys-Glu-Glu-X-Asp-X-X-Tyr
Serine (664)	Arg-X-Ser-X-X-X-X-Arg
Serine (725)	Lys-Arg-Ser-Ser-Lys
Threonine (698)	Arg-X-Thr-X-X-X-X-Lys

sult in the expression of a second sorting signal for the receptor to be routed to the apical plasma membrane.

8. Summary

The transport of polymeric immunoglobulins, predominantly IgA dimers, across the epithelia of mucous and exocrine glands, is of fundamental importance in the protection of mucosal surfaces from invasion by pathogenic organisms. Transepithelial transport of the pIg is mediated by a receptor known as the polymeric immunoglobulin receptor. This receptor is synthesized by the mucosal and exocrine epithelial cells as a transmembrane glycoprotein with an M_r of about 115,000. Analysis of the primary structure of the receptor reveals extensive homology with the immunoglobulin superfamily. The receptor is synthesized on the rER and is cotranslationally core-glycosylated. It is subsequently transported to the Golgi complex with a half-time of approximately 30 min and is terminally glycosylated. After maturation in the Golgi, where we propose that phosphorylation of its cytoplasmic tail occurs, the receptor is sorted to the basolateral plasma membrane where it encounters and binds its pIg ligand. The receptor–ligand complex is endocytosed, and the endocytic vesicles shuttle to the apical plasma membrane, avoiding degradation of their contents within lysosomes. By fusion of these vesicles with the apical plasma membrane and cleavage of the receptor's membrane anchoring domain, pIg bound to the ectoplasmic domain of the receptor can be released into exosecretions. The fate of the membrane anchoring domain is uncertain, but there is evidence to suggest that it too is released from the membrane into external secretions.

References

Adinolfi, M., Glynn, A.A., Lindsay, M., and Milne, C., 1966, IgA antibodies to *E. coli* present in human colostrum, *Immunology* **10:**517–526.

Akao, Y., Sasagawa, A., Shiga, S., and Kono, R., 1971, Comparative studies on the mode of neutralization reaction of poliovirus type 2, with serum IgG and secretory IgA from mother's milk and foetal extract, *Jpn. J. Med. Sci. Biol.* **24:**135–152.

Arny, M., Kelly-Hatfield, P., Lamm, M.E., and Phillips-Quagliata, J.M., 1984, T-cell help for the IgA response: The function of T cells from different lymphoid organs in regulating the proportions of plasma cells expressing various isotypes, *Cell. Immunol.* **89:**95–112.

Asofsky, R., and Small, P.A., 1967, Colostral Immunoglobulin-A: Synthesis in vitro of T-chain by rabbit mammary gland, *Science* **158:**932–933.

Bergeron, J.J.M., Borts, D., and Cruz, J., 1978, Passage of serum destined proteins through the Golgi apparatus of rat liver, *J. Cell Biol.* **76:**87–97.

Bienenstock, J., and Befus, A.D., 1980, Mucosal immunity, *Immunology* **41:**249–270.

Bienenstock, J., and Befus, A.D., 1983, Regulation of lymphoid traffic and localization in mucosal tissues, with emphasis on IgA, *Fed. Proc.* **42:**3213–3217.

Bienenstock, J., and Befus, A.D., 1984, Gut- and bronchus-associated lymphoid tissue, *Am. J. Anat.* **170:**437–445.

Birbeck, M.S.C., Cartwright, P., Hall, J.G., Orlans, E., and Peppard, J., 1979, The transport by hepatocytes of immunoglobulin A from blood to bile visualized by autoradiography and electron microscopy, *Immunology* **37:**477–484.

Bockman, D.E., and Cooper, M.D., 1973, Pinocytosis by epithelium associated with lymphoid follicles in the Bursa of Fabricius, appendix, and Peyer's patches. An electron microscopic study, *Am. J. Anat.* **136:**455–478.

Brandtzaeg, P., 1974, Mucosal and glandular distribution of immunoglobulin components: Different localization of free and bound SC in secretory epithelial cells, *J. Immunol.* **112:**1553–1559.

Brandtzaeg, P., 1981, Transport models for secretory IgA and secretory IgM, *Clin. Exp. Immunol.* **44:**221–232.

Brandtzaeg, P., 1983, The secretory immune system of lactating human mammary glands compared with other exocrine organs, *Ann. N.Y. Acad. Sci.* **409:**353–382.

Brown, W.R., Newcomb, R.W., and Ishizaka, K., 1970, Proteolytic degradation of exocrine and serum immunoglobulins, *J. Clin. Invest.* **49:**1374–1380.

Brown, W.R., Isobe, Y., and Nakane, P.K., 1976, Studies on translocation of immunoglobulins across intestine epithelium. II. Immunoelectron-microscopic localization of immunoglobulin and secretory component in human intestinal mucosa, *Gastroenterology* **71:**985–995.

Bye, W.A., Allan, C.H., and Trier, J.S., 1984, Structure, distribution, and origin of M cells in Peyer's patches of mouse ileum, *Gastroenterology* **86:**789–801.

Campbell, D., and Vose, B.M., 1985, T cell control of IgA production. I. Distribution activation conditions and culture of isotype specific regulating helper cells, *Immunology* **6:**81–91.

Capasso, J.M., Abeijon, C., and Hirschberg, C.B., 1985, Phosphoproteins and protein kinases of the Golgi apparatus membrane, *J. Biol. Chem.* **260:**14879–14884.

Cebra, J.J., and Small, P.A., 1967, Polypeptide chain structure of rabbit immunoglobulin. III. Secretory gamma-A-immunoglobulin from colostrum, *Biochemistry* **6:**503–512.

Courtoy, P.J., Quintart, J., and Baudhuin, P., 1984, Shift of equilibrium density induced by 3,3′-diaminobenzidine cytochemistry: A new procedure for the analysis and purification of perixodase-containing organelles, *J. Cell Biol.* **98:**870–876.

Crago, S.S., and Mestecky, J., 1984, Presence of antibodies to food antigens in human colostral cells, in: *Protides of the Biological Fluids,* Vol. 32 (H. Peters, ed.), Pergamon Press, New York, pp. 227–230.

Crago, S.S., Kulhavy, R., Prince, S.J., and Mestecky, J., 1978, Secretory component on epithelial cells is a surface receptor for polymeric immunoglobulins, *J. Exp. Med.* **147:**1832–1837.

Cruz, J.R., and Hanson, L.A., 1983, Specific immune response in human milk to oral immunisation with food proteins, *Ann. N.Y. Acad. Sci.* **409:**808–809.

Cunningham-Rundles, C., and Lamm, M.E., 1975, Reactive half-cysteine peptides of the Secretory Component of human exocrine immunoglobulin A, *J. Biol. Chem.* **250:**1987–1991.

Deitcher, D.L., Neutra, M.R., and Mostov, K.E., 1986, Functional expression of the polymeric immunoglobulin receptor from cloned cDNA in fibroblasts, *J. Cell Biol.* **102:**911–919.

Delacroix, D., Denef, A.M., Acosta, G.A., Montgomery, P.C., and Vaerman, J.P., 1982, Immunoglobulins in rabbit hepatic bile: Selective secretion of IgA and IgM and active plasma-to-bile transfer of polymeric IgA, *Scand. J. Immunol.* **16:**343–350.

Ducroc, R., Heyman, M., Beaufrere, B., Morgat, J.L., and Desjeux, J.F., 1983, Horseradish peroxidase transport across rabbit jejunum and Peyer's patches *in vitro, Am. J. Physiol.* **245:**G54–G58.

Dunn, W.A., Wall, D.A., and Hubbard, A.L., 1983, Use of isolated, perfused liver in studies of receptor-mediated endocytosis, *Methods Enzymol.* **98:**225–240.

Dunphy, W.G., and Rothman, J.E., 1983, Compartmentation of Asp-linked oligosaccharide processing in the Golgi apparatus, *J. Cell Biol.* **97:**270–275.

Dunphy, W.G., Brands, R., and Rothman, J.E., 1985, Attachment of terminal *N*-acetylglucosamine to asparagine-linked oligosaccharides occurs in the central cisternae of the Golgi stack, *Cell* **40:**463–472.

Ehrenreich, J.H., Bergeron, J.J.M., Siekevitz, P., and Palade, G.E., 1973, Golgi fractions prepared from rat liver homogenates. I. Isolation procedure and morphological characterization, *J. Cell Biol.* **59:**45–72.

Eiffert, H., Quentin, E., Decker, J., Hillemeir, S., Hufschmidt, M., Klingmuller, D., Weber, M., and Hilschmann, N., 1984, Die primarstruktur der menschlichen freien sekretkomponent und die anordnung der disulfidbrucken, *Hoppe Seylers Z. Physiol. Chem.* **365:**1489–1495.

Elder, J.H., Pickett, R.A. II, Hampton, J., and Lerner, R., 1977, Radioiodination of proteins in single polyacrylamide gel slides, *J. Biol. Chem.* **252:**6510–6515.

Elson, C.O., Heck, J.A., and Strober, W., 1979, T cell regulation of murine IgA synthesis, *J. Exp. Med.* **149:**632–643.

Fisher, M.M., Nagy, B., Underdown, B.J., and Bazin, H., 1979, Biliary transport of IgA: Role of secretory component, *Proc. Natl. Acad. Sci. USA* **76:**2008–2012.

Fuller, S.D., Bravo, R., and Simons, K., 1985, An enzymatic assay reveals that proteins destined for the apical or basolateral domains of an epithelial cell line share the same late Golgi compartments, *EMBO J.* **4:**297–307.

Geuze, H.J., Slot, J.W., Strous, G.J.A.M., Peppard, J., Von Figura, K., Hasilik, A., and Schwartz, A.L., 1984, Intracellular receptor sorting during endocytosis: Comparative immunoelectron microscopy of multiple receptors in rat liver, *Cell* **37:**195–204.

Goldberg, D.E., and Kornfeld, S., 1983, Evidence for extensive subcellular organization of asparagine-linked oligosaccharide processing and lysosomal enzyme phosphorylation, *J. Biol. Chem.* **258:**3159–3165.

Goldblum, R.M., Ahlstedt, S., Carlsson, B., Hanson, L.A., Jodal, U., Lidin-Hanson, G., and Sohl-Akerlund, A., 1975, Antibody-forming cells in human colostrum after oral immunization, *Nature* **257:**797–798.

Grey, H., Abel, C.A., and Zimmermann, B., 1971, Structure of IgA proteins, *Ann. N.Y. Acad. Sci.* **190:**37–48.

Halpern, M.S., and Koshland, M.E., 1970, Novel subunit in secretory IgA, *Nature* **228:**1276–1278.

Hanson, L.A., Carlsson, B., Cruz, J.R., Garcia, B., Holmgren, J., Shaukat, R. Khan, Lindblad, B.S., Svennerholm, A.-M., Svennerholm, B., and Urrutia, J., 1979, Immune response in the mammary gland, in: *Immunology of Breast Milk,* Raven Press, New York, pp. 145–157.

Hendrick, S.M., Cohen, D.I., Nielson, E.A., and Davis, M.M., 1984a, Isolation of cDNA clones encoding T cell-specific membrane-associated proteins, *Nature* **308:**149–153.

Hendrick, S.M., Nielsen, E.A., Kavaler, J., Cohen, D.I., and Davis, M.M., 1984b, Sequence relationships between putative T-cell receptor polypeptides and immunoglobulins, *Nature (London)* **308:**153–158.

Hodes, H.L., Berger, R., Ainbender, E., Hevizy, M.M., Zepp, H.D., and Kochwa, S., 1964, Proof that colostrum polio antibody is different from serum antibody, *J. Pediatr.* **65:**1017–1024.

Hoppe, C.A., Connolly, T.P., and Hubbard, A.L., 1985, Transcellular transport of polymeric IgA in the rat hepatocyte: Biochemical and morphological characterization of the transport pathway, *J. Cell Biol.* **101:**2113–2123.

Huang, S.W., Fogh, J., and Hong, R., 1976, Synthesis of Secretory Component by human colon cancer cells, *Scand. J. Immunol.* **5:**263–268.

Hunter, T., and Cooper, J.A., 1985, Protein-tyrosine kinases, *Annu. Rev. Biochem.* **54:**897–930.

Jackson, G.D.F., Lemaitre-Coelho, I., Vaerman, J.P., and Beckers, A., 1978, Rapid disappearance from serum of intravenously injected rat myeloma IgA and its secretion into bile, *Eur. J. Immunol.* **8:**123–126.

Jones, A.L., Renston, R.H., and Burwen, S.J., 1982, Uptake and intracellular disposition of plasma-derived proteins and apoproteins by hepatocytes, *Prog. Liver Dis.* **7:**51–69.

Kawanishi, H., Saltzman, L., and Strober, W., 1983, Mechanisms regulating IgA class-specific immunoglobulin production in murine gut-associated lymphoid tissues. I. T cells derived from Peyer's patches which switch sIgM B cells to sIgA cells in vitro, *J. Exp. Med.* **157:**433–445.

Kawanishi, H., and Strober, W., 1983, Regulatory T-cells in murine Peyer's patches directing IgA-specific isotype switching, *Ann. N.Y. Acad. Sci.* **409:**243–257.

Keljo, D.J., and Hamilton, J.R., 1983, Quantitative determination of macromolecular transport rate across intestinal Peyer's Patches, *Am. J. Physiol.* **244:**G637–G644.

Kiyonott, J.R., McGhee, L.M., Mostelter, J.H., Koopman, J.H., Kearney, J.K., and Michaelek, S.M., 1982, Murine Peyer's patch T cell clones. Characterization of antigen-specific helper T cells for IgA response, *J. Exp. Med.* **156:**1115–1121.

Knight, K.L., Vetter, M.L., and Malek, T.R., 1975, Distribution of covalently bound and non-covalently bound Secretory Component on subclasses of rabbit secretory IgA, *J. Immunol.* **115:**595–598.

Krebs, E.G., and Beavo, J.A., 1979, Phosporylation-dephosporylation of enzymes, *Annu. Rev. Biochem.* **48:**923–959.

Kuhn, L.C., and Kraehenbuhl, J.P., 1979a, Interaction of rabbit secretory component with rabbit IgA dimer, *J. Biol. Chem.* **254:**11066–11071.

Kuhn, L.C., and Kraehenbuhl, J.P., 1979b, Role of secretory component, a secreted glycoprotein, in the specific uptake of IgA dimer by epithelial cells, *J. Biol. Chem.* **254:**11072–11081.

Kuhn, L.C., and Kraehenbuhl, J.P., 1981, The membrane receptor for polymeric immunoglobulin is structurally related to secretory component, *J. Biol. Chem.* **256:**12490–12495.

Kuhn, L.C., and Kraehenbuhl, J.P., 1982, The sacrificial receptor—translocation of polymeric IgA across epithelia, *Trends Biochem. Sci.* **7:**299–302.

Kuhn, L.C., Kocher, H.P., Hanly, W.C., Cook, L., Jaton, J.-C., and Kraehenbuhl, J.-P., 1983, Structural and genetic heterogeneity of the receptor mediating translocation of immunoglobulin A dimer across epithelia in the rabbit, *J. Biol. Chem.* **258:**6653–6659.

Lamm, M.E., Weisz-Carrington, P., Roux, E.M., McWilliams, M., and Phillips-Quagliata, J.M., 1979, Mode of induction of an IgA response in the breast and other secretory sites by oral antigen, in: *Immunology of Breast Milk* (P.L. Ogra and D. Dayton, eds.), Raven Press, New York, pp. 105–109.

Larkin, J.M., Sztul E.S., and Palade, G.E., 1986, Phosphorylation of the rat hepatic polymeric IgA receptor, *Proc. Natl. Acad. Sci. USA* **83:**4759–4763.

Leferre, M.E., Olivo, R., Vanderhoff, J.W., and Joel, D.D., 1978, Accumulation of latex in Peyer's patches and its subsequent appearance in villi and mesenteric lymph nodes, *Proc. Soc. Exp. Biol. Med.* **159:**298–302.

Lemaitre-Coelho, I., Acosta, A.G., Barranco-Acosta, C., Meykens, R., and Vaerman, J.P., 1981, In vivo experiments involving secretory component in the rat hepatic transfer of polymeric IgA from blood to bile, *Immunology* **43:**261–270.

Limet, J.N., Schneider, Y.J., Vaerman, J.P., and Trouet, A., 1982, Binding uptake and intracellular processing of polymeric rat immunoglobulin A by cultured rat hepatocytes, *Eur. J. Biochem.* **125:**437–443.

Limet, J.N., Quintart, J., Schneider, Y.J., and Courtoy, P.J., 1985, Receptor-mediated endocytosis of polymeric IgA and galactosylated serum albumin in rat liver, *Eur. J. Biochem.* **146:**539–548.

Lincoln, T.M., and Corbin, J.D., 1977, Adenosine 3′:5′-cyclic monophosphate and guanosine 3′:5′-cyclic monophosphate dependent protein kinases: Possible homologous proteins, *Proc. Natl. Acad. Sci. USA* **74:**3239–3243.

Lindh, E., 1975, Increased resistance of immunoglobulin A dimers to proteolytic degradation after binding of secretory component, *J. Immunol.* **114:**284–286.

Lischwe, M.A., and Ochs, A., 1982, A new method for partial peptide mapping using *N*-chlorosuccinimide/urea and peptide silver staining in SDS-PAGE, *Anal. Biochem.* **127:**453–457.

Mestecky, J., McGhee, J.R., Russell, M.W., Michalek, S.M., Kutteh, W.H., Gregory, R.L., Scholler-Guinard, M., Brown, T.A., and Crago, S.S., 1984, Evidence for a common mucosal immune system in humans, in: *Protides of the Biological Fluids*, Vol. 32 (H. Peters, ed.), Pergamon Press, New York, pp. 25–29.

Montgomery, P.C., Connelly, K.M., Cohn, C., and Skandera, C.A., 1979, Remote-side stimulation of secretory IgA antibodies following bronchial and gastric stimulation, *Adv. Exp. Med. Biol.* **107:**113–122.

Montgomery, P.C., Skandera, C.A., and Majumdar, A.S., 1984, Evidence for migration of IgA bearing lymphocytes between peripheral mucosal sites, in: *Protides of the Biological Fluids*, Vol. 32 (H. Peters, ed.), Pergamon Press, New York, pp. 43–46.

Mostov, K.E., Kraehenbuhl, J.P., and Blobel, G., 1980, Receptor mediated transcellular transport of immunoglobulin: Synthesis of secretory component as multiple and larger transmembrane forms, *Proc. Natl. Acad. Sci. USA* **77:**7257–7261.

Mostov, K.E., and Blobel, G., 1982, A transmembrane precursor of secretory component, *J. Biol. Chem.* **257:**11816–11821.

Mostov, K.E., Friedlander, M., and Blobel, G., 1984, The receptor for transepithelial transport of IgA and IgM contains multiple immunoglobulin-like domains, *Nature* **308:**37–43.

Mostov, K.E., and Deitcher, D.L., 1986, Polymeric immunoglobulin receptor expressed in MDCK cells transcytoses IgA, *Cell.* **46:**613–621.

Mullock, B.M., Hinton, R.H., Dobrota, M., Peppard, J., and Orlans, E., 1979, Endocytic vesicles in liver carry polymeric IgA from serum to bile, *Biochim. Biophys. Acta* **587:**381–391.

Mullock, B.M., Hinton, R.H., Dobrota, M., Peppard, J., and Orlans, E., 1980a, Distribution of secretory component in hepatocytes and its mode of transfer into bile, *Biochem. J.* **190:**819–826.

Mullock, B.M., Jones, R.S., and Hinton, R.H., 1980b, Movement of endocytic shuttle vesicles from the sinusoidal to the bile canalicular face of hepatocytes does not depend on the occupation of receptor sites, *FEBS Lett.* **113:**201–205.

Mullock, B.M., Jones, R.S., Peppard, J., and Hinton, R.H., 1980c, Effect of colchicine on the transfer of IgA across hepatocytes into bile in isolated perfused rat livers, *FEBS Lett.* **120:**278–282.

Mullock, B.M., Luzio, J.P., and Hinton, R.H., 1983, Preparation of a low density species of endocytic vesicles containing immunoglobulin A, *Biochem. J.* **214:**823–827.

Nagura, H., Nakane, P.K., and Brown, W.R., 1979, Translocation of dimeric IgA through neoplastic colon cells in vitro, *J. Immunol.* **123:**2359–2368.

Neutra, M.R., Guerina, N.G., Hall, T.L., and Nicolson, G.L., 1982, Transport of membrane-bound macromolecules by M cells in rabbit intestine, *Gastroenterology* **82**(2)**:**1137.

Nigg, E.A., Schafer, G., Hilz, H., and Eppenberger, H.M., 1985, Cyclic-AMP-dependent protein kinase type II is associated with the Golgi complex and with centrosomes, *Cell* **41:**1039–1051.

Ogra, P.L., Losonsky, G.A., and Fishaut, M., 1983, Colostrum-derived immunity and maternal–neonatal interactions, *Ann. N.Y. Acad. Sci.* **408:**82–95.

Orlans, E., Peppard, J., Reynolds, J., and Hall, J., 1978, Rapid active transport of immunoglobulin A from blood to bile, *J. Exp. Med.* **147:**588–592.

Orlans, E., Peppard, J.V., Payne, A.W.R., Fitzharris, B.M., Mullock, B.M., Hinton, R.H., and Hall, J.G., 1983, Comparative aspects of the hepatobiliary transport of IgA, *Ann. N.Y. Acad. Sci.* **409:**411–427.

Owen, R.L., and Jones, A.L., 1974, Epithelial cell specialization within human Peyer's patches: An ultrastructural study of intestinal lymphoid follicles, *Gastroenterology* **66:**189–203.

Owen, R.L., Pierce, N.F., and Cray, W.D. Jr., 1983, Autoradiographic analysis of M cell uptake and transport of *cholera vibrio* into follicles of rabbit Payer's patches, *Gastroenterology* **84:**1267.

Peppard, J.V., Orlans, E., Andrew, E., and Payne, W.R., 1982, Elimination into bile of circulating antigen by endogenous IgA antibody in rats, *Immunology* **45:**467–472.

Phillips-Quagliata, J.M., Roux, M.E., Arny, M., Kelly-Hatfield, P., MacWilliams, M., and Lamm, M., 1983, Migration and regulation of B-cells in the mucosal immune system, *Ann. N.Y. Acad. Sci.* **409:**194–203.

Porter, P., 1973, Intestinal defence in the young pig—a review of the secretory antibody systems and their possible role in oral immunization, *Vet. Rec.* **92:**658–664.

Porter, P., 1979, Adoptive immunization of the neonate by breast factors, in: *Immunology of Breast Milk* (P.L. Ogra and D. Dayton, eds.), Raven Press, New York, pp. 197–206.

Renston, R.H., Jones, A.L., Christiansen, W.D., and Hradek, G.T., 1980, Evidence for a vesicular transport mechanism in hepatocytes for biliary secretion of immunoglobulin A, *Science* **208:**1276–1278.

Rindler, M.J., Ivanov, I.E., Plesken, H., Rodriguez-Boulan, E.J., and Sabatini, D.D., 1984, Viral glycoproteins destined for apical or basolateral plasma membrane domains transverse the same Golgi apparatus during their intracellular transport in Madin-Darby canine kidney cells, *J. Cell Biol.* **98:**1304–1319.

Rindler, M.J., Ivanov, I.E., Plesken, H., and Sabatini, D.D., 1985, Polarized delivery of viral glycoproteins to the apical and basolateral plasma membranes of Madin-Darby canine kidney cells infected with temperature-sensitive viruses, *J. Cell Biol.* **100:**136–151.

Roux, M.E., McWilliams, M., Phillips-Quagliata, J.M., Weisz-Carringtron, P., and Lamm, M.E., 1977, Origin of IgA secreting plasma cells in the mammary gland, *J. Exp. Med.* **146:**1311–1322.

Russell, M.W., Brown, T.A., and Mestecky, J., 1982, Preferential transport of IgA and IgA-immune complexes to bile compared with other external secretions, *Mol. Immunol.* **19:**677–682.

Saif, L.J., and Bohl, E.H., 1979, Role of secretory IgA in passive immunity of swine to enteric viral infections, in: *Immunology of Breast Milk* (P.L. Ogra and D. Dayton, eds.), Raven Press, New York, pp. 237–255.

Schiff, M.J., Fisher, M.M., and Underdown, B.J., 1984, Receptor-mediated bilary transport of immunoglobulin A and asialoglycoprotein: Sorting and missorting of ligands revealed by two radiolabeling methods, *J. Cell Biol.* **98:**79–89.

Schiff, M.J., Fischer, M.M., Jones, A.L., and Underdown, B.J., 1986, Human IgA as a heterovalent ligand: Switching from the asialoglycoprotein receptor to secretory component during transport across the rat hepatocyte, *J. Cell Biol.* **102:**920–931.

Sheldrake, R.F., Husband, A.J., Watson, D.L., and Cripps, A.W., 1984, Selective transport of serum-derived IgA into mucosal secretions, *J. Immunol.* **132:**363–368.

Shimizu, Y., and Andrew, W., 1967, Studies on the rabbit appendix. I. Lymphocytoepithelial relations and the transport of bacteria from lumen to lymphoid nodule, *J. Morphol.* **123:**231–250.

Socken, D.J., Khursheed, N., Jeejeebhoy, K.N., Bazin, H., and Underdown, B.J., 1979, Identification of secretory component as an IgA receptor on rat hepatocytes, *J. Exp. Med.* **150:**1538–1548.

Solari, R., and Kraehenbuhl, J.P., 1984, Biosynthesis of the IgA antibody receptor: A model for the transepithelial sorting of a membrane glycoprotein, *Cell* **36:**61–71.

Solari, R., and Kraehenbuhl, J.P., 1987, Phosphorylation of the polymeric Ig receptor in the rat hepatocyte, submitted.

Solari, R., Kuhn, L.C., and Kraehenbuhl, J.P., 1985, Antibodies recognizing different domains of the polymeric immunoglobulin receptor, *J. Biol. Chem.* **260:**1141–1145.

Solari, R., Racine, L., Tallichet, C., and Kraehenbuhl, J.P., 1986, Distribution and processing of the polymeric immunoglobulin receptor in the rat hepatocyte: Morphological and biochemical characterization of subcellular fractions, *J. Histochem. Cytochem.* **34:**17–23.

South, M.A., Cooper, M.D., Wollheim, F.A., Hong, R., and Good, R.A., 1966, The IgA system. I. Studies of the transport and immunochemistry of IgA in the saliva, *J. Exp. Med.* **123:**615–627.

Speicher, D.W., Morrow, J.S., Knowles, W.J., and Marchesi, V.T., 1982, A structural model of human erythrocyte spectrin, *J. Biol. Chem.* **257:**9093–9101.

Stockert, R.J., Kressner, M.S., Collins, J.C., Sternlieb, I., and Morell, A.G., 1982, IgA interaction with the asialoglycoprotein receptor, *Proc. Natl. Acad. Sci. USA* **79:**6229–6231.

Strominger, J.L., Engelhard, V.H., Guild, B.C., Kostyk, T.G., Lancet, D., Lopez De Castro, J.A., Orr, H.T., Parham, P., Ploegh, H.L., and Pober, J.S., 1980, Complete primary structure of human histocompatibility antigen HLA-B7; evolutionary and functional implications, *Top. Dev. Biol.* **14:**97–113.

Sztul, E.S., Howell, K.E., and Palade, G.E., 1983, Intracellular and transcellular transport of secretory component and albumin in rat hepatocytes, *J. Cell. Biol.* **97:**1582–1591.

Sztul, E.S., Howell, K.E., and Palade, G.E., 1985a, Biogenesis of the polymeric IgA receptor in rat hepatocytes. I. Kinetic studies of its intracellular forms, *J. Cell Biol.* **100:**1248–1254.

Sztul, E.S., Howell, K.E., and Palade, G.E., 1985b, Biogenesis of the polymeric IgA receptor in rat hepatocytes. II. Localization of its intracellular forms by cell fractionation studies, *J. Cell Biol.* **100:**1255–1261.

Takahashi, I., Nakane, P.K., and Brown, W.R., 1982, Ultrastructural events in the translocation of polymeric IgA by rat hepatocytes, *J. Immunol.* **128:**1181–1187.

Tomasi, T.B., and Zigelbaum, S., 1963, The selective occurrence of gamma 1A globulins in certain body fluids, *J. Clin. Invest.* **42:**1552–1560.

Tomasi, T.B., Tan, E.M., Soloman, A., and Pendergast, R.A., 1965, Characteristics of an immune system common to certain external secretions, *J. Exp. Med.* **121:**101–124.

Tomasi, T.B., and Grey, H.M., 1972, Structure and function of immunoglobulin A, *Prog. Allergy* **16:**81–213.

Tseng, J., 1982, Expression of immunoglobulin heavy chain isotypes by Peyer's patch lymphocytes stimulated with mitogens in culture, *J. Immunol.* **128:**2719–2725.

Underdown, B.J., and Dorrington, K.J., 1974, Studies on the structure and conformational basis for the relative resistance of serum and secretory immunoglobulin A to proteolysis, *J. Immunol.* **112:**949–959.

Underdown, B.J., Schiff, M.J., Nagy, B., and Fisher, M.M., 1983, Differences in processing of polymeric IgA and asialoglycoproteins by the rat liver, *Ann. N.Y. Acad. Sci.* **409:**402–410.

Warren, R.J., Lepow, M.S., Bartsch, C.T.E., and Robbins, F.C., 1964, The relationship of maternal antibody, breast feeding and age to the susceptibility of newborn infants to infection with attenuated polio-viruses, *Pediatrics* **34:**4–12.

Weisz-Carrington, P., Roux, M.E., and Lamm, M.E., 1977, Plasma cells and epithelia immunoglobulins in the mouse mammary gland during pregnancy and lactation, *J. Immunol.* **119:**1306–1309.

Weisz-Carrington, P., Roux, M.E., McWilliams, M., Phillips-Quagliata, J.M., and Lamm, M.E., 1978, Hormone induction of the secretory immune system in the mammary gland, *Proc. Natl. Acad. Sci. USA* **75:**2928–2932.

Wilde, C.E., and Koshland, M.E., 1973, Molecular size and shape of the J chain from polymeric immunoglobulins, *Biochemistry* **12:**3218–3224.

Williams, A.F., and Gagnon, J., 1982, Neuronal cell Thy-1 glycoprotein: Homology with immunoglobulin, *Science* **216:**696–703.

Wolf, J.L., Rubin, D.H., Finberg, R., Kauffman, R.S., Sharpe, A.M., Trier, J.S., and Fields, B.N., 1981, Intestine M cells: A pathway for entry of retrovirus into the host, *Science* **212:**471–472.

Yanagi, Y., Yoshikai, Y., Leggett, K., Clark, S.P., Aleksander, I., and Mak, T., 1984, A human T cell-specific cDNA clone encodes a protein having extensive homology to immunoglobulin chains, *Nature* **308:**145–149.

III

Molecular Biology of the Mammary Gland

9

Milk Protein Gene Structure and Expression

Jeffrey M. Rosen

1. Introduction

The abundant milk proteins, the caseins and major whey proteins, α-lactalbumin, and whey acidic protein, are of interest because they provide specific molecular markers for studying the hormonal and developmental regulation of mammary gland gene expression. Prior to the advent of recombinant DNA technology, the mammary gland was a particularly attractive system for studying the mechanisms by which peptide and steroid hormones regulate gene expression. It was possible to purify partially the highly abundant casein mRNAs, to synthesize specific cDNA probes, and to study the effects of hormones in explant cultures using a chemically defined medium (Matusik and Rosen, 1978). More recently, it has been possible to isolate both cDNA and genomic clones specifying many of the individual milk protein mRNAs (Richards et al., 1981; Jones et al., 1985). This permitted a detailed comparison of gene and protein structures and an understanding of the evolution of these genes. It also has provided evidence for their differential regulation by hormones and during mammary development. These studies of milk protein gene structure are just beginning to provide insight into the mechanisms regulating milk protein gene expression.

Progress in the identification of *cis*-acting DNA sequences important for milk protein gene regulation has been disappointingly slow.

Jeffrey M. Rosen • Department of Cell Biology, Baylor College of Medicine, Houston, Texas 77030.

Only a few laboratories have reported the isolation and detailed characterization of these genes, so extensive sequence comparisons have not been possible. More importantly, the functional analysis of *cis*-acting DNA sequences requires the availability of hormonally responsive, preferably clonal cell lines that are amenable to gene transfection. Although a variety of breast tumor cell lines maintaining both hormone receptors and responsiveness exist, these cell lines usually do not retain specific milk protein synthesis. The expression of milk protein synthesis in primary mammary epithelial cell cultures has been shown to be dependent on cell–cell and cell–substratum interactions, as well as hormonal signals (Lee et al., 1985; Levine and Stockdale, 1985). Thus, it may be difficult to reproduce these conditions in transformed cell lines. An alternate approach that should eventually permit the identification of *cis*-acting sequences important for the hormonal and tissue-specific expression of the milk protein genes is the analysis of entire genes and their flanking DNA, as well as gene fusions in transgenic mice (Palmiter and Brinster, 1986).

In this chapter, recent information about milk protein gene structure and evolution, as well as evidence for the differential regulation of the individual casein and whey protein genes, is reviewed. These studies have led to the identification of a potential mammary consensus sequence that provides a target for future functional analyses. Readers are referred to several earlier reviews for information about the roles of individual hormones in regulating milk protein gene expression and attempts to define regulatory sequences by gene transfer experiments (Rosen et al., 1985,1986).

2. Casein Gene Structure

The caseins are a family of milk phosphoproteins that form calcium-dependent micelles (Waugh, 1971). The α- and β-caseins are described as calcium sensitive, because they precipitate in the presence of low concentrations of calcium (Waugh, 1971). These calcium-sensitive caseins are maintained in stable suspension in milk because of their interaction with κ-casein (Mackinlay and Wake, 1971). The bovine caseins have been studied extensively at the protein level and their amino acid sequences are known (Ribadeau-Dumas et al., 1972). Extensive nucleotide sequence analysis of a number of casein mRNAs from rat (Blackburn et al., 1982; Hobbs and Rosen, 1982), mouse (Hennighausen and Sippel, 1982a), guinea pig (Hall et al., 1984a,b), and cow (Stewart et al., 1984, 1987) has revealed a considerable species divergence among the casein nucleotide sequences. This divergence was expected: The caseins represent one of the most rapidly diverging protein families yet studied. Three regions of the calcium-sensitive casein mRNAs, however, are highly conserved. These include the 5′ noncoding region, signal peptide, and casein kinase phosphorylation sequences.

The unusual conservation of the 5′ noncoding region of the casein mRNAs may be related to the formation of a potentially stable secondary structure, which in turn may have a role in the posttranscriptional regulation of casein synthesis. The signal peptides of the calcium-sensitive caseins are all 15 amino acids in length and contain an invariant lysine residue in position 2 and a cysteine residue in position 8. These residues may play a role in the efficient translocation of the molecule into the endoplasmic reticulum and the recognition and removal of the signal sequence. The conservation of the signal peptide sequences is also unexpected because they usually diverge more rapidly than the coding regions of their respective proteins. In the casein proteins, phosphorylation commonly occurs on a serine residue, when it is in the sequence Ser-X-Glu or Ser-X-SerP, which constitutes a minor phosphorylation site. Addition of a second Glu residue to a (Ser)*n*-Glu sequence converts a minor to a major phosphorylation site, $(\text{Ser})_n$-Glu-Glu. The conservation of the casein phosphorylation site is of critical importance for its function in the transport and sequestering of calcium phosphate in milk.

Our laboratory was the first to characterize the structure of any of the casein genes (Yu-Lee and Rosen, 1983; Jones et al., 1985; Yu-Lee et al., 1986). We have focused our attention on the structure of the genes encoding the rat calcium-sensitive caseins, which were designated the α-, β-, and γ-caseins. By sequence analysis, these have been shown to be analogous to the better characterized bovine α_{s1}-, β-, and α_{s2}-caseins, respectively. The 7.2-kb rat β-casein gene contains 9 exons ranging in size from 21 to 525 base pairs (Jones et al., 1985). As shown in Fig. 1, there is an interesting relation between the β-casein gene and protein structures. Gilbert (1978) and Blake (1978) proposed that proteins are composed of functional domains, and these domains are encoded by an exon or a group of exons. Thus, new proteins could easily be assembled from previously evolved functional domains by recruitment of the corresponding exons to form a new gene. To fulfill their nutritional role, the caseins must perform three functions: (1) be secreted, (2) form protein aggregrates termed micelles, and (3) be phosphorylated to allow calcium binding and transport. When the exon structure of the β-casein gene was examined, the expected relation between exon structure and functional domains was observed. Exon II was shown to encode the entire amino terminal signal peptide domain and the first two amino acids of

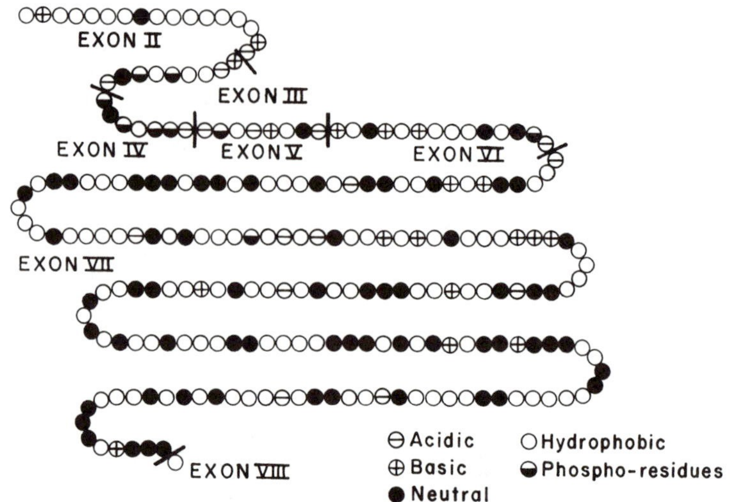

Figure 1. Relation of β-casein gene and protein structures. Each amino acid residue is designated by a circle. Solid lines designate the positions of the exon boundaries.

the mature protein. Exons III–VI each encode regions of the protein that contain minor phosphorylation sites or vestiges of these sites. Exon VII encodes the majority of the coding region of the protein, which is characterized by its hydrophobicity. Casein proteins aggregate and form micelles by the interaction of their carboxy-terminal hydrophobic domains (Waugh, 1971). Exon VIII encodes the carboxy terminus of the protein as well as a portion of the 3′ noncoding region of the casein mRNA. The two exons not included in Fig. 1, exons I and IX, contain the 5′ and 3′ noncoding regions, respectively, of β-casein mRNA.

The conserved major phosphorylation site of β-casein is not encoded by a single exon but rather is formed by an RNA splicing event. The conserved sequence of the major phosphorylation site is split with the Ser-Ser-Glu residues, the equivalent of a minor phosphorylation site, encoded by the 3′ region of exon IV and the final glutamic acid residue encoded by the 5′ end of exon V. Exons that have junctions between codons and that conform to the known RNA splice junction consensus sequences frequently encode Glu-Glu residues at their exon–intron junctions. The positioning of introns within the phosphorylation coding region may explain the complete conservation of the glutamate codons of the phosphorylation site. The amino-terminal glutamate codon is always GAG, while that of the carboxy-terminus is GAA such that they form part of the exon–intron consensus sequence. Thus, these codons are under selective pressure not only to maintain the phosphorylation site but also to maintain correct splicing.

The split architecture of the conserved phosphorylation site may reveal a relation between the exon structure of the β-casein gene and the structure of the β-casein protein. Craik et al. (1983) has hypothesized that exon–intron junctions often encode peptides found at the surface of the native protein. If this is true for β-casein, the phosphorylation sites would exist at its surface, allowing the polar residues, serines, and glutamic acids to be more accessible to the Golgi casein kinase activity, as well as for calcium binding.

3. Casein Gene Evolution

The sequence, size, and clustering of exons III–VI all support the hypothesis that they have arisen by intragenic exon duplication (Fig. 2). This had been suggested earlier based on the analysis of both casein protein and cDNA sequences (Ribadeau-Dumas et al., 1972; Hobbs and Rosen, 1982; Stewart et al., 1987). The four exons are quite similar in sequence, expecially at their 3′ ends. In addition to the sequence homology, the small sizes and the grouping of the exons, that is, two sets of small exons separated by a small intron, suggest that they are the result of two duplication events as illustrated in Fig. 2. One small exon encod-

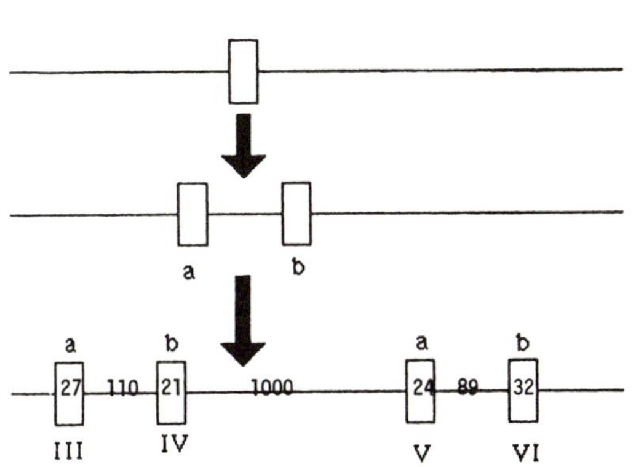

NUCLEOTIDE HOMOLOGY COMPARISONS

a	b	%
III	IV	52%
III	VI	52%
V	IV	52%
V	VI	50%
a	a	
III	V	58%
b	b	
IV	VI	71%

Figure 2. Intragenic duplication of the β-casein gene phosphorylation exon. The duplication of a primordial exon into an exon pair designated "a" and "b" followed by the reduplication of this pair to form the four exons, III, IV, V, and VI, in the rat β-casein gene is shown. The numbers in the boxes represent the sizes of the exons in base pairs, while those in between are the sizes of the introns.

ing the primordial phosphorylation site may have been duplicated to give two small exons separated by a small intron. Later, this pair of exons reduplicated to give the two pairs of exons observed today.

The calcium-sensitive casein gene family is believed to have evolved from an ancestral gene containing a site for phosphorylation and calcium binding. To test this hypothesis, we isolated and characterized regions of the rat α-, β-, and γ-casein genes (Yu-Lee and Rosen, 1983; Yu-Lee et al., 1986). In all three rat casein genes, a conserved 5′ exon structure was observed (Fig. 3) with exon I containing the 5′ noncoding sequences, ending with AAG at the 3′ terminus, exon II containing the 63-base-pair signal peptide domain, and exons III–V containing the small minor phosphorylation exon or a vestige thereof. In contrast to their exon structure, neither the size nor sequence of the introns has been conserved among the three rat genes. A similar 5′ exon I structure is also found in the bovine α_{S1}-gene and guinea pig α_{s2}-gene (Yu-Lee et al., 1986; L. Hall and R. Craig, personal communication).

Based on these observations, a model of casein gene evolution has been proposed (Fig. 4; Jones et al., 1985): The casein gene is composed of several distinct regions, each encoded by its own exon or exons. These exons appear to have arisen as the result of exon recruitment or shuffling to form a primitive casein gene followed by both intra- and intergenic duplications. Based on the rates of divergence of the casein signal peptides (Hobbs and Rosen, 1982), a calcium-sensitive casein-like gene appears to have originated 300 million years ago at the time of the appearance of primitive mammals. This casein-like gene may have been the result of exon shuffling bringing together the basic elements of the modern caseins: a 5′ noncoding region exon, a signal peptide exon, an exon with a minor phosphorylation site at its 3′ end, and a hydrophobic domain exon. Between 300 million years ago and the mammalian radiation 75 million years ago, two types of duplication appear to have occurred. The phosphorylation exon was duplicated intragenically to create the several small exons observed in the modern day genes. These exons encode several minor phosphorylation sites, one of which may have been converted to a major phosphorylation site by mutating the first codon of the downstream exon to a glutamate codon. Intergenic duplications also occurred creating the individual members of the casein gene family.

It is unlikely that the κ-casein gene, which encodes a noncalcium-sensitive casein with a distinct signal peptide sequence, is a product of these intragenic duplications. In fact, both protein and cDNA sequences obtained for the bovine (Stewart et al., 1984) and rat (Nakhasi et al., 1984) κ-caseins have indicated that it has a totally different evolutionary

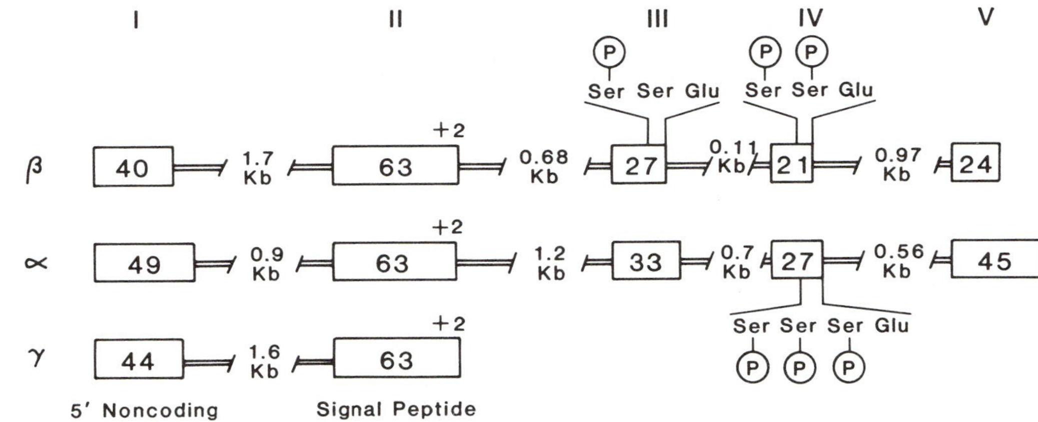

Figure 3. Conserved 5′ exon structure of the rat casein genes. Numbers within boxes indicate exon sizes in base pairs, and those in between the boxes represent approximate intron sizes in kilobases. The position of the second amino acid in the caseins is indicated by +2. The position and the typical amino acid sequence of the phosphorylation sites (Ser-Ser-Glu) are as indicated, where Ⓟ indicates that the residue is phosphorylated.

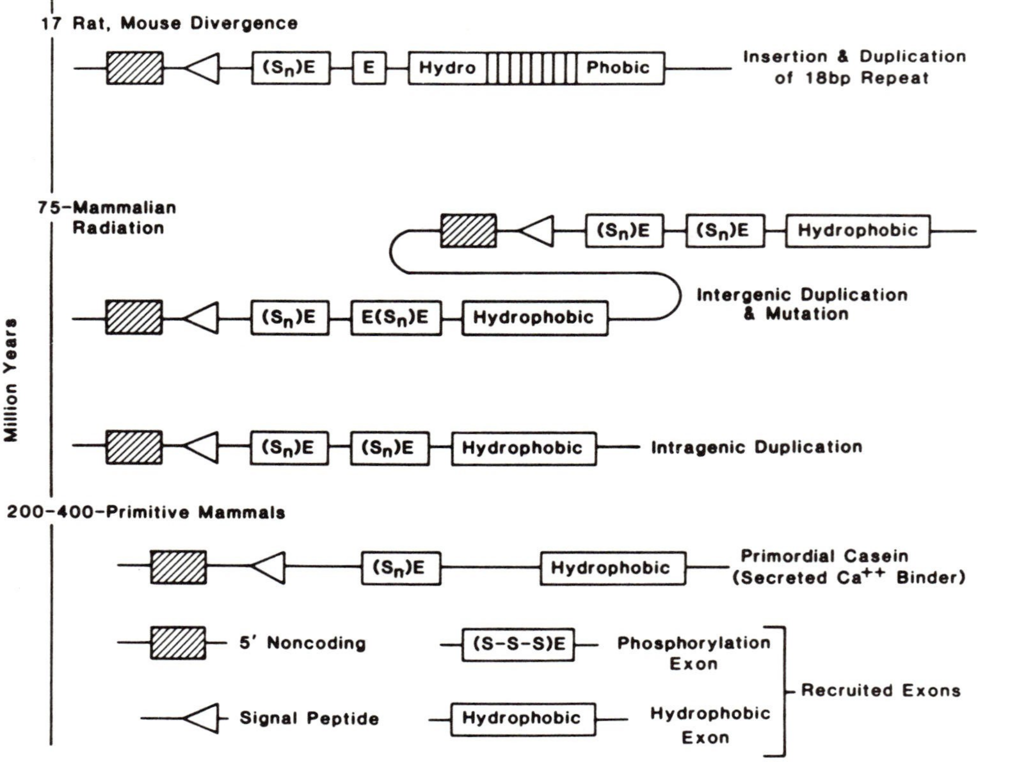

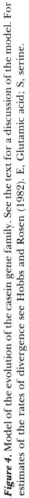

Figure 4. Model of the evolution of the casein gene family. See the text for a discussion of the model. For estimates of the rates of divergence see Hobbs and Rosen (1982). E, Glutamic acid; S, serine.

history. Considerable homology has been observed between two regions of κ-casein and human γ-fibrinogen cDNAs (Thompson et al., 1985), suggesting that κ-casein, a milk clotting protein, and γ-fibrinogen, a blood clotting protein, may have evolved from a common ancestor. It is therefore curious that the calcium-sensitive and κ-caseins have been reported to be clustered based on genetic data (Matyukov and Urnysher, 1980).

A final aspect of the model of casein gene evolution deals with the presence of $9\frac{1}{2}$ copies of an 18-base-pair repeat sequence, which is flanked by a direct repeat, CCAA (Hobbs and Rosen, 1982), in the rat α-casein. This insertion appears to be the result of a transpositional event based on both the observation that a similar sequence is lacking in the bovine α_{s1}-casein mRNA (Stewart et al., 1984) and the presence of a direct repeat flanking the insertion. The inserted repetitive sequence encodes a relatively hydrophobic peptide and is inserted within the hydrophobic region of rat α-casein as strikingly illustrated by the "nine fingers" present in the hydrophobicity plot between residues 130 and 190 shown in Fig. 5. The presence of this rather large hydrophobic peptide does not appear to affect the ability of the α-casein to form micelles. The repeat units have diverged to a very limited extent, and it is probable that they are due to a recent insertion into the rat gene. Assuming the repeat region is diverging at the same rate as the rest of the protein or the carboxy-terminal part, the insertion of this region into the rat α-casein may have occurred 10–20 million years ago, or just prior to the divergence of the rat and mouse. The insertion of this sequence

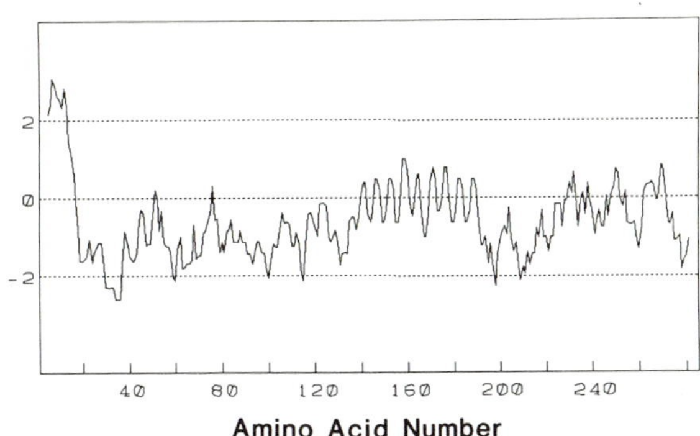

Figure 5. Hydropathy analysis of rat α-casein. The amino acid sequence of a rat α-casein was derived from the nucleic acid sequence published in Hobbs and Rosen (1982). The hydropathy analysis was performed using the Baylor Molecular Biology Information Resource program "hydropath."

before the divergence of these two rodent species would explain the larger size of the homologous mouse α-casein, as well as the rat α-casein, when compared to other mammalian α-caseins by gel electrophoresis. The functional significance of this hydrophobic insertion in these two rodent species remains to be established, but it may relate to the more concentrated protein composition of rodent milk as compared to the milks of other mammals.

Although little information is available concerning the structure of other mammalian casein genes, the complete sequences of the bovine α_{s1}-,α_{s2}-, and β-caseins have been reported by Mackinlay and his colleagues (Stewart et al., 1984, 1986). A comparison of the rat α- and bovine α_{s1}-casein mRNA sequences has revealed several interesting features. First, the percentage of replacement substitutions in the mature protein coding sequence is quite high (36–39%) and, uncharacteristically, is as high as the percentage of silent substitutions (33–44%). This is consistent with the high percentage divergence between the two proteins. The most conserved region of the protein and nucleic acid sequences is that encoding the signal peptide, which displays only an 8.8% divergence at the nucleotide level. As mentioned previously, the 5′ noncoding nucleic acid sequences are more conserved (21.3–24.5% divergence) than those encoding the mature protein (36.5% divergence). Finally, the evolutionary histories of the α- and β-casein coding sequences can be contrasted. Comparison of the bovine and rat β-caseins shows that their divergence has involved a high rate of nucleotide substitution but that no major insertions or deletions of sequence have occurred. On the other hand, alignment of the rat, bovine, guinea pig, and mouse α_{s2}-like sequences shows that the divergence of their translated regions has been characterized by duplication and deletion of discrete segments of sequences, which probably correspond to exons. This observation is consistent with the role of these proteins in the casein micelle; β-casein is important in determining the surface properties of casein micelles and is essential for curd formation (Pearse et al., 1986), while the α-caseins, by contrast, occur in varying amounts or may be absent altogether as appears to be the case for human milk.

4. Whey Protein Gene Structure and Evolution

α-Lactalbumin is the major whey protein in most mammalian species (Brew and Hill, 1975). It interacts with the enzyme galactosyltransferase, modifying its substrate specificity, promoting the transfer of galactose to glucose, and resulting in the synthesis of lactose. Both α-lactalbumin and lysozyme, an enzyme that catalyzes the hydrolysis of a glycosidic linkage in polysaccharides, have been proposed to have arisen from a common ancestral gene (Brew et al., 1967). This hypothesis has been confirmed by a comparison of the structures of both the rat and human α-lactalbumin genes with the structure of the chicken egg white lysozyme gene (Qasba and Safaya, 1984; Hall et al., 1986). Both the α-lactalbumin and lysozyme genes contain three introns at similar positions, and the first three exons are quite similar in sequence (ranging from 43 to 56%). While the positions of the introns are conserved between the human and rat α-lactalbumin genes, the sizes of the introns differ markedly between these two species.

In contrast to other species, the major whey protein in mice and rats is neither α-lactalbumin nor β-lactoglobulin, but an acidic, cysteine-rich protein with a molecular weight of 14 kDa, termed whey acidic protein or WAP (Hennighausen and Sippel, 1982b). WAP has so far been identified only in the milk of rats, mice, and rabbits (Hennighausen et al., 1982) and not in the more completely characterized ruminant milks. Although the function of WAP is unknown, certain features of its primary structure derived from the mRNA sequences (Hennighausen et al., 1982) allow comparisons with other proteins of known function. The arrangement of cysteines in each of the two domains of WAP is similar to that seen in other "four disulfide core" proteins (Drenth et al., 1980). These proteins, which include wheat germ agglutinin, several snake venom toxins, and the neurophysins, share a common pattern of cysteines (Fig. 6), which in some cases have been shown to form specific intramolecular disulfide bonds and folding patterns. As illustrated in Fig. 6, the arrangement of the cysteines is quite similar in the two domains of WAP and not much different from the arrangement observed in bovine neurophysin. There is, however, no similarity in other amino acid or nucleotide sequences of the two domains in WAP or between WAP and neurophysin.

All four disulfide core proteins with known functions interact with membrane receptors. It is possible that the WAP interacts with an unknown receptor in the digestive system or mammary gland. Alternatively, the large number of cysteines suggests either a metal-carrying function analogous to that of the metallothioneins, possible with a role in binding and carrying trace metals in the milk, or a direct role in providing cysteine for nutritional use.

Cloned WAP cDNAs from mouse and rat have been sequenced and the respective protein sequences deduced (Hennighausen et al., 1982). The mouse protein contains 134 amino acid residues, while the rat protein contains 137. The signal peptide and cysteine domain I of the rat

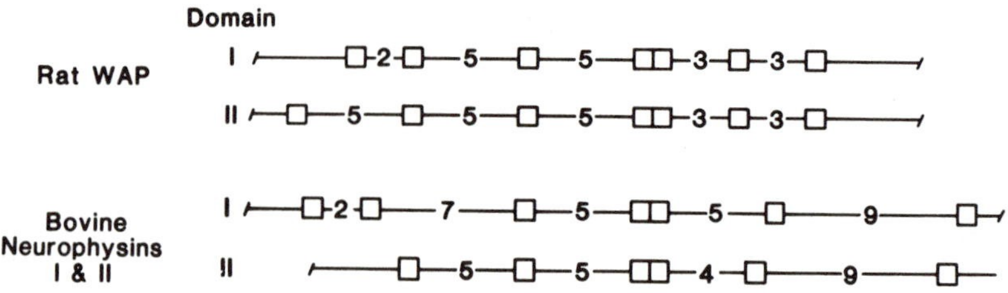

Figure 6. Two domain structures of the rat whey acidic protein as compared to bovine neurophysin. The positions of the cysteines are shown by the boxes and the numbers of amino acids between each cysteine are as indicated.

and mouse WAP are more conserved at the amino acid level than cysteine domain II. Additionally, the 3′ noncoding region is better conserved than the coding portions of the mRNA. A putative rabbit WAP cDNA sequence is only 28% homologous with the rat sequence at the nucleic acid level (L. Houdebine, personal communication), and significant protein homologies are limited to some conservation between the second cysteine domains of the rat gene, composed mostly of cysteine residues. The overall protein homology is only 15% between rat and rabbit WAP, suggesting that there is little constraint on the evolution of functional sequences within this milk protein. This could also explain the failure to identify WAP analogs in the well-characterized ruminant milks.

The characterization and sequence of the rat and mouse WAP genes have been reported (Campbell et al., 1984). The WAP gene extends over 2.8 kb in the rat and 3.3 kb in the mouse and is composed of four exons divided by three introns (Fig. 7). The difference in the sizes of the genes is primarily due to a difference between the third introns: In the mouse the size is 1.1 kb, while in the rat this intron is 0.5 kb. The first exon of the rat WAP gene encodes 41 nucleotides of the 5′ untranslated region of the mRNA plus the 19 amino acid signal peptide and the first 10 amino acids of the mature protein. It has been hypothesized that the second and third exons of the WAP gene arose via an intragenic duplication of a primordial gene in which each contained a single cysteine domain (Hennighausen et al., 1982). Each of these exons encodes precisely one cysteine domain; additionally, the 3′ ends of the second and third exons are both located at analogous positions with respect to the cysteine clusters; the splice junction splits the 14th codon 3′ to the double cysteine in each domain (Fig. 7). The fourth exon consists of 161

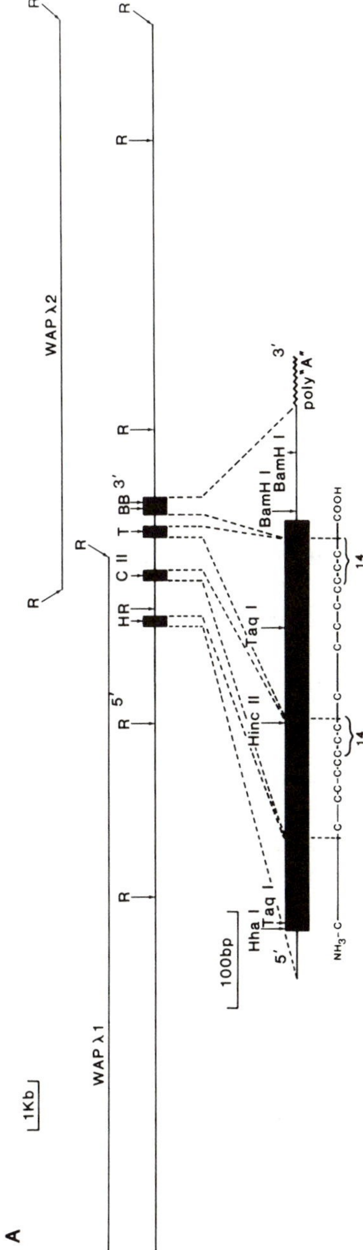

Figure 7. Structure of the rat WAP gene as compared to its mRNA. Solid boxes in the genomic portion of the figure represent exons. The heavy line in the mRNA diagram represents the protein coding portion of the mRNA. The following abbreviations for restriction endonucleases are used: R = EcoRI, H = Hha I, C II = Hinc II, T = Tag I, B = Bam HI.

nucleotides in the rat encoding the last eight amino acids, the stop codon, and the conserved 3′ noncoding region of the mRNA. Thus, exon multiplication seems to have played a role in the evolution of both the casein and WAP genes.

5. Differential Regulation of Milk Protein Gene Expression

Studies of milk protein gene expression during mammary development and in explant and cell cultures have indicated that the accumulation of the individual mRNAs can be differentially regulated (Hobbs et al., 1982). Using specific cloned DNA probes, scientists have been able to quantitate the levels of the individual casein and whey protein mRNAs during mammary development (Hobbs et al., 1982). As illustrated in Fig. 8, there are markedly different basal levels of α-, β-, and γ-casein and WAP mRNAs observed in the virgin mammary gland, with α-casein mRNA present at levels of several hundred molecules per cell, and WAP mRNA at only a few molecules per cell. During early gestation, the levels of these mRNAs increase noncoordinately, such that by midgestation β-casein mRNA is the predominant rat casein mRNA. WAP mRNA levels increase more slowly in early gestation but by late gestation appear to increase coordinately with the three calcium-sensitive casein mRNAs. Recent studies in the mouse have also reported differences in the kinetics of κ- and α-casein mRNA accumulation during mammary development (Vonderhaar and Nakhasi, 1986). The levels of κ-casein are low but detectable until midgestation and then increase markedly in concert with α-casein mRNA, maintaining a relative level two to threefold less than α-casein mRNA at later stages of gestation and lactation. Likewise, several studies have indicated that the levels of α-lactalbumin and casein increase in a noncoordinate fashion during pregnancy and lactation (Nakhasi and Qasba, 1979).

Studies using primary mammary epithelial cell cultures and explant cultures have also revealed marked differences in the regulation of the casein and whey protein genes. For example, in explant cultures, where some form of heterotypic and homotypic interactions between cells remains, expression of all the casein mRNAs as well as WAP mRNA can be detected (Hobbs et al., 1982). In primary cultures of mouse mammary epithelial cells maintained on floating collagen gels, with or without the addition of other extracellular matrix components, casein mRNAs are hormonally regulated, but WAP and α-lactalbumin are still not expressed (Lee et al., 1984, 1985). Coculture of mouse mammary epithelial cells with Swiss 3T3-L1 adipocytes allows hormone-dependent differ-

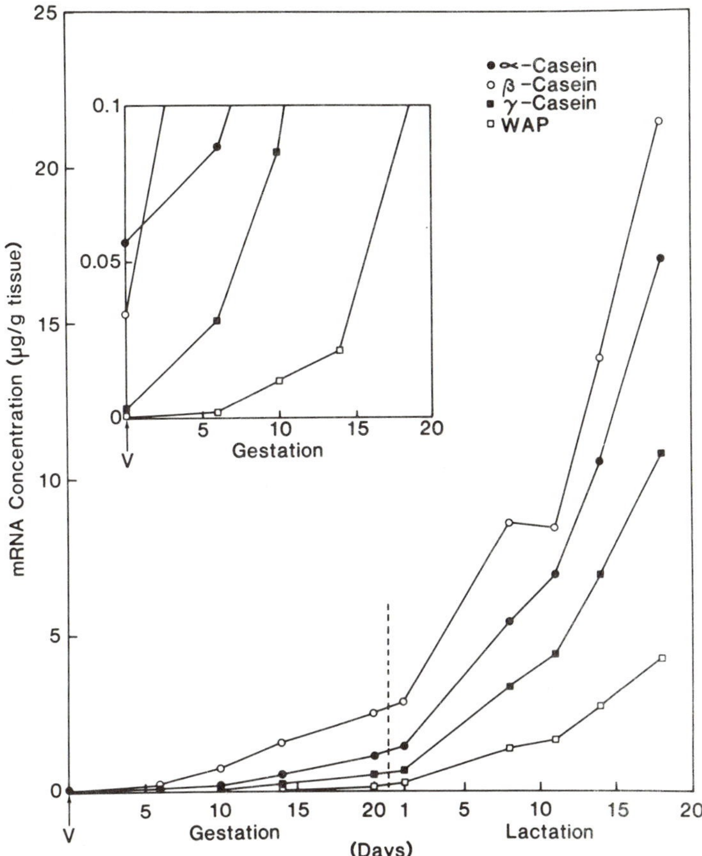

Figure 8. Differential accumulation of casein and WAP mRNAs during rat mammary development. Details are provided in Hobbs et al. (1982). The inset shows the same results for the period of gestation, but with the ordinate axis magnified 100-fold.

entiation and expression of α-lactalbumin, as well as the casein genes (Levine and Stockdale, 1985). Finally, differential effects of prolactin and hydrocortisone alone and in combination have been observed on the accumulation of the casein and WAP mRNAs (Hobbs et al., 1982). Thus, cell–cell, cell–substratum, and hormonally induced factors all play a critical role in the regulation of milk protein gene expression. Furthermore, these factors may not always act in a concerted fashion to regulate the expression of the individual milk protein genes. These observations should be considered when regulatory sequences are compared between the individual milk protein genes as discussed in the following section.

6. Regulatory Sequences Involved in Milk Protein Gene Expression

With the recent availability of genomic sequences of several of the milk protein genes, it has been possible to analyze the DNA sequences immediately upstream or 5′ to the site of the initiation of transcription of these genes. These sequence comparisons have yielded some interesting insights into the promoter regions of these genes and have identified a putative conserved sequence that may be involved in the tissue-specific expression of the milk protein genes. The initial comparison of 5′ flanking sequences of the three rat casein (α-, β-, and γ-) and the bovine α_{s1}-casein genes revealed several regions that are more highly conserved than both the entire mature coding and intron regions of these genes (Yu-Lee et al., 1986). As shown in Fig. 9, these sequences reside within the first 200 base pairs of the 5′ flanking DNA and extend beyond the TATA- and CAAT-box sequences known to be important for promoter function in many other eukaryotic genes. In the rat and bovine α-casein

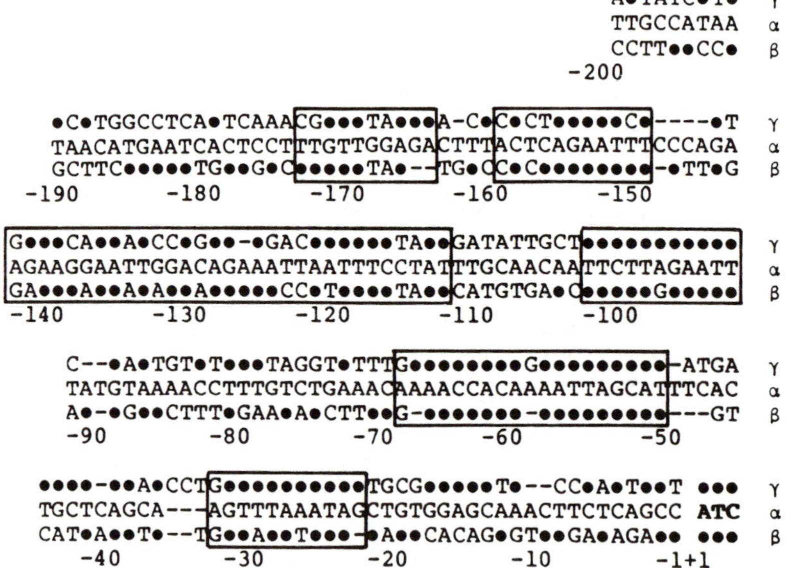

Figure 9. Conservation of the 5′ flanking regions of the casein genes. The sequences of the rat α-, β-, and γ-casein 5′ flanking DNA were aligned to give maximum homology. +1 designates the start of exon I in the α-casein gene, which is shown in boldfaced leters. All numbering refers to the α-casein gene sequence. Dots indicate similarities in the γ- or β-casein genes. Gaps (- - -) were introduced to maximize homology. The TATA box and five conserved regions are enclosed by boxes.

genes, significant homology is observed extending up to 550 base pairs upstream of the site of transcription initiation.

There are several noteworthy features of the 5′ flanking regions of the casein genes. First, these sequences are particularly AT rich (Fig. 10). The 200-base-pair region proximal to the site of transcription initiation has a mean melting temperature of only 65°C, almost 10°C less than the comparable globin gene promoter region (Myers et al., 1985) and considerably less than many housekeeping genes with highly GC-rich promoter regions (Ishii et al., 1985). Second, both the α- and γ-casein genes have the unusual TATA sequence, TTTAAAT. The transition of an A to a C,T, or G in the second position of the TATA sequence has been shown to reduce the in vitro efficiency of the promoter sequence in other genes (Conchino et al., 1983). The same altered TATA sequence is also found in both the mouse and rat WAP promoter regions (Campbell et al., 1984). Third, the rat α-casein gene contains a repeating sequence, $(CA)_{39}$, at −650 base pairs (as illustrated in the peak in Fig. 10). This sequence may act as an enhancer of gene transcription (Hamada et al., 1984) and may account for the higher basal level of α-casein gene expression in the absence of hormonal induction or virgin tissue (Fig. 8).

Recent sequence analyses of the 5′ flanking regions of several whey

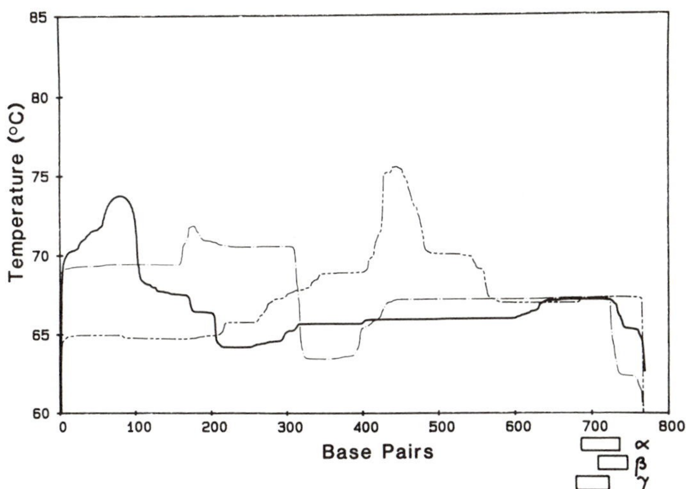

Figure 10. DNA melting profiles of the 5′ flanking regions of the rat casein genes. The positions of exon I for each of the three rat casein genes are illustrated by the open boxes below the abscissa axis. α-casein (—); β-casein (·-·-); γ-casein (- - —). The melting analyses were kindly performed by Zane Brittingham and Leonard Lerman at the Genetics Institute, Cambridge, MA (Myers et al., 1985).

protein genes have permitted comparison with the casein 5′ flanking sequences. Hall et al. (1987) first observed a region of approximately 30 base pairs, extending from −110 to −140 upstream of the site of transcription initiation, that was reasonably well conserved between the two α-lactalbumin genes and five casein genes (Fig. 11). This was the same region that was previously reported to be conserved between the casein genes in our laboratory (Fig. 9). When this putative mammary consensus sequence was aligned to the rat and mouse WAP 5′ flanking regions, the only significant similarities observed were between −279 and −309 on the noncoding DNA strand (Fig. 11). An exact 9 base pair similarity was observed, however, between the rat α-casein and mouse WAP genes at −140 and −109, respectively, but the remainder of the consensus was absent in this region of mouse WAP. No significant homologies were

```
Overall Consensus:       RGAAGRAAANTGGACAGAAA-TCAACGTTTCTA    Mismatches
 Consensus Gaps (-)            -                 --
Rat α-casein             ••••••••T-•••••••••••-•T••--••••CT       4
Rat β-casein             •A•••••••-•A••A•••••-C••T--••••••        5
Rat γ-casein             ••••C••••-•CC•G•••G•--•••--••••••        6
Bovine αs1-casein        •••G•••CT--•A••••••CA•TG•--••••CT       11
G.P. αs2-casein          ••••C-•G•-•••--•••••--•••--••••••        6
Human α-lactalbumin      ••••••••GC•••-•••GC--•••GCG•••••G        9
Rat α-lactalbumin        •••G••••GT•••-•••GC--••GGCG••••••       10
(usual position)         -140                             -110

Mouse WAP                ••TGA••••TGT••••AGTG-•••C--•••GAG       14
Rat WAP                  T•T•A••••TGT••••••T•-•••C--•••GA•       10
(position in rat)        -279                             -309
```

Figure 11. Identification of a consensus sequence present in several milk protein genes. The guinea pig (G.P.) α_{s2}-casein and human α-lactalbumin sequences are from Hall et al. (1986), the rat α-lactalbumin sequence is from Quasba and Sayafa (1984), the WAP sequences are from Campbell et al. (1984), and the other casein gene sequences are from Yu-Lee et al. (1986). Gaps (- - -) were introduced where necessary and were counted as single mismatches unless included as consensus gaps; bases introduced where there were required gaps in the consensus were also scored as single mismatches. Dots indicate bases that match the consensus. The numbers indicate the positions relative to the sites of transcription initiation.

observed with the sheep β-lactoglobulin 5′ flanking DNA kindly provided by Dr. J. Clark in Edinburgh. These results suggest that this sequence may be important in either the hormonal control or tissue-specific expression of the milk protein genes in the mammary gland (Hall et al., 1987). The latter of these possibilities seems more probable, especially because of the evidence for the differential regulation of milk protein gene expression reviewed previously.

To assay for hormone-dependent promoter and enhancer function, a series of constructions, in which the 5′ flanking regions of the β- and γ-casein genes have been cloned into the Simian virus 40-based expression vector designated SV_0CAT, have been generated (Bisbee and Rosen, 1986). These have been tested by DNA-mediated gene transfection into several different mammary and nonmammary derived cell lines. Several conclusions can be drawn from these experiments using casein-fusion genes. First, no effect of hormones (prolactin, insulin, and hydrocortisone) on CAT induction has yet been observed with up to 2.3 kb of 5′ flanking DNA. Thus, the important *cis*-acting regulatory sequences lie either further 5′ to the site of transcription initiation, or, alternatively, the sequences within and 3′ to the genes may be important in permitting the correct interaction of transcriptional and posttranscriptional regulatory signals. Second, the 5′ regions of the β- and γ-casein genes are relatively weak promoters, as compared to the SV 40 promoter and enhancer, usually yielding only 1–10% of the activity observed with SV_2CAT. The activity of these promoters was also shown to be orientation dependent; that is, they are considerably more active in the 5′ to 3′ orientation than in the opposite orientation. Finally, constructions that contain the first noncoding exon of the casein genes are more active than those containing the 5′ flanking DNA alone in mouse mammary cells. This may suggest that the 5′ noncoding exon may be important for the posttranscriptional regulation of casein gene expression observed previously (Rosen et al., 1986).

In conclusion, while DNA sequence comparisons have provided some insight into potential regulatory regions important for mammary-specific gene regulation, further studies are required to prove definitively the functional importance of these sequences. These studies will entail the analysis of milk protein fusion genes in transgenic mice, which is currently underway in our laboratory. These studies should be coordinated with specific deletion and point mutagenesis analyses, which hopefully can also be accomplished by DNA-mediated transfection in cell culture. Once the location and functional analysis of important *cis*-acting regulatory sequences is accomplished, it should be possible to identify specific *trans*-acting proteins interacting with these sequences. In this regard, preliminary experiments by Hennighausen and his colleagues have identified several protein-binding sites in the proximal 5′ flanking region of the mouse WAP gene (Lubon and Hennighausen, 1987). Several of the proteins interacting with these regions also appear to interact with similar regions in the rat casein genes (L. Hennighausen, personal communication). These combined approaches should help elucidate the mechanisms by which hormones and other factors regulate milk protein gene expression.

ACKNOWLEDGMENTS: I would like to thank a number of investigators for communicating their results prior to publication. These include Lothar Hennighausen, Louis-Marie Houdebine, Len Hall, Roger Craig, John Clark, and Tony Mackinlay. Without their assistance, this chapter would not have been possible. I would also like to thank Li Yu-Lee for help in assembling the background information for this chapter. The thermal melting profile of the rat casein genes 5′ flanking region was kindly performed by Zane Brittingham and Leonard Lerman at the Genetics Institute. Finally, Dan Goldman and Charlie Lawrence helped in the hydrophobicity analysis of rat α-casein performed using the Baylor Molecular Biology Information Resource. Research in my laboratory described herein was supported by NIH grant CA 16303 and a grant from the Welch Foundation Q-969.

References

Bisbee, C.A., and Rosen, J.M., 1986, DNA sequence elements regulating casein gene expression, in: *Transcriptional Control Mechanisms* (D.K. Granner, G. Rosenfeld, and S. Chang, eds.), UCLA Symposium on Molecular and Cellular Biology, New Series, Vol. 52, Alan R. Liss, New York.

Blackburn, D.E., Hobbs, A.A., and Rosen, J.M., 1982, Rat β-casein: Sequence analysis and evolutionary comparisons, *Nucleic Acids Res.* **10:**2295–2306.

Blake, C.C.F., 1978, Do genes-in-pieces imply proteins-in-pieces? *Nature* **273:**267.

Brew, K., and Hill, R.L., 1975, Lactose biosynthesis, *Rev. Physiol. Biochem. Pharmacol.* **72:**105–157.

Brew, K., Vanaman, T., and Hill, R.L., 1967, Comparison of the amino acid sequence of bovine α-lactalbumin and hen egg white lysozyme, *J. Biol. Chem.* **242:**3747–3749.

Campbell, S.M., Rosen, J.M., Hennighausen, L.C., Strech-Jurk, U., and Sippel, A.E., 1984, Comparison of the whey acidic protein genes of the rat and mouse, *Nucleic Acids Res.* **12:**8685–8697.

Conchino, M., Goldman, R.A., Caruthers, M.H., and Weinmann, R., 1983, Point mutations of the adenovirus major late promoter with different transcriptional efficiencies *in vitro, J. Biol. Chem.* **258:**8493–8496.

Craik, C.S., Rutter, W.J., and Fletterick, R., 1983, Splice junctions: Association with variation in protein structure, *Science* **220:**1125–1129.

Drenth, J., Low, B.W., Richardson, J.S., and Wright, C.S., 1980, The toxin–agglutinin fold, *J. Biol. Chem.* **255:**2652–2655.

Gilbert, W., 1978, Why genes-in-pieces? *Nature* **271:**501.

Hall, L., Emery, D.C., Davies, M.S., Parker, D., and Craig, R.K., 1987, Organisation and sequence of the human α-lactalbumin gene, *Biochem. J.*, (in press).

Hall, L., Laird, J.E., and Craig, R.K., 1984a, Nucleotide sequence determination of guinea-pig casein B mRNA reveals homology with bovine and rat α_{s2}-caseins and conservation of the non-coding regions of the mRNA, *Biochem. J.* **222:**561–570.

Hall, L., Laird, J.E., Pascall, J.C., and Craig, R.K., 1984b, Guinea-pig casein A cDNA. Nucleotide sequence analysis and comparison of the deduced protein sequence with that of bovine α_{s2}-casein, *Eur. J. Biochem.* **138:**585–589.

Hamada, H., Seidman, M., Howard, B.H., and Gorman, C.M., 1984, Enhanced gene expression by the poly(dT-dG)·poly(dC-dA) sequence, *Mol. Cell. Biol.* **4:**2622–2630.

Hennighausen, L.G., and Sippel, A.E., 1982a, Characterization and cloning of the mRNAs specific for the lactating mouse mammary gland, *Eur. J. Biochem.* **125:**131–141.

Hennighausen, L.G., and Sippel, A.E., 1982b, Mouse whey acidic protein is a novel member of the family of "four-disulfide core" proteins, *Nucleic Acids Res.* **10:**2677–2684.

Hennighausen, L.G., Sippel, A.E., Hobbs, A.A., and Rosen, J.M., 1982, Comparative sequence analysis of the mRNAs coding for mouse and rat whey acidic protein, *Nucleic Acids Res.* **10:**3733–3744.

Hobbs, A.A., and Rosen, J.M., 1982, Sequence of the rat α- and γ-casein mRNAs: Evolutionary comparison of the calcium-dependent casein multigene family, *Nucleic Acids Res.* **10:**8079–8098.

Hobbs, A.A., Richards, D.A., Kessler, D.J., and Rosen, J.M., 1982, Complex hormonal regulation of casein gene expression, *J. Biol. Chem.* **257:**3598–3605.

Ishii, S., Merlino, G.T., and Pastan, I, 1985, Promoter region of the human Harvey *ras* proto-oncogene: Similarity to the EGF receptor proto-oncogene promoter, *Science* **230:**1378–1381.

Jones, W.K., Yu-Lee, L.-Y., Clift, S.M., Brown, T.L., and Rosen, J.M., 1985, The rat casein multigene family. III. Fine structure and evolution of the β-casein gene, *J. Biol. Chem.* **260:**7042–7050.

Lee, E.Y.-H., Parry, G., and Bissell, M.J., 1984, Modulation of secreted proteins of mouse mammary epithelial cells by the collagenous substrata, *J. Cell Biol.* **98:**146–155.

Lee, E.Y.-H., Lee, W.-H., Kaetzel, C.S., Parry, G., and Bissell, M.J., 1985, Interaction of mouse mammary epithelial cells with collagen substrata: Regulation of casein gene expression and secretion, *Proc. Natl. Acad. Sci. USA* **82:**1419–1423.

Levine, J.F., and Stockdale, F.E., 1985, Cell–cell interactions promote mammary epithelial cell differentiation, *J. Cell Biol.* **100:**1415–1422.

Lubon, H., and Hennighausen, L., 1987, Nuclear proteins from lactating mammary glands bind to the promoter of a milk protein gene, *Nucleic Acids Res.* **15:**2103–2121.

Mackinlay, A.C., and Wake, R.G., 1971, κ-casein and its attack by rennin (chymosin), in: *Milk Proteins: Chemistry and Molecular Biology II* (H.A. McKenzie, ed.), Academic Press, New York, pp. 175–215.

Matusik, R.J., and Rosen, J.M., 1978, Prolactin induction of casein mRNA in organ culture: A model system for studying peptide hormone action on gene expression, *J. Biol. Chem.* **253:**2343–2347.

Matyukov, V.S., and Urnysher, A.P., 1980, Linkage between cattle milk α_{s1}-, β-, κ-casein loci, *Genetika* **16:**884–886.

Myers, R.M., Fischer, S.C., Maniatis, T., and Lerman, L.S., 1985, Modivication of the melting properties of duplex DNA by attachment of a GC-rich DNA sequence as determined by denaturing gradient gel electrophoresis, *Nucleic Acids Res.* **13:**3111–3129.

Nakhasi, H.L., and Qasba, P.K., 1979, Quantitation of milk proteins and their mRNAs in rat mammary gland at various stages of gestation and lactation, *J. Biol. Chem.* **254:**6016–6025.

Nakhasi, H.L., Granthan, F.H., and Gullino, P.M., 1984, Expression of κ-casein in normal and neoplastic rat mammary gland is under the control of prolactin, *J. Biol. Chem.* **259:**14894–14898.

Palmiter, R.D., and Brinster, R.L., 1986, Germline transformation of mice, *Ann. Rev. Genet.* **20:**465–499.

Pearse, M.J., Linklater, P.M., Hall, R.J., and Mackinlay, A.G., 1987, Effect of casein micelle composition and casein dephosphorylation on coagulation and syneresis, *J. Dairy Res.*, in press.

Qasba, P., and Safaya, S.K., 1984, Similarity of the nucleotide sequences of rat α-lactalbumin and chicken lysozyme genes, *Nature* **308:**377–380.

Ribadeau-Dumas, B., Brignon, G., Grosclaude, F., and Mercier, J.-C., 1972, Structure primaire de la caseine β bovine, *Eur. J. Biochem.* **25:**505–514.

Richards, D.A., Rodgers, J.R., Supowit, S.C., and Rosen, J.M., 1981, Construction and preliminary characterization of the rat casein and α-lactalbumin cDNA clones, *J. Biol. Chem.* **256:**526–532.

Rosen, J.M., Jones, W.K., Campbell, S.M., Bisbee, C.A., and Yu-Lee, L.-Y., 1985, Structure and regulation of peptide hormone responsive genes, in: *Membrane Receptors and Cellular Regulation* (M.P. Czech and C.R. Kahn, eds.), Alan R. Liss, New York, pp. 385–396.

Rosen, J.M., Rodgers, J.R., Couch, C.H., Bisbee, C.A., David-Inouye, Y., Campbell, S.M., and Yu-Lee, L.-Y., 1986, Multi-hormonal regulation of milk protein gene expression, in: *Metabolic Regulation: Application of Recombinant DNA Techniques,* New York Academy of Science, New York.

Stewart, A.F., Willis, I.M., and Mackinlay, A.G., 1984, Nucleotide sequences of bovine α_{s1}- and κ-casein cDNAs, *Nucleic Acids Res.* **12:**3895–3907.

Stewart, A.F., Bonsing, J., Beattie, C.W., Shah, F., Willis, I.M., and Mackinlay, A.G., 1987, Complete nucleotide sequences of bovine α_{s2}- and β-casein cDNAs: Comparisons with related sequences in other species, *Mol. Biol. Evol.* **4:**231–241.

Thompson, M.D., Dave, J.R., and Nakhasi, H.L., 1985, Molecular cloning of mouse mammary gland κ-casein: Comparison with rat κ-casein and rat and human γ-fibrinogen. *DNA* **4:**263–271.

Vonderhaar, B.K., and Nakhasi, H.L., 1986, Bifunctional activity of epidermal growth factor on α- and κ-casein gene expression in rodent mammary glands *in vitro, Endocrinology* **119:**1178–1184.

Waugh, D.F., 1971, Formation and structure of casein micelles, in: *Milk Proteins: Chemistry and Molecular Biology II* (H.A. McKenzie, ed.), Academic Press, New York, pp. 3–85.

Yu-Lee, L.-Y., and Rosen, J.M., 1983, The rat casein multigene family: I. Fine structure of the γ-casein gene, *J. Biol. Chem.* **258:**10794–10804.

Yu-Lee, L.-Y., Richter-Mann, L., Couch, C.H., Stewart, A.F., Mackinlay, A.G., and Rosen, J.M., 1986, Evolution of the casein multigene family: Conserved sequences in the 5′ flanking and exon regions, *Nucleic Acids Res.* **14:**1883–1902.

10

Retrovirus and Proto-oncogene Involvement in the Etiology of Breast Neoplasia

Robert Callahan

1. Introduction

The etiology of breast cancer is thought to involve a complex interplay of genetic, hormonal, and dietary factors that are superimposed on the physiological status of the host (Harris et al., 1982; Gompel and van Kerkem, 1983; Lynch et al., 1984). Extensive studies have been undertaken to determine the relation between these factors and tumor development in humans and experimental rodent models. Attempts to derive a cohesive picture of how these factors participate in mammary tumorigenesis have been hampered, in part, by a lack of information on the specific genetic lesions that contribute to the initiation and/or evolution of tumor development.

The study of experimentally induced mammary tumors has focused primarily on various high-incidence strains of inbred mice infected with the mammary mouse tumor virus (MMTV) as well as chemical carcinogen-induced tumors in mice and rats (reviewed by Weiss et al., 1982; Welsch, 1985). The demonstration that MMTV, like other retroviruses, can act as an insertion mutagen (Varmus, 1982) represents a significant advance, since the viral genome, unlike chemical carcinogens, can be used as a tag to identify the relevant mutagenic events. The association

Robert Callahan • Laboratory of Tumor Immunology and Biology, National Cancer Institute, National Institutes of Health, Bethesda, Maryland 20892.

between MMTV and mammary tumorigenesis has provided a conceptual basis to consider a similar etiology in human breast cancer (reviewed by Sarkar, 1980). In earlier studies, it had been claimed that MMTV-related nucleotide sequence and proteins are present in human breast tumors. However, these results were difficult to interpret because of the nature of the reagents used for detection. The availability of recombinant DNA clones of the MMTV genome and more sensitive detection techniques have led to a reexamination of this question (Callahan et al., 1982a; May et al., 1983; Deen and Sweet, 1986).

There is substantial evidence in neoplasias of several tissues that either the expression of certain cellular genes has been activated or the gene product has been altered by mutation (Klein, 1981). In many cases, these cellular genes are related to the acute tumorigenic retroviruses and are referred to as proto-oncogenes (Bishop, 1985). The particular proto-oncogene and type of genetic alteration (chromosomal translocation, gene amplification, point mutation, or deletion) are often specific to the type of tumor (Aaronson and Tronick, 1985). At the present time, there is little direct evidence that these cellular mutations are responsible for tumorigenesis (Duesberg, 1985). However, the high frequency with which they are altered in a particular type of cancer has been taken as evidence that they provide the tumor cell with a selective growth advantage that contributes to the evolution of the tumor (Klein, 1981).

The purpose of this chapter is to review recent advances in the identification of cellular genes that are frequently activated or genetically altered in breast carcinomas. It focuses primarily on three areas: (1) MMTV-induced tumorigenesis in mice; (2) the current status of MMTV-related sequences in human cellular DNA; and (3) cellular proto-oncogenes that are frequently altered in human breast cancer. Chemical carcinogen-induced mammary tumorigenesis has recently been reviewed (Welsch, 1985) and therefore is not discussed in detail.

2. MMTV-Induced Mammary Tumorigenesis in Mice

2.1. Biological Aspects of Tumor Development

Spontaneous mammary tumorigenesis in mice is frequently associated with a chronic infection of the host mammary tissue by the MMTV (Teich et al., 1982). The association between MMTV and mammary tumor development was first recognized in inbred strains of mice that have a high incidence of tumors (Bitner, 1942). In these mice, MMTV is transmitted congenitally through the milk. The development of the disease appears to involve a multistep process. In the high-incidence C3H strain, the earliest detectable stage of tumor development is the appearance of hyperplastic alveolar nodules (DeOme et al., 1959; Nandi, 1963). These lesions are considered premalignant precursors to the later developing (8–12 months) pregnancy-independent adenocarcinomas. In the absence of milk-borne MMTV(C3H), C3H mice develop mammary tumors at a later age (14–24 months) (Boot and Muhlbock, 1956; Pitelka et al., 1964). These tumors are also associated with MMTV infection by the genetically transmitted or endogenous MMTV genome defined by the *Mtv*-1 locus (van Nie and Verstraeten, 1975; Verstraeten and van Nie, 1978). The BR-6 inbred mouse strain contains an independent strain of milk-borne MMTV [designated MMTV(RIII)] that induces pregnancy-dependent mammary tumors (Foulds, 1949). These tumors regress at parturition and, after two or more pregnancies, progress to hormone independence (Lee, 1968).

2.2. The MMTV LTR and orf Protein

Attempts to define the link between MMTV infection and mammary tumor development have focused on a unique coding sequence within the viral genome and the potential induction of cellular mutations as a consequence of viral replication. Early studies by Hilgers and Bentvelzen (1978) led them to speculate that MMTV contains a gene that contributes to tumorigenesis. The long terminal repeat (LTR) sequence of MMTV became an attractive candidate when it was found to contain an open reading frame (orf) capable of encoding a 36,000-dalton protein (Dickson and Peters, 1981; Donehower et al., 1981; Kennedy et al., 1982). At the present time, it seems unlikely that the orf protein by itself has oncogenic potential. Pregnant and lactating BALB/c mice produce high levels of a MMTV LTR-related 1.6-kb species of RNA but rarely develop spontaneous mammary adenocarcinomas (Donehower et al., 1981). However, until more is understood about the biological properties of the orf protein, it cannot be ruled out as a contributing factor in the etiology of virally induced mammary tumors. For example, by analogy with several infectious retroviruses (human T-cell leukemia virus, human immunodeficiency virus, and the bovine leukemia virus), the orf protein could have a *trans*-acting effect on the expression of host cellular genes (Haseltine et al., 1985).

2.3. MMTV as an Insertional Mutagen

MMTV, like other retroviruses, can act as an insertional mutagen (Varmus, 1982). The retroviral genome can integrate at numerous, perhaps random, sites in the cellular genome. Indeed, the integration of a retroviral genome at a common integration locus in several tumors of the same type has been reported in avian B-cell lymphomas induced by two unrelated type C retroviruses (Hayward et al., 1981; Noori-Daloii et al., 1981), avian erythroleukemia induced by a type C retrovirus (Fung et al., 1983), and T-cell lymphomas induced by the murine leukemia virus (Tsichlis et al., 1983; Cuypers et al., 1984). In each case, the consequence of viral integration at a common locus in tumor DNA is the activation of expression of an adjacent cellular gene. The common integration loci in B-cell lymphomas and avian erythroleukemia are, respectively, the c-*myc* and c-*erb* B proto-oncogenes. Each of these genes is a progenitor of an acute tumorigenic retroviral oncogene. Based on these observations, it has been proposed as a general hypothesis that cellular genes, whose expression is activated or augmented as a result of retroviral integration in many tumors of the same type, probably contribute to tumorigenesis (Varmus, 1982).

2.4. Characteristics of the int Loci

Cohen et al. (1979), using restriction enzyme analysis, observed that MMTV-induced mammary tumors are clonal, that is, descendants of a single viral-infected mammary gland cell. Nusse and Varmus (1982) obtained recombinant DNA clones of a restriction fragment containing host–viral junction sequences from a C3H tumor DNA containing a single new MMTV proviral genome. They were able to show that this region (designated *int*-1) of the cellular genome was occupied by an MMTV provirus in 80% of the C3H mammary tumors. Using a similar strategy, Peters et al. (1983) identified a second unrelated common integration locus (designated *int*-2) that is frequently occupied by an MMTV provirus in BR-6 strain mammary tumors. The insertion of a viral genome at either locus activates the expression of a previously silent gene within the affected locus (Nusse and Varmus, 1982; Dickson et al., 1984). These activated cellular genes are highly conserved among vertebrates and are unrelated to each other or to the known proto-oncogenes (Nusse et al., 1984; van Ooyen and Nusse, 1984; Casey et al., 1986; Moore et al., 1986). They are located, respectively, on mouse chromosomes 15 and 7 (Nusse et al., 1984; Peters et al., 1984a).

The frequent insertion of a MMTV genome at the *int*-1 and *int*-2 loci is not limited to mammary tumors of high-incidence inbred mouse strains (Escot et al., 1986a). Previous surveys of feral *M. musculus domesticus* demonstrated the presence of poorly infectious MMTV in the milk of breeding females (Andervont, 1952). In general, the incidence of mammary tumors in feral breeding females is low and tumor development occurs late in life (Andervont and Dunn, 1962; Rongey et al., 1973). Recently, pedigreed breeding colonies of several species of *Mus* from different geographical regions of the world have been established (Callahan and Todaro, 1978; Callahan et al., 1982b). With few exceptions, all transmit a milk-borne MMTV (Gallahan et al., 1986b), each of which can be distinguished by immunological (Horan Hand et al., 1980; Teramoto et al., 1980) and molecular biological (Callahan et al., 1982b; Escot et al., 1986a; Gallahan and Callahan, 1986) criteria from one another or from laboratory strains of MMTV. A survey of 20 pregnancy-independent tumors from *M. cervicolor popaeus* mice was made to determine whether MMTV insertion into either the *int*-1 or *int*-2 locus is a common feature of MMTV-induced mammary tumors (Escot et al., 1986a). Tumor DNA from 10 mice contained an altered *int*-1, while one tumor had an altered *int*-2 locus. In the case of the *int*-1-positive tumors, it was possible to show that the expression of *int*-1 RNA had been activated. In contrast, a survey of 16 mammary tumors from the Czech II strain of *M. musculus musculus* revealed no cases of MMTV integration at the *int*-1 or *int*-2 loci (Gallahan and Callahan, 1986). However, an MMTV genome was found within a 0.5-kb region of the cellular genome in five out of 16 Czech II mammary tumors. MMTV (Czech II) insertion at these sites activated the expression of a previously silent gene that is adjacent to the integration locus. This region of the cellular genome has been designated *int*-3, since it is unrelated to the *int*-1 and *int*-2 loci. The *int*-3 locus is located on mouse chromosome 17, 11 cM distal to the H-2 (major histocompatibility complex) locus (Gallahan et al., 1986a). Like the other *int* loci, *int*-3 is unrelated to the known proto-oncogenes but is well conserved among avian and mammalian species.

The different strains of MMTV isolated from inbred and feral *M. musculus* are all highly related. Thus, it seems a paradox that the frequency with which the different *int* loci are activated varies with the particular strain of MMTV (Nusse and Varmus, 1982; Escot et al., 1986a; Gallahan and Callahan, 1986; Peters et al., 1986). Since different strains of mice were used in these studies, it is not possible to evaluate the potential contribution of the host's genetic background to the apparent specificity. It is known, however, that the kind of tumor (pregnancy-dependent or -independent) induced by MMTV is associated with the particular strain of virus and is independent of the mouse strain (Squartini et al., 1963). Similarly, it could be that the relative frequency with which different *int* loci are activated reflects a property of the virus which distinguishes different target cell populations in the developing mammary gland. It will be of interest to determine whether the mammary tumors induced by new strains of MMTV from feral mice (Escot et al.,

1986a; Gallahan and Callahan, 1986; Gallahan et al., 1986b) reveal the existence of additional *int* loci in tumor DNA.

The topology of the *int*-1 and *int*-2 loci is very similar (Fig. 1). The insertion of viral genomes occurs around a central core of cellular DNA that contains the respective activated cellular genes. The transcriptional orientation of the viral genomes integrated at the 5′ end of the activated gene is generally in the opposite direction. Those integrated at the 3′ end of the gene are generally in the same transcription orientation. Less is known about the *int*-3 locus. In the five tumors containing viral insertions in this region of the cellular genome, the transcriptional orientation of the viral genomes are all in the same direction. The cellular transcribed region is located 5′ to the integrated viral genomes and encodes a 2.4-kb species of RNA. It seems unlikely that the activation of these *int* loci is the result of transcription initiation from the MMTV LTR. Nusse et al. (1984) and Dickson et al. (1984) have proposed that the MMTV LTR contains sequences with enhancer-like activity in addition to the signal sequences for RNA transcription. Enhancer sequences can exert, at a considerable distance (21.0 kb), a positive *cis*-acting influence on the expression of adjacent cellular genes (de Villiers et al., 1982; Banerji et al., 1983; Gillies et al., 1983; Queen and Baltimore, 1983; Spandidos and Wilkie, 1983). The effect of the enhancer element is independent of its orientation to the transcribed gene. The near uniform orientation of the proviral genomes can be explained if enhancers

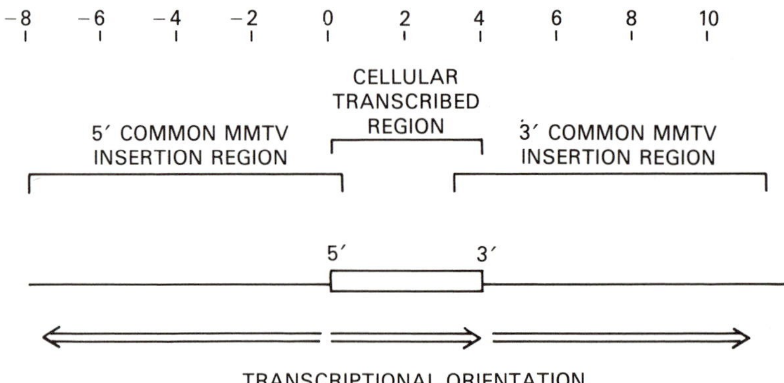

Figure 1. The organization of the *int*-1 or *int*-2 loci in MMTV-induced mammary tumors (Nusse and Varmus, 1982; Peters et al., 1983; Dickson et al., 1984). The arrows indicate the transcriptional orientation of the integrated MMTV genomes and the central cellular transcribed region. The cellular transcribed region is indicated by an open box.

act only, or preferentially, upon proximal transcriptional promoters (de Villiers et al., 1982; Wasylyk et al., 1983). Thus, only cellular genes that are 5′ to the proviral genome would be affected by the enhancer sequences in the MMTV LTR.

The nucleotide sequence of the *int*-1 and *int*-2 transcribed regions has been determined (van Ooyen and Nusse, 1984; Fung et al., 1985; Moore et al., 1986). Although the 5′ end of the *int*-1 locus has not been defined precisely, there appear to be at least four exons that are transcribed into a 2.6-kb species of poly A+ RNA. In some tumors, viral insertions have occurred in the nontranslated portion of exon 4. In these cases, it seems unlikely that a chimeric peptide composed of the *int*-1 and MMTV orf protein is expressed, since the site of viral insertion occurs 3′ to the translation stop signal within the *int*-1 exon. In vitro translation of *int*-1 RNA results in the production of a 41,000-dalton protein (Fung et al., 1985; Rijsewijk et al., 1986). The N-terminus of the protein is rich in hydrophobic amino acids, suggesting that it could be bound to or secreted from the cellular membrane. In addition, it contains four potential sites for N-linked glycosylation and a cysteine-rich carboxy terminus. These properties are reminiscent of growth factors or membrane-associated receptors. The *int*-2 transcribed region is 8.0 kb and encodes major 3.2- and 2.9-kb species of RNA composed of three exons (Moore et al., 1986). Minor species of 1.8- and 1.4-kb RNA have also been detected (Jakobovits et al., 1986). The multiple species of *int*-2 RNA probably reflect alternate promoters, splicing patterns, or novel polyadenylation signals. This remains to be determined. The protein deduced from the translated amino acid sequence encoded by the 3.2-kb RNA is 27,000 daltons. It is relatively basic but, like the *int*-1 protein, is enriched for hydrophobic amino acids near the N-terminus.

It seems probable that multiple MMTV-induced and/or stochastic mutations are required for tumor development. Indeed, the activation of *int*-1 and *int*-3 is associated with the development of virally induced pregnancy-independent mammary adenocarcinomas. The activation of the *int*-2 locus occurs very early in the pregnancy-dependent stage of MMTV (RIII)-induced mammary tumors (Peters et al., 1984b). Additional mutations are probably required for the progression to hormone independence. Peters et al. (1986) have found in 30 MMTV (RIII)-induced mammary tumors 15 with viral insertions in both the *int*-1 and *int*-2 loci, six tumors with an insertion at *int*-1 only, and six tumors with an insertion at *int*-2 only. Recently, they have shown that two of the three remaining tumors that lack viral insertions at *int*-1 or *int*-2 contain a viral insertion at *int*-3 (G. Peters, personal communication). Whether the activation of *int*-1 and *int*-3 occurs early during the pregnancy-dependent stage of tumor development or later in the progression to hormone independence is not known.

Attempts to determine the biological activity of the activated *int* locus are being pursued. Recently, a functional assay has been developed for *int*-1 (Rijsewijk et al., 1986; H. Varmus, personal communication). The *int*-1 gene, when placed in a retroviral shuttle vector, alters the morphology and growth properties of an infected mammary epithelial cell line but not the NIH 3T3 fibroblast culture. In related experiments, Sonnenberg et al. (1986) have developed a cell line (designated RAC) from an MMTV (RIII)-induced BALB/c mammary tumor. Three phenotypically different cell types can be distinguished: polygonal, cuboidal, and elongated cells. Polygonal cells retain many characteristics of epithelial cells and induce differentiated adenocarcinomas when implanted in mice. Cuboidal cells are poorly tumorigenic. Elongated cells induce highly malignant carcinosarcomas when implanted in mice and appear to be stable after many passages in culture. Analysis of the developmental relation between these cell types suggests that they progress linearly from polygonal→cuboidal→elongated. The cells of the RAC clone contain an integrated MMTV (RIII) genome within the *int*-2 locus; however, only polygonal cells express *int*-2 RNA. Although addition of the glucocorticoid hormone dexamethasone results in elevated levels of MMTV RNA in each cell type, expression of *int*-2 remains unaffected. These observations suggest the following: (1) MMTV-induced *int* gene expression and its biological consequences may be restricted to mammary cells that retain differentiation characteristics of epithelial cells; (2) expression of at least *int*-2 is caused by an enhancing activity in the MMTV LTR that is not dependent on steroid hormones; and (3) expression of *int*-2 may be important in the early stages of tumor development (i.e., polygonal cells) but not necessary in the later stages of tumor progression (cuboidal and elongated cells).

Earlier studies demonstrated that the *int*-1 and *int*-2 loci are not expressed in normal mammary tissue from pregnant or lactating mice (Dickson et al., 1984; Nusse et al., 1984). Moreover, unlike many other proto-oncogenes (Varmus, 1984; Marshall, 1985), their activation has only been implicated in mammary tumorigenesis. Jakobovits et al. (1986) reasoned that this might be characteristic of genes that normally function only in specific cell types or at defined times during embryogenesis. They have found that *int*-1 is expressed in midgestational embryos (8.5–11.5 days) and in postpuberal testes. The *int*-2 RNA is found earlier during embryogenesis, with the highest levels in cells of the primitive endoderm lineage. Expression of *int*-2 has not been detected in several adult tissues tested (liver, kidney, mammary gland, brain, muscle, spleen, and testes). Relative to the known proto-oncogenes, the expression of *int*-1 and *int*-2 appears to be restricted to short periods during embryogenesis and suggests that they might play a crucial role in mammalian development.

2.5. Summary

The use of different strains of MMTV has led to the identification of three cellular genes whose expression is frequently activated by viral integration in mammary tumor DNA. The association between different strains of MMTV and the frequency with which a particular *int* locus is activated suggests that additional *int* loci may be identified by using other strains of MMTV or different virus–host strain combinations. The frequent activation of the *int* loci in MMTV-induced tumors provides a strong argument for their involvement in tumor development. However, direct evidence demonstrating their oncogenic potential is limited. Moreover, it is unclear whether they can act in a complementary manner or are functionally independent in their contribution to tumor development. The likely availability, in the near future, of retroviral shuttle vectors containing each of the *int* loci should make it possible to address these issues in vivo as well as in the RAC and mammary epithelial cell lines.

3. Other Studies on Mouse Mammary Tumorigenesis Involving the c-myc and c-ras Proto-oncogenes

3.1. Transgenic Mice Containing Activated c-myc

Activation of members of the *myc* and *ras* proto-oncogene families by genetic mutation has been observed in a variety of neoplasias (Aaronson and Tronick, 1985). Recently, Stewart et al. (1984) have introduced recombinant DNA containing c-*myc* linked to the MMTV (C3H) LTR into the germline of the CD-1 mouse strain. This strain lacks infectious MMTV and has a low spontaneous incidence of mammary tumors. One of the transgenic sublines (designated 141-3) develops a high incidence of mammary adenocarcinomas, suggesting deregulation of c-*myc* expression contributes to tumorigenesis. In this respect, it is pertinent that c-*myc* has not been identified as a common integration site for MMTV in mammary tumor DNA (Nusse et al., 1985; Escot et al., 1986b). Possibly, there is a subpopulation of cells in the developing mammary gland that are sensitive to overexpression of c-*myc* but are resistant to MMTV infection.

3.2. Chemical Carcinogenesis

Deregulation of c-*myc* expression itself is not sufficient for tumorigenesis, since not every mammary epithelial cell is tumorigenic. Thus, at a minimum, secondary mutations are required for tumorigenesis. The identity of the affected genes that might complement activated c-*myc* is at the present time unknown. However, one obvious candidate might be a member of the *ras* proto-oncogene family (K, H, or N). Cotransfection of primary rat embryo fibroblasts with the c-*myc* and H-*ras* oncogenes is sufficient to induce a malignant phenotype, whereas either gene alone lacks this ability (Land et al., 1983; Lee et al., 1985). Consistent with this possibility, it has been found that chemical carcinogen-induced rat mammary tumors frequently contain an activated c-H-*ras*-1 oncogene (Sukumar et al., 1983; Zarbl et al., 1985). These activated genes, depending on the chemical carcinogen used (nitrosomethyl urea [NMU] and 7,12-dimethylbenzanthracene [DMBA], respectively), contain a point mutation within either the amino acid 12 or 61 codon. More recently, Dandekar et al. (1986) have found that DMBA-induced BALB/c mouse mammary tumors arising from a transplantable hyperplastic outgrowth line each contain a point mutation within the amino acid 61 codon. In related experiments, Sonnenberg et al. (1986) have shown that cuboidal cells derived from the RAC cell line transform into elongated cells when transfected with the H-*ras* oncogene. In contrast, point mutations in c-H-*ras*-1 have not been reported in spontaneous mammary adenocarcinomas arising in MMTV-infected mice, HPO, or the RAC cell line (Lane et al., 1981; Dandekar et al., 1986; Sonnenberg et al., 1986). Thus, although it may be possible that complete tumorigenic transformation of mammary epithelial cells might occur in transgenic mice containing both an activated c-*myc* and H-*ras*-1 oncogene, it is more likely that other mutational events are responsible for mammary tumor development in the c-*myc* transgenic mouse.

3.3. Summary

The development of transgenic mice containing proto-oncogenes linked to the MMTV LTR offers an attractive new approach to identify cellular genes that, when mutated or activated, complement the recombinant gene in the development of mammary tumors. However, the general feasibility of this approach will depend on several factors, including the effect of deregulated expression of the particular proto-oncogene on embryonic development. This may be a particularly relevant problem with the *int* genes. A second and far more difficult problem to overcome will be the identification of the secondary mutations in the tumor DNA. The NIH 3T3 transfection assay is probably inadequate, since it detects primarily mutated *ras* genes (Aaronson and Tronick, 1985). Infection of the transgenic mouse strains with MMTV may offer a solution, since the viral genome could be used as a tag to identify new common insertion sites in tumor DNA.

4. MMTV-Related Sequences in Human Cellular DNA

4.1. Review of Early Studies

Several laboratories have searched for a common element associated with human breast cancer. The potential involvement of members of the Retroviridae family of viruses has represented a major focus of investigation (reviewed in Sarkar, 1980). This was primarily influenced by studies of mammary cancer in high-incidence strains of laboratory mice. Early studies suggested that a retrovirus resembling MMTV is expressed in human mammary tumors. These viral-like particles were reported to have the expected density (1.16 g/ml) and size (600S) and to contain an associated reverse transcriptase activity complexed with single-stranded RNA. Immunological studies using antisera raised against the MMTV envelope protein gp52 suggested that a related antigen could be detected by immunoperoxidase staining of paraffin sections of primary breast tumor specimens. The T47D cell line, derived from the pleural effusion of a patient with breast cancer, was reported to release retroviral-like particles which contain the MMTV gp52-related antigen (Keydar et al., 1982, 1984; Segev et al., 1985).

However, attempts to identify MMTV-related RNA in human breast tissue met with variable success because of the poor quality of available DNA probes and the insensitivity of the techniques used to quantitate or detect DNA–RNA hybrids (Axel et al., 1972; Vaidya et al., 1974). In recent years, using recombinant MMTV DNA and low-stringency blot hybridization conditions, sequences homologous to MMTV have been detected in human DNA (Callahan et al., 1982a; May et al., 1983; Deen and Sweet, 1986). The major region of homology was with the MMTV *gag* and *pol* genes. A weaker signal with human DNA was reported with the MMTV *env* gene and LTR probes.

4.2. Characteristics of the HLM-2 Proviral Genome

Recombinant clones of human cellular DNA containing MMTV-related sequences have been isolated (Callahan et al., 1982a; May et al., 1983; Deen and Sweet, 1986). The majority of these clones share se-

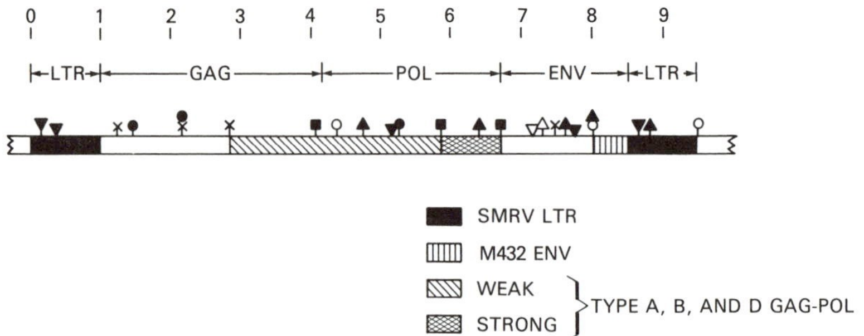

Figure 2. The organization of the human endogenous proviral genome in the HLM-2 recombinant DNA clone. Sequences related to other classes of infectious or endogenous retroviruses are indicated with hatched or shaded boxes. A partial restriction map of the proviral genome is shown. ▼, SST I; ○, ECO RI; ●, BGL II; ▲, PST I; △, AVA I; X, HIND III; ■, ECO RV; ▽, XHO I; ▼, BAM HI.

quence homology with the MMTV *gag* and *pol* genes. These sequences are organized within genetic loci that resemble endogenous proviral genomes. One of these, HLM-2 (Callahan et al., 1982a), is illustrated in Fig. 2. The *gag-pol*-related sequences in the HLM-2 proviral genome are bounded by two LTR-like elements that are approximately 1.0 kb in size. Nucleotide sequence analysis of these demonstrated that they are 95% related (R. Callahan, unpublished data). However, they share no significant sequence homology with the MMTV LTR. The HLM-2 LTRs do contain the transcription signal sequences characteristic of retroviral LTRs. The U-3 portion of the LTR, unlike the MMTV LTR, does not contain an orf capable of encoding a protein (see Section 2). Nucleotide sequence analysis of the MMTV-related structural genes within the HLM-2 provirus demonstrated significant homology with the 3′ end of the MMTV *gag* gene, the 5′ and 3′ ends of the *pol* gene, and no homology with the MMTV *env* genes. The HLM-2 proviral genome is probably not biologically active, since the structural genes contain numerous stop codons as well as small deletions and insertions (R. Callahan, unpublished data).

4.3. Frequency of HLM-2-Related Proviral Genomes in Human DNA

There are approximately 50 copies of HLM-2-related proviral genomes in human cellular DNA (R. Callahan, unpublished data). Comparative restriction enzyme analysis and heteroduplex analysis of several of these proviral genomes have demonstrated extensive nucleotide sequence heterogeneity among members of this family of endogenous retroviruses. Human–mouse somatic cell hybrids have been used to determine the distribution of these proviral genomes among the human chromosomes (Horn et al., 1986). It is no surprise that most, perhaps all, of the human chromosomes contain HLM-2-related restriction fragments. The HLM-2 and related HLM-25 proviruses are located, respectively, on chromosomes 1 and 5. Using unique cellular sequences flanking the HLM-2 and HLM-25 proviruses, we have observed similar size host–viral junction restriction fragments in chimpanzee cellular DNA (unpublished data). This suggests that these proviruses entered the germline prior to the divergence of the two species.

In contrast to the HLM-2 viral-related structural genes, the LTR-like sequences are reiterated 1000 times in human cellular DNA (R. Callahan, unpublished data). These sequences appear to be unassociated with viral structural genes. Preliminary analysis of two recombinant clones containing these sequences revealed that they are adjacent to, or perhaps within, members of the *kpn*-1 family of repetitive cellular DNA sequences. Like the viral structural genes, they appear to be distributed throughout the cellular genome (Horn et al., 1986). The origin of these elements and mechanism by which they have been amplified are unknown. One possibility is that, during the evolution of the species, the LTRs became separated from the viral structural genes by cellular recombinational events and then subsequently amplified. Such a mechanism seems likely for the origin of solitary type C retroviral LTRs in murine and human DNA (Wirth et al., 1983; Steele et al., 1984). Alternatively, viral RNA may have been spliced inappropriately, such that the structural genes were lost but the signals for reverse transcription were preserved. This structure might then have reinserted into the germline. A similar phenomenon may have occurred with the MMTV LTR in BALB/c mice (Donehower et al., 1981). In either case, these solitary LTRs may act as itinerant sequences or transposons.

4.4. Relation of the HLM-2 Provirus to Infectious Retroviruses

The existence of two major *pol* gene families in the evolution of retroviruses has been established (Chiu et al., 1984; Ono et al., 1985). One family consists of mammalian type C retroviruses. The second family includes type A (intracisternal A particles, IAP), type B (MMTV), type D (squirrel monkey retrovirus, SMRV), and avian type C viruses (Rous sarcoma virus and avian myeloblastosis-associated virus). Because of the promiscuous nature of retroviruses (Chiu et al., 1984), we explored the possibility that other members of Retroviridae might also share homology with the HLM-2 provirus (Callahan et al., 1985). The results of reciprocal low-stringency blot hybridization analysis are summarized in Fig. 2. A major region of homology exists between the type A, B, and D retroviral *pol* genes and the *pol* region of HLM-2 DNA. In the case of SMRV, a type D retrovirus, the homology includes the 3′ half of the *gag* gene as well as the *pol* gene. The SMRV LTR also hybridizes weakly with the HLM-2 LTR-like elements. In addition to the *pol* region, the IAP-related retrovirus M432 hybridizes to an area of the HLM-2 putative *env* gene that is immediately adjacent to the 3′ LTR. No homology was detected with a number of different mammalian type C proviral genomes. The findings show that (1) the HLM-2 *pol* gene probably arose from the same progenitor that gave rise to the *pol* genes of the infectious type A, B, D, and avian type C retroviral genera, and (2) the HLM-2 provirus appears to be a mosaic of sequences related to different classes of Retroviridae. This conclusion has been reinforced by the recent characterization of IAP-related recombinant clones of human cellular DNA (Ono, 1986). Probes derived from these clones detect the same restriction fragments that the HLM-2 proviral fragments detect in restricted human cellular DNA.

To determine whether there are tumor-specific amplifications of the HLM-2 proviral sequences and how conserved these sequences are between individuals, we have begun to screen cellular DNA from normal and breast tumor tissue. Our results to date (unpublished data) provide no evidence for the amplification of proviral sequences in primary breast tumor DNA. This may reflect the limited number of tumors tested or the variability in the fraction of the material that contains tumor cells. In this connection, May et al. (1983) have shown that the MCF-7 human breast tumor cell line contains two MMTV-related *Eco*RI restriction fragments not seen in a normal human placenta cellular DNA. The significance of this finding is difficult to assess, since the karyotype of the MCF-7 cell line is very different from that of normal cells, indicating several genetic rearrangements that may have been incurred during the passage in tissue culture. In addition, we have observed several restriction site polymorphisms in cellular DNA from normal human tissues. Whether these polymorphisms reflect the presence or absence of specific proviral genomes in individual cellular DNAs or the highly diverged nature of this family of proviral genomes will require further study.

4.5. MMTV env-Related Sequences in Human DNA

The organizational relation between MMTV *gag-pol-* and MMTV *env*-related human DNA sequences remains unclear. The HLM-2 recombinant clone contains MMTV *env*-related sequences, but these are located outside the proviral genome (Callahan et al., 1982a). We have determined the nucleotide sequence of a 1.8-kb *Eco*RI fragment from HLM-2 which reacts with the MMTV *env* probe (unpublished data). Weak nucleotide sequence homology (36%) between the gp52 region of the *env* gene and a 690-bp region of the *Eco*RI fragment was observed. However, it is in the opposite transcriptional orientation relative to the HLM-2 provirus and contains no significant orf for peptide synthesis. No homology with the gp36 portion of the *env* gene was detected. A second human recombinant clone (HLM-46A) was initially detected using the entire MMTV genome as a probe. This clone contains only MMTV *env*-related sequences and shares no homology with the HLM-2 proviral genome. Again, the region of homology corresponds to the gp52 portion of the *env* gene but contains no orf for protein synthesis. At present, it is an open question as to whether the MMTV *env*-related sequences detected so far in human DNA represent bona fide viral-related genes or reflect a potential artifact involved in the use of low-stringency blot hybridization to detect highly diverged genes.

4.6. Expression of HLM-2 Proviral-Related RNA

A major issue is whether the MMTV-related genes detected in human DNA are expressed in breast tumors (Sarkar, 1980; Keydar et al., 1982, 1984; Segev et al., 1985). In a preliminary screening of 20 primary breast tumors, one was found to express a 6.7-kb species of poly A+ RNA that hybridized to the HLM-2 *pol-env* probe (R. Callahan, unpublished data). However, it did not hybridize with the HLM-2 LTR. In addition, we have not been able to detect HLM-2 proviral-related RNA in MCF-7, BT20, or T47D tissue culture cells. In the case of the primary breast tumors, one complicating factor is the variable extent of cellular heterogeneity resulting from the amount of adjacent normal tissue and lymphoplasma cellular infiltrates in the tumor specimen. A solution to this problem is suggested by the use of RNA : RNA in situ hybridization on frozen or paraffin sections of tumor tissue to detect gene expression at the cellular level. The availability of recombinant clones of human MMTV-related sequences makes this approach feasible.

4.7. Summary

The MMTV *gag-*, *pol-*, and *env*-related sequences have been identified in human cellular DNA. These sequences do not appear to be organized in a manner expected for a human MMTV-related endogenous proviral genome. Instead, the MMTV *gag-pol*-related sequences are found within a new class of human endogenous retroviral genomes that appear to be a mosaic of sequences related to different retroviral genera. This is consistent with accumulating evidence that genetic interactions between retrovirus genera have played an important role in their evolution (reviewed in Chiu et al., 1984). The LTR-like element of this class of human proviral genomes is also found unassociated with viral structural genes and is highly reiterated in cellular DNA. The effect that these "solitary" LTR elements have on the expression of adjacent cellular genes and their potential role in carcinogenesis will provide a provocative new avenue for future research. With respect to MMTV *env*-related sequences in human cellular DNA, there is currently no evidence that they are associated with a complete proviral genome. It seems probable that the existence of MMTV gp52-related genes in human breast tumors and their possible relation to viral genes must await the isolation of recombinant cDNA clones that encode the antigenic determinants detected by the anti-gp52 sera.

5. Genetic Alterations of Cellular Proto-oncogenes in Human Breast Cancer

5.1. Methods Used to Identify Genetic Alterations

The activation of cellular proto-oncogenes by point mutation, genetic rearrangement, or amplification has been implicated in the development of solid tumors and leukemias (Aaronson and Tronick, 1985). At least two general strategies involving biological assays or cytogenetic and molecular genetic analyses have been used to identify the location and nature of genetic lesions associated with tumor development. Transfection of NIH 3T3 fibroblasts with cellular DNA from tumor-derived tissue culture cell lines has been the primary biological assay. The activated oncogene causes morphological changes as well as an increased tumorigenic potential of NIH 3T3 cells. A human carcinosarcoma cell line (HS578T) derived from a rare form of breast cancer was found to contain an activated c-H-*ras*-1 oncogene with an amino acid 12 mutation (Kraus et al., 1984). The MCF-7 breast tumor cell line has been reported to contain at least two activated oncogenes (Fasano et al., 1984; Graham et al., 1985). One of these represents an amplification of N-*ras*. However, using this approach, scientists have found the identification of activated oncogenes in primary breast tumors elusive. This may be the result of cellular heterogeneity in the tumor tissue or may reflect the inability of the relevant activated oncogenes to transform NIH 3T3 fibroblasts to the tumorigenic phenotype.

5.2. Cytogenetic Analysis of Primary Breast Tumors

Cytogenetic analysis of primary breast tumors using chromosome banding techniques has only recently begun (reviewed in Trent, 1985). The majority of primary and metastatic breast cancers contain an abnormal karyotype that includes unidentified "marker" chromosomes, homogeneously stained regions, and extrachromosomal double minutes. Frequent genetic alterations involving chromosomes 1q (translocations), 6q (deletions and translocations), 7p (translocations, paracentric inversions, and isochromosomes), and 11q (translocations) have been observed. It may be pertinent that cellular proto-oncogenes are located on each of these chromosomes (1q, c-*sis*; 6q, c-*myb*; 7p, c-*erb*B; and 11q, *int*-2 and c-*ets*-1). However, at present there is no information on whether these genetic alterations are associated with specific cellular genes.

5.3. c-H-ras-1 in Breast Cancer Patients and Primary Breast Tumors

A systematic study of primary breast tumors representing different histological types has been initiated to determine which of the known proto-oncogenes have been genetically altered or are aberrantly expressed in tumor cells (Escot et al., 1986b; Lidereau et al., 1986; Theillet et al., 1986). One aim of these studies was to attempt to correlate the findings with various clinicopathological parameters, characteristics of the tumor, and the patient's prognosis. The initial focus of the studies was on the *ras* and *myc* proto-oncogene families, since they have been implicated in several other neoplasms (see Secfion 3). Horan Hand et al. (1984) prepared monoclonal antibodies against a synthetic peptide reflecting amino acids 10–17 of the human T24 H-*ras* p21. This monoclonal antibody reacts with normal and point-mutated *ras* p21 from all three members of the *ras* proto-oncogene family. They observed, using immunohistochemical techniques, that 63% of invasive ductal carcinomas demonstrated enhanced expression of *ras* p21. In contrast, only 10% (2 of 21) benign lesions were equally reactive. Subsequent studies (Ohuchi et al., 1986) showed that invasive carcinomas contained the highest levels of *ras* p21 (percentage of reactive cells) with decreasing expression in carcinomas in situ, hyperplasias with atypia, and nonatypical hyperplasias, respectively. Comparison of the levels of *ras* p21 expression with a variety of clinicopathological variables suggested that carcinomas from postmenopausal and nulliparous women generally demonstrated higher *ras* p21 expression than tumor specimens from premenopausal women.

In a separate study, H-*ras* RNA was detected by Northern blot analysis in 16 of 22 invasive ductal carcinomas (Theillet et al., 1986). The K-

and N-*ras* proto-oncogenes were either not expressed or expressed at low levels. These results, as well as others (Spandidos and Agnantis, 1984; Slamon et al., 1984), strongly suggest that the H-*ras* p21 is primarily, if not exclusively, expressed in breast tumors. The tumor-specific expression of *ras* p21 is not the result of gene amplification or rearrangement of the three *ras* genes, since none was observed in 104 tumor DNAs tested (Theillet et al., 1986).

The c-H-*ras*-1 proto-oncogene is polymorphic in human cellular DNA (Capon et al., 1983; Krontiris et al., 1985). Different alleles can be recognized by a restriction fragment length polymorphism resulting from the variable tandem reiteration of a 28 base pair sequence (designated VTR) adjacent to the c-H-*ras*-1 gene. Krontiris et al. (1985) surveyed a limited number of several different tumor types and found that, collectively, cancer patients seem to have a higher frequency of rare c-H-*ras*-1 restriction fragments or alleles than an unaffected population. However, no correlation could be made between the frequency of rare alleles or of specific rare alleles and different types of solid tumors. In a more extensive study of 104 breast cancer patients and 56 unaffected individuals, four common and 19 rare c-H-*ras*-1 alleles were detected in the combined population (Lidereau et al., 1986). The distribution of common and rare alleles differed significantly between the cancer patient and normal populations. The common restriction fragments represented 91% of the allele pool in the unaffected population. In breast cancer patients, these common alleles represented only 59% of the allele pool ($p < 0.001$). More specifically, the frequency of two of the common fragments (the 6.5- and 8.0-kb fragments) was significantly diminished in the breast cancer population ($p < 0.001$ and $p < 0.02$, respectively). The frequency of rare c-H-*ras*-1 alleles and hence genotypes composed of two rare alleles was increased in the breast cancer population ($p < 0.001$). One of the rare alleles had a significant ($p < 0.05$) association with these breast cancer patients. Attempts to correlate the rare c-H-*ras*-1 alleles with several clinical and biochemical characteristics of the breast tumors or aspects of the patient's medical history have so far been uninformative.

A similar study of 132 lung cancer patients also demonstrated an abnormal distribution of c-H-*ras*-1 alleles compared with a control population (Heighway et al., 1986). Although no comparable increase in rare alleles was observed in these patients, there was a significant increase in the frequency of one common allele in non-small-cell lung carcinoma patients compared with small-cell lung carcinoma patients ($p < 0.004$) or controls ($p < 0.05$). These results, taken together with those observed in breast cancer patients, suggest that genotype analysis of the c-H-*ras*-1 locus, in combination with other clinical parameters, may be of prognostic value in assessing the potential for certain cancers. Epidemiological studies have implicated an inheritable genetic component in the etiology of breast cancer in families with a high incidence of the disease (Lynch et al., 1984). Genetic linkage analysis of several of these families failed to reveal a consistent correlation between breast cancer incidence and genetic markers on chromosomes 1, 2, 4, 6, 9, 13, 14, 16, 19, or 22 (King et al., 1983). These results suggest that future analysis of c-H-*ras*-1 in these populations may be informative.

5.4. Genetic Instability of Human Chromosome 11

The molecular and biological consequences of the high frequency of rare c-H-*ras*-1 alleles in breast cancer patients are at present unknown. However, there are two pertinent observations that can be considered. First, Krontiris et al. (1985) have claimed that the deletion of the VTR in the EJ *ras* oncogene decreases the transforming potential five- to 10-fold. This suggests that the VTR region affects the regulation of expression of c-H-*ras*-1. The similarity between the frequency of rare genotypes in breast cancer patients (50%) and the frequency of tumors expressing H-*ras* p21 (60%) (Horan Hand et al., 1984) raises the possibility that the expression of rare c-H-*ras*-1 alleles may be aberrantly regulated. Second, c-H-*ras*-1 is located on chromosome 11; thus, the high frequency of rare alleles in breast cancer patients may be symptomatic of increased genetic instability in this region of the chromosome. In this regard, it is pertinent that, in tumor DNAs from 14 of 51 patients heterozygous for c-H-*ras*-1-related *Bam*HI restriction fragments, one allele was lost (Theillet et al., 1986). This allele loss did not seem to alter *ras* p21 expression. Correlation with clinicopathological data showed, however, that the loss of one c-H-*ras*-1 allele in breast carcinoma DNA is significantly linked to histological grade III tumors ($p < 0.02$), the lack of estrogen and/or progesterone receptors ($p < 0.01$), and the subsequent occurrence of distal metastasis ($p < 0.05$). These results thus indicate that the loss of one c-H-*ras*-1 allele correlates with the aggressive primary carcinomas of the breast.

Genetic instability of the short arm of chromosome 11 (11p) is not uncommon. The loss of a c-H-*ras*-1 allele has also been observed in carcinomas of the colon, lung, esophagus, ovary, and bladder (Fearon et al., 1985; Krontiris et al., 1985; Yokota et al., 1986), as well as Wilms' tumor/aniridia/gonadoblastoma/retardation complex (Fearon et al., 1984; Koufos et al., 1984; Orkin et al., 1984; Reeve et al., 1984). In another study, c-H-*ras*-1 allele loss was reported to occur twice as frequently in metastases as in primary tumors of the above tissues, including the breast (Yokota et al., 1986). In general, it is unclear whether allele loss represents random changes associated with aneuploidy, which occur during the evolution of the tumor, or is a selected event. The observation that homozygosity at a number of genes on different chromosomes is a common occurrence in 24 melanoma cell lines favors the random loss concept (Dracopoli et al., 1985). Other studies are more consistent with the proposal that loss of normal regulatory or suppressor genes may be associated with tumor development (Knudson and Strong, 1972; Cavenee et al., 1983). This scenario would require two genetic alterations: (1) inactivation of a suppressor gene by mutation on one chromosome 11p and (2) deletion of the normal suppressor gene on the other chromosome 11p. The region of chromsome 11p most frequently lost in Wilms' tumors (11p13) is located near the gene for the β subunit of follicle-stimulating hormone (Glaser et al., 1986). Our own preliminary studies suggest that c-H-*ras*-1 allele loss is not a random event, since most cells in an affected tumor contain the deletion. However, the region of chromosome 11p that is most frequently deleted appears to be closer to the centromere than c-H-*ras*-1. Thus, some tumors contain both c-H-*ras*-1 alleles but are deleted at the β-globin locus. Further analysis will be required to determine whether or not a putative breast tumor locus is separate from the Wilms' tumor locus.

5.5. Amplification and Rearrangements of c-myc

Amplification of the c-*myc* proto-oncogene has been reported in one breast carcinoma cell line (Kozbor and Croce, 1984) and in tumors induced in nude mice by the SWGB-S human breast carcinoma cell line (Modjtahedi et al., 1985). In the latter case, double minute chromosomes and homogeneously staining regions were associated with c-*myc* amplification. In a study of 101 solid tumors from various tissues (including 10 breast carcinomas), 17% contained an amplified c-*myc* (Yokota et al., 1986). More recently, Escot et al. (1986b) have surveyed 121 primary breast carcinomas. Two types of genetic alteration were observed: (1) a two- to 15-fold amplification of c-*myc* in 32% of the carcinoma DNAs and (2) a novel c-*myc*-related restriction fragment in five carcinoma DNAs. In one tumor, the novel fragment was shown to reflect a genetic rearrangement (probably a translocation) that occurred near the 3′ end of the third exon. A similar type of rearrangement has been observed in some Burkitt's lymphomas (Hollis et al., 1984; Taub et al., 1984). Since all the tumors tested correspond to an advanced stage of the disease, it is possible that amplification of c-*myc* reflects polyploidy. However, three observations argue against this as an explanation. First, the c-*mos* proto-oncogene, which is linked to c-*myc* on chromosome 8, was not amplified or rearranged in these tumor DNAs (Lidereau et al., 1985). Second, no amplification or rearrangement of proto-oncogenes located on other chromosomes (N-*myc*, the *ras* proto-oncogene family, c-*sis*, c-*erb*B, as well as eight anonymous cellular DNA fragments) was observed. Third, cytogenetic studies of breast cancer have shown that these tumor cells are usually not more than hyperdiploid (Trent, 1985). Moreover, because of the variability of the tumor tissue-to-stroma ratio and the potential presence of normal breast tissue in the tumor samples, our assessment of the frequency and magnitude of c-*myc* amplification is probably an underestimate. Amplification or rearrangement of c-*myc* was significantly correlated ($p < 0.02$) with tumors from patients 51 years of age or greater. The women composing this group of patients were either postmenopausal or had an earlier hysterectomy (25–30 years of age). In addition, the only two tumors from male patients examined each contained an amplified c-*myc*.

Amplification or rearrangement of proto-oncogenes is generally associated with their enhanced expression. Indeed, using Northern blot analysis, high levels of c-*myc* RNA were observed in six invasive ductal carcinomas bearing an amplified c-*myc* (Escot et al., 1986b). However, elevated levels of c-*myc* expression have also been observed in four of eight tumors in which the gene appeared unaltered. It is conceivable that more subtle genetic alterations affecting RNA stability or genetic rearrangements outside the regions examined (Taub et al., 1984) are responsible for the enhanced levels of c-*myc* RNA in these tumors. Another possibility is that other cellular gene(s) that regulate the expression of c-*myc* have been altered. Little is known about the factors that normally regulate the expression of c-*myc* in epithelial cells of the breast. Recent studies of c-*myc* expression in developing human embryos suggest that the expression of this gene is not simply linked to cell proliferation but rather is under cell type specific and developmental control (Ohlsson et al., 1985). Examination of c-*myc* RNA expression at the cellular level in frozen tissue sections should provide more information on the possible relation between enhanced expression and clinicopathological parameters, including stage of tumor development.

5.6. Summary

Statistically, significant correlations have been found between specific genetic lesions and various aspects of the patient's history or properties of the tumor. It is likely that these studies will be extended to other proto-oncogenes (including the human homologs of the murine *int* loci), as well as the genes encoding various hormones, growth factors, and their respective receptors. The focus of the current studies has been primarily on the advanced, moderately to poorly differentiated ductal carcinomas which represent a late stage in the development of the disease. Although this histiotype is the most common, several others are recognized. In addition, we do not know whether these mutations are associated with the initial stages of neoplastic transformation or if it is a late phenomenon that is positively selected during the evolution of the disease. The development of techniques that lead to the recovery of high-molecular-weight DNA from formalin-fixed tissue specimens embedded in paraffin (Goelz et al., 1985; Dubeau et al., 1986) should provide an additional resource to obtain adequate samples of rare histiotypes and early tumors. Moreover, the vast archives of tumor specimens in pathology departments throughout the world could be used in retrospective studies to determine the prognostic significance of specific genetic mutations.

In a related area, 5% (Lynch et al., 1984) of all breast cancer patients have an inheritable component in the etiology of their disease. It has been proposed that autosomal dominant mutations cosegregate with the inheritable breast cancer syndrome. Their relation to somatic mutations that occur during the evolution of sporadic (noninheritable) breast cancer is unknown. Moreover, there is at present very little information on the identity or chromosomal location of these mutations. The increasing availability of large numbers of recombinant clones of human DNA, which can be used to detect restriction site polymorphisms in the human genome, has made it experimentally feasible to approach these questions.

Although systematic studies of inheritable, as well as tumor-specific, mutations will provide a great deal of valuable information for the determination of genetic risk factors in the development of breast cancer and the prognosis for the future course of the disease, there are significant limitations in this approach. For example, point mutations and small deletions or insertions in breast tumor DNA will more than likely go undetected. Similarly, the mutations to cellular genes that are strictly associated with breast tumors, such as the mouse mammary tumor *int* loci, will also probably go undetected. Thus, the development of functional assays for the tumor-associated genetic mutations, in the context of mammary epithelial cells, still remains the most formidable challenge.

Acknowledgments: I thank Drs. G. Peters, A. Sonnenberg, S. Sukumar, and H. Varmus for helpful discussions and communication of results before publication.

References

Aaronson, S.A., and Tronick, S.R., 1985, The role of oncogenes in human neoplasia, in: *Important Advances in Oncology 1985* (V.T. DeVita, S. Hellman, and S.A. Rosenberg, eds), J.B. Lippincott Company, Philadelphia, pp.3–15.

Andervont, H.B., 1952, Biological studies on the mammary tumor inciter in mice, *Ann. N.Y. Acad. Sci.* **54:**1004–1011.

Andervont, H.B., and Dunn, T.B., 1962, Occurrence of tumors in wild house mice, *J. Natl. Cancer Inst.* **28:**1153–1163.

Axel, R., Schlom, J., and Spieglman, S., 1972, Presence in human breast cancer of RNA homologous to mouse mammary tumor virus RNA, *Nature* **235:**32–36.

Banerji, J., Olson, L., and Schaffner, W., 1983, A lymphocyte specific cellular enhancer is located downstream of the joining region of immunoglobulin heavy chain genes, *Cell* **33:**729–740.

Bishop, J., 1985, Viral oncogenes, *Cell* **42:**23–38.

Bitner, J.J., 1942, The milk influence of breast tumors in mice, *Science* **95:**462–463.

Boot, L.M., and Muhlbock, O., 1956, The mammary tumor incidence in the C3H mouse strain with and without the agent (C3H, C3Hf, C3He), *Acta Unio Int. Contra Cancrum* **12:**569–581.

Callahan, R., and Todaro, G., 1978, Four major endogenous retrovirus classes each genetically transmitted in various species of *Mus*, in: *Origins of Inbred Mice* (H.C. Morse III, ed.), Academic Press, New York, pp. 689–713.

Callahan, R., Drohan, W., Tronick, S., and Schlom, J., 1982a, Detection and cloning of human DNA sequences related to the mouse mammary tumor virus genome, *Proc. Natl. Acad. Sci. USA* **79:**5503–5507.

Callahan, R., Drohan, W., Gallahan, D., D'Hoostelaere, L., and Potter, M., 1982b, Novel class of mouse mammary tumor virus-related DNA sequences found in all species of *Mus*, including mice lacking the virus proviral genome, *Proc. Natl. Acad. Sci. USA* **79:**4113–4117.

Callahan, R., Chiu, I.M., Wong, J.F.H., Tronick, S.R., Roe, B., Aaronson, S.A., and Schlom, J., 1985, A new class of endogenous human retroviral genomes, *Science* **228:**1208–1211.

Capon, D.J., Chen, E.Y., Levinson, A.D., Seeburg, P.H., and Goeddel, D.B., 1983, Complete nucleotide sequences of the T24 human bladder carcinoma oncogene and its normal homologue, *Nature* **302:**33–37.

Casey, G., Smith, R., McGillivray, D., Peters, G., and Dickson, C., 1986, Characterization and chromosome assignments of the human homolog of *int*-2, a potential proto-oncogene, *Mol. Cell. Biol.* **6:**502–510.

Cavenee, W.K., Dryja, T.P., Phillips, R.A., Benedict, W.F., Godbort, R., Gallie, B.L., Murphee, A.L., Strong, L.C., and White, R.L., 1983, Expression of recessive alleles by chromosomal mechanism in retinoblastoma, *Nature* **305:**779–784.

Chiu, I.M., Callahan, R., Tronick, S.R., Schlom, J., and Aaronson, S.A., 1984, Major *pol* gene progenitors in the evolution of oncoviruses, *Science* **223:**364–370.

Cohen, J.C., Shank, P.R., Morris, V.L., Cardiff, R., and Varmus, H., 1979, Integration of the DNA of mouse mammary tumor virus in virus-infected normal and neoplastic tissue of the mouse, *Cell* **16:**333–345.

Cuypers, H.T., Selten, G., Quint, W., Zijstra, M., Maandag, B.R., Boelens, W., Van Wezenbeek, P., Melief, C., and Berns. A., 1984, Murine leukemia virus induced T-cell lymphomagenesis: Integration of proviruses in a distinct chromosomal region, *Cell* **37:**141–150.

Dandekar, S., Sukumar, S., Zarbl, H., Young, L.J.T., and Cardiff, R.D., 1986, Specific activation of the cellular Harvey *ras* oncogene in dimethylbenzanthracene induced mouse mammary tumors, **6:**4104–4108.

Deen, K.C., and Sweet, R.W., 1986, Murine mammary tumor virus *pol*-related sequences in human DNA: Characterization and sequence comparison with the complete murine mammary tumor virus *pol* gene, *J. Virol.* **57:**422–432.

DeOme, K.B., Faulkin, L.J., Bern, H.H., and Blair, P.B., 1959, Development of mammary tumors from hyperplastic alveolar nodules transplanted into gland free mammary fat pads of female C3H mice, *Cancer Res.* **19:**515–520.

de Villiers, J., Olson, L., Banerji, J., and Schaffner, W., 1982, Analysis of the transcriptional enhancer effect, *Cold Spring Harbor Symp. Quant. Biol.* **46:**911–919.

Dickson, C., and Peters, G., 1981, Protein coding potential of mouse mammary tumor virus genome RNA as examined by *in vitro* translation, *J. Virol.* **37:**36–47.

Dickson, C., Smith, R., Brookes, S., and Peters, G., 1984, Tumorigenesis by mouse mammary tumor virus: Proviral activation of a cellular gene in the common integration region *int*-2, *Cell* **37:**529–536.

Donehower, L.A., Huang, A.L., and Hager, G.L., 1981, Regulatory and coding potential of the mouse mammary tumor virus long terminal redundancy, *J. Virol.* **37:**226–238.

Dracapoli, N.C., Houghton, A.N., and Lloyd, J.O., 1985, Loss of polymorphic restriction fragments in malignant melanoma: Implication for tumor heterogeneity, *Proc. Natl. Acad. Sci. USA* **82:**1470–1474.

Dubeau, L., Chandler, L.A., Gralow, J.R., Nichols, P.W., and Jone, P.A., 1986, Southern blot analysis of DNA extracted from formalin fixed pathology specimens, *Cancer Res.* **46:**2964–2969.

Duesberg, P.H., 1985, Activated proto-oncogenes sufficient or necessary for cancer, *Science* **228:**669–677.

Escot, C., Hogg, E., and Callahan, R., 1986a, Mammary tumorigenesis in feral *Mus cervicolor popaeus, J. Virol.* **58:**619–625.

Escot, C., Theillet, C., Lidereau, R., Spyratos, F., Champeme, M.H., Gest, J., and Callahan, R., 1986b, Genetic alteration of the c-*myc* protooncogene in human primary breast carcinoma, *Proc. Natl. Acad. Sci. USA,* **83:**4834–4838.

Fasano, O., Birnbaum, D., Edlund, L., Fogh, J., and Wigler, M., 1984, New human transforming genes detected by a tumorigenicity assay, *Mol. Cell. Biol.* **4:**1695–1705.

Fearon, E.R., Vogelstein, B., and Feinberg, A.P., 1984, Somatic deletion and duplication of genes on chromosome 11 in Wilms' tumors, *Nature* **309:**176–178.

Fearon, E.R., Feinberg, A.P., Hamilton, S.H., and Vogelstein, B., 1985, Loss of genes on the short arm of chromosome 11 in bladder cancer, *Nature* **318:**377–380.

Foulds, L., 1949, Mammary tumors in hybrid mice: The presence and transmission of the mammary tumor agent, *Br. J. Cancer* **3:**230–239.

Fung, Y.K., Lewis, W.G., Crittenden, L.B., and Kung, H.J., 1983, Activation of the cellular oncogene c-*erb* B by LTR insertion: Molecular basis for induction of erythroblastosis by avian leukosis virus, *Cell* **33:**357–368.

Fung, Y.K.T., Shackleford, G.M., Brown, A.M.C., Sanders, G.S., and Varmus, H.E., 1985, Nucleotide sequence and expression in vitro of cDNA derived from mRNA of *int*-1, a provirally activated mouse mammary oncogene, *Mol. Cell. Biol.* **5:**3337–3344.

Gallahan, D., and Callahan, R., 1986, Mammary tumorigenesis in feral mice: Identification of a new *int* locus in MMTV(Czech II)-induced mammary tumors, *J. Virol.,* **61:**66–74.

Gallahan, D., Kozak, C., and Callahan, R., 1986a, A new common integration region (*int*-3) for the mouse mammary tumor virus on mouse chromosome 17, *J. Virol.,* **61:**218–220.

Gallahan, D., Escot, C., Hogg, E., and Callahan, R., 1986b, Mammary tumorigenesis in feral species of the genus *Mus, Curr. Top. Microbiol. Immunol.,* **127:**354–361.

Gillies, S.D., Morrison, S.L., Oi, V.T., and Tonegawa, S., 1983, A tissue specific transcription enhancer element is located in the major intron of a rearranged immunoglobulin heavy chain gene, *Cell* **33:**717–728.

Glaser, T., Lewis, W.H., Bruns, G.A.P., Watkins, P.C., Rogler, C.E., Shows, T.B., Power, V.E., Willard, H.F., Goguen, J.M., Simola, O.J., and Housman, D.E., 1986, The β subunit of follicle-stimulating hormone is deleted in patients with aniridia and Wilms' tumor, allowing a further definition of the WAGR locus, *Nature* **321:**882–887.

Goelz, S.E., Hamilton, S.R., and Voelstein, B., 1985, Purification of DNA from formaldehyde-fixed and paraffin-embedded human tissue, *Biochem. Biophys. Res. Commun.* **130:**118–126.

Gompel, G., and van Kerkem, C., 1983, The breast, in: *Principles of Surgical Pathology*, Vol. I (S. Silverberg, ed.), Wiley Medical, New York, pp. 245–255.

Graham, K.A., Richardson, C.L., Minden, M.D., Trent, J.M., and Buick, R.N., 1985, Varying degrees of amplification of the N-*ras* oncogene in the human breast cancer cell line MCF7, *Cancer Res.* **45:**2201–2205.

Harris, J.R., Hellman, S., Canellos, G.P., and Fisher, B., 1982, Cancer of the breast, in: *Cancer Principles and Practice of Oncology* (V.T. DeVita, S. Hellman, and S.A. Rosenberg, eds.), J.B. Lippincott Company, Philadelphia, pp. 1119–1178.

Haseltine, W.A., Sodroski, J., and Rosen, C., 1985, The *lor* gene and pathogenesis of HTLV II, II, and III, *Cancer Res.* **45:**4545–4549.

Hayward, W., Neel, B., and Astrin, S., 1981, Activation of a cellular *onc* gene by promotion, insertion in ALV-induced lymphoid leukosis, *Nature* **290:**475–480.

Heighway, J., Thatcher, N., Cerny, T., and Hasleton, P.S., 1986, Genetic predisposition to human lung cancer, *Br. J. Cancer* **53:**453–457.

Hilgers, J., and Bentvelzen, P., 1978, Interaction between viral and genetic factors in murine mammary cancer, *Adv. Cancer Res.* **26:**143–195.

Hollis, G.F., Mitchell, K.F., Battey, J., Potter, H., Taub, R., Lenoir, G.M., and Leder, P., 1984, A variant translocation places the λ immunoglobulin gene 3′ to the c-*myc* oncogene in Burkitt's lymphoma, *Nature* **307:**752–755.

Horan Hand, P., Teramoto, Y.A., Callahan, R., and Schlom, J., 1980, Interspecies radioimmunoassay for the major internal protein of mammary tumor viruses, *Virology* **101:**61–71.

Horan Hand, P., Thor, A., Wunderlich, D., Muraro, R., Caruso, A., and Schlom, J., 1984, Monoclonal antibodies of predefined specificity detect activated *ras* gene expression in human mammary and colon carcinomas, *Proc. Natl. Acad. Sci. USA* **81:**5227–5231.

Horn, T.M., Huebner, K., Croce, C., and Callahan, R., 1986, Chromosomal locations of members of a family of novel endogenous human retroviral genomes, *J. Virol.* **58:**955–959.

Jakobovits, A., Shackleford, G.M., Varmus, H.E., and Martin, G.R., 1986, Two proto-oncogenes implicated in mammary carcinogenesis, *int*-1 and *int*-2, are independently regulated during mouse development, *Proc. Natl. Acad. Sci. USA* **83:**7806–7810.

Kennedy, N., Knedlitschek, G., Groner, B., Hynes, N.E., Herrlich, P., Michalides, R., and Van Ooyen, A.J.J., 1982, Long terminal repeats of endogenous mouse mammary tumor virus contain a long open reading frame which extends into adjacent sequences, *Nature* **295:**622–624.

Keydar, I., Selzer, G., Chaitchik, S., Harcuveni, M., Karby, S., and Hizi, A., 1982, A viral antigen as a marker for the prognosis of human breast cancer, *Eur. J. Cancer Clin. Oncol.* **18:**1321–1328.

Keydar, I., Ohno, T., Nayak, R., Sweet, R., Simoni, F., Weiss, F., Karby, S., Mesa-Tejada, R., and Spiegelman, S., 1984, Properties of retrovirus-like particles produced by a human breast carcinoma line: Immunological relationship with mouse mammary tumor virus proteins, *Proc. Natl. Acad. Sci. USA* **81:**4188–4192.

King, M.C., Rodney, C.P. Go, Lynch, H.T., Elston, R.C., Terasaki, P.I., Petrakis, N.L., Rodgers, G.C., Lattenzio, D., and Wilson, J.B., 1983, Genetic epidemiology of breast cancer and associated cancers in high risk families II. Linkage analysis, *J. Natl. Cancer Inst.* **71:**463–467.

Klein, G., 1981, The role of gene dosage and genetic transposition in carcinogenesis, *Nature* **294:**290–293.

Knudson, A.G., and Strong, L.C., 1972, Mutation and cancer: A model for Wilms' tumor of the kidney, *J. Natl. Cancer Inst.* **48:**313–324.

Koufos, A., Hausen, M.F., Lampkin, B.C., Wakman, M.L., Copeland, N.G., Jenkins, N.A., and Cavenee, W.K., 1984, Loss of allele at loci on human chromosome 11 during genesis of Wilms' tumor, *Nature* **309:**170–172.

Kozbor, D. and Croce, C., 1984, Amplification of the c-*myc* oncogene in one of five human breast carcinoma cell lines, *Cancer Res.* **44:**438–441.

Kraus, M.H., Yuasa, Y., and Aaronson, S.A., 1984, A position 12-activated H-*ras* oncogene in all HS 578T mammary carcinoma cells but not normal mammary cells of the same patient, *Proc. Natl. Acad. Sci. USA* **81:**5384–5388.

Krontiris, T.G., DiMartino, N.A., Colb, M., and Parkinson, D.R., 1985, Unique allelic restriction fragments of the human Ha-*ras* locus in leukocyte and tumor DNAs of cancer patients, *Nature* **313:**369–374.

Land, H., Parada, L., and Weinberg, R.A., 1983, Cellular oncogenes and multistep carcinogenesis, *Nature* **304:**596–602.

Lane, M.A., Sainten, A., and Cooper, G.M., 1981, Activation of related transforming genes in mouse and human mammary carcinomas, *Proc. Natl. Acad. Sci. USA* **78:**5185–5189.

Lee, A.E., 1968, Genetic and viral influences on mammary tumors in BRG mice, *Br. J. Cancer* **22:**77–82.

Lee, W.M., Schwab, M., Westaway, D., and Varmus, H.E., 1985, Augmented expression of normal c-*myc* is sufficient for cotransfection of rat embryo cells with a mutant *ras* gene, *Mol. Cell. Biol.* **5:**3345–3356.

Lidereau, R., Mathieu-Mahul, D., Theillet, C., Renaud, M., Manchauffe, M., Gest, J., and Larsen, C.J., 1985, Presence of allelic *Eco*RI restriction fragment of the c-*mos* locus in leukocyte and tumor cell DNAs of breast cancer patients, *Proc. Natl. Acad. Sci. USA* **82:**7068–7070.

Lidereau, R., Escot, C., Theillet, C., Champeme, M.H., Brunet, M., Gest, J., and Callahan, R., 1986, High frequency of rare alleles of the human c-Ha-*ras*-1 protooncogene in breast cancer patients, *J. Natl. Cancer Inst.,* **77:**697–701.

Lynch, H.T., Albano, W.A., Danes, S., Layton, M.A., Kimberling, W.J., Lynch, J.F., Cheng, S.C., Costello, K.A., Mulcahy, G.M., Wagner, C.A., and Tindall, S.L., 1984, Genetic predisposition to breast cancer, *Cancer* **53:**612–622.

Marshall, C., 1985, Human oncogenes, in: *Molecular Biology of Tumor Viruses, RNA Tumor Viruses* (R. Weiss, N. Teich, H. Varmus, and J. Coffin, eds.), Cold Spring Harbor Laboratory, Cold Spring Harbor, NY, pp. 487–558.

May, F.E.B., Westley, B.R., Rochefort, H., Buetti, E., and Diggelmann, H., 1983, Mouse mammary tumor virus related sequences are present in human DNA, *Nucleic Acids Res.* **11:**4127–4139.

Modjtahedi, N., Lavielle, C., Poupon, M.-F., Landin, R.M., Cassingena, R., Monier, R., and Brison, O., 1985, Increased level of amplification of the c-*myc* oncogene in tumors induced in nude mice by a human breast carcinoma cell line, *Cancer Res.* **45:**4372–4379.

Moore, R., Casey, G., Brookes, S., Dixon, M., Peters, G., and Dickson, C., 1986, Sequence, topography and protein coding potential of mouse *int*-2: A putative oncogene activated by mouse mammary tumor virus, *EMBO J* **5:**919–924.

Nandi, S., 1963, New method for detection of mouse mammary tumor virus. I. Influence of foster nursing on the incidence of hyperplastic mammary nodules in BALB/c Crgl mice, *J. Natl. Cancer Inst.* **31:**57–73.

Noori-Daloii, M.R., Swift, R.A., Kung, N.J., Crittenden, L.B., and Witter, R.L., 1981, Specific integration of REV proviruses in avian bursal lymphomas, *Nature* **294:**574–576.

Nusse, R., and Varmus, H., 1982, Mammary tumor induced by the mouse mammary tumor virus: Evidence for a common region for provirus integration in the same region of the host genome, *Cell* **31:**99–109.

Nusse, R., van Ooyen, A., Cox, D., Fung, Y.-K., and Varmus, H., 1984, Mode of proviral activation of a putative mammary oncogene (*int*-1) on mouse chromosome 15, *Nature* **307:**131–136.

Nusse, R., van Ooyen, A., Schuuring, E., van Lohuizen, M., and Rijsewijk, F., 1985, Structural and biological properties of the *int*-1 mammary oncogene, in: *Breast Cancer: Origins, Detection, and Treatment* (M.A. Rich, J.C. Hagen, and J. Taylor-Papadimitriou, eds.), Martinus Nijhoff, London, pp. 167–177.

Ohlsson, S.P., Rydnert, J., Goustin, A.S., Larsson, E., Betholtz, C., and Ohlsson, R., 1985, Cell type-specific pattern of c-*myc* protooncogene expression in human developing embryos, *Proc. Natl. Acad. Sci. USA* **82:**5050–5054.

Ohuchi, N., Thor, A., Page, D.L., Horan Hand, P., Halter, S.A., and Schlom, J., 1986, Expression of the 21,000 molecular weight *ras* protein in a spectrum of benign and malignant human mammary tumors, *Cancer Res.* **46:**2511–2519.

Ono, M., 1986, Molecular cloning and long terminal repeat sequences of human endogenous retroviral genes related to type A and B retroviral genes, *J. Virol.* **58:**937–944.

Ono, M., Toh, H., Miyata, T., and Awaya, T., 1985, Nucleotide sequence of the Syrian hamster intracisternal A-particle gene: Close evolutionary relationship of type A particle gene to type B and D oncovirus genes, *J. Virol.* **54:**764–772.

Orkin, S.H., Goldman, D.S., and Sallan, S.E., 1984, Development of homozygosity for chromosome 11p markers in Wilms' tumor, *Nature* **309:**172–178.

Peters, G., Brookes, S., Smith, R., and Dickson, C., 1983, Tumorigenesis by mouse mammary tumor virus: Evidence for a common region for provirus integration in mammary tumors, *Cell* **33:**369–377.

Peters, G., Kozak, C., and Dickson, C., 1984a, Mouse mammary tumor virus integration region *int*-1 and *int*-2 map on different mouse chromosomes, *Mol. Cell. Biol.* **4:**375–378.

Peters, G., Lee, A.E., and Dickson, C., 1984b, Activation of cellular gene by mouse mammary tumor virus may occur early in mammary tumor development, *Nature* **309:**273–275.

Peters, G., Lee, A.E., and Dickson, C., 1986, Concerted activation of two potential protooncogenes in carcinomas induced by mouse mammary tumor virus, *Nature* **320:**628–631.

Pitelka, D.R., Bern, H.A., Nandi, S., and De Ome, K.B., 1964, On the significance of virus-like particles in mammary tissue of C3Hf mice, *J. Natl. Cancer Inst.* **33:**867–885.

Queen, C., and Baltimore, D., 1983, Immunoglobulin gene transcription is activated by downstream elements, *Cell* **33:**741–748.

Reeve, A.E., Harsiaux, P.J., Gardner, R.J.M., Chewings, W.E., Grindley, R.M., and Millow, L.J., 1984, Loss of Harvey *ras* allele in sporadic Wilms' tumour, *Nature* **309:**174–176.

Rijsewijk, R.A.M., van Lohuizen, M., Van Ooyen, A., and Nusse, R., 1986, Construction of a retroviral cDNA version of the *int*-1 mammary oncogene and its expression *in vitro, Nucleic Acids Res.* **14:**693–702.

Rongey, R.W., Hlavackova, A., Lara, S., Estes, J., and Gardner, M.B., 1973, Type B and cRNA virus in breast tissue and milk of wild mice, *J. Natl. Cancer Inst.* **50:**1581–1589.

Sarkar, N., 1980, Type B virus and human breast cancer, in: *The Role of Viruses in Human Cancer,* Vol. I (G. Giraldo and E. Beth, eds.), Elsevier North-Holland, New York, pp. 207–235.

Segev, N., Hizi, A., Kirenberg, F., and Keydar, I., 1985, Characterization of a protein released by the T47D cell line immunologically related to the major envelope protein of mouse mammary tumor virus, *Proc. Natl. Acad. Sci. USA* **82:**1531–1535.

Slamon, D.J., de Kernion, J.B., Verma, I.M., and Cline, M.J., 1984, Expression of cellular oncogenes in human malignancies, *Science* **224:**256–262.

Sonnenberg, A., van Balen, P., Hilgers, J., Schuuring, E., and Nusse, R., 1986, Oncogene expression during progression of mouse mammary tumor cells, activity of a proviral enhancer and the resulting expression of *int*-2 is influenced by the state of differentiation, (submitted).

Spandidos, D.A., and Wilkie, N.M., 1983, Host specificities of papilloma virus, Moloney murine sarcoma virus, and simian virus 40 enhancer sequences, *EMBO J.* **2:**1193–1199.

Spandidos, D.A., and Agnantis, N.J., 1984, Human malignant tumors of the breast, as compared to their respective normal tissue, have elevated expression of the Harvey-*ras* oncogene, *Anticancer Res.* **4:**269–279.

Squartini, F., Rossi, G., and Paoletti, J., 1963, Characters of mammary tumors in BALB/c female mice foster nursed by C3H and RIII mothers, *Nature* **197:**505–506.

Steele, P.E., Rabson, A.B., Bryan, T., and Martin, M.A., 1984, Distinctive termini characterize two families of human endogenous retroviral sequences, *Science* **225:**943–947.

Stewart, T., Pattengale, P., and Leder, P., 1984, Spontaneous mammary adenocarcinomas in transgenic mice that carry and express MTV/*myc* fusion genes, *Cell* **38:**627–637.

Sukumar, S., Notario, V., Martin-Zanca, D., and Barbacid, M., 1983, Induction of mammary carcinomas in rats by nitroso-methyl-urea involves the malignant activation of the H-*ras*-1 locus by single point mutations, *Nature* **306:**658–661.

Taub, R., Kelly, F., Battey, J., Latt, S., Lenoir, G.M., Tantravahi, U., Tu, Z., and Leder, P., 1984, A novel alteration in the structure of an activated c-*myc* gene in a variant t(2;8) Burkitt lymphoma, *Cell* **37:**511–520.

Teich, N., Wyke, J., Mak, T., Bernstein, A., and Hardy, W., 1982, Pathogenesis of retrovirus induced disease, in: *Molecular Biology of Tumor Viruses, RNA Tumor Viruses* (R. Weiss, N. Teich, H.E. Varmus, and J. Coffin, eds.), Cold Spring Harbor Laboratory, Cold Spring Harbor, NY, pp. 845–856.

Teramoto, Y.A., Hand, P.H., Callahan, R., and Schlom, J., 1980, Detection of novel murine mammary tumor viruses by interspecies immunoassays, *J. Natl. Cancer Inst.* **64:**967–975.

Theillet, C., Lidereau, R., Escot, C., Hutzell, P., Brunet, M., Gest, J., Schlom, J., and Callahan, R., 1986, Frequent loss of a H-*ras*-1 allele correlates with aggressive human primary breast carcinomas, *Cancer Res.* **46:**4776–4781.

Trent, J.M., 1985, Cytogenetic and molecular biologic alterations in human breast cancer: A review, *Breast Cancer Res. Treat.* **5:**221–229.

Tsichlis, P., Strauss, P.G., and Hu, L.F., 1983, A common region for proviral DNA integration in Mo MuLV-induced rat thymic lymphomas, *Nature* **302:**445–449.

Vaidya, A.B., Black, M.M., Dion, A.S., and Moore, D., 1974, Homology between human breast tumor RNA and mouse mammary tumor virus genome, *Nature* **249:**565–567.

van Nie, R., and Verstraeten, A.A., 1975, Studies of genetic transmission of mammary tumor virus by C3Hf mice, *Int. J. Cancer* **16:**922–931.

van Ooyen, A., and Nusse, R., 1984, Structure and nucleotide sequence of the putative mammary oncogene *int*-1: Proviral insertions leave the protein-encoding domain intact, *Cell* **39:**233–240.

Varmus, H.E., 1982, Recent evidence for oncogenesis by insertion mutagenesis and gene activation, *Cancer Surveys* **1:**309–319.

Varmus, H.E., 1984, The molecular genetics of cellular oncogenes, *Annu. Rev. Genet.* **18:**553–612.

Verstraeten, A.A., and van Nie, R., 1978, Genetic transmission of mammary tumor virus in the DBAf mouse strain, *Int. J. Cancer* **21:**473–475.

Wasylyk, B., Wasylyk, C., Augereau, P., and Chambon, P., 1983, The SV40 72 bp repeat preferentially potentiates transcription starting from proximal natural or substitute promoter elements, *Cell* **32:**503–514.

Weiss, R.N., Teich, N., Varmus, H., and Coffin, J., 1982, Origins of contemporary RNA virus research, in: *Molecular Biology of Tumor Viruses, RNA Tumor Viruses* (R. Weiss, N. Teich, H. Varmus, and J. Coffin, eds.), Cold Spring Harbor Laboratory, Cold Spring Harbor, NY, pp. 16–20.

Welsch, C.W., 1985, Host factors affecting the growth of carcinogen-induced rat mammary carcinomas: A review and tribute to Charles Brenton Huggins, *Cancer Res.* **45:**3415–3443.

Wirth, T., Gloggler, K., Baumruker, T., Schmidt, M., and Horak, I., 1983, Family of middle repetitive sequences in the mouse genome with structural features of solitary retroviral long terminal repeats, *Proc. Natl. Acad. Sci. USA* **80:**3327–3330.

Yokota, J., Tsunetsugu-Yokota, Y., Battifora, H., LeFevre, C., and Cline, M.J., 1986, Alterations of *myc*, *myb* and ras^{Ha} proto-oncogenes in cancers are frequent and show clinical correlation, *Science* **231:**261–265.

Zarbl, H., Sukumar, S., Arthur, A.V., Martin-Zanca, D., and Barbacid, M., 1985, Direct mutagenesis of Ha-*ras*-1 oncogenes by *N*-nitroso-*N*-methyl urea during initiation of mammary carcinogenesis in rats, *Nature* **315:**382–385.

IV

Hormonal Control of Mammary Growth and Function

11

Growth Factors in Mammary Gland Development and Function

Thomas C. Dembinski and Robert P.C. Shiu

1. Introduction

Hormones, neural input, cell–cell contacts, and extracellular matrix are some of the important influences affecting the mammary gland during its growth and differentiation. Prominent among these are a heterogeneous group of polypeptides known as growth factors, which may be generally defined as hormones with poorly understood physiological significance in the context of mammary biology.

This chapter is devoted to an examination of our current knowledge as to what extent growth factors are (or appear to be) important in regulating mammary gland function. In the first section, we review present knowledge of "Classical" endocrine multihormonal control of mammary gland development and function, in as far as this relates to current observations of growth factor interactions within this regulation. Recent reviews are available that extensively and specifically cover classical endocrine hormone regulation of the developmental biology and function of the mammary gland (Topper and Freeman, 1980; Neville and Neifert, 1983; Houdebine et al., 1985). In addition to these classical endocrine hormones, an increasing number of tissue growth factors have been identified that influence both the growth and function of normal and neoplastic mammary cells. The remaining sections therefore focus on the potential role of several growth factors in normal mammary

---

Thomas C. Dembinski and Robert P. C. Shiu • Department of Physiology, Faculty of Medicine, University of Manitoba, Winnipeg, Manitoba R3E OW3, Canada.

gland development and function. Available data are evaluated from studies (both human and animal) on normal breast cells and/or by inference from studies on breast cancer, owing to the sparsity of information on normal mammary gland physiology.

Interactions that may occur between different cell types of the mammary gland are not discussed here in detail. The recent review by Oka and Yoshimura (1986) specifically focuses on studies of cell–cell interactions in culture, the effects of several growth factors and conditioned media of component cells of mammary tissue, and the implications such studies may have on our understanding of growth, morphological development, and differentiation in the mammary gland.

2. Multihormonal Regulation of Mammary Gland Development and Function

During the lifetime of a female animal, profound changes occur in the mammary tissue, which can be divided into several distinct developmental and functional stages: (1) mammogenesis, the growth and differentiation of mammary ductal and alveolar tissue, (2) lactogenesis, the onset of copious milk secretion around parturition, (3) lactation, the continuing production of milk, and (4) involution, the return of the mammary gland to a less differentiated state at cessation of lactation. These stages are profoundly influenced by several ovarian, pituitary, and placental hormones from the time of embryogenesis through adolescence to maturity. Similarly, changes associated with the mature nonpregnant mammary gland throughout the menstrual cycle and at the time of menopause are intricately regulated by hormones.

Multiple hormonal interactions coordinate each stage. In vivo mammogenesis appears to require sex steroids, lactogenic hormones (prolactin and placental lactogen), and probably one or more growth factors. In addition, interactions between the mammary epithelial elements and the stroma in which they are situated, possibly mediated by locally produced growth factors, are clearly of importance although poorly understood.

Evidence for multiple hormonal involvement in the induction of mammary growth became available in the 1950s. Lyons (1958) performed extensive experiments injecting replacement hormones into "triply operated" rats (animals from which ovaries, pituitary, and adrenal glands had been removed) and was able to obtain ductal proliferation with the injection of estrogen, desoxycorticosterone acetate, and growth hormone. Addition of progesterone, prolactin, and prednisolone to this regimen produced the degree of lobuloalveolar development typically seen in the late pregnant animal.

The hormones responsible for growth of the mammary epithelium remain controversial, largely because no entirely satisfactory in vitro system for the study of mammary proliferation has been available. In animals, estrogens given in vivo bring about ductal proliferation and appear to stimulate secretory activity with very little lobuloalveolar development (Cowie, 1978). A correlation between mammary growth at puberty and the onset of ovarian function in women was clearly recognized by Halban in 1905. By the 1930s, it was well known that estrogen injections produced mammary development in a variety of mammals (Folley and Malpress, 1948). The treatment generally produced only ductal proliferation. These observations, plus the clear association of estrogen receptors with growth of a significant proportion of human mammary tumors (Leclerg and Heuson, 1979; Edwards et al., 1979), has led to wide acceptance of the idea that estrogens promote proliferation of mammary epithelium, particularly the ductal portions of the gland.

It is of interest to note that in human breast cancer cells transplanted into athymic nude mice, supplemental estrogen administration is frequently required to sustain progressive epithelial tumor cell growth (Soule and McGrath, 1980; Shafie and Grantham, 1981; Leung and Shiu, 1981), and evidence has been presented for a direct growth-stimulating effect of estrogen on human breast cancer cells in vivo (Huseby et al., 1984). However, the exact role of estrogen and other hormones in relation to normal mammary gland development is not yet precisely known because each hormone, besides having actions of its own, regulates the secretion and activity of other hormones. It appears that estrogen is a potent stimulant of normal breast epithelium but is ineffective in the absence of pituitary and placental hormones, and probably other growth factors. Progesterone has some effects similar to those of estrogen, although this hormone predominantly influences the differentiation of mammary tissue. Both insulin and the adrenal corticosteroids, on the other hand, appear to be necessary for most phases of breast growth, maintenance, and function.

During pregnancy, the high blood levels of estrogen and progesterone, as well as prolactin (which increases steadily throughout gestation in women), have profound effects on the breasts. Both the ductal and lobular elements in the gland undergo dramatic proliferation. Furthermore, because it was possible to induce mammary growth in animals during pregnancy with either placental lactogen or prolactin in the absence of steroids both in vivo (Talwalker and Meites, 1961) and in vitro (Turkington and Topper, 1966; Peters et al., 1979), a primary role in the regulation of human mammogenesis during pregnancy has been assigned to these lactogenic hormones. However, because placental lactogen is secreted only in pregnancy, its physiological role in mammary function must be limited to the stimulation of mammary growth and differentiation at this time. At present, the physiological role of placental lactogen in human mammary development is still undefined. The documentation (Nielsen et al., 1979; Sideri et al., 1983) that women who failed to express placental lactogen during pregnancy delivered normal babies and had normal mammary gland function may suggest that placental lactogen has little function in the human. In addition, many species (such as rabbit, pig, and dog) have no detectable placental lactogen during pregnancy (Kelly et al., 1976). However, since immunoreactive and not biologically active placental lactogen was measured in these studies, a cautious conclusion on the importance of placental lactogen in mammary gland function is appropriate.

Although it would appear that much is known about hormonal control of mammary gland function, the regulation of both mammogenesis and lactogenesis has been a confused issue for many decades. The currently emerging picture from studies at the cellular and molecular levels, for example, is at considerable variance with that often found in current textbooks. The ideas in these texts, developed prior to 1960, were based on a central role for ovarian steroids in stimulating mammogenesis and for a prolactin surge that stimulated lactogenesis. More recent work suggests that a key role should be assigned to growth factors of various sources. It would be fair therefore to state that our knowledge of the mechanisms by which hormones and growth factors regulate the growth and activities of the mammary gland is still evolving. Major advances in concepts can be expected within the decade, especially if the remaining, as yet undiscovered, active growth factors and hormone-like biomolecules can be identified and their mode of action elucidated.

A number of lines of evidence suggest that factors such as epidermal growth factor (EGF) (Tonelli and Sorof, 1980; Yang et al., 1980) or a specific mammary growth factor (Ptashne et al., 1979) are required for mammary growth. The possibility that estrogens stimulate secretion of these or other factors by extramammary organs was suggested by the experiments of Sirbasku (1978), in which extracts of uterus, kidney, brain, and platelets from estrogen-treated animals stimulated growth of a mammary tumor line. The mechanism by which estrogens sensitize the mammary cell to mitogenic factors is unknown. Apart from their direct interaction with estrogen receptors on the mammary cell, the possibility should seriously be considered that estrogen-inducible tissue growth factors (estromedins) (Ikeda et al., 1982; Sirbasku et al., 1984) or pituitary-derived mammary mitogens (Dembinski et al., 1985; Shiu et al., 1986a) are mediators or potentiators, respectively, of estrogen's growth-promoting action on the normal mammary epithelium. When progesterone is injected with estrogen, secretion is inhibited and lobuloalveolar development promoted. Because these steroids have no effect in hypophysectomized animals (Cowie et al., 1966; Stoudemire et al., 1975), it has been suggested that a pituitary hormone, possibly prolactin, and/or a growth factor, other than a traditional hormone, is responsible for mammary growth in the estrogen- and progesterone-treated animal.

3. Pituitary Factors

There is increasing evidence to indicate that the intact pituitary gland supplies poorly characterized, as well as known, growth factors and hormones for normal mammary gland development. Observations indicating direct mitogenic stimulation of the mammary gland by estrogen are few (Jacobsohn, 1954; Traurig and Morgan, 1964; Norgren, 1968; Klevjer-Anderson and Buehring, 1980; Stampfer et al., 1980) and the extent of the observed stimulation has been limited. Moreover, most of the observed effects of estrogens in whole animals require that the pituitary gland be intact (Lyons, 1958; Meites, 1966; Haslam and Shyamala, 1979), suggesting either that the hormone acts indirectly by stimulating secretion of a pituitary growth factor or that a pituitary hormone acts synergistically with the steriod to induce mammary growth.

A wealth of convincing in vitro and in vivo evidence exists showing that estrogens promote pituitary prolactin secretion. That this estrogen effect occurs under physiological conditions in humans is suggested by the correlation between plasma estradiol-17β levels and the levels of prolactin at puberty (Robyn et al., 1977), during pregnancy (Del Pozo, 1977; Hertz et al., 1978), and at the menarch (Robyn et al., 1977). Furthermore, increases in estradiol levels in pubertal boys with gynecomastia were correlated with increases in plasma prolactin levels (Large et al., 1980). Thus, from a physiological standpoint in humans, increases in plasma estrogen and prolactin levels go hand-in-hand, raising the possibility that estrogen effects on mammary growth may be mediated, at least in part, by prolactin. In addition, hyperprolactinemia due to pituitary tumors in human males produces mammary growth (gynecomastia) only when plasma estrogen levels are manipulated (Antunes et al., 1977; Sultan et al., 1979), suggesting that estrogens act synergistically with prolactin to produce mammary growth.

On the other hand, there is evidence suggesting that estrogens have growth-promoting actions of their own in mammary tissue. Mitogenic activity in several human breast cancer cell lines is stimulated by estradiol-17β in vitro (reviewed by Lippman et al., 1977). However, it is still unclear whether (1) estrogens act as primary mitogens in mammary tissue, (2) estrogens are permissive agents that sensitize mammary tissue to the action of lactogenic hormones and growth factors, or (3) estrogen action is entirely indirect, being mediated through stimulation of secretion of other hormones and growth factors (see Section 7). Furthermore, the idea of a synergistic and/or mediating *pituitary mammogen*, other than prolactin, has persisted. Turner (1939) was one of the first to suggest that the ovarian hormones may exert their effect indirectly, their action being mediated by the pituitary gland. The idea that steroid hormone action could be mediated by pituitary hormones was given considerable support by the work of Reece and Leonard (1941), who found that hypophysectomy prevented the stimulation of mammary growth with estrogen and progesterone. Similarly, two clinical studies showed that estrogen injected into breast cancer patients stimulated the growth of the tumors, whereas it failed to do so when injected into the same patients after hypophysectomy (Pearson and Bronson, 1959; Lipsett and Bergenstal, 1960). Indeed, the authors of these clinical studies suggested that a pituitary factor, distinct from prolactin and growth hormone, was required for estrogen action in breast cancer patients. The identity of this factor is unknown, but may in all likelihood be one of the mammary mitogens involved in normal growth.

More direct experiments suggesting a positive growth-promoting role for pituitary factors were provided by Clifton and Furth (1960), who implanted a pituitary mammotropic tumor secreting prolactin, growth hormone, and ACTH into adrenogonadectomized rats. They obtained good mammary growth in the complete absence of steroid hormones. These findings led Meites (1966) to conclude that "the anterior pituitary hormones are the primary stimulators of mammary growth even in normal 'physiological states'." Moreover, implantation studies of recent years, similar to those of Clifton and Furth (1960), using normal and tumorous pituitary and mammary tissue and cells (Leung and Shiu, 1981; McManus and Welsch, 1981; Welsch et al., 1981; Dembinski et al., 1985), together with studies in which purified pituitary hormones were injected in the absence and presence of estrogens (Dembinski et al., 1985), have provided strong support for a pituitary mammary growth factor for both normal and neoplastic mammary epithelial cells. Although the identity of the active pituitary-derived growth factor has not been firmly established, several candidates have recently emerged.

Estrogen-potentiating factor (EPF) has been characterized as a pituitary growth factor for estrogen-responsive breast cancer cells (Dembinski et al., 1985; Shiu et al., 1986a). The pituitary factor was shown to potentiate growth of estrogen-responsive human breast cancer cells in the presence of estradiol both in vivo and in a serum-free medium in vitro (Dembinski et al., 1985). Our studies on the pituitary-derived EPF for human breast cancer epithelial cells suggested that it is an endocrine growth factor secreted by normal human and rat pituitaries, as well as being present in conditioned media of some pituitary tumor cell lines (Dembinski et al., 1985). It appears to be unrelated to any of the known anterior pituitary hormones. Furthermore, EPF appears to stimulate and potentiate specifically the effect of estrogen on the proliferation of estrogen receptor-positive human breast cancer cells in vitro.

Recent work from our laboratory concerning EFP has revealed that it is probably related to insulin-like growth factor 2 (IGF-2) (Shiu et al., 1986b). Studies with normal and tumorous rat pituitary cells using antibodies to rat IGF-2 showed that there was a strong correlation between the presence of IGF-2 immunoreactive peptides and the ability to stimulate the proliferation of human breast cancer cells. Extracts of normal human pituitary also stimulated the growth of human breast cancer cells. The normal human anterior pituitary has been shown to possess the highest amounts of IGF-2-like immunoreactivity, representing a 100-fold increase in comparison to other brain regions (Haselbacher et al., 1985). In our studies, highly purified rat IGF-2 was potent in stimulating the growth of T-47D human breast cancer cells in culture (Myal et al., 1984). Therefore, our observations strongly suggest that the pituitary gland secretes IGF-2-like peptides, which are potent mitogens for breast tumor cells. The concept that IGF-2 is important for estrogen action is supported by the work of Evans et al. (1981), which showed that an IGF-like peptide was required during estrogen-mediated induction of ovalbumin gene transcription in the chick oviduct. The potential influence of IGF-2 on normal mammary epithelial cells therefore warrants investigation.

Interestingly, addition of bovine pituitary extract to a hormone-supplemented serum-free defined medium has been found to support optimal growth and maintenance of the differentiated state of normal human mammary epithelial cells and results in their rapid clonal proliferation and greatly extended serial passage (10–20 passages) in culture (Hammond et al., 1984). These authors, however, have not further characterized the pituitary growth factor(s) present in this extract. It should also be noted that Ptashne et al. (1979) and Rudland et al. (1977, 1979) demonstrated that mitogenic activity for normal mammary cells of rodents was present in both plasma and the pituitary gland. The pituitary activity has been partially purified; pituitary-derived mammary growth factor (PMGF) appears to stimulate specifically the division of cuboidal mammary epithelial cells (Smith et al., 1984).

Mittra (1980a,b) has previously identified a modified form of prolactin that has a specific cleavage site in its large disulfide loop and is synthesized and secreted by rat pituitary glands. This *cleaved* prolactin is made up of two chains; the two component polypeptides are separable into an N-terminal 16-kDa fragment and a C-terminal 8-kDa fragment by the reduction of the intervening disulfide bridge. The 16-kDa N-terminal fragment was reported to be capable of stimulating mitosis of mammary epithelial cells both in vivo and in vitro, whereas the intact prolactin was inactive. Moreover, the production of this cleaved prolactin was regulated by physiological stimuli normally associated with increased mammary growth and was estrogen dependent. It was not produced in pituitaries of ovariectomized rats, but its production was resumed if ovariectomized rats were injected with estrogen. Unfortunately, no new information concerning the further characterization of this estrogen-regulated modified prolactin moiety has appeared in the literature since the first publication. The potential significance of this cleaved prolactin for mammary cell growth therefore remains to be established.

4. Insulin-like Growth Factor Family

The physiological role of insulin in mammary alveolar cell growth and differentiation is presently not well understood, although insulin has long been known to stimulate cell replication in mammary explants (Juergens et al., 1965; Friedberg et al., 1970; Martel and Houdebine, 1982) and to potentiate the lactogenic effect of prolactin (Devinoy et al., 1978; Bolander et al., 1981). Largely based on the observation that supraphysiological doses (usually at μg/ml or 10^{-6} M) of insulin have generally been found necessary in culture systems to maintain mammary tissues and to enhance the differentiation response to prolactin and cortisol, a role for this hormone was proposed in the regulation of mammary cell development. However, there is little evidence for a physiological role for insulin as a mitogen for mammary cells. Insulin levels were found to vary randomly during a course of estrogen- and progesterone-induced lactation in goats (Hart and Morant, 1980), and alloxan-induced diabetes did not interfere with estrogen-stimulated mammary growth in hypophysectomized male rabbits (Norgren, 1968). Streptozotocin diabetes did not prevent estrogen- and progesterone-induced mammary growth in male mice (Topper and Freeman, 1980). In vitro,

Errick and Kano-Sueoka (1983) were able to obtain prolactin stimulation of rat mammary alveolar cell proliferation in the absence of insulin. A possible interpretation of these findings is that insulin at high concentrations serves as a mammary growth factor in vitro by mimicking insulin-like growth factor(s).

First described as a *sulfation factor* by Salmon and Daughaday (1957), somatomedin C is the best known member of a family of insulin-like peptides, ancestrally related to proinsulin (Blundell and Humbel, 1980); other members of the family include IGF-1 and IGF-2. Supraphysiological concentrations of insulin (of the order of 100 n*M*) can replace the IGF requirement in defined media through cross-reaction with ubiquitous IGF receptors (Van Wyk et al., 1975). It has been speculated that IGF-1 may be an adult somatomedin, whereas IGF-2 would be its embryonic counterpart (Adams et al., 1983). IGF-1 and IGF-2 share 62% homology with each other and 47% homology with insulin. Both are potent mitogens, not only for mesenchymal cells, but also for human mammary tumor cells (Furlanetto and DiCarlo, 1984; Myal et al., 1984).

There is no direct information available to indicate whether IGFs are important for growth and development of the mammary gland in vivo. However, because of their role as progression factors in the cell cycle of target cells and their ubiquitous nature, in that they are present in a variety of organs and cell types (D'Ercole et al., 1980; Perkins et al., 1986), one may expect that they are involved in the development of the mammary gland. More importantly, however, the IGFs share common biological activities with insulin, presumably because of their structural similarity (Rinderknecht and Humbel, 1978), and insulin can influence the growth of the human mammary gland in organ cultures (Ceriani et al., 1972). In general, however, because the mitogenic effect of insulin on in vitro cultures is only observed with supraphysiological concentrations, it has been speculated that the weak mitogenic effect of insulin is due primarily to the structural similarity to the IGFs. Distinct cell membrane receptors for IGF-1 and IGF-2 are present on several lines of human breast cancer cells (Furlanetto and DiCarlo, 1984; Myal et al., 1984), and physiological levels of somatomedins are mitogenic for these cultured human breast tumor cells. Furthermore, it has been shown that Somatomedin C/IGF-1 immunoreactive material is synthesized by human and rat fibroblasts (Atkison et al., 1980; Clemmons et al., 1981; Adams et al., 1983) and human breast cancer cells themselves (Lippman et al., 1986a,b). Also, in explant cultures of mouse mammary glands, IGF-1 can substitute for insulin in the development of the high basal rate of carrier-mediated glucose transport observed in mammary cells from lactating mice (Prosser and Topper, 1986). Such findings suggest therefore that the somatomedins may act on epithelial cells of the mammary gland in vivo via paracrine and autocrine routes.

Another member of the insulin-like growth factor family is relaxin. After a long period of relative obscurity since its initial discovery some 60 years ago, relaxin has again been hailed as a *new* hormone (Bryant-Greenwood, 1982). Interest, however, has been rather sporadic in the mammary gland as a target tissue for relaxin. It is unique in being the only well-characterized peptide hormone produced by the corpus luteum of the ovary. It is not confined to the ovary and is produced in lower concentrations in several other distinct body sites such as the placenta (Bryant-Greenwood, 1982), implying a potential role for relaxin as a local reproductive or connective tissue growth factor. Effects of relaxin include softening the cervix, relaxing pubic ligaments, increasing uterine growth, decreasing uterine contractility, and stimulating mammary gland development (Schwabe et al., 1978; Bryant-Greenwood, 1982; Wright and Anderson, 1983; Bani and Bigazzi, 1984). Previous studies have demonstrated the potential importance of relaxin in synergizing with estrogen and progesterone (Harness and Anderson, 1975), or with prolactin or ovarian steroids (Harness and Anderson, 1977), in stimulating the proliferation and lobulation of mammary ducts and in depressing the secretory activity of the mammary gland of the rat (Harness and Anderson, 1975); relaxin alone had no effect on growth of mammary tissue in the absence of prolactin or ovarian steroids. It has been speculated that the action of relaxin may be directed more to the loosening of the connective tissue matrix to allow mammary duct penetration than upon the ducts themselves (Bryant-Greenwood, 1982). This would be in keeping with relaxin's actions on the interpubic ligament, uterus, and cervix. Relaxin appears to behave, based on these studies, not only as a *classical* endocrine hormone, but also as a growth factor with potential importance for mammary gland function.

5. Epidermal Growth Factor and Related Growth Factors

Epidermal growth factor (EGF) is a single-chain polypeptide consisting of 53 amino acid residues, with a molecular weight and structure similar to insulin and relaxin (Carpenter and Cohen, 1979). Functional receptors for EGF exist on normal mouse mammary epithelial cells (Taketani and Oka, 1983c). Further receptor levels in mammary tissues from cycling, gestating, and lactating mice have been shown to correlate with the physiological state of the animal (Edery et al., 1985). Epidermal growth factor has been shown to exert a dual function, stimulating proliferation and inhibiting functional differentiation (milk protein synthesis) in normal mouse mammary epithelial cells in vitro (Tonelli and Sorof, 1980; Yang et al., 1980; Taketani and Oka, 1983a,b). Tonelli and Sorof (1980) obtained two full cycles of development and regression in whole mammary glands in culture, from estrogen- and progesterone-primed BALB/c mice. After a first cycle of 9 days in a medium containing insulin, prolactin, aldosterone, and hydrocortisone (each at 5 μg/ml), glands showed extensive lobuloalveolar development. On transfer to a medium containing insulin alone for 15 days, regression occurred. A second cycle of development was then obtained only if EGF (10 n*M*) was added to the four hormones in the combination medium. Hydrocortisone was also necessary for development in these cultures. In experiments of this type, the significance of each hormone has not been fully clarified. In all probability, EGF acts as a cell cycle early progression factor on competent mammary epithelial cells.

Epidermal growth factor may also be involved in the synthesis of type IV collagen by mammary epithelium. Mammary epithelial cells in vivo are in contact with type IV collagen, a component of the basal lamina. Basement membrane collagen (type IV collagen) synthesis by mammary cells is important for the growth and/or survival, both in vivo and in vitro, of the epithelium of the normal rodent mammary gland and of well-differentiated tumors derived from it (Wicha et al., 1979, 1980; Kidwell et al., 1980; Lewko et al., 1981). There is also considerable evidence indicating that collagen production is tightly coupled to a mitogenic response of these cells. Salomon et al. (1981) found that the ability to synthesize and accumulate type IV collagen was important for proliferation of rat mammary epithelial cells. In these studies, cells maintained on plastic or collagen type I required EGF and glucocorticoids to promote the accumulation of type IV collagen, for attachment and growth. Cells grown on type IV collagen, however, did not require these factors for proliferation.

Some in vivo evidence exists to indicate that EGF may be physiologically important for mammary gland function during pregnancy (Okamoto and Oka, 1984). These authors found that pregestational sialoadenectomy (removal of submandibular glands, a source of EGF in mice) of virgin mice resulted in decreased growth of the mammary gland and in its ultimate ability to produce milk, in addition to an increase in offspring mortality during lactation. Administration of EGF to sialoadenectomized pregnant mice partially reversed the trend, in that it was effective in enhancing the survival rate of their pups during the nursing period. However, these results should be interpreted cautiously. Previous studies (Byyny et al., 1974) have demonstrated that sialoadenectomy leaves basal plasma and urine levels of EGF unchanged, a result later confirmed by Oka's laboratory itself (Kurachi and Oka, 1985). It appears that significant amounts of EGF are normally secreted by other mouse tissues, in addition to the contribution from the submandibular gland. In light of these paradoxical results, one may conclude that, in the mouse, EGF from the submandibular gland may in part be important for lactogenesis, although the possibility should be considered that in vivo growth and function of the mouse mammary gland during pregnancy and lactation are influenced not primarily by EGF but by an as yet uncharacterized (growth) factor present in the intact submandibular gland. Previous studies have shown that EGF added to cultured mammary cells acts as a potent mitogen and also inhibits casein and α-lactalbumin production (Tonelli and Sorof, 1980; Yang et al., 1980; Taketani and Oka, 1983a,b; Vonderhaar and Nakhasi, 1986). In addition, it has been reported (Gospodarowicz, 1981) that the circulating level of EGF was increased during pregnancy, whereas its level was low in nonpregnant states. These observations taken together suggest that EGF may be involved in the development of the mouse mammary gland during pregnancy, by stimulating growth and inhibiting precocious differentiation.

Transforming growth factor α (TGF-α) (Todaro et al., 1980) closely resembles EGF in structure and potency as a ligand for the EGF receptor. TGF-α was first purified from the conditioned media of malignant tumor cell lines and it may contribute to solid tumor growth by autocrine or paracrine mechanisms (Todaro et al., 1980; Sporn and Roberts, 1985). It is discussed further in Sections 7 and 8.

6. Fibroblast Growth Factor and Related Growth Factors

Recent studies have indicated that fibroblast growth factors (FGFs) and related factors belong to the larger group of heparin-binding growth factors (HBGFs), which can be subdivided into two main classes (Lobb et al., 1986). Within each class, growth factors are very closely related structurally and in some cases may be identical. For example, FGFs purified from several sources, such as pituitary, brain, and placenta, show strong identity with each other (Gospodarowicz et al., 1984). Class 1 HBGFs are anionic mitogens of molecular weight 15,000–17,000 found in high levels in neural tissue and include acidic brain FGF and retina-derived growth factor. Class 2 HBGFs are cationic mitogens of molecular weight 18,000–20,000 found in a wide variety of normal tissues and are typified by basic pituitary FGF and cartilage growth factor. Typical class 2 HBGFs have also been isolated from a rat chondrosarcoma, a human melanoma, and a human hepatoma (Lobb et al., 1986).

It was previously thought that FGFs were exclusive mesodermal and neuroectodermal cell mitogens that primarily affected three types of target cell in culture, namely, fibroblasts, endothelial cells, and chondrocytes. However, an increasing number of studies have shown that FGFs can also stimulate the growth of normal rat mammary cells and human breast cancer cells, suggesting both a potentially new function for the growth factor and a wider spectrum of target cells than previously thought. In one study, bovine pituitary FGF was shown to stimulate specifically the growth of cloned lines of stromal and myoepithelial-like cells, but not cuboidal epithelial cells, derived from normal and neoplastic rat mammary glands (Smith et al., 1984). Similarly, 10 ng/ml of bovine pituitary FGF stimulated the growth of T47D human breast cancer cells fourfold in a serum-free medium, in the absence of other hormones and growth factors, and twofold in a medium supplemented with 1% charcoal-treated fetal calf serum, after 7 days of culture (Shiu, 1981).

A human mammary tumor-derived growth factor (h.MTGF) has been purified by its affinity for heparin and copper. Therefore, the factor is apparently a class 2 HBGF related to basic human pituitary FGF by molecular weight, heat and acid lability, cationic nature, and FGF–target cell specificity for rabbit fetal chondrocytes, bovine corneal endothelial cells, human fibroblasts, and human breast cancer (T47D) cells (Rowe et al., 1986). It was therefore postulated that this factor (h.MTGF) may play a role in the autonomous growth and fibrovascular stromal changes associated with malignant breast tumors. Similar growth factors, which stimulate vascular endothelium and angiogenesis, have been isolated not only from a variety of neoplastic cells and solid tumors but also from normal tissue (Maciag et al., 1984).

Such studies therefore raise the possibility that both locally synthesized and systemic FGF/endothelial cell growth factor-like peptides are involved in the promotion of normal mammary gland growth, development, and function. If correct, proliferation of several types of normal mammary cell in the vicinity of FGF-producing cells may be expected to be stimulated in concert during a particular stage of mammary gland development. Unfortunately, virtually nothing is known about the physiology of FGF. The in situ function of FGF in any tissue may not necessarily be exclusively linked to the stimulation of cell growth; a nonmitogenic pituitary function of FGF in regulating prolactin and thyrotropin secretion has been described (Baird et al., 1985). Therefore, whether an FGF moiety is one of the principal mammotrophic factors responsible for regulated growth and function of the mammary gland in vivo remains to be determined.

7. Endocrine, Autocrine, and Paracrine Growth Factors

Primary cultures of nonmalignant human mammary epithelial cells have been shown to be responsive specifically to physiological concentrations of estradiol (see Section 2). However, the mechanism by which estradiol produces its mitogenic signal in target cells is poorly understood. In recent years, numerous studies have suggested that the action of estrogen may be mediated by growth factors acting through endocrine, paracrine, and autocrine modes. The endocrine hypothesis was based on the finding of increased growth of mammary tumor cells when incubated with extramammary tissues, such as pituitary, kidney, and uterus, which has previously been exposed to estrogen (Ikeda et al., 1982; Sirbasku and Leland, 1982). The putative growth factors are as yet poorly characterized, preventing further studies on their role in the in vivo growth of normal or neoplastic mammary cells.

Additional information is available, however, that indicates that the growth-promoting action of estrogen on mammary tissue may be mediated, at least in part, via an autocrine growth factor. Specific membrane receptors for EGF (to which TGF-α can bind) (Imai et al., 1982; Fitzpatrick et al., 1984; Salomon et al., 1984) and for IGFs (Myal et al., 1984; Furlanetto and DeCarlo, 1984) have been shown to exist on several lines of human breast cancer cells. Furthermore, in these cells, a variety of growth-promoting factors are induced and secreted in response to estradiol, such as EGF/TGF-α-related peptides (Salomon et al., 1984; Dickson et al., 1986a,b,c), IGF-1 (Dickson et al., 1986b), and a 52K glycoprotein (Vignon et al., 1986). In addition, TGF-α activities have been detected in extracts of solid human mammary tumors, in human breast milk (Salomon et al., 1984; Zwiebel et al., 1986), and in epithelium from bovine mammary gland (Eckert et al., 1985). The presence of TGFs in nonmalignant tissue suggests that these peptides may be important for the function of the normal mammary gland. TGF-β activity is also secreted by human breast cancer cells, although its production is not stimulated by estrogen; some evidence exists to suggest that it may be involved in inhibiting cell growth (Dickson et al., 1986a,b).

Recent studies have shown (Dickson et al., 1986b) that estrogen-induced growth factors (TGF-α-like and IGF-1-like peptides) present in conditioned medium can partially replace estrogen to promote human mammary tumor cell growth both in vitro and in vivo in nude mice. Because the neoplasms regressed after 2 weeks, additional mechanisms may maintain growth in estrogen-induced breast tumors. Such factors may be relevant in the control of normal mammary gland development and, in addition, may mediate the effect of estrogen on angiogenesis or expression of cell surface determinants such as growth factor receptors. In a recent study, Schreiber et al. (1986) have shown that TGF-α has potent angiogenic properties. Convincing direct evidence, however, for an autocrine mechanism that mediates the action of estrogen on the mammary gland requires demonstration that (1) the mammary epithelium elaborates a growth factor in response to estrogen, (2) specific receptors for the growth factor exist on these mammary cells, and (3) an antibody that blocks receptor binding of the growth factor also blocks the estrogen-induced growth of the mammary cell. These criteria have still to be applied and tested in the physiological situation.

8. Breast Milk Growth Factors

In the first few days after childbirth, the human produces not milk but colostrum, a thick yellow fluid rich in protein, fat-soluble vitamins, minerals, antibodies, and growth-promoting substances. The importance of colostrum for the health of the newborn has become more widely accepted but is not entirely agreed on. Studies with colostrum have revealed striking growth-promoting effects on intestinal tissue both in vivo and on cultured cells in vitro (Read at al., 1984), which exceed those found with mature milk. In early lactation, a wave of breast epithelial cell proliferation is observed (Traurig, 1967) and simultaneously colostrum is produced that contains larger amounts of growth-promoting activity than milk (Carpenter, 1980). A wide range of hormones has also been identified in milk, including prolactin, prostaglandins, thyroid hormones, glucocorticoids, thyroid-stimulating hormone, and adrenocorticotrophic hormone (Koldovsky, 1980). Although the role of these hormones and growth modulators is not entirely defined, it is possible that their presence in the milk may reflect their functions in the mammary gland.

The growth-promoting activity for human fibroblasts in vitro that is present in milk (Klagsbrun, 1978) has been attributed in part to the presence of an EGF-like polypeptide (Carpenter, 1980), which was later identified in human but not in bovine milk (Shing and Klagsbrun, 1984). The physiological significance of growth factor differences in various milks is not yet apparent.

Several putative growth factors—specifically insulin and epidermal growth factor (EGF)—were previously measured in human milk samples by radioimmunoassay and by competitive-binding radioreceptor assays, respectively (Read et al., 1984). Concentrations of bioactive insulin and EGF in mature milk were only 10% of those in colostrum, but still considerably higher than in serum. It has not been clearly established whether insulin, EGF, and other EGF-related polypeptides in milk originate from blood or are synthesized in the mammary gland itself. Cevreska et al. (1975) reported a close correlation between insulin concentrations in human plasma and milk. Less information is available on the origin of EGF, but it has been shown that radioactively labeled EGF can pass from the circulation into milk (Blakeley et al., 1982). The studies of Read et al. (1984) also suggest that insulin-like growth factors may occur in high concentrations in human and bovine colostrum and could be responsible for most of the growth-promoting activity of milk.

Human milk, apart from containing authentic EGF which is identical with urogastrone from human urine (Shing and Klagsbrun, 1984; Petrides et al., 1985), contains a considerable amount of both α and β TGF-like activities (Noda et al., 1984; Petrides et al., 1985; Zwiebel et al., 1986). These can be resolved into several major species, of which three bear similar identity to TGFs detected in both rat (Zwiebel et al., 1982) and human (Salomon et al., 1984; Zwiebel et al., 1986) mammary tumors.

One of these species, designated milk-derived growth factor-2 (MDGF-2) (Zwiebel et al., 1986), appears to be an α-TGF, based on its interaction via the EGF system and neutralization of normal rat kidney (NRK)–soft agar growth-promoting activity by an anti-EGF receptor antibody. Since a factor resembling MDGF-2 is released into the growth medium by a human mammary carcinoma cell line (Salomon et al., 1984) and human mammary tumors (Zwiebel et al., 1986) contain MDGF-2, this growth factor may be a reasonable candidate for a mammary autocrine or paracrine growth factor produced by and acting on both normal and neoplastic mammary epithelium. It is therefore possible that EGF and TGFs are physiologically important for mammary gland development and function during pregnancy and lactation.

In addition, recent studies suggest the presence of growth factors, other than EGF and TGF-related peptides, in milk. One of these is mammary-derived growth factor-1 (MDGF-1), with a molecular mass of 62 kDa and a p*I* of 4.8, which appears to be distinct from other known growth factors (Bano et al., 1985), including a bone marrow colony-stimulating factor found in milk (Sinha and Yunis, 1983). A factor apparently identical to milk-derived MDGF-1 was also isolated in the study of human mammary tumors (Bano et al., 1985), suggesting that MDGF-1 might act as an autocrine growth factor for mammary cells as suggested for MDGF-2. In support of this role, MDGF-1 was found to bind to specific high-affinity membrane receptors present on normal mouse mammary epithelium (Bano et al., 1985). Interestingly, MDGF-1 at picomolar levels stimulated the growth of normal mammary cells and greatly amplified their production of type IV collagen (Bano et al., 1983). The responsiveness of mammary epithelium to MDGF-1 was conditional. The cells responded if plated on type I collagen but not on a type IV collagen substratum. MDGF-1 thus may regulate the production of new basement membrane in vivo, since mammary epithelium is known to invade the stroma in response to a proliferative stimulus (Wicha et al., 1980). The presence of growth factors in colostrum and mature milk, however, does not by itself establish their importance in mammary gland function. The physiological significance of milk growth factors remains to be established.

9. Retinoids

Naturally occurring vitamin A derivatives are indispensable for growth, maintenance, and differentiation of epithelial tissues and are important in visual and reproductive functions (Underwood, 1984). However, the biological effects of vitamin A on the mammary gland are uncertain. Sankaran and Topper (1982) reported that the response to lactogenic hormones of the mammary glands from rats fed a vitamin A-free diet was similar to that of mammary glands from control rats. They concluded that vitamin A does not have a physiological role in either maintenance of the mammary epithelium or its potential for hormone-dependent phenotypic expression. Retinyl acetate is reported to stimulate formation of the mammary duct and alveolar growth in mice (Mariorana and Gullino, 1980) but to suppress ductal branching and alveolar growth in rats (Moon et al., 1979). Recent studies in rats have indeed confirmed that retinoids can significantly decrease normal mammary gland growth and development in vivo, regardless of the level of dietary fat (Aylsworth et al., 1986). Mehta et al. (1981) reported that hormone dependent mammary growth in vitro is inhibited by retinoids.

The possible interaction of vitamin A and EGF in the regulation of mammary gland development and function has been considered (Turkington, 1969; Tonelli and Sorof, 1980; Taketani and Oka, 1983a,b; Komura et al., 1986). Retinoic acid alone in these studies appeared to have no significant effect on mammary cell growth but enhanced the mitogenic effect of EGF in mammary explants and potentiated the EGF inhibition of the hormone-induced synthesis of casein and α-lactalbumin activity. The synergistic effect of retinoic acid was apparently due to its effect in increasing binding of EGF to mammary cells.

Retinoic acid exerts its influence through a retinoic acid-binding protein, isolated from several tissues including the mammary glands of rats and mice (Sani and Corbett, 1977). The cytosolic retinoic acid-binding protein was detected in mammary glands of virgin, pregnant, and lactating rats and the concentration of cytosolic retinoic acid-binding protein increased during pregnancy and decreased toward the time of lactation (Mehta and Moon, 1981). Therefore, it appears likely that retinoic acid has some effect on development of the mammary gland during pregnancy. One possibility suggested is that retinoic acid bound to retinoic acid-binding protein may enhance the development of mammary glands induced by a high level of circulating EGF and may inhibit precocious differentiation by increasing the capacity of mammary epithelium to bind EGF. The potential relevance of these findings to the human situation, however, is presently unknown.

10. Concluding Remarks

In this chapter, we have surveyed several families of hormones and growth factors that regulate many aspects of growth, development, and differentiation of the normal and cancerous mammary gland. From many of these studies, the concept that some growth factors act in a paracrine and/or autocrine manner within the mammary gland has gained popularity. However, one must keep in mind that the vast majority of the data have provided only circumstantial or even conjectural evidence that growth factors are physiologically significant molecules and that they indeed operate in vivo via autocrine/paracrine mechanisms. It is perhaps appropriate to quote Sporn and Roberts (1985): "Most of the [above] data provide only circumstantial evidence for the biological significance of an autocrine mechanism of growth factor action in [cancer] cells. A critical experiment would be to control the growth of [cancer] cells by an extracellular antagonist of a presumed autocrine peptide." We are not aware that such proof is available for the mammary gland system. Nevertheless, we hope that our critical viewpoint can stimulate future research to establish the biological importance of growth factors in mammary gland function. The many interesting studies so far performed can perhaps serve as a solid foundation toward achieving this goal. Finally, the excitement and attention focused on the relation between many oncogenes and growth factors may further our understanding not only of the role of growth factors on normal mammary gland function but also on the involvement of growth factor-mediated pathways in the pathophysiology of breast cancer.

ACKNOWLEDGMENTS: We appreciate the secretarial assistance of June McDougald and Cheryl Toews. The work done in our laboratory was supported by grants from the Medical Research Council of Canada and the National Cancer Institute of Canada. T.C. Dembinski is a postdoctoral fellow, supported by the St. Boniface Hospital Research Foundation, and R.P.C. Shiu is a Scientist of the Medical Research Council of Canada.

References

Adams, S.O., Nissley, S.P., Handwerger, S., and Rechler, M.M., 1983, Developmental patterns of insulin growth factor-I and -II synthesis and regulation in rat fibroblasts, *Nature* **302:**150–153.

Antunes, J.L., Housepian, E.M., Frantz, A.G., Holub, D.A., Hui, R.M., Carmel., P.W., and Quest, D.O., 1977, Prolactin-secreting pituitary tumors, *Ann. Neurol.* **2:**148–153.

Atkison, P.R, Weidman, E.R., Bhaumick, B., and Bala., R.M. 1980, Release of somatomedin-like activity by cultured WI-38 human fibroblasts, *Endocrinology* **106:**2006–2012.

Aylsworth, C.F., Cullum, M.E, Zile, M.H., and Welch, C.W., 1986, Influence of dietary retinyl acetate on normal rat mammary gland development and on the enhancement of 7,12-dimethylbenz[a]anthracene-induced rat mammary tumorigenesis by high levels of dietary fat, *J. Natl. Cancer Inst.* **76:**339–345.

Baird, A., Mormede, P., Ying, S-Y., Wehrenberg, W.B., Ueno, N., Ling, N., and Guillemin, R., 1985, A nonmitogenic pituitary function of fibroblast growth factor: Regulation of thyrotropin and prolactin secretion, *Proc. Natl. Acad. Sci. USA* **82:**5545–5549.

Bani, G., and Bigazzi, M., 1984, Morphological changes induced in mouse mammary gland by porcine and human relaxin, *Acta Anat.* **119:**149–154.

Bano, M., Salomon, D.S., and Kidwell, W.R., 1985, Purification of a mammary-derived growth factor from human milk and human mammary tumors, *J. Biol. Chem.* **260:**5745–5752.

Bano, M., Zwiebel, J.A., Salomon, D.S., and Kidwell, W.R., 1983, Detection and partial characterization of collagen synthesis stimulating activities in rat mammary adenocarcinomas, *J. Biol. Chem.* **258:**2729–2735.

Blakeley, D.M., Brown, K.D., and Fleet, I.R., 1982, Transfer of epidermal growth factor from blood to milk in lactating goats, *J. Physiol.* **326:**57P.

Blundell, T.L., and Humbel, R.E., 1980, Hormone families: Pancreatic hormones and homologous growth factors, *Nature* **287:**781–787.

Bolander, F.F., Nicholas, K.R., Van Wyck, J.J., and Topper, Y.J., 1981, Insulin is essential for accumulation of casein mRNA in mouse mammary epithelial cells, *Proc. Natl. Acad. Sci. USA* **78:**5682–5684.

Bryant-Greenwood, G.D., 1982, Relaxin as a new hormone, *Endoc. Rev.* **3**(1):62–90.

Byyny, R.L., Orth, D.N., Cohen, S., and Doyne, E.S., 1974, Epidermal growth factor: Effects of androgens and adrenergic agents, *Endocrinology* **95:**776–782.

Carpenter, G., 1980, Epidermal growth factor is a major growth promoting agent in human milk, *Science* **210:**198–199.

Carpenter, G., and Cohen, S. 1979, Epidermal growth factor, *Annu. Rev. Biochem.* **48:**193–216.

Ceriani, R.L., Contess, G.P., and Natoz, B.M.S., 1972, Hormone requirement for growth and differentiation of the human mammary gland in organ culture, *Cancer Res.* **32:**2190–2193.

Cevreska, S., Kovacev, V.P., Stankovski, M., and Kalamares, E., 1975, The presence of immunologically reactive insulin in milk of women, during the first week of lactation and its relation to changes in plasma insulin concentration, *God. Zb. Med. Fak. Skopje.* **21:**35–38.

Clemmons, D.R., Underwood, L.E., and Van Wyk, J.J., 1981, Hormonal control of immunoreactive somatomedin production by cultured human fibroblasts, *J. Clin. Invest.* **67:**10–19.

Clifton, K.H., and Furth, J., 1960, Ducto-alveolar growth in mammary glands of adrenogonadectomized male rats bearing mammotropic pituitary tumors, *Endocrinology* **66:**893–897.

Cowie, A.T., 1978, Backward glances, in: *Physiology of Mammary Glands* (A. Yokoyama, H. Mizuno, and H. Nagasawa, eds.), University Park Press, Baltimore, pp. 43–56.

Cowie, A.T., Tindal, J.S., and Yokoyama, A., 1966, The induction of mammary growth in the hypophysectomized goat, *J. Endocrinol.* **34:**185–195.

Del Pozo, E., Hiba, J., Lancranjan, I., and Kunzig, H.J., 1977, Prolactin measurements throughout the life cycle, in: *Prolactin and Human Reproduction* (P.G. Crosignani and C. Robyn, eds.), Academic Press, London, pp. 61–70.

Dembinski, T.C., Leung, C.K.H., and Shiu, R.P.C., 1985, Evidence for a novel pituitary factor that potentiates the mitogenic effect of estrogen in human breast cancer cells, *Cancer Res.* **45:**3083–3089.

D'Ercole, A.J., Applewhite, G.T., and Underwood, L.E., 1980, Evidence that somatomedin is synthesized by multiple tissues in the fetus, *Dev. Biol.* **75:**315–328.

Devinoy, E., Houdebine, L.M., and Delouis, C., 1978, Role of prolactin and glucocorticoids in the expression of casein genes in rabbit mammary gland organ culture, *Biochim. Biophys. Acta* **517:**360–366.

Dickson, R.B., Bates, S.E., McManaway, M., and Lippman, M.E., 1986a, Characterization of estrogen responsive transforming activity in human breast cancer cell lines, *Cancer Res.* **46:**1707–1713.

Dickson, R.B., McManaway, M.E., and Lippman, M.E., 1986b, Estrogen-induced factors of breast cancer cells partially replace estrogen to promote tumor growth, *Science* **232:**1540–1543.

Dickson, R.B., Huff, K.K., Spencer, E.M., and Lippman, M.E., 1986c, Induction of epidermal growth factor-related polypeptides by 17 beta-estradiol in MCF-7 human breast cancer cells, *Endocrinology* **118:**138–142.

Eckert, K., Lubbe, L., Schon, R., and Grosse, R., 1985, Demonstration of transforming growth factor activity in mammary epithelial tissues, *Biochem. Int.* **11:**441–451.

Edery, M., Pang, K., Larson, L., Colosi, T., and Nandi, S., 1985, Epidermal growth factor receptor levels in mouse mammary glands in various physiological states, *Endocrinology* **117:**405–411.

Edwards, D.P., Chamness, G.C., and McGuire, W.L., 1979, Estrogen and progesterone receptor proteins in breast cancer, *Biochim. Biophys. Acta* **560:**457–486.

Errick, J.E., and Kano-Sueoka, T., 1983, *In vitro* model systems for the study of hormonal control of mammary gland growth and differentiation, in: *Lactation—Physiology, Nutrition and Breast-Feeding* (M.C. Neville and M.R. Neifert, eds.), Plenum Press, New York, pp. 179–194.

Evans, M.I., Hager, L.J., and McKnight, G.S., 1981, A somatomedin-like peptide hormone is required during the estrogen-mediated induction of ovalbumin gene transcription, *Cell* **25:**187–193.

Fitzpatrick, S., LaChance, M.P., and Schultz, G.S., 1984, Characterization of epidermal growth factor receptor and action on human breast cancer cells in culture, *Cancer Res.* **44:**3442–3447.

Folley, S.J., and Malpress, F.H., 1948, Hormonal control of lactation, in: *The Hormones,* Vol. 1 (G. Pincus, ed.), Academic Press, New York, pp. 745–805.

Friedberg, S.H., Oka, T., and Topper, Y.J., 1970, Development of insulin-sensitivity by mouse mammary gland *in vitro, Proc. Natl. Acad. Sci. USA* **67:**1493–1500.

Furlanetto, R.W., and DiCarlo, J.N., 1984, Somatomedin-C receptors and growth effects in human breast cells maintained in long-term tissue culture, *Cancer Res.* **44:**2122–2128.

Gospodarowicz, D., 1981, Epidermal and nerve growth factors in mammalian development, *Annu. Rev. Physiol.* **43:**251–263.

Gospodarowicz, D., Cheng, J., Liu, G-M., Baird, A., and Bohlent, P., 1984, Isolation of brain fibroblast growth factor by heparin-Sepharose affinity chromatography: Identity with pituitary fibroblast growth factor, *Proc. Natl. Acad. Sci. USA* **81:**6963–6967.

Halban, J., 1905, Die innere Sekretion von Ovarium und Placenta und ihre Bedeutug fur die Funktion der Milchdruse, *Arch. Gynaekol.* **75:**353–441.

Hammond, S.L., Ham, R.G., and Stampfer, M.R., 1984, Serum-free growth of human mammary epithelial cells: Rapid clonal growth in defined medium and extended serial passage with pituitary extract, *Proc. Natl. Acad. Sci. USA* **81:**5435–5439.

Harness, J.R., and Anderson, R.R., 1975, Effects of relaxin on mammary gland growth and lactation in the rat, *Proc. Soc. Exp. Biol. Med.* **148:**933–936.

Harness, J.R., and Anderson, R.R., 1977, Effects of relaxin in combination with prolactin and ovarian steroids on mammary growth in hypophysectomized rats, *Proc. Soc. Exp. Biol. Med.* **156:**354–358.

Hart, I.C., and Morant, S.V., 1980, Roles of prolactin, growth hormone, insulin and thyroxine in steroid-induced lactation in goats, *J. Endocrinol.* **84:**343–351.

Haselbacher, G.K., Schwab, M.E., Pasi, A., and Humbel, E., 1985, Insulin-like growth factor 2 (IGF-2) in human brain: Regional distribution of IGF-2 and of higher molecular mass forms, *Proc. Natl. Acad. Sci. USA* **82:**2153–2157.

Haslam, S.Z., and Shyamala, G., 1979, Progesterone receptors in normal mammary glands of mice: Characterization and relationship to development, *Endocrinology* **105:**786–795.

Hertz, J., Andersen, A.N., and Larsen, J.F., 1978, Correlation between prolactin and progesterone, oestradiol 17-beta and oestriol during early human pregnancy, *Clin. Endocrinol.* **9:**97–100.

Houdebine, L.M., Djiane, J., Dusanter-Fourt, I., Martel, P., Kelly, P.A., Devinoy, E., and Servely, J.L., 1985, Hormonal action controlling mammary activity, *J. Dairy Sci.* **68:**489–500.

Huseby, R.A., Maloney, T.M., and McGrath, C.M., 1984, Evidence for a direct growth-stimulating effect of estradiol on human MCF-7 cells *in vivo, Cancer Res.* **44:**2654–2659.

Ikeda, T., Liu, Q.F., Danielpour, D., Officer, J.B., Ho, M., Leland, F.E., and Sirbasku, D.A., 1982, Identification of estrogen-inducible growth factors (estromedins) for rat and human mammary tumor cells in culture, *In Vitro* **18:**961–975.

Imai, Y., Leung, C.K.H., Friesen, H.G., and Shiu, R.P.C., 1982, Epidermal growth factor receptors and effect of epidermal growth factor on growth of human breast cancer cells in long-term tissue culture, *Cancer Res.* **42:**4394–4398.

Jacobsohn, D., 1954, Action of estradiol monobenzoate on the mammary glands of hypophysectomized rabbits, *Acta Physiol. Scand.* **32:**304–313.

Juergens, W.F., Stockdale, F.E., Topper, Y.J., and Elias, J.J., 1965, Hormone-dependent differentiation of mammary gland *in vitro, Proc. Natl. Acad. Sci. USA* **54:**629–634.

Kelly, P.A., Tsushima, T., Shiu, R.P.C., and Friesen, H.G., 1976, Lactogenic and growth hormone-like activities in pregnancy determined by radioreceptor assays, *Endocrinology* **99:**765–774.

Kidwell, W.R., Wicha, M.S., Salomon, D.S., and Liotta, L.A., 1980, Hormonal controls of collagen substratum formation by cultured mammary cells: Implications for growth and differentiation, in: *Control Mechanisms in Animal Cells* (L. Jimenez de Asua, R. Levi-Montalcini, R. Shields, and S. Iacobelli, eds.), Raven Press, New York, pp. 333–340.

Klagsbrun, M., 1978, Human milk stimulates DNA synthesis and cellular proliferation in cultured fibroblasts, *Proc. Natl. Acad. Sci. USA* **75:**5057–5061.

Klevjer-Anderson, P., and Buehring, G.C., 1980, Effect of hormones on growth rates of malignant and nonmalignant human mammary epithelia in cell culture, *In Vitro* **16:**491–501.

Koldovsky, O., 1980, Hormones in milk, *Life Sci.* **26:**1833–1836.

Komura, H., Wakimoto, H., Chu-Fung, C., Terakawa, N., Aono, T., Tanizawa, O., and Matsumoto, K., 1986, Retinoic acid enhances cell responses to epidermal growth factor in mouse mammary gland in culture, *Endocrinology* **118:**1530–1536.

Kurachi, H., and Oka, T., 1985, Changes in epidermal growth factor concentrations of submandibular gland, plasma and urine of normal and sialoadenectomized female mice during various reproductive stages, *J. Endocrinol.* **106:**197–202.

Large, D.M., Anderson, D.C., and Laing, I., 1980, Twenty-four hour profiles of serum prolactin during male puberty with and without gynecomastia, *Clin. Endocrinol.* **12:**293–302.

Leclerg, G., and Henson, J.C., 1979, Physiological and pharmacological effects of estrogens in breast cancer, *Biochim. Biophys. Acta* **560:**427–455.

Leung, C.K.H., and Shiu, R.P.C., 1981, Required presence of both estrogen and pituitary factors for the growth of human breast cancer cells in athymic nude mice, *Cancer Res.* **41:**546–551.

Lewko, W.M., Liotta, L.A., Wicha, M.S., Vonderhaar, B.K., and Kidwell, W.R., 1981, Sensitivity of *N*-nitrosomethylurea-induced rat mammary tumors to *cis*-hydroxyproline, an inhibitor of collagen production, *Cancer Res.* **41:**2855–2862.

Lippman, M.E., Osborne, C.K., Knazek, R., and Young, N., 1977, *In vitro* model systems for the study of hormone-dependent human breast cancer, *N. Engl. J. Med.* **296:**154–159.

Lippman, M.E, Dickson, R.B., Kasid, A., Gelmann, E., Davidson, N., McManaway, M., Huff, K., Bronzert, D., Bates, S., Swain, S., and Knabbe, C., 1986a, Autocrine and paracrine growth regulation of human breast cancer, *J. Steroid Biochem.* **24:**147–154.

Lippman, M.E., Dickson, R.B., Gelman, E.P., Kasid, A., Bates, S., Knabbe, C., Swain, S.M., McManaway, M., Wilding, G., Davidson, N., Huff, K., and Bronzert, D., 1986b, Mechanisms of growth regulation of human breast cancer, in: *Advances in Gene Technology: Molecular Biology of the Endocrine System,* Vol. 4 (D. Puett, F. Ahmad, S. Black, D.M. Lopez, M.H. Melner, W.A. Scott, and W.J. Whelan, eds.), Cambridge University Press, New York, pp. 254–257.

Lipsett, M.B., and Bergenstal, D.M., 1960, Lack of effect of human growth hormone and ovine prolactin on cancer in man, *Cancer Res.* **20:**1172–1178.

Lobb, R., Sasse, J., Sullivan, R., Shing, Y., D'Amore, P., Jacobs, J., and Klagsbrun, M., 1986, Purification and characterization of heparin-binding endothelial cell growth factor, *J. Biol. Chem.* **261:**1924–1928.

Lyons, W.R., 1958, Hormonal synergism in mammary growth, *Proc. R. Soc. London Ser. B* **149:**303–325.

Maciag, T., Mehlman, T., Friesel, R., and Shreiber, A.B., 1984, Heparin binds endothelial cell growth factor, the principal endothelial cell mitogen in bovine brain, *Science* **225:**932–935.

Mariorana, A., and Gullino, P.M., 1980, Effect of retinyl acetate on the incidence of mammary carcinomas and hepatomas in mice, *J. Natl. Cancer Inst.* **64:**655–663.

Martel, P., and Houdebine, L.M., 1982, Effect of various drugs affecting cytoskeleton and plasma membranes on the induction of DNA synthesis by insulin, epidermal growth factor and prolactin in mammary explants, *Biol. Cell* **44:**111–118.

McManus, M.J., and Welsch, C.W., 1981, Hormone-induced ductal DNA synthesis of human breast tissues maintained in the athymic nude mouse, *Cancer Res.* **41:**3300–3305.

Mehta, R.G., and Moon, R.C., 1981, Hormonal regulation of retinoic acid-binding proteins in the mammary gland, *Biochem. J.* **200:**591–595.

Mehta, R.G., Cerny, W.L., Ronan, S.S., and Moon, R.C., 1981, Inhibition of prolactin-induced mammary gland differentiation by retinoids *in vitro, Abstr. 445, Proc. Am. Assoc. Cancer Res.* **22:**112.

Meites, J., 1966, Control of mammary growth and lactation, in: *Neuroendocrinology,* Vol. 1 (L. Martin and W.F. Ganong, eds.), Academic Press, New York, pp. 669–701.

Mittra, I., 1980a, A novel "cleaved prolactin" in the rat pituitary: Part I, Biosynthesis, characterization and regulatory control, *Biochem. Biophys. Res. Commun.* **95:**1750–1759.

Mittra, I., 1980b, A novel "cleaved prolactin" in the rat pituitary: Part II, *In vivo* mammary mitogenic activity of its N-terminal 16K moiety, *Biochem. Biophys. Res. Commun.* **95:**1760–1767.

Moon, R.C., Thompson, H.J., Becci, P.J., Grubbs, C.J., Gander, R.J., Newton, D.L., Smith, J.M., Phillips, S.L., Henderson, W.R., Mullen, L.T., Brown, C.C., and Sporn, M., 1979, *N*-(4-Hydroxyphenyl) retinamide, a new retinoid for prevention of breast cancer in the rat, *Cancer Res.* **39:**1339–1346.

Myal, Y., Shiu, R.P.C., Bhaumick, B., and Bala, M., 1984, Receptor binding and growth-promoting activity of insulin-like growth factors in human breast cancer cells (T-47D) in culture, *Cancer Res.* **44:**5486–5490.

Neville, M.C., and Neifert, M.R., 1983, An introduction to lactation and breast-feeding, in: *Lactation—Physiology, Nutrition and Breast-Feeding* (M.C. Neville and M.R. Neifert, eds.), Plenum Press, New York, pp. 3–18.

Nielsen, P.V., Pedersen, H., and Kampmann, E.-M., 1979, Absence of human placental lactogen in an otherwise uneventful pregnancy, *Am. J. Obstet. Gynecol.* **135:**322–326.

Noda, K., Umeda, M., and Ono, T., 1984, Transforming growth factor activity in human colostrum, *Gann* **75:**109–112.

Norgren, A., 1968, Modification of mammary development in rabbits injected with ovarian hormones, *Acta Univ. Lund. Sect. 2* **4:**4–42.

Oka, T., and Yoshimura, M., 1986, Paracrine regulation of mammary gland growth, *Clin. Endocrinol. Metab.* **15:**79–97.

Okamoto, S., and Oka, T., 1984, Evidence for physiological function of epidermal growth factor: Pregestational sialoadenectomy of mice decreases milk production and increases offspring mortality during lactation period, *Proc. Natl. Acad. Sci. USA* **81:**6059–6063.

Pearson, O.H. and Bronson, S.R., 1959, Results of hypophysectomy in the treatment of metastatic mammary carcinoma, *Cancer* **12:**85–92.

Perkins, S.N., Zangger, I., Eberwine, J.H., Barchas, J.D., Jansen, M., Hintz, R., and Hoffman, A.R., 1986, Tissue distribution of insulin-like growth factor I and insulin-like growth factor II messenger RNA, *68th Annual Meeting of the Endocrine Society,* Abstract 252, p. 94.

Peters, J.M., van Marle, J., and Ariens, A.T., 1979, Hormonal effects on rat mammary gland *in vitro, Acta Endocrinol.* **92** (suppl. 228):1–190.

Petrides, P.E, Hosang, M., Shooter, E., Esch, F.S., and Bohlen, P., 1985, Isolation and characterization of epidermal growth factor from human milk, *FEBS Lett.* **187:**89–95.

Prosser, C.G., and Topper, Y.J., 1986, Changes in the rate of carrier-mediated glucose transport by mouse mammary epithelial cells during ontogeny: Hormone dependence delineated *in vitro, Endocrinology* **119:**91–96.

Ptashne, K., Hsueh, H.W., and Stockdale, F.E., 1979, Partial purification and characterization of mammary stimulating factor, a protein which promotes proliferation of mammary epithelium, *Biochemistry* **18:**3533–3539.

Read, L.C., Upton, F.M., Francis, G.L., Wallace, J.C., Dahlenburg, G.W., and Ballard, F.J., 1984, Changes in the growth-promoting activity of human milk during lactation, *Pediatr. Res.* **18:**133–138.

Reece, R.P., and Leonard, S.L., 1941, Effect of estrogens, gonadotropins and growth hormone on mammary glands of hypophysectomized rats, *Endocrinology* **29:**297–305.

Rinderknecht, E., and Humbel, R.E., 1978, Primary structure of human insulin-like growth factor II, *FEBS Lett.* **89:**283–286.

Robyn, C., Delvoye, P., Van Exter, C., Vekemans, M., Caufriez, A., de Nayer, P., Delogne-Desnoeck, J., and L'Hermite M., 1977, Physiological and pharmacological factors influencing prolactin secretion and their relation to human reproduction, in: *Prolactin and Human Reproduction* (P.G. Crosignani and C. Robyn, eds.), Academic Press, London, pp. 17–96.

Rowe, J.M., Kasper, S., Shiu, R.P.C., and Friesen, H.G., 1986, Purification and characterization of a human mammary tumor-derived growth factor, *Cancer Res.* **46:**1408–1412.

Rudland, P.S., Hallowes, P.C., Durbin, H., and Lewis, D., 1977, Mitogenic activity of pituitary hormones on cell cultures of normal and carcinogen-induced tumor epithelium from rat mammary glands, *J. Cell. Biol.* **73:**561–577.

Rudland, P.S., Bennett, D.C., and Warburton, M.J., 1979, Hormonal control of growth and differentiation of cultured rat mammary gland epithelial cells, *Cold Spring Harbor Conf. Cell Proliferation* **6:**677–688.

Salmon, W.D., Jr., and Daughaday, W.H., 1957, A hormonally controlled serum factor which stimulated sulfate incorporation by cartilage *in vitro, J. Lab. Clin. Med.* **49:**825–829.

Salomon, D.S., Liotta, L.A., and Kidwell, W.R., 1981, Differential response to growth factors by rat mammary epithelium plated on different collagen substrata in serum-free medium, *Proc. Natl. Acad. Sci. USA* **78:**382–386.

Salomon, D.S., Zwiebel, J.A., Bano, M., Losonczy, I., Fehnel, P., and Kidwell, W.R., 1984, Presence of transforming growth factors in human breast cancer cells, *Cancer Res.* **44:**4069–4077.

Sani, B.P., and Corbett, T.H., 1977, Retinoic acid-binding protein in normal tissues and experimental tumors, *Cancer Res.* **37:**209–213.

Sankaran, L., and Topper, Y.J., 1982, Effect of vitamin A deprivation on maintenance of rat mammary tissue and on the potential of the epithelium for hormone-dependent milk protein synthesis, *Endocrinology* **111:**1061–1067.

Schreiber, A.B., Winkler, M.E., and Derynck, R., 1986, Transforming growth factor-alpha: A more potent angiogenic mediator than epidermal growth factor, *Science* **232:**1250–1253.

Schwabe, C., Steinetz, B., Weiss, G., Segaloff, A., McDonald, J.K., O'Byrne, E., Hochmann, J., Carriere, B., and Goldsmith, L., 1978, Relaxin, *Recent Prog. Horm. Res.* **34:**123–198.

Shafie, S.M., and Grantham, F.H., 1981, Role of hormones in the growth and regression of human breast cancer cells (MCF-7) transplanted into athymic nude mice, *J. Natl. Cancer Inst.* **67:**51–56.

Shing, Y.W., and Klagsbrun, M., 1984, Human and bovine milk contain different sets of growth factors, *Endocrinology* **115:**273–282.

Shiu, R.P.C., 1981, Prolactin, pituitary hormones and breast cancer, in: *Hormones and Breast Cancer,* Banbury Report 8 (M.C. Pike, P.K. Siiteri, and C.W. Welsch, eds.), Cold Spring Harbor Laboratory, Cold Spring Harbor, NY, pp. 185–196.

Shiu, R.P.C., Lima, G., Leung, C.K.H., and Dembinski, T.C., 1986a, Intrinsic and extrinsic factors in estrogen action in human breast cancer: Role of polamines and pituitary factors, *J. Steroid Biochem.* **24:**133–138.

Shiu, R.P.C., Myal, Y., Leung, C.K.H., Dembinski, T.C., and Iwasiow, B., 1986b, Relationship between a pituitary-derived growth factor for breast cancer and insulin-like growth factor 2 (IGF-2), Institute Scientifique Roussel Symposium on Hormones, Oncogenes and Growth Factors, Paris, June 1986.

Sideri, M., Virgilis, G., Guidobono, F., Borgese, N., Sereni, L.P., Nicolini, U., and Remotti, G., 1983, Immunologically undetectable human placental lactogen in a normal pregnancy. Case Report, *Br. J. Obstet. Gynaecol.* **90:**771–773.

Sinha, S.K., and Yunis, A.A., 1983, Isolation of colony stimulating factor from human milk, *Biochem. Biophys. Res. Commun.* **114:**797–803.

Sirbasku, D.A., 1978, Estrogen induction of growth factors specific for hormone-responsive mammary, pituitary, and kidney tumor cells, *Proc. Natl. Acad. Sci. USA* **75:**3786–3790.

Sirbasku, D.A., and Leland, F.E., 1982, Growth factors for hormone-sensitive tumor cells, in: *Hormonal Regulation of Mammary Tumors,* Vol. II, *Peptide and Other Hormones* (B.S. Leung, ed.), Eden Press, St. Albans, VT, pp. 88–122.

Sirbasku, D.A., Ikeda, T., and Danielpour, D., 1984, Endocrine and autocrine estromedins for mammary and pituitary tumor cells, *Symp. Fundam. Cancer Res.* **37:**213–232.

Smith, J.A., Winslow, D.P., and Rudland, P.S., 1984, Different growth factors stimulate cell division of rat mammary epithelial, myoepithelial and stromal cell lines in culture, *J. Cell. Physiol.* **119:**320–326.

Soule, H.D., and McGrath, C.M., 1980, Estrogen responsive proliferation of clonal human breast carcinoma cells in athymic mide, *Cancer Lett.* **10:**177–189.

Sporn, M.D., and Roberts, A.B., 1985, Autocrine growth factors and cancer, *Nature* **313:**745–747.

Stampfer, M., Hallowes, R.C., and Hackett, A.J., 1980, Growth of normal human mammary cells in culture, *In Vitro* **16:**415–425.

Stoudemire, G.A., Stumpf, W.E., and Sar, M., 1975, Synergism between prolactin and ovarian hormones on DNA synthesis in rat mammary gland, *Proc. Soc. Exp. Biol. Med.* **149:**189–192.

Sultan, C., Descomps, B., Garandeau, P., Bressot, N., and Jean, R., 1979, Pubertal gynecomastia due to an estrogen-producing adrenal tumor, *J. Pediatr.* **95:**744–746.

Taketani, Y., and Oka, T., 1983a, Possible physiological role of epidermal growth factor in the development of the mouse mammary gland during pregnancy, *FEBS Lett.* **152:**256–260.

Taketani, Y., and Oka, T., 1983b, Epidermal growth factor stimulates cell proliferation and inhibits functional differentiation of mouse mammary epithelial cells in culture, *Endocrinology* **113:**871–877.

Taketani, Y., and Oka, T., 1983c, The functional receptors of epidermal growth factor in normal mammary epithelial cells, *Proc. Natl. Acad. Sci. USA* **80:**2647–2650.

Talwalker, P.K., and Meites, J., 1961, Mammary lobulo-alveolar growth induced by anterior pituitary hormones in adreno-ovariectomized-hypophysectomized rats, *Proc. Soc. Exp. Biol. Med.* **107:**880–883.

Todaro, G.J., Fryling, C., and DeLarco, J.E., 1980, Transforming growth factors produced by certain human tumor cells: Polypeptides that interact with epidermal growth factor receptors, *Proc. Natl. Acad. Sci. USA* **77:**5258–5262.

Tonelli, Q.J., and Sorof, S., 1980, Epidermal growth factor requirement for development of cultured mammary gland, *Nature* **285:**250–252.

Topper, Y.J., and Freeman, C.S., 1980, Multiple hormone interactions in the developmental biology of the mammary gland, *Physiol. Rev.* **60:**1049–1106.

Traurig, H.H., 1967, Cell proliferation in the mammary gland during late pregnancy and lactation, *Anat. Rec.* **157:**489–504.

Traurig, H.H., and Morgan, C.F., 1964, The effect of ovarian and hypophyseal hormones on mammary gland epithelial cell proliferation, *Anat. Rec.* **150:**423–434.

Turkington, R.W., 1969, The role of epidermal growth factor in mammary gland development *in vitro, Exp. Cell. Res.* **57:**79–85.

Turkington, R.W., and Topper, Y.J., 1966, Stimulation of casein synthesis and histological development of mammary gland by human placental lactogen *in vitro, Endocrinology* **79:**175–181.

Turner, C.W., 1939, The mammary glands, in: *Sex and Internal Secretions,* 2nd ed. (E. Allen, ed.), Williams and Wilkins, Baltimore, pp. 740–803.

Underwood, B.A., 1984, Vitamin A in animal and human nutrition, in: *The Retinoids,* Vol. 1 (M.B. Sporn, A.B. Roberts, and D.S. Goodman, eds.), Academic Press, New York, pp. 281–294.

Van Wyk, J.J., Underwood, L.E., Baseman, J.B., Hintz, R.L., Clemmons, D.R., and Marshall, R.N., 1975, Explorations of the insulin-like and growth promoting properties of somatomedin by membrane assays, *Adv. Metab. Disord.* **8:**127–150.

Vignon, F., Capony, F., Chambon, M., Freiss, G., Garcia, M., and Rochefort, H., 1986, Autocrine growth stimulation of the MCF-7 breast cancer cells by the estrogen-regulated 52K protein, *Endocrinology* **118:**1537–1545.

Vonderhaar, B.K., and Nakhasi, H.L., 1986, Bifunctional activity of epidermal growth factor on α- and κ-casein gene expression in rodent mammary glands *in vitro, Endocrinology* **119:**1178–1184.

Welsch, C.W., Swim, E.L., McMagnus, M.J., White, A.C., and McGrath, C.M., 1981, Estrogen induced growth of human breast cancer cells (MCF-7) in athymic nude mice is enhanced by secretions from a transplantable pituitary tumor, *Cancer Lett.* **14:**309–316.

Wicha, M.S., Liotta, L.A., Garbisa, S., and Kidwell, W.R., 1979, Basement membrane collagen requirements for attachment and growth of mammary epithelium, *Exp. Cell. Res.* **124:**181–190.

Wicha, M.S., Liotta, L.A., Vonderhaar, B.K., and Kidwell, W.R., 1980, Effects of inhibition of basement membrane collagen deposition on rat mammary gland development, *Dev. Biol.* **80:**253–266.

Wright, L.C., and Anderson, R.R., 1983, Effect of relaxin on mammary growth in the hypophysectomized rat, in: *Relaxin* (R.R. Anderson, ed.), Plenum Press, New York, pp. 341–355.

Yang, J., Guzman, R., Richards, J., Imagawa, W., McCormick, K., and Nandi, S., 1980, Growth factor and cyclic-nucleotide induced proliferation of normal and malignant mammary epithelial cells in primary culture, *Endocrinology* **107:**35–41.

Zwiebel, J.A., Davis, M.R., Kohn, E., Salomon, D.S., and Kidwell, W.R., 1982, Anchorage-independent growth-conferring factor production by rat mammary tumor cells, *Cancer Res.* **42:**5117–5125.

Zwiebel, J.A., Bano, M., Nexo, E., Salomon, D.S., and Kidwell, W.R., 1986, Partial purification of transforming growth factors from human milk, *Cancer Res.* **46:**933–939.

12

Prolactin

Transport, Function, and Receptors in Mammary Gland Development and Differentiation

Barbara Kay Vonderhaar

1. Introduction

While no single hormone or growth factor can be said to be the "controlling" or the "most important" in growth, development, and differentiation of the mammary gland, it is abundantly clear that prolactin plays a key and pivotal role in these processes. This conclusion is drawn from the cumulative research efforts of many scientists using a variety of techniques to examine this hormone's actions both in vivo and in vitro under a variety of culture conditions. Since the mammary gland is acted on by many hormones and growth factors, it is not possible to isolate prolactin action from other multiple hormonal events. Hormonal manipulations in vivo may alter direct actions of prolactin on the mammary gland but also can greatly influence synthesis, processing, and secretion of the hormone itself. While studies in vitro may appear less complex, the endogenous hormones introduced by the tissue in primary culture, the hormonal components of serum if this is used with the culture medium, and the effects that other exogenously added hormones have on the sensitivity of the tissue to prolactin are all of concern. In addition, the

Barbara Kay Vonderhaar • Laboratory of Tumor Immunology and Biology, National Cancer Institute, National Institutes of Health, Bethesda, Maryland 20892.

well-known facts of species and even strain differences make generalization concerning prolactin action difficult. This is further complicated by the fact that prolactin itself varies with the source and exists in several forms [e.g., dimers (Meuris et al., 1983), glycosylated versus nonglycosylated (Lewis et al., 1984), isoelectric point variants (Cheng et al., 1981; Nyberg et al., 1982)] and sizes [e.g., big-big, big, monomer (von Werder and Clemm, 1974; Frantz, 1977; Cheng et al., 1981; Nyberg et al., 1982; Meuris et al., 1983), cleaved (Sinha and Baxter, 1979; Mittra, 1984)]. Which of these is biologically active or relevant for the physiological response under study is not clear. The biological versus immunological activities of the various prolactins have been compared in recent studies where it was found that the two assays do not always give comparable results (Leung et al., 1978; Sinha and Baxter, 1979; Talamantes et al., 1984; Subramanian and Gala, 1986). Despite all this, certain basic observations concerning prolactin's function and mode of action in mammary gland biology can be emphasized.

2. Prolactin Gene Family

2.1. Structure

Prolactin is an ancient hormone (Wallis, 1981, 1984; Nicoll, 1982), one of a group of related peptide hormones within a multigene family (Moore et al., 1982). Using the human species as an example, at least eight members of the family have been identified (Wallis, 1981; Moore et al., 1982; Linzer et al., 1985). These are human growth hormone (hGH), human placental lactogen (hPL), prolactin, and several variants (both hGH-like and hPL-like) that show high homology with hGH at the gene level (Moore et al., 1982). If the sequences of growth hormone and prolactin from any one mammalian species are aligned, they are identical at about 25% of all amino acids (Bewley et al., 1972; Wallis, 1984). Moreover, many of the differing amino acids reflect conservative replacements. At the level of protein sequences, hGH is 85% homologous with hPL (Niall et al., 1971; Wallis, 1975). In addition, the members of the prolactin gene family have two or three similarly positioned disulfide bonds, reflecting very similar secondary structures (see Fig. 1) (Li, 1980; Colosi et al., 1982; Kohmoto et al., 1984).

Several laboratories have used cDNA clones to show that the mRNA sequences of hGH and hPL are very similar; the two cDNA clones are 92% homologous and completely cross-hybridize with one another under all but the most stringent conditions (Shine et al., 1977; Martial et al.,

1979). hGH, in fact, appears structurally much more similar to hPL and to human prolactin than it is to nonprimate growth hormones (Niall et al., 1971).

Pituitary prolactin and related peptides predominantly exist as 22–25-kDa monomeric proteins. In addition to the 22-kDa monomer, hGH also exists as a 20-kDa single-chained variant peptide first described by Lewis et al. (1979, 1980) and believed to arise from an internal deletion at the position of the second intervening sequence of the growth hormone mRNA (Wallis, 1980). Thus, this 20-kDa form differs from the normal 22-kDa monomer only by the internal deletion of 15 amino acids. This variant makes up 10–15% of the hGH in the normal human pituitary (Lewis et al., 1980). The 20-kDa variant retains full growth-promoting activity in the human, as well as full lactogenic activity (Lewis et al., 1980; Sigel et al., 1981; Hughes et al., 1985). A similar small form has not been definitively identified for any nonprimate growth hormones or for prolactins.

Rat prolactin, however, has been reported to exist as a two-chained enzymatically cleaved form (Mittra, 1980a,b, 1984). Using pituitary glands from animals in various physiological states, it was found that the range of cleavage was precisely regulated and specific for prolactin since growth hormone secreted by the same pituitaries was not cleaved (Mittra, 1980a). The two chains of molecular weight 16 and 8 kDa could be separated after S–S reduction. The 16-kDa N-terminal fragment increased DNA synthesis and cell division in the rat mammary gland in vivo, while the native 22-kDa monomer, similarly injected, was inactive (Mittra, 1980b). Similarly, experimental proteolysis of both hGH and hPL, using a variety of enzymes, has resulted in fragments of these hormones, some of which retain full biological activity and others of which acquire enhanced bioactivity in a mammary differentiation assay (Yadley and Chrambach, 1973; Singh et al., 1974; Lewis et al., 1975, 1977; Russell et al., 1979). A 16-kDa form of human prolactin has been identified in crude human pituitary homogenates (Meuris et al., 1983). In addition to the existence of possibly biologically relevant fragments of the lactogenic hormones, both hGH and prolactin from several species have been reported to exist in the circulation in forms larger than the monomer (von Werder and Clemm, 1974; Frantz, 1977; Meuris et al., 1983). The physiological significance of any of these cleaved forms, as well as of the other size and charge variants, is not yet clear.

The newest putative member of the prolactin growth hormone family, that is, the 25-kDa glycosylated protein *proliferin,* which is found in mouse placenta and is immunologically distinct from mouse placental lactogen (Linzer et al., 1985; Nathans et al., 1986), has not yet been

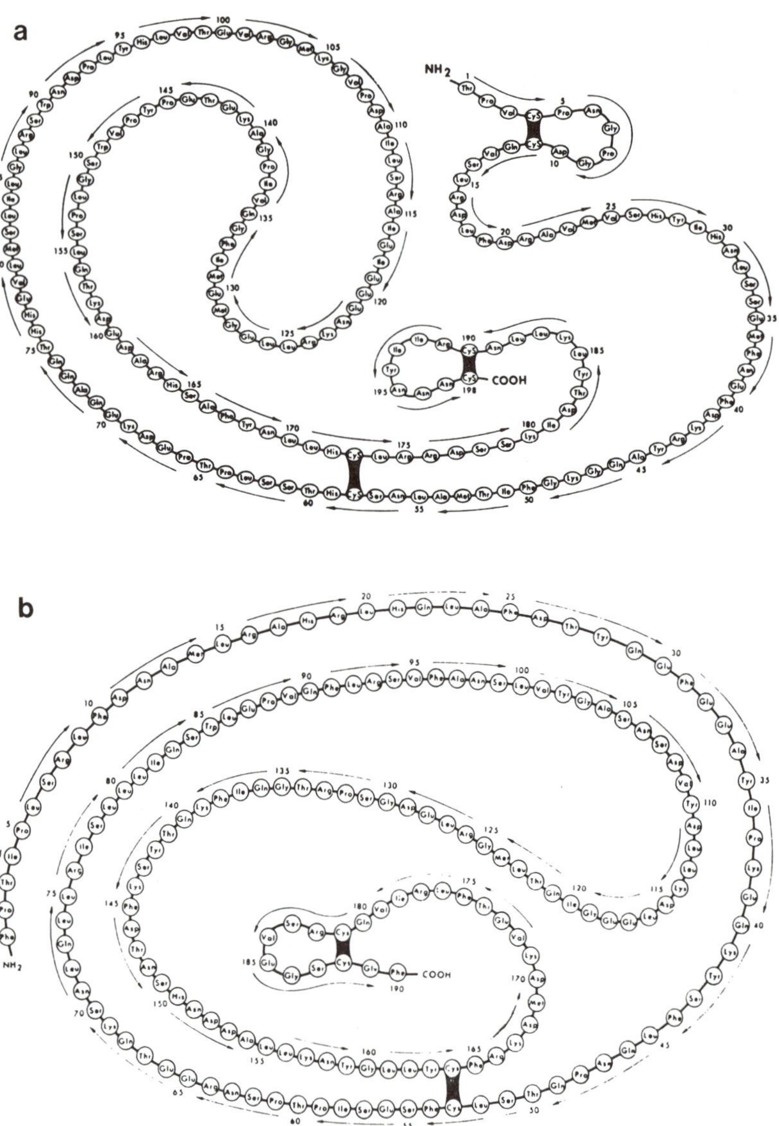

Figure 1. Amino acid sequence of (a) ovine prolactin, (b) human growth hormone, and (c) human placental lactogen. From Li (1972).

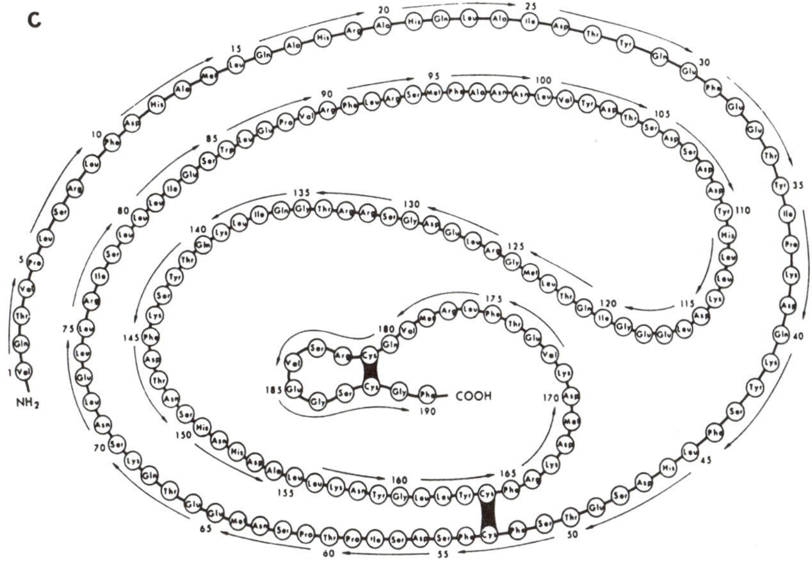

Figure 1. *(Continued)*

found to possess biological activity similar to that of prolactin in the mammary gland or any other lactogen-responsive system. However, its gene is structurally similar to that of prolactin and has 55% nucleotide sequence homology with bovine prolactin (Linzer and Nathans, 1984). The amino acid sequence homology between mouse proliferin and bovine or mouse prolactin is 46 and 32%, respectively (Linzer and Nathans, 1984; Kohmoto et al., 1984); bovine growth hormone and bovine prolactin have only 37% amino acid homology.

All other members of the prolactin hormone family in their native monomeric form that have been tested can function within the mammary gland system in vitro to promote development and differentiation (Forsyth, 1969; Rivera, 1969; Doneen, 1976; Leung et al., 1978; Talamantes et al., 1984). However, the biological potency of the various lactogens may vary with the species of origin for the hormone and/or the mammary tissue. Each active hormone is believed to function through the same receptor system, that is, the lactogenic hormone receptor. However, the possible existence of variants of the receptor, like those of the hormone, and their relation to biological response represent an area only now coming under investigation.

2.2. Control of Secretion

2.2.1. Diurnal Rhythm and Hormones

Secretion of prolactin is controlled by a variety of physiological (Amenomori et al., 1970; Morishige et al., 1973; Murr et al., 1974; Frantz, 1977; Barkley, 1979; Parkening et al., 1980; Michael et al., 1980), neuroendocrinological (Gluckman et al., 1981), and hormonal factors (Chen and Meites, 1970; Boot et al., 1973; Michael, 1976; Jacques and Gala, 1979; Blank et al., 1986), as well as aspects of life-style such as beer consumption (Carlson et al., 1985) and exercise (DeMeirleir et al., 1985). Manipulation of any of these regulatory systems can profoundly affect the subsequent response to prolactin by the mammary glands either in vivo or in vitro in primary culture. In humans, prolactin secretion is higher in women with normal functioning ovaries than in men (Frantz, 1977). Similar results have been reported in rodents (Barkley, 1979; Michael et al., 1980). Secretion of prolactin is subject to diurnal variation; during sleep, there is a rise in serum prolactin concentration (Sassin et al., 1972; Frantz, 1978). Prolactin secretion is regulated in vivo by a negative influence of dopamine, which reaches the pituitary in portal venous blood (Frantz, 1977). Separate prolactin release-inhibiting factor (PIF) and prolactin-releasing factors have also been proposed as regulators of the hormone's secretion (Nicoll et al., 1970; Valverde et al., 1972; Lu and Meites, 1973).

Recent work from Seeburg's laboratory showed that the carboxy-terminus of human placental gonadotropin-releasing hormone percursor, termed GAP for gonadotropin-releasing hormone-associated peptide, inhibited prolactin secretion in primary cultures of anterior pituitary cells, thus clearly establishing the existence of PIF (Nikolics et al., 1985). A polyclonal antibody raised against a synthetic polypeptide comprised of 14 internal amino acids of the 10-kDa GAP protein also recognized a substance in secretory granules of nerve terminals in the rat median eminence (Phillips et al., 1985). Cloned hypothalamic cDNAs for the GAP protein of humans and rats display 70% nucleotide sequence homology, and the 56-amino-acid-long PIF peptides from humans and rats have 17 substitutions, half of which are conservative (Adelman et al., 1986).

Thyrotropin-releasing hormone (TRH), given by injection, is a potent stimulator of prolactin secretion in both males and females (Bowers et al., 1971; Jacobs et al., 1971; Noel et al., 1974a; Frantz, 1977), but it is not known whether TRH in portal venous blood is physiologically important in modifying prolactin secretion. Hypothyroidism may increase circulating prolactin levels by altering the levels of TRH (Frantz, 1977).

2.2.2. *Estrous (Menstrual) Cycle*

Using rodent models, fluctuations in serum prolactin have been evaluated throughout the estrous cycle. Prolactin levels, determined by both radioimmunoassay and bioassay (Michael, 1976; Blank et al., 1986), peak in rats and mice on the afternoon of proestrus. A similar rise at midcycle and during the luteal phase has been reported in the human menstrual cycle (Vekemans et al., 1972). This fluctuation in prolactin secretion may be due in part to the actions of the female sex hormones estradiol and progesterone which also vary with the cycle. Estrogens cause hyperplasia and probably hypertrophy of the pituitary lactotrope cells and stimulate prolactin synthesis and secretion (Jacobs, 1977; Peillon et al., 1983). This effect is dependent on both the dose and the duration of exposure to the estrogens. Using ovariectomized rats, Chen and Meites (1970) showed that daily injections of estradiol benzoate resulted in increases in serum prolactin levels from two- to 10-fold. Daily injections of progesterone alone were without effect. However, when given simultaneously with estradiol, progesterone markedly counteracted its stimulatory action.

2.2.3. *Pregnancy and Lactation*

In addition to changes in prolactin secretion that occur during the estrous or menstrual cycle and the diurnal variations during the day, circulating prolactin, but not growth hormone, is increased by pregnancy [usually after the appearance of placental lactogen (Friesen et al., 1972; Li, 1980)], nursing, and breast stimulation (Amenomori et al., 1970; Morishige et al., 1973; Murr et al., 1974; Frantz, 1977). During pregnancy in the monkey, estradiol-17β levels increase two- to fourfold, followed by a similar small increase in prolactin (Friesen et al., 1972). In the human, estradiol increases several hundred-fold, while circulating prolactin levels increase 10- to 20-fold (Hwang et al., 1971; Jacobs et al., 1972). Negative feedback by prolactin on its own secretion occurs in animals (Boot et al., 1973).

3. Prolactin Uptake and Processing

3.1. Internalization and Transport into Milk

Radioimmunodetectable as well as bioactive (Gala et al., 1980) pituitary prolactin is abundant in the milk of several species, including humans (Gala et al., 1975; Jacobs, 1977), sheep (Erb et al., 1977), pigs (Mulloy and Malven, 1979), rats (McMurtry and Malven, 1974a), goats

(McMurtry and Malven, 1974b), and cows (Malven and McMurtry, 1974; Malven, 1983; Pennington and Malven, 1985). The concentration approximates that in blood plasma, and in some cases, such as immediately before parturition in the cow, the concentration greatly exceeds that in blood (Malven, 1983). Prepartum removal of the milk with the prolactin it contains does not result in a decrease in the prolactin content of the mammary alveoli (Pennington and Malven, 1985). In fact, more prolactin is subsequently transferred into the alveolar cells and the milk to replace that which is removed by milking. Malven (1983) has proposed that this trafficking of the prolactin through the gland to the milk may provide a physiological advantage to the animal. Hence, prepartum milking frequently induces premature lactogenesis with total cumulative prolactin transferred from blood into mammary secretions greatly exceeding the amounts found with control animals (Pennington and Malven, 1985). Depletion of pituitary and serum prolactin by treatment of the animals with ergot drugs does not significantly deplete subsequent prolactin levels in milk (Malven, 1983). Thus, when blood-borne prolactin is inadequate to initiate or sustain lactogenesis, intramammary transfer of prolactin may confer lactational benefits.

Since it is generally accepted that this hormone is not synthesized by the mammary gland to any great extent, its appearance in the secretion product of the gland must be accounted for by some physiological mechanism. It is not clear whether the hormone arrives in the milk via intracellular, paracellular, or intercellular transfer or by a combination of the above (Malven and Keenan, 1983). That at least part of the milk-borne prolactin results from the intracellular route and the association with specific hormone receptors (to be discussed later in the chapter) is supported by the work from several laboratories that examined localization of endogenous prolactin within the alveolar cells. Malven and Keenan (1983) fractionated lactating bovine mammary tissue into subcellular compartments and examined each for prolactin content by radioimmunoassay. Immunoreactive prolactin was found in rough endoplasmic reticulum, Golgi apparatus, and secretory vesicles in concentrations ranging from 10 to 25 ng/mg protein. These values exceed that of milk (about 3 ng/mg protein).

3.2. Localization within the Gland

The above findings are consistent with the immunocytochemical studies of Nolin and co-workers (Nolin and Witorsch, 1976; Nolin, 1979) using lactating rat mammary tissue and of Purnell et al. (1982) and Marchetti et al. (1984) using normal human breast and human breast cancer specimens, respectively. In addition to the localized staining on the plasma membranes believed to be the initial hormone-receptor interaction site (Marchetti et al., 1984), immunologically detectable prolactin was localized to the nuclei and the cytoplasm, suggesting intracellular uptake of the hormone (Nolin and Witorsch, 1976). Nolin (1979) also reported that the more lactationally active alveolar cells in the rat mammary gland contained more intracellular prolactin, especially in the nuclei. Resting milk secretory cells lining fully distended alveoli, which are present at the end of the lactational cycle, did not contain prolactin, even though this hormone was present in the milk in the lumen. When the milk was removed, the resting cells reentered an active phase of the lactational cycle, progressed from tall columnar to cuboidal cells, and accumulated immunoreactive intracellular prolactin. The correlation of cyclic prolactin incorporation into the cells and the cycle of lactational activity might suggest a function for the intracellular hormone. However, whether or not the intracellular prolactin is physiologically important is not clear at this time. Likewise, whether the uptake of the hormone is through a receptor-mediated endocytosis pathway followed by an intracellular delivery to subcellular components by receptosomes (Pastan and Willingham, 1981) and whether the prolactin remains associated with the receptor or a portion of the receptor remain to be established.

3.3. Processing

In addition, what proportion of the intracellular prolactin is ultimately transferred to the milk is not known. It is clear, however, that not all the prolactin taken up by the cells is secreted intact and biologically active (Gala et al., 1980) into the milk. Using human breast cells (Shiu, 1980) and rat livers (Basset et al., 1984), processing of internalized prolactin by target tissues has been examined. Shiu (1980) found that the human cells, whether "normal" or cancerous, degraded from 15 to 40% of the biologically active exogenously added hormone depending on the cell line used. The prolactin was degraded to at least three small molecular weight peptides that were subsequently secreted by the cells. These peptides were biologically inactive in that they did not bind to cellular receptors, and they also were no longer recognized by antiprolactin antibodies. Based on studies using a variety of protease inhibitors and lysosomotropic agents, he concluded that the prolactin was degraded by an energy-dependent internalization process such as pinocytosis and that degradation probably took place in the lysosomes. In similar studies with liver, Basset et al. (1984) concluded that prolactin internalized to the lysosomes was extensively degraded, whereas that associated with low-density membranes such as the Golgi and endoplasmic reticulum remains intact. In the mammary gland, whether this trafficking of prolactin into the cell, followed by degradation or secretion into the milk, may result in physiologically significant events beneficial to the growth, development, and differentiation of the gland remains to be clarified. At present, the postreceptor event(s) responsible for prolactin's action in mammary tissue, as well as any other target tissue, is unclear.

4. Prolactin Function

4.1. Growth and Lobuloalveolar Development

As a result of its interaction with, and possibly internalization by, the mammary gland, prolactin along with other hormones and growth factors exerts a variety of physiological effects. One of its first and most fundamental actions is at the level of growth and maintenance of the morphology of the gland. In general, ductal growth and branching are controlled by the ovarian steroids estrogen and progesterone (Nandi, 1958; Vonderhaar, 1984). Lobuloalveolar development and extensive growth of the alveolar epithelial cells during pregnancy require prolactin. Cyclic growth of the mature gland during the estrous or menstrual cycle may require prolactin to maintain responsiveness to estrogen and progesterone. In this case, prolactin itself may not serve as a mitogen but only function in a permissive role (Tucker, 1981).

Early work of Lyons and co-workers (Lyons, 1958; Lyons et al., 1952, 1958), later confirmed by Talwalker and Meites (1961), using doubly (hypophysectomized–ovariectomized) and triply (hypophysectomized–ovariectomized–adrenalectomized) operated rats, demonstrated that the only minimal combination of hormones that produced lobuloalveolar growth was estrogen plus progesterone plus prolactin. The extent of development with these three hormones, however, was only equivalent to that seen in early pregnancy (i.e., small lobules). When growth hormone was also given along with the three hormones, full lobuloalveolar development, equivalent to that of late pregnancy, was obtained. However, growth hormone did not substitute for prolactin in that no lobuloalveolar growth occurred with estrogen plus progesterone plus growth hormone. In these surgically ablated animals, prolactin itself or in any combination that did not also include the ovarian steroids did not promote glandular development.

That the effects of the various hormones were direct was strongly supported by studies from these same researchers (Lyons et al., 1958) using pellets of hormonal combinations implanted directly on the mammary glands of hypophysectomized female rats. Again, the minimal hormonal combination for lobuloalveolar development was estrogen plus progesterone plus prolactin. The effects were direct in that only those portions of the gland immediately adjacent to the pellet showed development, while distal portions of the same gland and the contralateral glands remained undeveloped.

Similar observations on the role of prolactin in lobuloalveolar development in the mouse have shown that mature virgin C3H mice that are either ovariectomized or hypophysectomized completely lose their alveoli, whereas adrenalectomy causes little decrease in alveolar content. In addition, full development in triply operated mice required estrogen plus progesterone plus either growth hormone or prolactin (Nandi, 1958). Figure 2 shows that, in ovariectomized C3H mature virgin mice, alveolar buds are absent (Fig. 2a). When prolactin is administered (2 mg/day for 1 week) along with estrogen and progesterone, extensive lobuloalveolar development occurs (Fig. 2b), resulting in a gland that is morphologically similar to that from a midpregnant animal (Vonderhaar, 1984). Prolactin administration alone has little or no effect on lobuloalveolar development in these animals (Fig. 2c). Nagasawa and coworkers (1985) showed that pituitary isografts in mature virgin SHN mice stimulated mammary gland growth and end bud formation in endocrinologically intact, but not ovariectomized, animals. Progesterone pellet implantation alone in ovariectomized mice was without effect, but when done in combination with the pituitary isograft, full restoration of mammary growth was achieved. These data suggested that prolactin's effect on mammary development is both direct and indirect through its luteotropic action (i.e., through its stimulation of ovarian progesterone secretion). During pregnancy, however, hypophysectomy does not affect mammary cell number or lobuloalveolar development, suggesting that the structurally similar placental lactogen is an important lactogen at this time. Indeed, injection of saline extracts of rat placenta into doubly operated rats stimulated lobuloalveolar development considerably (Ray et al., 1955).

In ruminants, Cowie and Tindal (1971) have shown that prolactin is necessary for udder growth and for the initiation of lactation. In doubly operated goats, estrogen, progesterone, prolactin, growth hormone, and adrenocorticotrophin are required in combination to induce lobuloalveolar development similar to that of midpregnancy. After milk secretion is established, it appears that growth hormone is essential for maintaining lactation, and prolactin is relatively less important.

The role played by prolactin in human mammogenesis remains

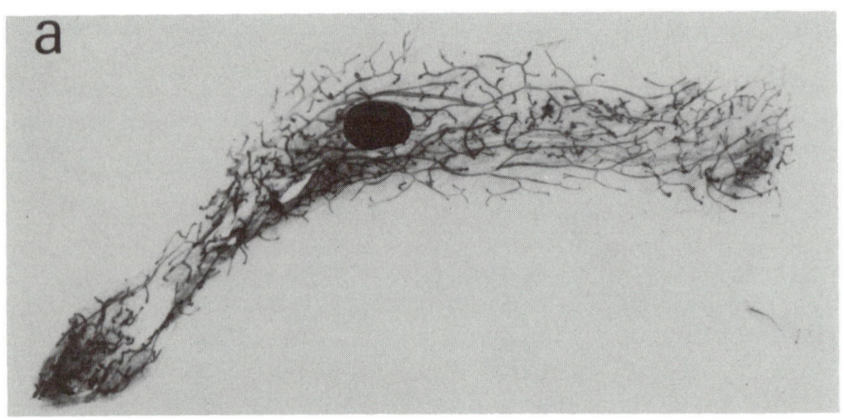
a

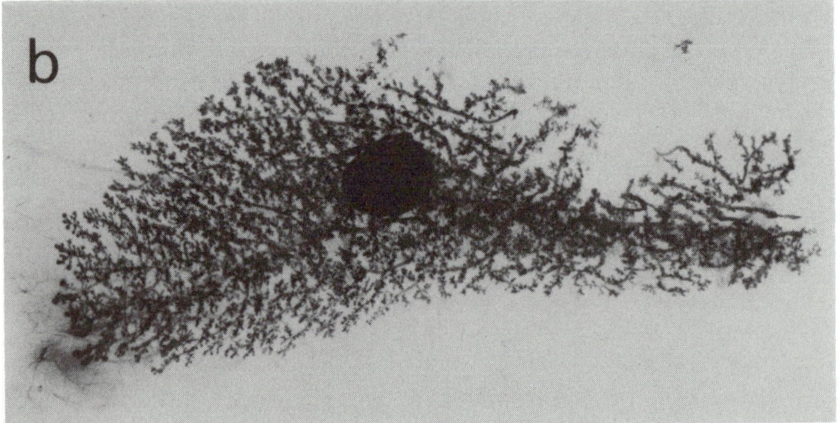
b

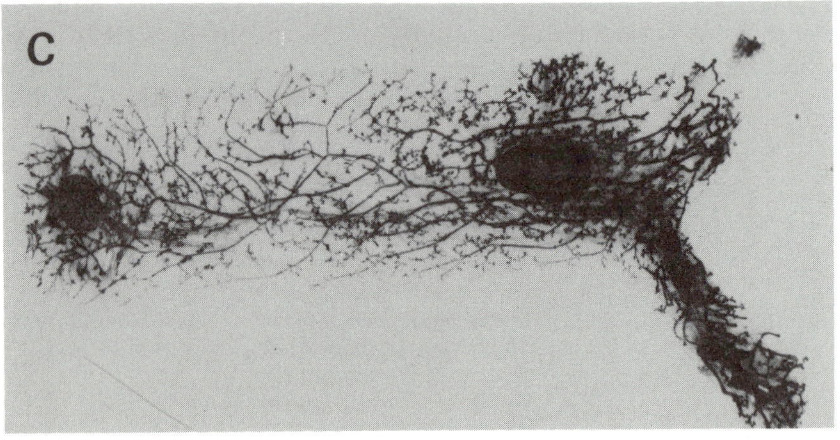
c

unclear. Levels of circulating prolactin in adult women are only slightly higher than those in similarly aged men, while measurements in prepubertal children generally are similar to those in men and are not different for boys and girls (Foley et al., 1972; Friesen et al., 1972). The rise of both estrogen and prolactin during puberty in females is gradual (Friesen et al., 1972; Ehara et al., 1975), while the majority of breast growth in girls occurs relatively early in puberty. Jacobs (1977) suggested that certain minimal levels of prolactin are required in a permissive way for breast development to occur under the influence of the sex steroids.

The growth and development of the human breast during pregnancy can be attributed to combined effects of elevated levels of estrogen, progesterone, and prolactin. In late pregnancy, estrogen and progesterone levels are several hundred-fold higher than in the follicular phase of the menstrual cycle. Circulating hPL is as high as 10–12 μg/ml, while circulating levels of pituitary prolactin are about 20 times higher than nonpregnancy levels (i.e., about 200 ng/ml average at term) (Jacobs, 1977). A physiological role for placental lactogen in mammary development has not been established. While hPL can elicit differentiative effects on breast tissue in vitro (Turkington and Topper, 1966; Vonderhaar and Topper, 1974), many species lack placental lactogen during pregnancy (Kelly et al., 1976). In addition, women who do not synthesize immunoreactive placental lactogen can have normal term pregnancies with normal breast function (Nielsen et al., 1979; Sideri et al., 1983).

Several laboratories have attempted to confirm and clarify the role of lactogenic hormones in mammary gland growth using a variety of in vitro techniques. Using in vivo–ex vivo studies, Welsch et al. (1979b) implanted mammary tissue from midpregnant cows subcutaneously in the backs of female athymic nude mice. After treating the mice with various hormonal combinations, the tissue slices were removed and incubated for 4 h with [^{3}H]thymidine to determine the thymidine labeling index (TLI), a measure of DNA synthesis. The most effective combination of hormones was growth hormone plus prolactin plus estrogen plus progesterone, which resulted in a nearly fourfold increase in TLI over control (no hormones) and a twofold increase over estrogen plus progesterone alone.

Similarly, rabbit mammary tissue from pseudopregnant animals

***

Figure 2. Whole mounts of mammary glands of 4-month-old female virgin mice: (a) ovariectomized; (b) ovariectomized, treated with prolactin plus estrogen plus progesterone; and (c) ovariectomized, treated with prolactin only. All hormone supplements were begun 1 week after ovariectomy.

showed an increase in TLI and mitotic index within 6 h after intraductal injection of prolactin (Bourne et al., 1974). Mammary epithelial cells from midpregnant rabbits prepared by collagenase digestion of the tissue and cultured for up to 6 days on floating collagen gels required insulin, hydrocortisone, prolactin, estrogen, and progesterone for optimal DNA synthesis. When the cells were grown on extracellular matrix from the same rabbit mammary tissue, optimal DNA synthesis required only insulin, hydrocortisone, and prolactin, with estrogen and progesterone having an inhibitory effect (Wilde et al., 1984).

Human breast tissue from the periphery of excised benign tumors was transplanted into nude mice and examined for response to mitogenic stimuli. Ductal epithelium in the transplanted specimens responded maximally to a combination of exogenously administered estrogen and hPL with enhanced DNA synthesis in situ (McManus et al., 1978; McManus and Welsch, 1981) and with an increase in TLI ex vivo (McManus and Welsch, 1984). A similar increase of TLI was obtained using benign human breast tumor slices cultured with human prolactin (Welsch et al., 1979a).

Normal epithelial cells isolated from human breast and placed in primary culture are stimulated to grow by combinations of estrogen, human prolactin, and human growth hormone (Klevjer-Anderson and Buehring, 1980) and insulin, aldosterone, hydrocortisone, and hPL (Yang et al., 1980b). Multiple serial passages of human mammary epithelial cells in serum-free conditions require the presence of bovine pituitary extract. Replacement of the extract with prostaglandin E_1 and ovine prolactin yields a defined medium that allows for up to four serial passages (Hammond et al., 1984). Primary and secondary cultures of epithelial cells from rat mammary tissues grown on plastic require prolactin for stimulation of DNA synthesis. Cultures of epithelial cells derived from tumors responded to prolactin alone while normal breast tissue required insulin and hydrocortisone in addition to prolactin for maximal DNA synthesis and cell growth (Rudland et al., 1977).

Mammary tissues in organ culture exhibit diurnal changes in TLI patterns which reflect the diurnal variations in circulating prolactin levels (Borst and Mahoney, 1980). Monodisperse suspensions of midpregnancy mouse mammary epithelial cells prepared by collagenase plus hyaluronidase and pronase digestion, grown in monolayers on tissue culture plastic, responded to prolactin (200 ng/ml) with a three- to fourfold increase in thymidine incorporation compared with control cultures lacking hormones. Addition of estradiol (1 ng/ml) and progesterone (1 μg/ml) to the culture medium enhanced prolactin's effect and resulted in DNA synthesis five- to sixfold over control levels (Ceriani and Blank,

1977). When enzymatically dissociated midpregnancy mammary epithelial cells were grown inside collagen gels, the cell number increased three- to fivefold after 6–8 days in the presence of 3% porcine serum, insulin, hydrocortisone, transferrin, epidermal growth factor, and prolactin (Flynn et al., 1982). When this culture system was further defined (Imagawa et al., 1985) in terms of hormonal requirements, a two- to fourfold increase in cell growth was obtained in cells from mature virgin mice grown in the presence of ovine prolactin (1 μg/ml). The cells responded to progesterone (10^{-6}–10^{-8} M) with a similar increase, while together, prolactin and progesterone gave as much as a 17-fold increase in cell number. This work directly confirms the observations in vivo of Nagasawa et al. (1985).

The essential role of prolactin in lobuloalveolar development has been confirmed in vitro by culturing the whole organ in a chemically defined hormonally supplemented medium using the technique originally developed by Ichinose and Nandi (1964, 1966) and refined by Banerjee and colleagues (1973). This method, which has been described extensively elsewhere (Wood et al., 1975; Banerjee et al., 1976; Vonderhaar, 1984), uses the whole second thoracic gland of 3–4-week old immature BALB/c female mice primed with a mixture of estradiol and progesterone for 9 days. The priming with steroids in vivo is essential for subsequent lobuloalveolar development in vitro; as yet, no hormonal combination in culture that promotes full development of the glands from unprimed mice (Vonderhaar, 1984) has been identified. The glands from primed mice undergo a single round of lobuloalveolar development in serum-free medium under the influence of a combination of insulin, aldosterone, hydrocortisone, and prolactin. The presence of prolactin is absolutely essential (Ichinose and Nandi, 1964, 1966) and can be enhanced by the addition of thyroid hormones to the medium (Singh and Bern, 1969). In addition, prolactin is essential for maintenance of the morphologically developed state. If prolactin is removed after full lobuloalveolar development is achieved in the presence of the four-hormone mammogenic combination mentioned above, complete regression of the alveolar structures occurs, leaving only a ductal parenchyma (Banerjee et al., 1983).

4.2. Lactogenesis

4.2.1. Osmoregulation

In addition to its role in general growth and morphological development of the gland, prolactin is vital in the induction of functional differentiation and lactogenesis. The lactogenic action of prolactin in no small part may be one of osmoregulation, because lactogenesis involves large quantities of water and electrolytes (Nicoll and Bern, 1972). Prolactin's action in osmoregulation in the mammary gland may be to promote retention of fluid rather than of salts (Clarke and Bern, 1980), although secretion of milk is linked to ion transport (Linzell and Peaker, 1971; Taylor et al., 1975). The enzyme Na^{+}/K^{+}ATPase, which is associated with transport, is very active in the mammary gland (Vreeswijk et al., 1973) in times when prolactin is active. Prolactin has been shown to stimulate active secretion of the Na^{+} ion by the mammary gland (Falconer and Rowe, 1975, 1977), while ouabain has been shown to inhibit prolactin-induced lactogenesis (Falconer et al., 1978). In a series of experiments designed to assess directly the role of prolactin in osmoregulation and the electrophysiology of the mammary gland, Bisbee and coworkers (Bisbee et al., 1979; Bisbee, 1981a,b) showed that prolactin stimulates active uptake of Na^{+} from the fluid bathing the apical poles of midpregnant mouse mammary cells comprising an artificial membrane. They then examined the electrophysiological changes in cultured mouse mammary epithelium under hormonal influence. Ovine prolactin at concentrations as low as 1 ng/ml, but not growth hormone, significantly increased short-circuit current and decreased resistance of the cells. Bisbee (1981b) concluded that prolactin may have effects on passive permeability properties in addition to its documented effects on active transport.

4.2.2. *Secretory Immune System*

In addition to its role in ion transport and water balance, prolactin is essential for the induced synthesis and secretion of the macromolecular components of milk. Among these are the components of the secretory immune system, milk lipids, and specific proteins. The secretory immune system and its hormonal regulation are covered extensively in Chapter 8 in this volume. Binding of IgA dimer to intact mammary cells is mediated by secretory component, a family of glycoproteins produced by the secretory epithelial cells and expressed at the cell surface (Kühn and Kraehenbuhl, 1979, 1981; Kühn et al., 1983; Solari and Kraehenbuhl, 1984). To be secreted intact, dimeric IgA must be translocated across the epithelial cells by binding to secretory component (Lamm, 1976). Using monolayers of epithelial cells from lactating mouse mammary glands cultured on collagen-coated petri dishes, Weisz-Carrington et al. (1984) found that selective binding and internalization of dimer serum IgA was hormonally induced. Insulin alone was without effect, while the addition of estrogen and progesterone along with insulin gave a slight increase. When prolactin was added to the medium with the other three hormones, a further 25-fold increase in dimeric IgA binding was obtained.

4.2.3. Fatty Acid Uptake and Synthesis

Another aspect of lactogenesis subject to regulation by prolactin is the synthesis of milk-specific fatty acids and the uptake of fatty acids by mammary epithelial cells. This latter effect of prolactin results in vivo in an increase in glandular unsaturated (epithelial cell growth-promoting) relative to saturated (epithelial cell growth-inhibiting) fatty acids (Wicha et al., 1979). In vitro studies further demonstrated that prolactin (300 ng/ml) stimulates a fourfold increase in release of free fatty acids within 24 h in explant cultures of mammary glands from mature virgin mice (Kidwell et al., 1982). Similar results on prolactin-enhanced secretion of fatty acids were obtained within 4 h in cultured slices of mammary glands from lactating ewes and rabbits (Daudet et al., 1981). The cell of origin of the fatty acids was probably the adipocyte, since isolated mammary epithelial cells took up unsaturated fatty acids selectively when prolactin was added to the growth medium (Kidwell et al., 1982). Secretion into the milk of mammary-specific medium-chain fatty acids by the epithelial cells is also sensitive to the presence of prolactin. The enzyme thioesterase II is found exclusively in mammary glands, with highest levels in glands of lactating rabbits (Carey and Dils, 1973; Strong et al., 1973; Knudsen et al., 1976), rats (Smith and Abraham, 1975; Smith, 1977), and mice (Smith and Stern, 1981). It has a molecular weight of 29–32 kDa and is required for the synthesis of the medium chain (C8–C12) fatty acids. Its activity increases during gestation, plateaus in lactation, and then decreases directly parallel to the circulating levels of prolactin (Smith and Stern, 1981). Low levels of thioesterase II are present in the cells lining the lumen of the ductal and end bud structures of immature virgin rats and the lumen of the ductal and alveolar structures from glands of the mature virgin and midpregnant rat (Pasco et al., 1983). This enzyme has also been detected immunocytochemically in normal breast epithelial cells derived from both lactating and nonlactating tissue grown in primary cultures in the presence of prolactin (Smith et al., 1984).

The role of prolactin in medium-chain fatty acid synthesis and secretion was confirmed by in vitro studies in several laboratories. Explants of mammary glands from pregnant rabbits, cultured with insulin and prolactin, showed an increase in fatty acid synthesis within 20 h of onset of culture with a subsequent enrichment in the medium-chain variety (50% of the total at 48 h). Prolactin is essential for these changes (Forsyth et al., 1972; Speake et al., 1975) and works through induction of the thioesterase II enzyme. Similar results were obtained with physiological concentrations of prolactin (50 ng/ml) in the presence of insulin and corticosterone under serum-free primary culture conditions using alveolar structures liberated from the pseudopregnant rabbit mammary gland by collagenase–hyaluronidase digestion (Carrington et al., 1981). Mayer (1978) proposed that in the rabbit prolactin, alone or possibly in concert with insulin, is responsible for selective formation of the medium-chain fatty acids characteristic of milk secretions. In the mouse mammary gland, prolactin alone is ineffective, but it is an absolute requirement in the presence of insulin and corticosterone to enhance synthesis of the medium-chain fatty acids (Wang et al., 1972).

4.2.4. Milk Proteins

4.2.4a. Protein Synthesis and Secretion. Besides its role in mammary cell growth, probably the most studied function of prolactin in mammary tissue is that of regulation of synthesis and secretion of milk proteins. Accumulation of rough endoplasmic reticulum (RER, the site of protein synthesis) within secretory epithelial cells from midpregnant and virgin mouse mammary glands is dependent on the concerted actions of insulin and glucocorticoids (Oka and Topper, 1971). The addition of prolactin to the medium results in enhanced RNA content in the RER (Oka and Topper, 1971) and complete ultrastructural development characterized by translocation of the RER, Golgi apparatus, and nucleus and the appearance of secretory protein granules within the cytoplasm (Mills and Topper, 1970; Topper and Freeman, 1980; Vonderhaar and Smith, 1982).

These initial observations in organ culture on the role of prolactin in development of the secretory cell confirmed earlier in vivo observations from several laboratories assessing a necessary involvement of prolactin in milk protein synthesis and secretion. Very early studies had demonstrated that injections of pituitary prolactin into intact animals stimulated lactogenesis but failed to do so in hypophysectomized animals (Nelson and Gaunt, 1936; Gomez and Turner, 1936). Cowie (1969) demonstrated that hypophysectomy of goats causes a rapid decline in milk yield. Glucocorticoids, thyroid hormones, and growth hormone injections restored lactation to about one-third of the normal level, with full lactation restored only when prolactin was added to the three-hormone combination.

In ruminants, ergot drugs given just before parturition to suppress prolactin secretion reduced but did not completely suppress subsequent lactation (Schams et al., 1972). If exogenous prolactin was given along with the ergot drug, lactation occurred at normal levels (Akers et al., 1981). However, suppression of prolactin secretion with ergot drugs during an established lactation in cows did not affect milk production (Smith et al., 1974). By contrast, treatment of rodents with these same drugs before onset of lactation and during established lactation completely suppressed milk production (Tucker, 1979). In hypophysectomized rats, doses of prolactin and cortisol that are themselves too small to produce milk secretion can do so when given together (Meites et al., 1963). Exogenous prolactin shortens the time required for the mammary gland to refill with milk in rats (Grosvenor et al., 1970). In rabbits, prolactin alone may be all that is necessary for lactogenesis, although other hormones may play a key role in the normal physiological preparation of the gland for subsequent prolactin action. Lyons (1942) clearly demonstrated this when he injected prolactin into individual mammary ducts of rabbits whose glands had been developed to the lobuloalveolar stage with estrogen and progesterone. Milk secretion occurred only in the prolactin-treated portion of the gland. After hypophysectomy, prolactin injections restored milk yields to normal in pseudopregnant rabbits (Kilpatrick et al., 1964; Cowie et al., 1969). Injecting prolactin into adrenalectomized and adrenalectomized–ovariectomized pseudopregnant rabbits resulted in a full lactogenic response (Cowie and Watson, 1966).

In the human, as in the dairy cow, it appears that prolactin is required for the initiation of lactation, but it is not as critical for maintenance of an established lactation (Jacobs, 1977). Tactile stimulation of the breast and nipple results in release of prolactin (Kolodny et al., 1972; Noel et al., 1974b). In endocrinologically normal but nonpregnant women, lactogenesis can be induced by administration of estrogen and a regular program of tactile manipulation of the breast and nipple, followed by abrupt cessation of the estrogen treatment (Tyson et al., 1975). Early in lactation, suckling results in dramatic rises in serum prolactin levels, but as nursing continues, a slow decline in prolactin to the basal level occurs, as well as a lack of response to the suckling stimulus (Tyson et al., 1972). Thus, normal lactation appears to occur in the absence of accelerated prolactin secretion.

Further confirmaton of the essential role of prolactin in the induction of specific milk protein synthesis was initially described using organ culture techniques and chemically defined medium (Elias, 1957; Elias and Rivera, 1959; Juergens et al., 1965). Following these initial studies in the mouse, similar prolactin-dependent stimulation of milk protein synthesis and secretion has been established in a variety of different kinds of culture of the tissue from various species. In all cases, including mice (Elias, 1957; Elias and Rivera, 1959; Juergens et al., 1965; Vonderhaar et al., 1973; Ono et al., 1981; Bolander, 1983, 1984), rats (Ray et al., 1981; Sankaran and Topper, 1982, 1983; Quirk et al., 1986; Vonderhaar and Nakhasi, 1986), guinea pigs (Fairhurst et al., 1971), cows (Anderson and Larson, 1970; Goodman et al., 1983), humans (Kleinberg, 1975; Wilson et al., 1980), sheep (Gaye and Denamur, 1970), and goats (Skarda et al., 1982a,b), with the possible exception of the rabbit which requires only prolactin (DeLouis and Denamur, 1972; Houdebine, 1979, 1980; Al-Sarraj et al., 1979; Teyssot and Houdebine, 1981; Suard et al., 1983; Sankaran and Toper, 1984), prolactin stimulates milk protein synthesis in vitro in concert with other hormones such as insulin and glucocorticoids (Juergens et al., 1965; Banerjee, 1976; Topper et al., 1984; Quirk et al., 1986), as well as the sex steroids (Bolander and Topper, 1980, 1981) and thyroid hormones (Vonderhaar, 1975, 1977; Ray et al., 1981; Terada and Oka, 1982; Goodman et al., 1983; Bhattacharjee and Vonderhaar, 1984; Vonderhaar and Bhattacharjee, 1985). Progesterone inhibits the action of prolactin on the induction of milk protein synthesis (Vonderhaar, 1977). The action of prolactin on the mammary epithelial cells in culture is influenced by the other components of the system, such as cell shape (Hauptle et al., 1983b), collagenous substrata (Emerman and Pitelka, 1977; Emerman et al., 1977; Flynn et al., 1982; Lee et al., 1984; Rocha et al., 1985), mesenchymal cells in coculture (Levine and Stockdale, 1985), and components of the extracellular matrix (Wicha et al., 1982; Bissell et al., 1986).

4.2.4b. Gene Expression. Using the techniques of molecular biology, hormonal regulation of (and the role of prolactin in) the expression of the genes for the milk proteins can be studied in great detail. The casein genes in particular have been subjected to extensive investigation. Regulation of gene expression for α-lactalbumin in several species (Campbell et al., 1973; Craig et al., 1976; Nakhasi and Qasba, 1979; Takemoto et al., 1980; Hall et al., 1982; Qasba et al., 1982; Nagamatsu and Oka, 1983; Terada et al., 1983) and for whey acidic protein in rats and mice (Hennighausen and Sippel, 1982a,b; Hennighausen et al., 1982; Banerjee et al., 1983; Motojima and Oka, 1983; Vonderhaar and Nakhasi, 1986) has also been explored. The expression of these genes appears to be regulated by the same hormonal complement as are milk protein synthesis and secretion [i.e., insulin (Kulski et al., 1983), glucocorticoids (Terry et al., 1977; Devinoy et al., 1978; Ganguly et al., 1979, 1980;

Banerjee et al., 1983; Nagamatsu and Oka, 1983; Terada et al., 1983), and prolactin (Devinoy et al., 1978; Nakhasi and Qasba, 1979; Rosen et al., 1979; Ganguly et al., 1980; Kulski et al., 1983; Vonderhaar and Nakhasi, 1986)], with thyroid hormones enhancing prolactin's effect on α-lactalbumin mRNA synthesis (Terada and Oka, 1982; Herber and Vonderhaar, 1986) and progesterone blocking milk protein gene expression (Rosen et al., 1979). Early work from Rosen's laboratory (Matusik and Rosen, 1978, 1980; Rosen et al., 1979, 1980; Guyette et al., 1979) using explant cultures of mammary glands from midpregnant rats showed that incubation with prolactin resulted in a sevenfold increase in casein mRNA accumulation within 24 h of hormone addition. This was shown to be due to both an enhanced rate of synthesis and a decreased degradation (i.e., increased half-life) of the casein mRNA under prolactin's influence. A more detailed examination of the nature of the casein genes is dealt with in Chapter 9 in this volume.

5. Mechanism of Action

5.1. Receptors

5.1.1. Distribution

The actual means by which prolactin elicits its responses in the mammary tissue is in large part unknown. It is generally accepted that, to act at the cellular level, peptide hormones such as prolactin must first interact with receptors associated with the surface membrane of the target cells (Fig. 3). The mechanism by which prolactin interaction with the receptor results in the distinctive biological effects is still largely unknown but has been the subject of intensive study during the past decade. The specific high affinity binding sites for prolactin, which are distinct from growth hormone receptors (Hughes et al., 1985), were first described in mouse and rabbit mammary glands (Frantz and Turkington, 1972; Shiu et al., 1973). These sites appear to reside exclusively in the epithelial cells, since lactogen binding sites cannot be demonstrated in mammary fat pads cleared of epithelium (Bhattacharya and Vonderhaar, 1979a). However, they are clearly present in dispersed mammary epithelial cells prepared by collagenase digestion of the gland (Sakai et al., 1978; Suard et al., 1979).

Subsequent to their identification in mammary tissue, prolactin receptors have been found in a variety of other mammalian target tissues, including liver, adrenals, mammary tumors, kidney, prostate, ovaries, chorion of placenta, and lymphocytes (Hughes et al., 1985). In all tissues

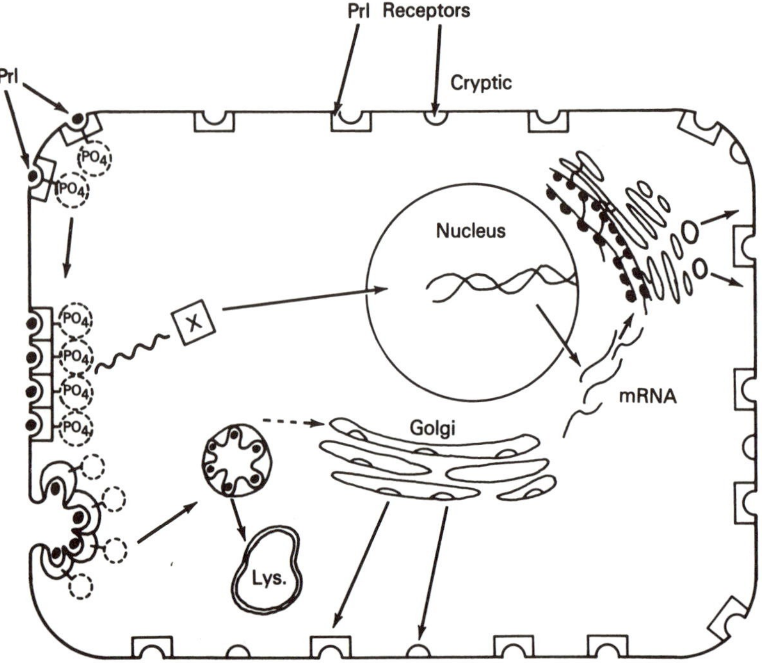

Figure 3. Schematic representation of the mechanism of prolactin (Prl) action on target cells. From Vonderhaar et al. (1985).

studied, the characteristics of the prolactin receptor appear to be similar. Prolactin binding proteins have been identified in plasma and Golgi membranes as well as endoplasmic reticulum and lysosomes (Bergeron et al., 1978; Josefsberg et al., 1979; Djiane et al., 1981b; Kahn et al., 1981; Rae-Venter and Dao, 1983; Kelly et al., 1984; Vonderhaar et al., 1985; Costlow, 1986). Whether any or all of these intracellular sites are involved in the triggering of the biological actions of prolactin is not as yet clear.

5.1.2. Purification and Characterization

During the past several years, considerable effort from several laboratories has been directed toward isolation, purification, and characterization of the lactogenic hormone receptor. Using a variety of target tissues and isolation techniques, specific lactogen binding entities have been identified with reported molecular weights ranging from 21 to 320 kDa (Shiu and Friesen, 1974a; Friesen, 1979; Carr and Jaffe, 1981; Liscia and Vonderhaar, 1982; Church and Ebner, 1982; Hauptle et al., 1983a; Necessary et al., 1984; Djiane et al., 1985; Katoh et al., 1985a; Vonderhaar et al., 1985; Smith et al., 1986; Mitani and Dufau, 1986). The higher molecular weight forms may be the result of aggregation of the receptor and/or incomplete dissociation of the receptor from the particulate membrane (Vonderhaar et al., 1985). The 21-kDa unit may be a result of partial degradation, oxidation, or deglycosylation (Necessary et al., 1984). Using the zwitterionic detergent CHAPS (3-[3-cholamidopropyl-dimethylammonio]-1-propanesulfonate), we first isolated and purified, by prolactin affinity chromatography, a receptor with an apparent molecular weight of 37 kDa (Liscia and Vonderhaar, 1982). This receptor was believed to be a *core binding unit.* It retained its specificity for lactogenic hormones and bound ^{125}I-labeled ovine prolactin with a K_a of 2–6 × 10^9 M^{-1}, which is similar to the association constant of the hormone for the native, membrane-bound receptor. Subsequently, 35-kDa (Hauptle et al., 1983a) and 42-kDa (Necessary et al., 1984) prolactin receptors were isolated from rabbit mammary glands using a hGH and an ovine prolactin affinity column, respectively.

Crosslinking studies have confirmed the core binding unit (termed the 40-kDa unit) as a prolactin receptor. ^{125}I-prolactin (22 kDa) covalently crosslinked to the receptor (40 kDa) from rat liver membranes yielded a 60-kDa band of radioactivity on sodium dodecyl sulfate (SDS) gels (Borst and Sayare, 1982). Similar crosslinking studies have indicated molecular weights of 45 and 40 kDa for the prolactin receptors from rat liver and rabbit mammary glands, respectively (Hughes et al., 1983). Another study determined the molecular weight of the rabbit mammary gland receptor to be 32 kDa by the same method (Djiane et al., 1985; Katoh et al., 1985a). Photoaffinity labeling of solubilized rabbit mammary lactogenic hormone binding sites suggested a molecular weight of 35 kDa (Hauptle et al., 1983a). Antireceptor antibodies precipitate a 35-kDa protein solubilized from membranes of late pregnant or early lactating rabbit mammary glands and livers (Haputle et al., 1983a).

More recently, an additional 85–90-kDa form of the receptor (termed the 85-kDa unit) has been purified from the membranes of lactating bovine mammary glands (Smith et al., 1986), rat ovaries (Mitani and Dufau, 1986), and by our laboratory from human chorion-decidua, MCF-7 human breast cancer cells grown as solid tumors in nude mice, and lactating mouse mammary glands and livers (unpublished data). This higher molecular weight form was confirmed as a receptor by its ability to bind ^{125}I-hGH specifically after SDS gel electrophoresis (Mitani and Dufau, 1986). The relation of the 40-kDa core binding unit to the larger molecular weight form, as well as their possible identification as *active* and/or *cryptic* forms, is of fundamental importance.

Hauptle et al. (1983a) and Mitani and Dufau (1986) indicated that the lactogenic hormone receptors form multimeric complexes in the membranes which are crosslinked via disulfide bridges. The lower molecular weight form does not aggregate with itself through S–S linkages (Katoh et al., 1985a), and the higher molecular weight form does not dissociate to yield the lower molecular weight form on reduction of the S–S bonds (Smith et al., 1986; Mitani and Dufau, 1986; and B. K. Vonderhaar, unpublished data). The two units, however, are related structurally since the 85-kDa form of the receptor is recognized by a polyclonal antibody raised against the 40-kDa unit (E. Ginsburg and B. K. Vonderhaar, unpublished data).

The solubilized holoreceptors from rat ovaries resolve into three isoforms on chromatofocusing with p*I* values of 4.0, 5.0, and 5.3 (Mitani and Dufau, 1986). These forms may reflect differences in glycosylation. Previous studies (Vonderhaar et al., 1985) have shown that binding of lactogenic hormones to mammary gland membranes is sensitive to addition of the lectin concanavalin A (ConA) to the binding reaction. Neuraminidase, an enzyme that cleaves sialic acid residues, does not inhibit lactogenic hormone binding to rabbit membranes (Shiu and Friesen, 1974b). Cleavage of sialic acid from rat liver membranes, however, stimulated prolactin receptor activity (Silverstein and Richards, 1979). CHAPS solubilized (Vonderhaar et al., 1985) and Zwittergent 3-12 affinity purified (Necessary et al., 1984) 40-kDa lactogen binding units do not bind to ConA–Sepharose or Lens culinaris–agarose columns, both of which are specific for recognizing glucose and/or mannose residues. The biochemical nature of the various isoforms of both the core binding unit and the 85-kDa unit and their relation to various biological functions of prolactin remain to be elucidated.

5.1.3. Regulation

5.1.3a. Antireceptor Antibodies. Regulation of the number of receptors on the target cell is a complex phenomenon. Until proper antibodies are exploited to study the actual synthesis of the receptor molecule and the gene cloned, regulation studies must rely on binding activity as the end point. Such studies are predicated on the assumption that changes in the binding activity reflect changes in the synthesis of the receptor molecule.

Several antibodies have been prepared against partially purified lactogenic hormone receptors (Shiu and Friesen, 1976c; Shiu et al., 1983; Katoh et al., 1984; Vonderhaar et al., 1985), but they are only now beginning to prove useful for studies on regulation of the receptor molecule. The polyclonal antibodies react across species lines and react with receptors from a variety of target tissues (Katoh et al., 1984; Vonderhaar et al., 1985). In explants of midpregnant rabbit mammary glands, polyclonal antireceptor antibodies were shown to block prolactin binding to its receptor (Shiu and Friesen, 1976c) and also to inhibit prolactin-stimulated casein synthesis and ^{14}C-aminoisobutyric acid transport (Shiu and Friesen, 1976b; Hughes et al., 1985). This same antibody reduces milk yield when injected into lactating rats (Bohnet et al., 1978). Shiu et al. (1983) subsequently showed partial prolactin agonist activity by an IgG fraction of the antireceptor preparation in explant cultures of rabbit mammary glands. This prolactin-mimicking action of the antireceptor antibodies was also observed by Djiane et al. (1981a). The antiserum, as well as its IgG fraction, inhibited prolactin-stimulated DNA and casein synthesis in rabbit mammary gland explants but initiated synthesis in the absence of the hormone. The stimulatory effect was augmented by the presence of glucocorticoids in the medium just as the prolactin-induced effects were. Colchicine, which is capable of blocking prolactin action in these explants, also prevented their induction by the antibody. The lysosomotropic agents, chloroquine and NH_4Cl, which do not interfere with prolactin action, likewise did not alter the response observed with the antibody. Bivalent fragments (Fab′2) of the antiprolactin receptor antibodies prepared by pepsin cleavage, as well as monovalent fragments (Fab′) prepared by dithiothreitol reduction of the Fab′2 fragments, were as potent as whole antiserum in inhibition of prolactin binding to its receptor and receptor down regulation in mammary gland explants (Djiane et al., 1985). Fab′2 fragments as well as whole antiserum were about 50–60% as effective as prolactin in inducing β-casein and DNA synthesis in explant culture. The Fab′ fragments were completely devoid of prolactin-mimicking activity (Dusanter-Fourt et al., 1984). The IgG fraction of the whole antireceptor serum also effectively induced β-casein synthesis when injected into pseudopregnant rabbits for 4 days (Dusanter-Fourt et al., 1982).

These studies used polyclonal antibodies prepared against partially purified receptors and hence must be cautiously interpreted. Pillion et al. (1980) have shown that hormonal-mimicking effects can also be obtained with antibodies that interact with nonreceptor components of the plasma membrane. This problem, however, should be minimized or eliminated by the use of either anti-idiotypic (Marx, 1985) or monoclonal antibodies that can be selected for direct and specific interaction with the prolactin binding domain of the receptor.

Anti-idiotypic antibodies have been raised against ovine prolactin and rat prolactin which subsequently recognize the prolactin receptor (Amit et al., 1986). The antiserum specifically inhibits binding of ^{125}I-

prolactin to its receptors in a dose-dependent manner. Species-specific monoclonal antibodies against the receptor were prepared using a partially purified (5000-fold) 32-kDa unit from rabbit mammary gland as immunogen (Djiane et al., 1985; Katoh et al., 1985b). These monoclonal antibodies completely inhibited binding of prolactin to both particulate and solubilized receptors from mammary glands as well as other target tissues from rabbit. Monoclonals were prepared that were either hormone binding site specific or that bind a domain partially but not entirely distinct from the hormone binding site. With these latter reagents in hand, regulation of the synthesis and insertion into membranes of the receptor molecule itself can now be examined more readily.

5.1.3b. Variation with Gestation. Various physiological factors influencing the amount of prolactin binding and hence by inference the number of lactogenic hormone receptors have been examined in the mammary gland. These studies show that the prolactin receptor is subject to both up and down regulation by prolactin itself (Kelly et al., 1974, 1980; Fellows and Soltysiak, 1980). This is reflected by changes in receptor levels during gestation and lactation (Kelly et al., 1974, 1979; Nagasawa and Yanai, 1978; Hayden et al., 1979; Suard et al., 1979; Dave et al., 1983; Soltysiak and Fellows, 1983; Emane et al., 1986) that parallel the changes in prolactin and placental lactogen secretion (Shiu and Friesen, 1976a). It is supported by experiments both in vivo (Bohnet et al., 1977; Djiane and Durand, 1977; Sheth et al., 1978; Djiane et al., 1979a; Dave et al., 1982) and in vitro (Djiane et al., 1979b, 1980, 1981b, 1982; Fellows and Soltysiak, 1980) using exogenous prolactin. Using an exchange radioreceptor assay that allows for assessment of total hormone binding sites (not just unoccupied sites), Kelly et al. (1979) showed that the level of lactogen binding in rat mammary gland membranes rises during gestation and peaks at late pregnancy (day 17–20). Likewise, prolactin receptor content in the ewe mammary gland (Emane et al., 1986) increases during pregnancy up to day 100 and remains stable during the last trimester. A second increase in prolactin receptor content occurs during early lactation. The studies are complicated by the presence of cryptic or masked binding sites on the cell membranes. The cryptic sites are subject to up and down regulation by prolactin (Costlow and Hample, 1984) as are the active sites.

5.1.3c. Up and Down Self-Regulation. Direct positive (or up) regulation by prolactin of its own receptor in mammary glands was first shown in vivo by Djiane and Durand (1977). When pseudopregnant rabbits were injected with 100 IU of ovine prolactin, a marked long-lasting increase in prolactin receptor levels was achieved. This positive effect was confirmed in vitro using primary monolayer cultures of mammary epithelial cells from 18- to 19-day pregnant rabbits (Fellows and Soltysiak, 1980). Within 24 h of addition of ovine prolactin or rabbit prolactin (10–100 ng/ml) to the culture medium in the absence of serum, increased levels of total prolactin receptors were achieved. Maximal stimulation (200% of control) was elicited by 10 ng/ml of ovine prolactin and 50 ng/ml of rabbit prolactin. At 48 h, increased binding (150–190% of control) was produced by both prolactins at concentrations as low as 1–10 ng/ml. At 1000 ng/ml, rabbit and ovine prolactins caused limited (20–60% of control, respectively) down regulation of the prolactin receptors in these same cell preparations.

Down regulation of the receptor has also been demonstrated in rabbits in vivo (Kelly et al., 1980). Lactating rabbits, injected with CB154 (2-bromo-α-ergocryptine) for 36 h to lower serum prolactin levels, were given bovine prolactin intravenously for 30 h, and mammary gland biopsies were taken throughout treatment. Using an exchange assay, total prolactin receptors in the biopsy samples were assayed and found to decrease progressively up to 6 h after onset of prolactin injections and only returned to normal levels at 24–30 h. Subcellular localization (Djiane et al., 1981b) showed that injections of ovine prolactin to lactating rabbits resulted in down regulation of the total prolactin receptors in the plasma membrane-rich fraction of the mammary gland and not in the Golgi.

5.1.3d. Other Hormones and Growth Factors. In addition to self-regulation by prolactin, the lactogen receptor on mammary epithelial cells is regulated by a variety of other hormones and growth factors. Among these are the steroid hormones. Harigaya et al. (1982) showed that ovariectomy increased the number of receptors per cell with no effect on the dissociation constant. This effect requires the presence of glucocorticoids. The number of prolactin receptors on mammary cells is also regulated by progesterone. In pseudopregnant rabbits, the self-regulation of the receptor by prolactin is antagonized by progesterone (Djiane and Durand, 1977). The number of prolactin receptors on mammary cells of rabbits (Suard et al., 1979) and mice (Sakai et al., 1978) in different developmental states varies in an inverse relation to serum progesterone levels. The opposite effect of progesterone on prolactin receptors was recently reported in cultured human breast cancer cells (Murphy et al., 1985, 1986). A 24-h incubation of T47D and MCF-7 human breast cancer cells with a synthetic progestin (R5020), progesterone, or medroxyprogesterone acetate, but not testosterone, estradiol, or hydrocortisone, resulted in a 200–250% increase in the specific binding of lactogenic hormones to these cells. No change in the affinity constant for the hormone–receptor interactions occurred. Receptors for other hormones such as insulin, calcitonin, transferrin, or ConA were unaffected.

The apparent contradiction between the effects of progesterone in the normal gland and tumor cells may reflect the difference in the action of prolactin in the different cells and correlates well with the observed biological effects of progesterone. While prolactin is regulating growth, as it does in the MCF-7 human breast cancer line (Biswas and Vonderhaar, 1986; Vonderhaar and Biswas, 1986), progesterone will stimulate prolactin binding. This is consistent with the work of Nagasawa et al. (1985) in vivo and Imigawa et al. (1985) in vitro, showing a synergism between prolactin and progesterone on mammary cell growth. When prolactin is regulating initiation of lactogenesis (i.e., induction of milk protein gene expression), progesterone is antilactogenic (Vonderhaar, 1977; Rosen et al., 1979) and acts by decreasing the number of prolactin binding sites.

Epidermal growth factor, which may also have the dual functions of promoting growth and inhibiting lactogenesis (Taketani and Oka, 1983a,b,c,d; Vonderhaar and Nakhasi, 1986), may produce this latter effect by suppressing binding of prolactin to secretory mammary epithelium (Taketani and Oka, 1983d).

The level of prolactin binding in membranes from glands from nulliparous as well as primiparous mice (Bhattacharya and Vonderhaar, 1979a) is sensitive to thyroid status in vivo. In addition, physiological levels of L-T_3 added along with insulin and hydrocortisone to serum-free explant cultures of midpregnancy mammary tissue results in a nearly twofold increase in lactogenic hormone binding to membranes. This induction of prolactin binding does not require protein synthesis, suggesting that thyroid hormones act, at least in part, by unmasking cryptic receptor sites (Vonderhaar and Bhattacharjee, 1985).

5.1.3e. Active Versus Cryptic Forms. The existence of such cryptic binding sites has been confirmed by a variety of techniques, including membrane solubilization with detergents (Aubert et al., 1978; Alhadi and Vonderhaar, 1982; Koppelman and Dufau, 1982; Liscia and Vonderhaar, 1982; Necessary et al., 1984; Vonderhaar et al., 1985), energy depletion (Costlow and Hample, 1982a,b, 1984), and changes in membrane lipid composition (Bhattacharya and Vonderhaar, 1979b; Knazek and Liu, 1980; Cave and Erickson-Lucas, 1982; Kidwell et al., 1982; Vonderhaar et al., 1985) and fluidity (Dave and Knazek, 1980, 1983;

Dave et al., 1982, 1983; Dave and Witorsch, 1986). Using crude microsomal membranes prepared from rabbit mammary glands removed 2 days postpartum, Aubert et al. (1978) found that solubilization with Triton X-100 resulted in a twofold increase in the number of femtomoles of prolactin bound per milligram membrane protein compared with the particulate membranes. However, use of Triton to solubilize the receptors also altered the affinity of the hormone for its binding unit. When zwitterionic detergents CHAPS (Liscia et al., 1982; Liscia and Vonderhaar, 1982; Alhadi and Vonderhaar, 1982; Vonderhaar et al., 1985) or Zwittergent 3-12 (Church and Ebner, 1982; Necessary et al., 1984) were used, a two- to threefold increase in prolactin binding activity was achieved without a change in affinity. The number of cryptic sites assessed by this method varied with the developmental state of the animal (Alhadi and Vonderhaar, 1982). The ratio of cryptic to active sites was lowest in tissue from virgin animals, rose after midpregnancy, and reached a peak just prior to parturition. After a small decrease, the level of cryptic sites remained high through midlactation and declined to nearly the original level after weaning of the pups.

The number of cryptic sites is also up and down regulated by prolactin itself (Costlow and Hample, 1984). Within 24 h of the addition of prolactin (0.1–0.5 ng/ml) to primary cultures of rat mammary tumor cells, cryptic receptor levels increased two- to threefold and were maintained for up to 6 days. Concentrations of 1–5 μg prolactin/ml caused a rapid dose-dependent down regulation of the cryptic sites. Down regulation was specific for lactogenic hormones and was completely reversed within 10 h of removal of the prolactin from the medium.

Lactogenic hormone receptor binding activity and the amount of cryptic binding sites are sensitive to the quality as well as the quantity of fatty acids in the diet (Knazek and Liu, 1980; Cave and Erickson-Lucas, 1982; Kidwell et al., 1982). Functionality of the cryptic prolactin receptors as well as the ability of the target cells to express newly synthesized receptors is dependent on the availability of essential fatty acids (Knazek and Liu, 1980; Kidwell et al., 1982). Cryptic binding sites in mouse mammary gland membranes become active through localized changes in phosphatidyl choline (PC) concentrations (Vonderhaar et al., 1985). Membranes of lactating mouse mammary glands contain the phospholipid-*N*-methyltransferase system (Vonderhaar et al., 1985), which transfers three methyl groups from the methyl donor S-adenosyl-methionine (SAM) to phosphatidyl ethanolamine to form PC (Crews et al., 1980). This process creates a local change in the PC concentration, alters membrane microviscosity (Hirata and Axelrod, 1978; Laggner, 1981; Vonderhaar et al., 1985), and, through local solvation, affects the expression of the prolactin receptor by changing cryptic to active forms (Vonderhaar et al., 1985). Addition of SAM to membranes of mammary glands from lactating mice (Bhattacharya and Vonderhaar, 1979b; Vonderhaar et al., 1985) results in a rapid, stable, and significant increase in the number of lactogen binding sites without a change in affinity, as determined by Scatchard analysis. In the same membrane preparations, addition of SAM was without effect on the binding of epidermal growth factor to its receptors.

The relevance of activation of cryptic sites to functionality of the receptor is emphasized by the fact that, in all three systems used to examine the subcellular localization of this process [i.e., energy depletion (Costlow and Rodgers, 1986), membrane fluidizers (Dave and Witorsch, 1986), and phospholipid methylation (Vonderhaar et al., 1985)], the effect is localized to the plasma membrane. Even though the majority of the prolactin receptors in some cases are located in Golgi membranes (Bergeron et al., 1978) and there are significant amounts of methyltransferase activity on the membranes, there is no SAM-mediated increase in binding. These data support the concept that receptors in the Golgi are nonfunctional precursors of plasma membrane receptors (Bergeron et al., 1978). Thus, it is the plasma membrane receptor, in its active form, which transmits the specific signal to the cell to elicit the hormonal response (see Fig. 3). Cryptic receptors may act as a buffer to allow the cells to respond rapidly to changes in prolactin concentrations at the cell surface.

5.2. Signal Transduction

5.2.1. Synlactin

Just how the receptors transmit the signal to the cell to elicit a given biological response once prolactin is bound is still largely unknown. Whether the receptor is autophosphorylated as are other peptide hormone receptors (Cohen et al., 1982; Zick et al., 1983) is not known. Much like other peptide hormones (Brown et al., 1983; Harrison and Kirchhausen, 1983; Schreiber et al., 1983), the prolactin–receptor complex is believed to form clusters before internalization (see Fig. 3). Which of these events is essential to the hormone's biological action is unknown. Nicoll and colleagues (Anderson et al., 1983, 1984; Mick and Nicoll, 1985; Nicoll et al., 1985) have proposed that the mitogenic effects of prolactin on target cells are mediated by the synergistic actions of prolactin and a prolactin-induced somatomedin-like molecule produced by the liver which they called *synlactin.* Thus, prolactin may work both directly and indirectly on target tissues. The signal from the receptor to the nucleus, which tells the cell to turn on DNA synthesis in response to prolactin as opposed to turning on specific differentiative functions, may not be a simple one but may be a composite of "signals" sent by prolactin and other hormones and growth factors acting in concert. The complexity of signal transduction in response to prolactin has recently been the subject of a comprehensive review by Rillema et al. (1986).

5.2.2. *Cyclic Nucleotides*

Unlike many other polypeptide hormones, prolactin does not stimulate adenylate cyclase activity in target cell membranes. Neither cyclic AMP (cAMP) nor dibutyryl cAMP (db-cAMP) mimic prolactin's differentiative function. In fact, db-cAMP inhibited prolactin-induced increases in the rate of synthesis of fatty acids, DNA, and RNA in rat mammary gland explants (Sapag-Hagar et al., 1974). In cultured guinea pig mammary glands, db-cAMP and phosphodiesterase inhibition reduced lactose production (Loizzi, 1978), while in rabbit mammary cultures, db-cAMP and theophylline decreased fatty acid synthetase activity (Speake et al., 1975). The prolactin-induced increase in α-lactalbumin in midpregnant mouse mammary explants was completely inhibited by 0.5 m*M* db-cAMP in the culture medium with partial inhibition of total casein synthesis (Perry and Oka, 1980). The levels of endogenous cAMP in these tissues decreased rapidly during culture, regardless of the presence of various combinations of insulin, hydrocortisone, and prolactin (Oka, 1983). Thus, if cAMP does play a role in prolactin signal transduction, it may be through the release of a negative influence. This is borne out by the fact that the levels of cAMP and adenylate cyclase activity rise during pregnancy but fall rapidly after parturition and the onset of lactogenesis (Sapag-Hagar and Greenbaum, 1974).

A possible positive role may be invoked for cGMP, since this agent mimics prolactin, at least partially, in stimulating RNA synthesis in cultured mouse mammary gland explants (Rillema, 1975) and the level of casein mRNA in cultured rat mammary tissue (Matusik and Rosen, 1980). However, cGMP had no effect on the rate of casein synthesis in the mouse mammary explants (Rillema, 1975), and prolactin does not directly stimulate the activity of guanylate cyclase in mammary tissue (Rillema, 1986). A limited effect on casein synthesis was seen when cGMP was added to the cultures along with spermidine (Rillema et al., 1977). Thus, cyclic nucleotides may play at least a partial role in prolactin-induced lactogenesis through stimulatory effects of cGMP and release of inhibitory effects of cAMP. This is consistent with the changes in the physiological levels of these molecules in the mammary gland at the onset of lactation. Unlike cAMP levels, intracellular cGMP levels increase immediately after parturition (Sapag-Hagar and Greenbaum, 1974).

As mentioned previously, cAMP levels in the mammary gland rise during pregnancy (Sapag-Hagar and Greenbaum, 1974), a period of intensive hormonally regulated growth and morphogenesis. Recent data have suggested that cholera toxin, a stimulator of adenylate cyclase, and cAMP can stimulate proliferation of mammary epithelial cells both in vivo (Silberstein et al., 1984) and in vitro (Yang et al., 1980a). Thus, it might appear that cAMP can have either a positive or a negative effect on the mammary cells depending on the end point of the prolactin action. Which effect is produced, however, may be the function of the concerted actions of a variety of other hormonal signals and the stage of the developmental cycle of the gland at the time it binds prolactin.

5.2.3. *Prostaglandins*

The prostaglandins affect cyclic nucleotide synthesis in cultured mammary cells (Burnstein et al., 1976, 1977). The onset of lactogenesis in rats was advanced by several hours when pregnant dams were injected with prostaglandin F2α (Vermouth and Deis, 1975). Prostaglandins B_2, E_2, and F2α caused prolactin-like increases in RNA synthesis but alone could not mimic prolactin's action on casein synthesis (Rillema, 1975). When combined with spermidine, however, prostaglandins and arachidonic acid could promote casein synthesis to a limited extent. In addition, indomethacin, an inhibitor of prostaglandin biosynthesis, blocked the stimulation of RNA and casein synthesis by prolactin (Rillema, 1976a,b). Terada et al. (1982) showed that prostaglandin E_2 added to cultured mouse mammary glands may play a role in hormonal regulation of α-lactalbumin production without affecting casein synthesis. However, prostaglandins were unable to replace prolactin in increasing casein mRNA accumulation in rat mammary cultures (Matusik and Rosen, 1980) or in inducing lactogenesis in cultured rabbit mammary tissue (Houdebine and Lacroix, 1980).

The prostaglandins in mammary glands are produced from arachidonic acid released from membrane phospholipids by the action of phospholipase A_2 (Rillema, 1980; Rillema et al., 1986). Phospholipase A_2 had a prolactin-like effect on RNA synthesis when added to the medium for mouse mammary gland explants but did not affect the rate of casein synthesis (Rillema and Anderson, 1976). Arachadonic acid and phospholipase A_2, however, did stimulate guanylate cyclase activity in broken cell preparations of mouse mammary glands (Rillema, 1978;

Rillema and Linebaugh, 1978). Thus, if prostaglandins play a role in mediating prolactin's effects in the mammary gland, it is most probably not a direct one but, rather, a supportive one for the other hormonally induced signals.

5.2.4. *Polyamines*

Several laboratories have proposed that polyamines may regulate lactogenic and proliferative effects of prolactin in the mammary gland. In the mammary glands of virgin mice (Oka et al., 1978) and rats (Russell and McVicker, 1972), the concentration of spermidine is relatively low. The intracellular concentration of this polyamine increases during pregnancy in parallel with increases in cell proliferation. The level of spermidine reaches maximum during midlactation. In mammary explant culture, prolactin in combination with insulin and hydrocortisone increased intracellular spermidine sevenfold before the induction of milk protein synthesis (Oka and Perry, 1974a; Rillema et al., 1977). The three-hormone lactogenic combination was shown to stimulate the whole series of enzymes involved in polyamine biosynthesis during the induction of lactogenesis in vitro, and specific inhibitors of the enzymes involved in spermidine biosynthesis were able to block milk protein synthesis in culture (Oka, 1983). However, they did not block prolactin-induced RNA synthesis (Oka and Perry, 1974b; Rillema et al., 1977). Spermidine, when added with other agents such as cGMP and prostaglandins, can stimulate the rate of RNA synthesis in mammary gland explants but not nearly to the extent that prolactin does (Rillema, 1976b; Rillema et al., 1977). In cultured rat (Matusik and Rosen, 1980) and rabbit (Houdebine et al., 1978) mammary tissues, spermidine was unable to stimulate casein mRNA accumulation. Thus, it would appear that spermidine (polyamines) may play a role in lactogenesis, but it is not solely responsible for mediating prolactin's actions.

5.2.5. *Calcium Binding Proteins and the Phosphatidyl Inositides (PI) Turnover Cycle*

Recently, several reports have suggested that protein kinase C and calcium ions may be involved in prolactin signal transduction in several target tissues (Gertler et al., 1985; Buckley et al., 1986; Caulfield and Bolander, 1986; Fabbro et al., 1986). Caulfield and Bolander (1986) found that protein kinase C activity in mouse mammary glands declined during pregnancy and remained low throughout lactation, suggesting an inverse relation with milk protein gene expression. Specific protein kinase C inhibitors added to culture medium with mouse mammary explants resulted in a doubling of the prolactin-stimulated levels of α-lactalbumin. Phorbol ester, an activator of protein kinase C, in the presence of elevated calcium levels, stimulated α-lactalbumin production 2.5-fold. Bolander (1985) previously had shown that the calcium channel blocker verapamil preferentially inhibited prolactin-induced differentiation of mouse mammary tissue in culture. In addition, prolactin stimulated calcium accumulation by this tissue. The calcium ionophore A23187 mimicked prolactin effects on calcium accumulation but was unable to induce differentiation in the absence of prolactin. Bolander (1985) thus concluded that the calcium–calmodulin system is involved in prolactin-induced differentiation of the mammary gland, but it is not the only mediator of prolactin's actions (i.e., it is necessary but not sufficient). Furthermore, he suggested that there also appears to be another separate action of calcium on casein synthesis, which involves prolactin sensitivity of the gland.

One possible, and yet unexplored, such function is that of stimulation of the turnover of PI in the plasma membranes of the target cells. This pathway is activated by a specific phospholipase C that hydrolyzes PI. The degradation products of the PI derivatives may be involved in cellular signal transduction in a variety of systems and may activate the calcium-dependent protein kinase C activity and increase intracellular calcium ion concentrations (Berridge and Irvine, 1984; Majerus et al., 1985). The prolactin-induced increase in intracellular calcium ion concentration (Bolander, 1985) may also be important in activation of phospholipase A_2 and hence the entire prostaglandin synthesis cycle. Rocha and colleagues (Braslau et al., 1984; Rocha et al., 1986) have identified novel calcium-dependent proteins associated with mammary epithelial cell migration and differentiation. These proteins have been identified as calelectrins (Hom et al., 1986), which have a very high homology with lipocortin, a phospholipase A_2 inhibitor (Wallner et al., 1986). The relation of these proteins to prostaglandin synthesis and PI turnover in the mammary gland, especially under the influence of prolactin, remains to be explored but raises exciting possibilities in unfolding the mechanism of prolactin action at the cellular level.

6. Concluding Statement

Prolactin is a multifaceted hormone that elicits a variety of responses in the mammary gland. The mechanism by which prolactin interaction with the surface membrane of the mammary epithelial cell results in the distinctive biological effects is still largely unknown. Although our current knowledge concerning the role of this hormone in breast development and differentiation is ever expanding, there remain large gaps in our understanding. As depicted in Fig. 3, receptors for prolactin on the cell membranes exist as both cryptic and active forms. Although the function of the cryptic sites remains largely unknown, whether the receptor is cryptic or active is influenced greatly by the lipid microenvironment in which it resides.

The prolactin receptor is subject to both up and down self-regulation, but its functionality is also influenced by the action of other hormones and growth factors, as well as by other membrane proteins with which it is associated. Whether the receptor is phosphorylated, as are a variety of other peptide hormone receptors, is not known. Much like other peptide hormones, the prolactin–receptor complex is believed to form clusters and is internalized by the target cell. However, it is not clear whether this complex is recycled through the Golgi apparatus or eventually completely degraded in the lysosomes. The physiological significance of intracellular and/or milk-borne prolactin in signal transduction remains to be explored.

One area of investigation that holds great promise for the immediate future is that of identification of the intracellular relay or second messenger for prolactin. A variety of candidates for this role have been proposed, many of which alone can account for part, but not all, of the events triggered by prolactin. Thus, the multiplicity of responses within the tissue may reflect the interaction of a variety of potential intracellular signals that can be generated when any given form of prolactin interacts with one of the heterogeneous receptor species present on the target cell membranes.

ACKNOWLEDGMENTS: The author thanks Mrs. Erika Ginsburg for her assistance in preparing this manuscript and her family and staff for their boundless patience.

References

Adelman, J.P., Mason, A.J., Hayflick, J.S., and Seeburg, P.H., 1986, Isolation of the gene and hypothalamic cDNA from the common precursor of gonadotropin-releasing hormone and prolactin release-inhibiting factor in human and rat, *Proc. Natl. Acad. Sci. USA* **83:**179–183.

Akers, R.M., Bauman, D.E., Capuco, A.V., Goodman, F.T., and Tucker, H.A., 1981, Prolactin regulation of milk secretion and biochemical differentiation on mammary epithelial cells in periparturient cows, *Endocrinology* **109:**23–30.

Alhadi, T., and Vonderhaar, B.K., 1982, Induction of cryptic lactogenic hormone binding in livers of adult female mice treated neonatally with estradiol or Nafoxidine, *Endocrinology* **110:**254–259.

Al-Sarraj, K., Newbury, J., White, D.A., and Moyer, R.J., 1979, Casein turnover in rabbit mammary explants in organ culture, *Biochem. J.* **182:**837–845.

Amenomori, Y., Chen, C.L., and Meites, J., 1970, Serum prolactin levels in rats during different reproductive states, *Endocrinology* **86:**506–510.

Amit, T., Barkey, R.J., Gavish, M., and Youdim, M.B.H., 1986, Antiidiotypic antibodies raised against anti-prolactin (PRL) antibodies recognize the PRL receptor, *Endocrinology* **118:**835–843.

Anderson, C.R., and Larson, B.L., 1970, Comparative maintenance of function in dispersed cell and organ culture of bovine mammary tissue, *Exp. Cell Res.* **67:**24–30.

Anderson, T.R., Rodriguez, J., Nicoll, C.S., and Spencer, E.M., 1983, The synlactin hypothesis: Prolactin's mitogenic action may involve synergism with a somatomedin-like molecule, in: *Insulin-Like Growth Factors/Somatomedins* (E.M. Spencer, ed.), Walter de Gruyter & Co., Berlin, pp. 71–78.

Anderson, T.R., Pitts, D.S., and Nicoll, C.S., 1984, Prolactin's mitogenic action on the pigeon crop-sac mucosal epithelium involves direct and indirect mechanisms, *Gen. Comp. Endocrinol.* **54:**236–246.

Aubert, M.L., Suard, Y., Sizonenko, P.C., and Kraehenbuhl, J.P., 1978, Receptors for lactogenic hormones: Study with dispersed cells from rabbit mammary gland, in: *Progress in Prolactin Physiology and Pathology* (C. Robyn and M. Harter, eds.), Elsevier-North Holland Biomedical Press, Amsterdam, pp. 45–57.

Banerjee, M.R., 1976, Response of mammary cells to hormones, *nt. Rev. Cytol.* **46:**1–97.

Banerjee, M.R., Wood, B.G., and Kinder, D.L., 1973, Whole mammary gland organ culture: Selection of appropriate gland, *In Vitro* **9:**129–133.

Banerjee, M.R., Wood, B.G., Lin, F.K., and Crump, L.R., 1976, Organ culture of the whole mammary gland of the mouse, *Tissue Culture Assoc. Man.* **2:**457–462.

Banerjee, M.R., Antoniou, M., Joshi, J.B., and Majumder, P.K., 1983, Recent advances in hormonal regulation of milk protein gene expression, in: *Understanding Breast Cancer: Clinical and Laboratory Concepts* (M.A. Rich, J.C. Hager, and P. Furmanski, eds.), Marcel Dekker, New York, pp. 335–364.

Barkley, M.S., 1979, Serum prolactin in the male mouse from birth to maturity, *J. Endocrinol.* **83:**31–33.

Basset, M., Smith, G.D., Pease, R., and Peters, T.J., 1984, Uptake and processing of prolactin by alternative pathways in rat liver, *Biochim. Biophys. Acta* **769:**79–84.

Bergeron, J.J.M, Posner, B.I., Josefsberg, Z., and Sikstrom, R., 1978, Intracellular polypeptide hormone receptors: The demonstration of specific binding sites for insulin and human growth hormone in Golgi fractions isolated from the liver of female rats, *J. Biol. Chem.* **253:**4058–4066.

Berridge, M.J., and Irvine, R.F., 1984, Inositol triphosphate, a novel second messenger in cellular signal transduction, *Nature* **312:**315–321.

Bewley, T.A., Dixon, J.S., and Li, C.H., 1972, Sequence comparison of human pituitary growth hormone, human chorionic somatomammotropin and ovine pituitary growth and lactogenic hormones, *Int. J. Pept. Protein Res.* **4:**281–287.

Bhattacharjee, M., and Vonderhaar, B.K., 1984, Thyroid hormones enhance the synthesis and secretion of α-lactalbumin by mouse mammary tissue *in vitro*, *Endocrinology* **115:**1070–1077.

Bhattacharya, A., and Vonderhaar, B.K., 1979a, Thyroid hormone regulation of prolactin binding to mouse mammary glands, *Biochem. Biophys. Res. Commun.* **88:**1405–1411.

Bhattacharya, A., and Vonderhaar, B.K., 1979b, Phospholipid methylation stimulates lactogenic binding in mouse mammary gland membranes, *Proc. Natl. Acad. Sci. USA* **76:**4489–4492.

Bisbee, C.A., 1981a, Prolactin effects on ion transport across cultured mouse mammary epithelium, *Am. J. Physiol.* **240**(*Cell Physiol.* 9)**:**C110–C115.

Bisbee, C.A., 1981b, Transepithelial electrophysiology of cultured mouse mammary epithelium: Sensitivity to prolactins, *Am. J. Physiol.* **241**(*Endocrinol. Metab.* 4)**:**E410–E413.

Bisbee, C.A., Machen, T.E., and Bern, H.A., 1979, Mouse mammary epithelial cells on floating collagen gels: Transepithelial ion transport and effects of prolactin, *Proc. Natl. Acad. Sci. USA* **76:**536–540.

Bissell, M.J., Lee, E.Y.H., Li, M.L., Chen, L.H., and Hall, H.G., 1986, Role of extracellular matrix and hormones in modulation of tissue specific functions in culture: Mammary gland as a model for endocrine sensitive tissues, The Second NIADDK Symposium on the Study of Benign Prostatic Hyperplasia, U.S. Government Printing Office, Washington, DC.

Biswas, R., and Vonderhaar, B.K., 1987, Role of serum in the prolactin responsiveness of MCF-7 human breast cancer cells in long-term tissue culture, *Cancer Res.*, (in press).

Blank, M.S., Ching, M.C., and Dufau, M.L., 1986, Bioactivity of serum and pituitary prolactin during the rat estrous cycle, *Endocrinology* **118:**1886–1891.

Bohnet, H.G., Gomez, F., and Friesen, H.G., 1977, Prolactin and estrogen binding sites in the mammary gland of the lactating and nonlactating rat, *Endocrinology* **101:**1111–1121.

Bohnet, H.G., Shiu, R.P.C., Grinwich, D., and Friesen, H.G., 1978, In vivo effects of antisera to prolactin receptors in female rats, *Endocrinology* **102:**1657–1661.

Bolander, F.F. Jr., 1983, Persistent alterations in hormonal sensitivities of mammary glands from parous mice, *Endocrinology* **112:**1796–1800.

Bolander, F.F. Jr., 1984, Enhanced endocrine sensitivity in mouse mammary glands: Hormonal requirements for induction and maintenance, *Endocrinology* **115:**630–633.

Bolander, F.F. Jr., 1985, Possible roles of calcium and calmodulin in mammary gland differentiation *in vitro, J. Endocrinol.* **104:**29–34.

Bolander, F.F. Jr., and Topper, Y.J., 1980, Stimulation of lactose synthetase activity and casein synthesis in mouse mammary explants by estradiol, *Endocrinology* **106:**490–495.

Bolander, F.F. Jr., and Topper, Y.J., 1981, Loss of differentiative potential of the mammary gland in ovariectomized mice: Identification of a biochemical lesion, *Endocrinology* **108:**1649–1653.

Boot, L.M., Kiva, A.G., and Röpcke, G., 1973, Radioimmunoassay of mouse prolactin: Prolactin levels in isograft-bearing orchidectomized mice, *Eur. J. Cancer* **9:**185–193.

Borst, D.W., and Mahoney, W.B., 1980, Diurnal changes in mouse mammary gland DNA synthesis, *J. Exp. Zool.* **214:**215–218.

Borst, D.W., and Sayare, M., 1982, Photoactivated cross-linking of prolactin to hepatic membrane binding sites, *Biochem. Biophys. Res. Commun.* **105:**194–201.

Bourne, R.A., Bryant, J.A., and Falconer, I.R., 1974, Stimulation of DNA synthesis by prolactin in rabbit mammary tissue, *J. Cell Sci.* **14:**105–111.

Bowers, C.Y., Friesen, H.G., Hwang, P., Guyda, H.J., and Folkers, K., 1971, Prolactin and thyrotropin release in man by synthetic pyroglutamyl-histidyl-prolinamide, *Biochem. Biophys. Res. Commun.* **45:**1033–1041.

Braslau, D.L., Ringo, D.L., and Rocha, V., 1984, Synthesis of novel calcium-dependent proteins associated with mammary epithelial cell migration and differentiation, *Exp. Cell Res.* **155:**213–221.

Brown, M.S., Anderson, R.G.W., and Goldstein, J.L., 1983, Recycling receptors: The round-trip itinerary of migrant membrane proteins, *Cell* **32:**663–667.

Buckley, A.R., Kibler, R., Putnam, C.W., and Russell, D.H., 1986, Prolactin signal transduction: Involvement of protein kinase C and Ca^{+2}, *Fed. Proc.* **45:**1736.

Burnstein, S., Gagnon, G., Hunter, S.A., and Maudsley, D.V., 1976, Prostaglandin biosynthesis and stimulation of cyclic AMP in primary monolayer cultures of epithelial cells from mouse mammary gland, *Prostaglandins* **11:**85–99.

Burnstein, S., Gagnon, G., Hunter, S.A., and Maudsley, D.V., 1977, Elevation of prostaglandin and cyclic AMP levels by arachidonic acid in primary epithelial cell cultures of C3H mouse mammary tumors, *Prostaglandins* **13:**41–53.

Campbell, P.N., McIlreavy, D., and Tarin, D., 1973, The detection of the messenger ribonucleic acid for the α-lactalbumin of guinea pig milk, *Biochem. J.* **134:**345–347.

Carey, E.M., and Dils, R., 1973, Fatty acid biosynthesis. X. Specificity for chain-termination of fatty acid biosynthesis in cell-free extracts of lactating rabbit mammary gland, *Biochim. Biophys. Acta* **306:**156–167.

Carlson, H.E., Wasser, H.L., and Reidelberger, R.D., 1985, Beer-induced prolactin secretion: A clinical and laboratory study of the role of salsolinol, *J. Clin. Endocrinol. Metab.* **60:**673–677.

Carr, F.E., and Jaffe, R.C., 1981, Solubilization and molecular weight estimation of prolactin receptors from *Rana catesbeiana* tadpole liver and tail fin, *Endocrinology* **109:**945–949.

Carrington, C.A., Hosick, H.L., Forsyth, I.A., and Dils, R.R., 1981, Novel multialveolar epithelial structures from rabbit mammary gland that synthesize milk specific fatty acids in response to prolactin, *In Vitro* **17:**363–368.

Caulfield, J.J., and Bolander, F.F., Jr., 1986, Involvement of protein kinase C in mouse mammary gland development, *J. Endocrinol* **109:**29–34.

Cave, W.T., Jr., and Erickson-Lucas, M.J., 1982, Effects of dietary lipids on lactogenic hormone receptor binding in rat mammary tumors, *J. Natl. Cancer Inst.* **68:**319–324.

Ceriani, R.L., and Blank, E.W., 1977, Response to prolactin and ovarian steroids of normal mammary epithelial cell cultures, *Mol. Cell. Endocrinol.* **8:**95–103.

Chen, C.L., and Meites, J., 1970, Effects of estrogen and progesterone on serum and pituitary prolactin levels in ovariectomized rats, *Endocrinology* **86:**503–505.

Cheng, C.H.K., Wong, T.M., Blake, J., and Li, C.H., 1981, Ovine prolactin: Isoelectric-focusing and characterization of the separated components, *Int. J. Pept. Protein Res.* **18:**343–347.

Church, W.R., and Ebner, K.E., 1982, Solubilization of prolactin receptor by a zwitterionic detergent, *Experientia* **38:**434–435.

Clarke, W.C., and Bern, H.A., 1980, Comparative endocrinology of prolactin, in: *Hormonal Proteins & Peptides,* Vol. VIII (C.H. Li, ed.), Academic Press, New York, pp. 106–197.

Cohen, S., Ushiro, H., Stoscheck, C., and Chinkers, M., 1982, A native 170,000 epidermal growth factor receptor–kinase complex from shed plasma membrane vesicles, *J. Biol. Chem.* **257:**1523–1531.

Colosi, P., Marr, G., Lopez, J., Haro, L., Ogren, L., and Talamantes, T., 1982, Isolation, purification, and characterization of mouse placental lactogen, *Proc. Natl. Acad. Sci. USA* **79:**771–775.

Costlow, M.E., 1986, Prolactin interaction with its receptors and the relationship to the subsequent regulation of metabolic processes, in: *Actions of Prolactin on Molecular Processes* (J.A. Rillema, ed.), CRC Press, Boca Raton, FL, (in press).

Costlow, M.E., and Hample, A., 1982a, Prolactin receptors in cultured rat mammary tumor cells: Unmasking of cell surface receptors by energy depletion, *J. Biol. Chem.* **257:**6971–6977.

Costlow, M.E., and Hample, A., 1982b, Prolactin receptors in cultured rat mammary tumor cells: Energy dependent uptake and degradation of hormone receptors, *J. Biol. Chem.* **257:**9330–9334.

Costlow, M.E., and Hample, A., 1984, Prolactin regulation of cryptic prolactin receptors in cultured rat mammary tumor cells, *J. Cell. Physiol.* **118:**247–252.

Costlow, M.E., and Rodgers, Q.E., 1986, Subcellular localization of cryptic prolactin receptors in mammary tumor cells, *Exp. Cell Res.* **163:**159–164.

Cowie, A.T., 1969, General hormonal factors involved in lactogenesis, in: *Lactogenesis: The Initiation of Milk Secretion at Parturition* (M. Reynolds and S.J. Foley, eds.), University of Pennsylvania Press, Philadelophia, pp. 157–169.

Cowie, A.T., and Tindal, J.S., 1971, *The Physiology of Lactation,* Monographs of the Physiology Society, U.K. #22, Williams and Wilkins, Baltimore, MD.

Cowie, A.T., and Watson, S.C., 1966, The adrenal cortex and lactogenesis in the rabbit, *J. Endocrinol.* **35:**213–214.

Cowie, A.T., Hartmann, P.E., and Turvey, A., 1969, The maintenance of lactation in the rabbit after hypophysectomy, *J. Endocrinol.* **43:**651–662.

Craig, R.K., Brown, P.A., Harrison, O.S., McIlreavy, D., and Campbell, P.N., 1976, Guinea pig milk-protein synthesis, *Biochem. J.* **160:**57–74.

Crews, F.T., Hirata, F., and Axelrod, J., 1980, Identification and properties of methyltransferases that synthesize phosphatidylcholine in rat brain synaptosomes, *J. Neurochem.* **34:**1491–1498.

Daudet, F., Augeron, C., and Ollivier-Bousquet, M., 1981, Early action of colchicine, ammonium chloride and prolactin, on secretion of milk lipids in the lactating mammary gland, *Eur. J. Cell Biol.* **24:**197–202.

Dave, J.R., and Knazek, R.A., 1980, Prostaglandin I_2 modifies both prolactin-binding capacity and fluidity of mouse liver membranes, *Proc. Natl. Acad. Sci. USA* **77:**6597–6600.

Dave, J.R., and Knazek, R.A., 1983, Changes in the prolactin-binding capacity of mouse hepatic membranes with development and aging, *Mech. Ageing Dev.* **23:**235–243.

Dave, J.R., and Witorsch, R.J., 1986, Modulation of prolactin binding sites *in vitro* by membrane fluidizers. IV. Differential effects on plasma membrane and Golgi fractions of male prostate and female liver in the rat, *Biochem. Biophys. Res. Commun.* **134:**1122–1128.

Dave, J.R., Brown, N.V., and Knazek, R.A., 1982, Prolactin modifies the prostaglandin synthesis, prolactin binding and fluidity of mouse liver membranes, *Biochem. Biophys. Res. Commun.* **108:**193–199.

Dave, J.R., Richardson, L.L., and Knazek, R.A., 1983, Prolactin-binding capacity, prostaglandin synthesis and fluidity of murine hepatic membranes are modified during pregnancy and lactation, *J. Endocrinol.* **99:**99–106.

DeLouis, C., and Denamur, R., 1972, Induction of lactose synthesis by prolactin in rabbit mammary gland explants, *J. Endocrinol.* **52:**311–319.

DeMeirleir, K.L., Baeyens, L., L'Hermite-Baleriaux, M., L'Hermite, M., and Hollman, W., 1985, Exercise-induced prolactin release is related to anaerobiosis, *J. Clin. Endocrinol Metab.* **60:**1250–1252.

Devinoy, E., Houdebine, L.M., and DeLouis, C., 1978, Role of prolactin and glucocorticoids in the expression of casein genes in rabbit mammary gland organ culture: Quantification of casein mRNA. *Biochim. Biophys. Acta* **517:**360–366.

Djiane, J., and Durand, P., 1977, Prolactin–progesterone antagonism in self-regulation of prolactin receptors in the mammary gland, *Nature* **266:**641–643.

Djiane, J., Clauser, H., and Kelly, P.A., 1979a, Rapid down-regulation of prolactin receptors in mammary gland and liver, *Biochem. Biophys. Res. Commun.* **90:**1371–1379.

Djiane, J., DeLouis, C., and Kelly, P.A., 1979b, Prolactin receptors in organ cultures of rabbit mammary gland: Effect of cycloheximide and prolactin, *Proc. Soc. Exp. Biol. Med.* **162:**342–345.

Djiane, J., Kelly, P.A., and Houdebine, L.M., 1980, Effects of lysosomotropic agents cytochalasin B and colchicine on the "down regulation" of prolactin receptors in mammary gland explants, *Mol. Cell. Endocrinol.* **18:**87–98.

Djiane, J., Houdebine, L.M., and Kelly, P.A., 1981a, Prolactin-like activity of anti-prolactin receptor antibodies on casein and DNA synthesis in the mammary gland, *Proc. Natl. Acad. Sci. USA* **78:**7445–7448.

Djiane, J., Houdebine, L.M., and Kelly, P.A., 1981b, Down-regulation of prolactin receptors in rabbit mammary gland: Differential subcellular localization, *Proc. Exp. Biol. Med.* **168:**378–381.

Djiane, J., Houdebine, L.M., and Kelly, P.A., 1982, Correlation between prolactin–receptor interaction, down regulation of receptors and stimulation of casein and deoxyribonucleic acid biosynthesis in rabbit mammary gland explants, *Endocrinology* **110:**791–795.

Djiane, J., Kelly, P.A., Katoh, M., and Dusanter-Fourt, I., 1985, Prolactin receptor: Identification of the binding unit by affinity labeling and characterization of poly- and monoclonal antibodies, *Horm. Res.* **22:**179–188.

Doneen, B.A., 1976, Biological activities of mammalian and teleostean prolactins and growth hormones on mouse mammary gland and teleost urinary bladder, *Gen. Comp. Endocrinol.* **30:**34–42.

Dusanter-Fourt, I., Djiane, J., Houdebine, L.M., and Kelly, P.A., 1982, *In vivo* lactogenic effects of anti-prolactin receptor antibodies in pseudopregnant rabbit, *Life Sci.* **32:**407–412.

Dusanter-Fourt, I., Djiane, J., Kelly, P.A., Houdebine, L.M., and Teyssot, B., 1984, Differential biological activities between mono- and bivalent fragments of anti-prolactin receptor antibodies, *Endocrinology* **114:**1021–1027.

Ehara, Y., Yen, S.S.C., and Siler, T.M., 1975, Serum prolactin levels during puberty, *Am. J. Obstet. Gynecol.* **121:**995–997.

Elias, J.J., 1957, Cultivation of adult mouse mammary gland in hormone-enriched synthetic medium, *Science* **126:**842–843.

Elias, J.J., and Rivera, E., 1959, Comparison of the responses of normal, precancerous, and neoplastic mouse mammary tissues to hormones *in vitro, Cancer Res.* **19:**505–511.

Emane, M.N., DeLouis, C., Kelly, P.A., and Djiane, J., 1986, Evolution of prolactin and placental lactogen receptors in ewes during pregnancy and lactation, *Endocrinology* **118:**695–700.

Emerman, J.T., and Pitelka, D.R., 1977, Maintenance and induction of morphological differentiation in dissociated mammary epithelium on floating collagen membranes, *In Vitro* **13:**316–328.

Emerman, J.T., Enami, J., Pitelka, D.R., and Nandi, S., 1977, Hormonal effects on intracellular and secreted casein in cultures of mouse mammary epithelial cells on floating collagen membranes, *Proc. Natl. Acad. Sci. USA* **74:**4466–4470.

Erb, R.E., Sitarz, N.E., and Malven, P.V., 1977, Blood plasma and milk prolactin, and effects of sampling technique on composition of milk from suckled ewes, *J. Dairy Sci.* **60:**197–203.

Fabbro, D., Regazzi, R., Costa, S.D., Borner, C., and Eppenberger, U., 1986, Protein kinase C desensitization by phorbol esters and its impact on growth of human breast cancer cells, *Biochem. Biophys. Res. Commun.* **135:**65–73.

Fairhurst, E., McIlreavy, D., and Campbell, P.N., 1971, The protein-synthesizing activity of ribosomes isolated from the mammary gland of lactating and pregnant guinea pigs, *Biochem. J.* **123:**865–874.

Falconer, I.R., and Rowe, J.M., 1975, Possible mechanism for action of prolactin on mammary cell sodium transport, *Nature* **256:**327–328.

Falconer, I.R., and Rowe, J.M., 1977, Effect of prolactin on sodium and potassium concentrations in mammary alveolar tissue, *Endocrinology* **101:**181–186.

Falconer, I.R., Forsyth, I.S., Wilson, B.M., and Dils, R., 1978, Inhibition by low concentrations of ouabain of prolactin-induced lactogenesis in rabbit mammary-gland explants, *Biochem. J.* **172:**509–516.

Fellows, R.E., and Soltysiak, R.M., 1980, Prolactin binding sites of rabbit mammary epithelial cells in primary monolayer culture, in: *Central and Peripheral Regulation of Prolactin Function* (R.M. MacLeod and U. Scapagnini, eds.), Raven Press, New York, pp. 159–171.

Flynn, D., Yang, J., and Nandi, S., 1982, Growth and differentiation of primary cultures of mouse mammary epithelium embedded in collagen gel, *Differentiation* **22:**191–194.

Foley, T.P., Jr., Jacobs, L.S., Hoffman, W., Daughaday, W.H., and Blizzard, R.M., 1972, Human prolactin and thyrotropin concentrations in the serums of normal and hypopituitary children before and after the administration of synthetic thyrotropin-releasing hormone, *J. Clin. Invest.* **51:**2143–2150.

Forsyth, I.A., 1969, The role of primate prolactins and placental lactogens in lactogenesis, in: *Lactogenesis: The Initiation of Milk Secretion at Parturition* (M. Reynolds and S.J. Foley, eds.), University of Pennsylvania Press, Philadelphia, pp. 195–205.

Forsyth, I.A., Strong, C.R., and Dils, R., 1972, Interactions of insulin, corticosterone and prolactin in promoting milk-fat synthesis by mammary explants from pregnant rabbits, *Biochem J.* **129:**929–935.

Frantz, A.G., 1977, The assay and regulation of prolactin in humans, in: *Advances in Experimental Medicine and Biology*, Vol. 80, *Comparative Endocrinology of Prolactin* (H.D. Dellman, J.A. Johnson, and D.M. Klachko, eds.), Plenum Press, New York, pp. 95–133.

Frantz, A.G., 1978, Prolactin, *N. Engl. J. Med.* **298:**201–207.

Frantz, W.L., and Turkington, R.W., 1972, Formation of biologically active ^{125}I-prolactin by enzymatic radioiodination, *Endocrinology* **91:**1545–1548.

Friesen, H.G., 1979, Prolactin and growth hormone receptors: Regulation and characterization, *Fed. Proc.* **38**·2610.

Friesen, H.G., Belanger, C., Guyda, H.J., and Hwang, P., 1972, The synthesis and secretion of placental lactogen and pituitary prolactin, in: *Lactogenic Hormones* (G.F.W. Wolstenholme and J. Knight, eds.), Churchill-Livingstone, London, pp. 83–103.

Gala, R.R., Singhakowinta, A., and Brennan, M.J., 1975, Studies on prolactin in human serum, urine, and milk, *Horm. Res.* **6:**310–320.

Gala, R.R., Forsyth, I.A., and Turvey, A., 1980, Milk prolactin is biologically active, *Life Sci.* **26:**987–993.

Ganguly, R., Mehta, N.M., Ganguly, N., and Banerjee, M.R., 1979, Glucocorticoid modulation of casein gene transcription in mouse mammary gland, *Proc. Natl. Acad. Sci. USA* **76:**6466–6470.

Ganguly, R., Ganguly, N., Mehta, N.M., and Banerjee, M.R., 1980, Absolute requirement of glucocorticoid for expression of the casein gene in the presence of prolactin, *Proc. Natl. Acad. Sci. USA* **77:**6003–6006.

Gaye, P., and Denamur, R., 1970, Preferential synthesis of β lactoglobulin by the bound polyribosomes of the mammary gland, *Biochem. Biophys. Res. Commun.* **41:**266–272.

Gertler, A., Walker, A., and Friesen, H.G., 1985, Enhancement of human growth hormone-stimulated mitogenesis of Nb2 node lymphoma cells by 12-O-tetradecanoyl-phorbol-13-acetate, *Endocrinology* **116:**1636–1644.

Gluckman, P.D., Grumbach, M.M., and Kaplan, S.L., 1981, The neuroendocrine regulation and function of growth hormone and prolactin in the mammalian fetus, *Endocr. Rev.* **2:**363–395.

Gomez, E.T., and Turner, C.W., 1936, Effect of hypophysectomy and replacement therapy on lactation in guinea pigs, *Proc. Soc. Exp. Biol. Med.* **35:**365–367.

Goodman, G.T., Akers, R.M., Friderici, K.H., and Tucker, H.A., 1983, Hormonal regulation of α-lactalbumin secretion from bovine mammary tissue cultured *in vitro, Endocrinology* **112:**1324–1330.

Grosvenor, C.E., Maiwig, H., and Mena, F., 1970, Effect of non-suckling interval on ability of prolactin to stimulate milk secretion in rats, *Am. J. Physiol.* **219:**403–408.

Guyette, W.A., Matusik, R.J., and Rosen, J.M., 1979, Prolactin-mediated transcriptional and post-transcriptional control of casein gene expression, *Cell* **7:**1013–1023.

Hall, L., Craig, R.K., Edbrooke, M.R., and Campbell, P.N., 1982, Comparison of the nucleotide sequence of cloned human and guinea-pig pre-α-lactalbumin cDNA with that of chick pre-lysozyme cDNA suggests evolution from a common ancestral gene, *Nucleic Acids Res.* **10:**3503–3515.

Hammond, S.L., Ham, R.G., and Stampfer, M.R., 1984, Serum-free growth of human mammary epithelial cells: Rapid clonal growth in defined medium and extended serial passage with pituitary extract, *Proc. Natl. Acad. Sci. USA* **81:**5435–5439.

Harigaya, T., Sakai, S., Kohmoto, K., and Shoda, Y., 1982, Influence of glucocorticoids on mammary prolactin receptors in pregnant mice after ovariectomy, *J. Endocrinol.* **94:**149–155.

Harrison, S.C., and Kirchhausen, T., 1983, Clathrin, cages and coated vesicles, *Cell* **33:**650–652.

Hauptle, M.T., Aubert, M.L., Djiane, J., and Kraehenbuhl, J.P., 1983a, Binding sites for lactogenic and somatogenic hormones from rabbit mammary gland and liver: Their purification by affinity chromatography and their identification by immunoprecipitation and photoaffinity labeling, *J. Biol. Chem.* **258:**305–314.

Hauptle, M.T., Suard, Y.L.M., Bogenmann, E., Reggio, H., Racine, L., and Kraehenbuhl, J.P., 1983b, Effect of cell shape change on the function and differentiation of rabbit mammary cells in culture, *J. Cell Biol.* **96:**1425–1434.

Hayden, T.J., Bonney, R.C., and Forsyth, I.A., 1979, Ontogeny and control of prolactin receptors in the mammary gland and liver of virgin, pregnant and lactating rats, *J. Endocrinol.* **80:**259–269.

Hennighausen, L.G., and Sippel, A.E., 1982a, Mouse whey acidic protein is a novel member of the family of four-disulfide core proteins, *Nucleic Acids Res.* **10:**2677–2684.

Hennighausen, L.G., and Sippel, A.E., 1982b, Characterization and cloning of the mRNAs specific for the lactating mouse mammary gland, *Eur. J. Biochem.* **125:**131–141.

Hennighausen, L.G., Sippel, A.E., Hobbs, A.A., and Rosen, J.M., 1982, Comparative sequence analysis of the mRNAs coding for mouse and rat when protein, *Nucleic Acids Res.* **10:**3733–3744.

Herber, R.L., and Vonderhaar, B.K., 1986, The isolation and examination of α-lactalbumin mRNA from mouse mammary glands, Iowa Academy of Science Annual Meeting 1986, abstract #14.

Hirata, F., and Axelrod, J., 1978, Enzymatic methylation of phosphatidyl-ethanolamine increases erythrocyte membrane fluidity, *Nature* **275:**219–220.

Hom, Y.K., Sudhof, T.C., and Rocha, V., 1986, Ca^{++}-binding (dependent) proteins associated with mammary epithelial cell spreading are calelectrins, *Fed. Proc.* **45:**1912.

Houdebine, L.M., 1979, Role of prolactin in the expression of casein genes in the virgin rabbit, *Cell Differ.* **8:**49–59.

Houdebine, L.M., 1980, Effect of various lysosomotropic agents and microtubule disrupting drugs on the lactogenic and the mammogenic action of prolactin, *Eur. J. Cell Biol.* **22:**755–760.

Houdebine, L.M., and Lacroix, M.C., 1980, Effect of indomethacin on the lactogenic action of prolactin, *Biochemie* **62:**441–444.

Houdebine, L.M., Devinoy, E., and DeLouis, C., 1978, Role of spermidine in casein gene expression in the rabbit, *Biochemie* **60:**735–741.

Hughes, J.P., Simpson, J.S.A., and Friesen, H.G., 1983, Analysis of growth hormone and lactogenic binding sites cross-linked to iodinated human growth hormone, *Endocrinology* **112:**1980–1985.

Hughes, J.P., Elsholtz, H.P., and Friesen, H.G., 1985, Growth hormone and prolactin receptors, in: *Polypeptide Hormone Receptors* (B.I. Posner, ed.), Marcel Dekker, New York, pp. 157–199.

Hwang, P., Guyda, H., and Friesen, H., 1971, A radioimmunoassay for human prolactin, *Proc. Natl. Acad. Sci. USA* **68:**1902–1906.

Ichinose, R.R., and Nandi, S., 1964, Lobulo-alveolar differentiation in mouse mammary tissue *in vitro, Science* **145:**496–497.

Ichinose, R.R., and Nandi, S., 1966, Influence of hormones on lobulo-alveolar differentiation of mouse mammary glands *in vitro, J. Endocrinol.* **35:**331–340.

Imagawa, W., Tomooka, Y., Hamamoto, S., and Nandi, S., 1985, Stimulation of mammary epithelial cell growth *in vitro:* Interaction of epidermal growth factor and mammogenic hormones, *Endocrinology* **116:**1514–1524.

Jacobs, L.S., 1977, The role of prolactin in mammogenesis and lactogenesis, in: *Advances in Experimental Medicine and Biology,* Vol. 80, *Comparative Endocrinology of Prolactin* (H.D. Dellman, J.A. Johnson, and D.M. Klachko, eds.), Plenum Press, New York, pp. 173–191.

Jacobs, L.S., Snyder, P.J., Wilber, J.F., Utiger, R.D., and Daughaday, W.H., 1971, Increased serum prolactin after administration of synthetic thyrotropin releasing hormone (TRH) in man, *J. Clin. Endocrinol. Metab.* **33:**996–998.

Jacobs, L.S., Mariz, I.K., and Daughaday, W.H., 1972, A mixed heterologous radioimmunoassay for human prolactin, *J. Clin. Endocrinol. Metab.* **34:**484–490.

Jacques, S., Jr., and Gala, R.R., 1979, The influence of oestrogen administration *in vivo* on *in vitro* prolactin release, *Acta Endocrinol.* **92:**437–447.

Josefsberg, Z., Posner, B.I., Patel, B., and Bergeron, J.J.M., 1979, The uptake of prolactin into female rat liver: Concentration of intact hormone in the Golgi apparatus, *J. Biol. Chem.* **254:**209–214.

Juergens, W.G., Stockdale, F.E., Topper, Y.J., and Elias, J.J., 1965, Hormonal-dependent differentiation of mouse mammary gland *in vitro, Proc. Natl. Acad. Sci. USA* **54:**629–634.

Kahn, M.N., Posner, B.I., Verma, A.K., Kahn, R.J., and Bergeron, J.J.M., 1981, Intracellular hormone receptors: Evidence for insulin and lactogen receptors in a unique vesicle sedimenting in lysosome fractions of rat liver, *Proc. Natl. Acad. Sci. USA* **78:**4980–4984.

Katoh, M., Djiane, J., LeBlanc, G., and Kelly, P.A., 1984, Characterization of antisera to a partially purified prolactin receptor: Effect on prolactin binding in different target tissues, *Mol. Cell. Endocrinol.* **34:**191–200.

Katoh, M., Djiane, J., and Kelly, P.A., 1985a, Prolactin-binding components in rabbit mammary gland: Characterization by partial purification and affinity labeling, *Endocrinology* **116:**2612–2620.

Katoh, M., Djiane, J., and Kelly, P.A., 1985b, Monoclonal antibodies against rabbit mammary prolactin receptors, *J. Biol. Chem.* **260:**11422–11429.

Kelly, P.A., Posner, B.I., Tsushima, T., and Friesen, H.G., 1974, Studies of insulin, growth hormone and prolactin binding: Ontogenesis, effects of sex and pregnancy, *Endocrinology* **95:**532–539.

Kelly, P.A., Tsushima, T., Shiu, R.P.C., and Friesen, H.G., 1976, Lactogenic and growth-hormone-like activities in pregnancy determined by radioreceptor assays, *Endocrinology* **99:**765–774.

Kelly, P.A., LeBlanc, G., and Djiane, J., 1979, Estimation of total prolactin binding sites after *in vitro* desaturation, *Endocrinology* **104:**1631–1638.

Kelly, P.A, Djiane, J., and DeLean, A., 1980, Interaction of prolactin with its receptor: Dissociation and down-regulation, in: *Central and Peripheral Regulation of Prolactin Function* (R.M. MacLeod and U. Scapagnini, eds.), Raven Press, New York, pp. 273–288.

Kelly, P.A., Djiane, J., Katoh, M., Ferland, L.H., Houdebine, L.M., Teyssot, B., and Dusanter-Fourt, I., 1984, The interaction of prolactin with its receptors in target tissues and its mechanism of action, *Recent Prog. Horm. Res.* **40:**379–439.

Kidwell, W.R., Knazek, R.A., Vonderhaar, B.K., and Losonczy, I., 1982, Effects of unsaturated fatty acids on the development and proliferation of normal and neoplastic breast epithelium, in: *Molecular Interrelations of Nutrition and Cancer* (M.S. Arnott, J. Van Eys, and Y.M. Wang, eds.), Raven Press, New York, pp. 219–236.

Kilpatrick, R., Armstrong, D.T., and Greep, R.O., 1964, Maintenance of the corpus luteum by gonadotrophins in the hypophysectomized rabbit, *Endocrinology* **74:**453–461.

Kleinberg, D.L., 1975, Human α-lactalbumin: Measurement in serum and in breast cancer organ cultures by radioimmunoassay, *Science* **190:**276–278.

Klevjer-Anderson, P., and Buehring, G.C., 1980, Effect of hormones on growth rates of malignant and nonmalignant human mammary epithelia in cell culture, *In Vitro* **16:**491–501.

Knazek, R.A., and Liu, S.C., 1980, Dietary essential fatty acids are required for the maintenance and induction of prolactin receptors, *Proc. Soc. Exp. Biol. Med.* **162:**346–350.

Knudsen, J., Clark, S., and Dils, R., 1976, Purification and some properties of a medium-chain acyl-thioester hydrolase from lactating-rabbit mammary gland which terminates chain elongation in fatty acid synthesis, *Biochem. J.* **160:**683–691.

Kohmoto, K., Tsunasawa, S., and Sakiyama, F., 1984, Complete amino acid sequence of mouse prolactin, *Eur. J. Biochem.* **138:**227–237.

Kolodny, R.C., Jacobs, L.S., and Daughaday, W.A., 1972, Mammary stimulation causes prolactin secretion in non-lactating women, *Nature* **238:**284–286.

Koppelman, M.C.S., and Dufau, M.L., 1982, Prolactin receptors in luteinizing rat ovaries: Unmasking of specific binding sites with detergent treatment, *Endocrinology* **111:**1350–1357.

Kühn, L.C., and Kraehenbuhl, J.P., 1979, Role of secretory component, a secreted glycoprotein, in the specific uptake of IgA dimer by epithelial cells, *J. Biol. Chem.* **254:**11072–11081.

Kühn, L.C., and Kraehenbuhl, J.P., 1981, The membrane receptor for polymeric immunoglobulin is structurally related to secretory component, *J. Biol. Chem.* **256:**12490–12495.

Kühn, L.C., Kocher, H.P., Hanly, W.C., Cook, L., Jaton, J.C., and Kraehenbuhl, J.P., 1983, Structural and genetic heterogeneity of the receptor mediating translocation of immunoglobulin and dimer antibodies across epithelia in the rabbit, *J. Biol. Chem.* **258:**6653–6659.

Kulski, J.K., Nicholas, K.R., Topper, Y.J., and Qaska, P., 1983, Essentiality of insulin and prolactin for accumulation of rat casein mRNAs, *Biochem. Biophys. Res. Commun.* **116:**994–999.

Laggner, P., 1981, Lateral diffusion of lipids in sarcoplasmic reticulum membranes is area limited, *Nature* **294:**373–374.

Lamm, M.E., 1976, Cellular aspects of immunoglobulin A, *Adv. Immunol.* **22:**223–290.

Lee, E.Y.H., Parry, G., and Bissell, M.J., 1984, Modulation of secreted proteins of mouse mammary epithelial cells by the collagenous substrata, *J. Cell Biol.* **98:**146–155.

Leung, F.C., Russell, S.M., and Nicoll, C.S., 1978, Relationship between bioassay and radioimmunoassay estimates of prolactin in rat serum, *Endocrinology* **103:**1619–1628.

Levine, J.F., and Stockdale, F.E., 1985, Cell–cell interactions promote mammary epithelial cell differentiation, *J. Cell. Biol.* **100:**1415–1422.

Lewis, U.J., Pence, S.J., Singh, R.N.P., and Vanderlaan, W.P., 1975, Enhancement of the growth promoting activity of human growth hormone, *Biochem. Biophys. Res. Commun.* **67:**617–623.

Lewis, U.J., Singh, R.N.P., Vanderlaan, W.P., and Tutwiler, G.F., 1977, Enhancement of the hyperglycemic activity of human growth hormone by enzymic modification, *Endocrinology* **101:**1587–1603.

Lewis, U.J., Singh, R.N.P., Bonewald, L.F., Lewis, L.J., and Vanderlaan, W.P., 1979, Human growth hormone: Additional members of the complex, *Endocrinology* **104:**1256–1265.

Lewis, U.J., Singh, R.N.P., Tutwiler, G.F., Sigel, M.B., Vanderlaan, E.F., and Vanderlaan, W.P., 1980, Human growth hormone: A complex of proteins, *Recent Prog. Horm. Res.* **36:**477–508.

Lewis, U.J., Singh, R.N.P., Lewis, L.J., Seavey, B.K., and Sinha, Y.N., 1984, Glycosylated ovine prolactin, *Proc. Natl. Acad. Sci. USA* **81:**385–389.

Li, C.H., 1972, Recent knowledge of the chemistry of lactogenic hormones, in: *Lactogenic Hormones* (G.E. Wolstenholme and J. Knight, eds.), London CIBA Foundation, Churchill-Livingstone, Edinburgh, pp. 7–22.

Li, C.H., 1980, The chemistry of prolactin, in: *Hormonal Proteins and Peptides,* Vol. III (C.H. Li, ed.), Academic Press, New York, pp. 1–36.

Linzell, U.L., and Peaker, M., 1971, Intracellular concentrations of sodium, potassium, and chloride in the lactating mammary gland and their relation to the secretory mechanism, *J. Physiol. (Lond.)* **216:**683–700.

Linzer, D.I., and Nathans, D., 1984, Nucleotide sequence of a growth-related mRNA encoding a member of the prolactin-growth hormone family, *Proc. Natl. Acad. Sci. USA* **81:**4255–4259.

Linzer, D.I., Lee, S.J., Ogren, L., Talamantes, F., and Nathans, D., 1985, Identification of proliferin mRNA and protein in mouse placenta, *Proc. Natl. Acad. Sci. USA* **82:**4356–4359.

Liscia, D.S., and Vonderhaar, B.K., 1982, Purification of a prolactin receptor, *Proc. Natl. Acad. Sci. USA* **79:**5930–5934.

Liscia, D.S., Alhadi, T., and Vonderhaar, B.K., 1982, Solubilization of active prolactin receptors by a non-denaturing zwitterionic detergent, *J. Biol. Chem.* **257:**9401–9405.

Loizzi, R.F., 1978, Cyclic AMP inhibition of mammary gland lactose synthesis: Specificity and potentiation by 1-methyl-3-isobutylxanthine, *Horm. Metab. Res.* **10:**415–419.

Lu, K.H., and Meites, J., 1973, Effects of serotonin precursors and melatonin on serum prolactin release in rats, *Endocrinology* **93:**152–155.

Lyons, W.R., 1942, The direct mammotrophic action of lactogenic hormone, *Proc. Soc. Exp. Biol. Med.* **51:**308–311.

Lyons, W.R., 1958, Hormonal synergism in mammary growth, *Proc. R. Soc. Lond. [Biol.]* **B149:**303–325.

Lyons, W.R., Li, C.H., and Johnson, R.E., 1952, The enhancing effect of somatotropin on the mammary growth induced in rats with estrin, progestin and mammotropin, *J. Clin. Endocrinol. Metab.* **12:**937.

Lyons, W.R., Li, C.H., and Johnson, R.E., 1958, The hormonal control of mammary growth and lactation, *Recent Prog. Horm. Res.* **14:**219–248.

Majerus, P.W., Wilson, D.B., Connolly, T.M., Bross, T.E., and Neufeld, E.J., 1985, Phosphoinositide turnover provides a link in stimulus–response coupling, *Trends Biochem. Sci.* **10:**168–171.

Malven, P.V., 1983, Transfer of prolactin from plasma into milk and associated physiological benefits to mammary cells, *Endocrinol. Exp. (Bratisl.)* **17:**283–299.

Malven, P.V., and Keenan, T.W., 1983, Immunoreactive prolactin in subcellular fractions from bovine mammary tissue, *J. Dairy Sci.* **66:**1237–1242.

Malven, P.V., and McMurtry, J.P., 1974, Measurement of prolactin in milk by radioimmunoassay, *J. Dairy Sci.* **57:**411–415.

Marchetti, E., Rimondi, A.P., Querzoli, P., Fabris, G., and Nenci, I., 1984, Prolactin and prolactin binding sites in human breast cancer cells, in: *Hormones and Cancer* (E. Gurpide, R. Calandra, C. Levy, and R.J. Soto, eds.), Alan R. Liss, New York, pp. 109–117.

Martial, J.A., Hallewell, R.A., Baxter, J.D., and Goodman, H.M., 1979, Human growth hormone: Complementary DNA cloning and expression in bacteria, *Science* **205:**602–607.

Marx, J.L., 1985, Making antibodies without the antigens, *Science* **228:**162–165.

Matusik, R.J., and Rosen, J.M., 1978, Prolactin induction of casein mRNA in organ culture, *J. Biol. Chem.* **253:**2343–2347.

Matusik, R.J., and Rosen, J.M., 1980, Prolactin regulation of casein gene expression: Possible mediators, *Endocrinology* **106:**252–259.

Mayer, R.J., 1978, Hormonal factors in lipogenesis in mammary gland, *Vitam. Horm.* **36:**101–163.

McManus, M.J., and Welsch, C.W., 1981, Hormone-induced ductal DNA synthesis of human breast tissues maintained in the athymic nude mouse, *Cancer Res.* **41:**3300–3305.

McManus, M.J., and Welsch, C.W., 1984, The effect of estrogen, progesterone, thyroxine, and human placental lactogen on DNA synthesis of human breast ductal epithelium maintained in athymic nude mice, *Cancer* **54:**1920–1927.

McManus, M.J., Dembroske, S.E., Pienkowski, M.M., Anderson, T.J., Mann, L.C., Shuster, J.S., Vollwiler, L.L., and Welsch, C.W., 1978, Successful transplantation of human benign breast tumors into the athymic nude mouse and demonstration of enhanced DNA synthesis by human placental lactogen, *Cancer Res.* **38:**2343–2349.

McMurtry, J.P., and Malven, P.V., 1974a, Radioimmunoassay of endogenous and exogenous prolactin in milk of rats, *J. Endocrinol.* **61:**211–217.

McMurtry, J.P., and Malven, P.V., 1974b, Experimental alterations of prolactin levels in goat milk and blood plasma, *Endocrinology* **95:**559–564.

Meites, J., Hopkins, T.F., and Talwalker, P.K., 1963, Induction of lactation in pregnant rabbits with prolactin, cortisol acetate or both, *Endocrinology* **73:**261–264.

Meuris, S., Svoboda, M., Vilamala, M., Christophe, J., and Robyn, C., 1983, Monomeric pituitary growth hormone and prolactin variants in man characterized by immunoperoxidase electrophoresis, *FEBS Lett.* **154:**111–115.

Michael, S.D., 1976, Plasma prolactin and progesterone during the estrous cycle in the mouse, *Proc. Soc. Exp. Biol. Med.* **153:**254–257.

Michael, S.D., Kaplan, S.B., and Macmillan, B.T., 1980, Peripheral plasma concentrations of LH, FSH, prolactin and GH from birth to puberty in male and female mice, *J. Reprod. Fertil.* **59:**217–222.

Mick, C.C.W., and Nicoll, C.S., 1985, Prolactin directly stimulates the liver *in vivo* to secrete a factor (synlactin) which acts synergistically with the hormone, *Endocrinology* **116:**2049–2053.

Mills, E.S., and Topper, Y.J., 1970, Some ultrastructural effects of insulin, hydrocortisone and prolactin on mammary gland explants, *J. Cell. Biol.* **44:**310–328.

Mitani, M., and Dufau, M.L., 1986, Purification and characterization of prolactin receptors from rat ovary, *J. Biol. Chem.* **261:**1309–1315.

Mittra, I., 1980a, A novel "cleaved prolactin" in the rat pituitary: Part I. Biosynthesis, characterization and regulatory control, *Biochem. Biophys. Res. Commun.* **95:**1750–1759.

Mittra, I., 1980b, A novel "cleaved prolactin" in the rat pituitary: Part II. *In vivo* mammary mitogenic activity of its N-terminal 16K moiety, *Biochem. Biophys. Res. Commun.* **95:**1760–1767.

Mittra, I., 1984, Somatomedins and proteolytic bioactivation of prolactin and growth hormones, *Cell* **38:**347–348.

Moore, D.D., Conkling, M.A., and Goodman, H.M., 1982, Human growth hormone: A multigene family, *Cell* **29:**285–286.

Morishige, W.K., Pepe, G.J., and Rothchild, I., 1973, Serum luteinizing hormone, prolactin and progesterone levels during pregnancy in the rat, *Endocrinology* **92:**1527–1530.

Motojima, K., and Oka, T., 1983, 5′ terminal sequence of the mRNA of mouse whey acidic protein contains three possible sites of interaction with 18S rRNA, *Biochem. Biophys. Res. Commun.* **116:**167–172.

Mulloy, A.L., and Malven, P.V., 1979, Relationships between concentrations of porcine prolactin in blood serum and milk of lactating sows, *J. Anim. Sci.* **48:**876–881.

Murphy, L.J., Sutherland, R.L., and Lazarus, L., 1985, Regulation of growth hormone and epidermal growth factor receptors by progestins in breast cancer cells, *Biochem. Biophys. Res. Commun.* **131:**767–773.

Murphy, L.J., Murphy, L.C., Stead, B., Sutherland, R.L., and Lazarus, L., 1986, Modulation of lactogenic receptors by progestins in cultured human breast cancer cells, *J. Clin. Endocrinol. Metab.* **62:**280–287.

Murr, S.M., Bradford, G.E., and Geschwind, I.I., 1974, Plasma luteinizing hormone, follicle-stimulating hormone and prolactin during pregnancy in the mouse, *Endocrinology* **94:**112–116.

Nagamatsu, Y., and Oka, T., 1983, The differential actions of cortisol on the synthesis and turnover of α-lactalbumin and casein and on accumulation of their mRNA in mouse mammary gland in organ culture, *Biochem. J.* **212:**507–515.

Nagasawa, H., and Yanai, R., 1978, Mammary gland prolactin receptor and pituitary prolactin secretion in lactating mice with different lactational performance, *Acta Endocrinol. (Copenh.)* **88:**94–98.

Nagasawa, H., Miur, K., Niki, K., and Namiki, H., 1985, Interrelationship between prolactin and progesterone in normal mammary gland growth in SHN virgin mice, *Exp. Clin. Endocrinol.* **86:**357–360.

Nakhasi, H.L., and Qasba, P.K., 1979, Quantitation of milk proteins and their mRNAs in rat mammary gland at various stages of gestation and lactation, *J. Biol. Chem.* **254:**6016–6025.

Nandi, S., 1958, Endocrine control of mammary gland development and function in the C3H/He Crgl mouse, *J. Natl. Cancer Inst.* **21:**1039–1063.

Nathans, D., Lau, L.F., Lee, S.-J., Linzer, D.I.H., 1986, Changes in gene expression following growth stimulation of cultured cells, in: *Advances in Gene Technology: Molecular Biology of the Endocrine System* (D. Puett, F. Ahmad, S. Black, D.M. Lopez, M.H. Melner, W.A. Scott, and W.J. Whelan, eds.), ICSU Press, Cambridge University, Cambridge, pp. 70–72.

Necessary, P.C., Humphrey, P.A., Mahajan, P.B., and Ebner, K.E., 1984, Purification of rabbit mammary prolactin receptor by acidic elution from a prolactin affinity column, *J. Biol. Chem.* **259:**6942–6946.

Nelson, W.O., and Gaunt, R., 1936, Initiation of lactation in hypophysectomized guinea pigs, *Proc. Soc. Exp. Biol. Med.* **34:**671–673.

Niall, H.D., Hogan, M.L., Saver, R., Rosenblum, I.Y., and Greenwood, F.C., 1971, Sequences of pituitary and placental lactogenic and growth hormones: Evolution from a primordial peptide by gene reduplication, *Proc. Natl. Acad. Sci. USA* **68:**866–891.

Nicoll, C.S., 1982, Prolactin and growth hormone: Specialists on one hand and mutual mimics on the other, *Perspect. Biol. Med.* **25:**369–381.

Nicoll, C.S., and Bern, H.A., 1972, On the actions of prolactin among the vertebrates: Is there a common denominator?, in *Lactogenic Hormones* (G.E.W. Wolstenholme and J. Knight, eds), Churchill-Livingstone, London, pp. 299–327.

Nicoll, C.S., Fiorindo, R.P., McKennee, C.T., and Parsons, J.A., 1970, Assay of hypothalamic factors which regulate prolactin secretion, in: *Hyphophysiotropic Hormones of the Hypothalamus: Assay and Chemistry* (J. Meites, ed.), Williams and Wilkins, Baltimore, pp. 115–144.

Nicoll, C.S., Hebert, N.J., and Russell, S.M., 1985, Lactogenic hormones stimulate the liver to secrete a factor that acts synergistically with prolactin to promote growth of the pigeon crop-sac mucosal epithelium *in vivo, Endocrinology* **116:**1449–1453.

Nielsen, P.V., Pedersen, H., and Kampmann, E.M., 1979, Absence of human placental lactogen in an otherwise uneventful pregnancy, *Am. J. Obstet. Gynecol.* **135:**322–326.

Nikolics, K., Mason, A.J., Szonyi, E., Ramachandran, J., and Seeburg, P.H., 1985, A prolactin-inhibiting factor within the precursor for human gonadotropin-releasing hormone, *Nature* **316:**511–517.

Noel, G.L., Dimond, R.C., Wartofsky, L., Earll, J.M., and Frantz, A.G., 1974a, Studies of prolactin and TSH secretion by continuous infusion of small amounts of thyrotropin-releasing hormone (TRH), *J. Clin. Endocrinol. Metab.* **39:**6–17.

Noel, G.L., Suh, H.K., and Frantz, A.G., 1974b, Prolactin release during nursing and breast stimulation in postpartum and non-postpartum subjects, *J. Clin. Endocrinol. Metab.* **38:**413–423.

Nolin, J.M., 1979, The prolactin incorporation cycle of the milk secretory cell, *J. Histochem. Cytochem.* **27:**1203–1204.

Nolin, J.M., and Witorsch, R.J., 1976, Detection of endogenous immunoreactive prolactin in rat mammary epithelial cells during lactation, *Endocrinology* **99:**949–958.

Nyberg, F., Roos, P., and Isaksson, O., 1982, Isolation of rat pituitary prolactin isohormones differing in charge size, and specific immunological activity, *Prep. Biochem.* **12:**153–173.

Oka, T., 1983, Intracellular mediators of lactogenic hormones, in: *Biochemistry of Lactation* (T.B. Mepham, ed.), Elsevier Science Publishers BV, New York, pp. 381–396.

Oka, T., and Perry, J.W., 1974a, Spermidine as a possible mediator of glucocorticoid effect on milk protein synthesis in mouse mammary epithelium *in vitro, J. Biol. Chem.* **249:**7647–7652.

Oka, T., and Perry, J.W., 1974b, Studies on the function of glucocorticoid in mouse mammary epithelial cell differentiation *in vitro, J. Biol. Chem.* **249:**7647–7652.

Oka, T., and Topper, Y.J., 1971, Hormone-dependent accumulation of rough endoplasmic reticulum in mouse mammary epithelial cells *In vitro*, *J. Biol. Chem.* **246:**7701–7707.

Oka, T., Sakai, T., Lundgren, D.W., and Perry, J.W., 1978, Polyamines in growth and development of mammary gland, in: *Hormones, Receptors and Breast Cancer* (W.L. McGuire, ed.), Raven Press, New York, pp. 301–323.

Ono, M., Perry, J.W., and Oka, T., 1981, Concentration-dependent differential effects of cortisol on synthesis of α-lactalbumin and of casein in cultured mouse mammary gland explants: Importance of prolactin concentration, *In Vitro* **17:**121–128.

Parkening, T.A., Collins, T.J., and Smith, E.R., 1980, Plasma and pituitary concentration of LH, FSH, and prolactin in aged female C57BL/6 mice, *J. Reprod. Fertil.* **58:**377–386.

Pasco, D., Smith, S., Quan, A., Richards, J., and Nandi, S., 1983, The use of thioesterase II as a rat mammary epithelial cell-specific marker, *Cell Tissue Res.* **234:**57–70.

Pastan, I.H., and Willingham, M.C., 1981, Receptor-mediated endocytosis of hormones in cultured cells, *Annu. Rev. Physiol.* **43:**239–250.

Peillon, F., Brandi, A.M., Bression, D., LeDefniet, M., Cesselin, F., Pichon, M.F., and Racadot, J., 1983, *In vitro* studies of human prolactin secretion with concomitant evaluation of dopamine and estrogen receptors from human pituitary adenomas, in: *Prolactin and Prolactinomas* (G. Tolis, C. Stefanis, T. Mountokalakis, and F. Labrie, eds.), Raven Press, New York, pp. 311–325.

Pennington, J.A., and Malven, P.V., 1985, Prolactin in bovine milk near the time of calving and its relationship to premature induction of lactogenesis, *J. Dairy Sci.* **68:**1116–1122.

Perry, J.W., and Oka, T., 1980, Cyclic AMP as a negative regulator of hormonally induced lactogenesis in mouse mammary gland organ culture, *Proc. Natl. Acad. Sci. USA* **77:**2093–2097.

Phillips, H.S., Nikolics, K., Branton, D., and Seeburg, P.H., 1985, Immunocytochemical localization in rat brain of a prolactin release-inhibiting sequence of gonadotropin-releasing hormone prohormone, *Nature* **316:**542–545.

Pillion, D.J., Carter-Su, C.A., Pilch, P.F., and Czech, M.P., 1980, Isolation of adipocyte plasma membrane antigens by immunoaffinity chromatography, *J. Biol. Chem.* **255:**9168–9176.

Purnell, D.M., Hillman, E.A., Heatfield, B.M., and Trump, B.F., 1982, Immunoreactive prolactin in epithelial cells of normal and cancerous human breast and prostate detected by the unlabeled antibody peroxidase–antiperoxidase method, *Cancer Res.* **42:**2317–2324.

Qasba, P.K., Dandekar, A.M., Horn, T.M., Losonczy, I., Siegel, M., Sobiech, K.A., Nakhasi, H.L., and Devinoy, E., 1982, Milk protein gene expression in the rat mammary gland, *CRC Crit. Rev. Food Sci. Nutr.* **16:**165–186.

Quirk, S.J., Gannell, J.E., Fullerton, M.J., and Funder, J.W., 1986, Specificity and mechanism of biphasic action of glucocorticoids on α-lactalbumin production by rat mammary gland explants, *Endocrinology* **118:**909–914.

Rae-Venter, B., and Dao, T.L., 1983, Hydrodynamic properties of rat hepatic prolactin receptors, *Arch. Biochem. Biophys.* **222:**12–21.

Ray, D.B., Horst, I.A., Jansen, R.W., Mills, N.C., and Kowal, J., 1981, Normal mammary cells in long term culture. II. Prolactin, corticosterone, insulin and triiodothyronine effects on α-lactalbumin production, *Endocrinology* **108:**584–590.

Ray, E.W., Anerill, S.C., Lyons, W.R., and Johnson, R.E., 1955, Rat placental hormonal activities corresponding to those of pituitary mammotropin, *Endocrinology* **56:**359–373.

Rillema, J.A., 1975, Cyclic nucleotides and the effect of prolactin on uridine incorporation in RNA in mammary gland explants in mice, *Horm. Metab. Res.* **7:**45–49.
Rillema, J.A., 1976a, Effects of prostaglandins on RNA and casein synthesis in mammary gland explants of mice, *Endocrinology* **99:**490–495.
Rillema, J.A., 1976b, Activation of casein synthesis by prostaglandins plus spermidine in mammary explants in mice, *Biochem. Biophys. Res. Commun.* **70:**45–49.
Rillema, J.A., 1978, Activation of guanylate cyclase by arachidonic acid in mammary gland homogenates from mice, *Prostaglandins* **15:**857–865.
Rillema, J.A., 1980, Mechanism of prolactin action, *Fed. Proc.* **39:**2593–2598.
Rillema, J.A. (ed.), 1986, *Actions of Prolactin on Molecular Processes,* CRC Press, Boca Raton, FL.
Rillema, J.A., and Anderson, L.D., 1976, Phospholipases and the effect of prolactin on uridine incorporation into RNA in mammary gland explants of mice, *Biochim. Biophys. Acta* **428:**819–824.
Rillema, J.A., and Linebaugh, B.E., 1978, Effects of phospholipase A and Triton X-100 on guanylate cyclase activity in mammary gland homogenates from mice, *Horm. Metab. Res.* **10:**331–336.
Rillema, J.A., Linebaugh, B.E., and Mulder, J.A., 1977, Regulation of casein synthesis by polyamine in mammary gland explants of mice, *Endocrinology* **100:**529–536.
Rillema, J.A., Etindi, R.N., Ofenstein, J.P., and Waters, S.B., 1986, Mechanism of prolactin actions, in: *The Physiology of Reproduction* (E. Knobil and J.D. Neill, eds.), Raven Press, New York, (in press).
Rivera, E.M., 1969, Some observations on the activities of hGH and hPL in mouse mammary organ cultures, in: *Lactogenesis: The Initiation of Milk Secretion at Parturition* (M. Reynolds and S.J. Folley, eds.), University of Pennsylvania Press, Philadelphia, pp. 217–221.
Rocha, V., Ringo, D.L., and Read, D.B., 1985, Casein production during differentiation of mammary epithelial cells in collagen gel culture, *Exp. Cell Res.* **159:**201–210.
Rocha, V., Hom, Y.K., and Marinkovich, M.P., 1986, Basal lamina inhibition suppresses synthesis of calcium-dependent proteins associated with mammary epithelial cell spreading, *Exp. Cell Res.,* **165:**450–460.
Rosen, J.M., Guyette, W.A., and Matusik, R.J., 1979, Hormonal regulation of casein gene expression in the mammary gland, in: *Ontogeny of Receptors and Reproductive Hormone Action* (T.H. Hamilton, J.H. Clark, and W.A. Sadler, eds.), Raven Press, New York, pp. 249–279.
Rosen, J.M., Matusik, R.J., Richards, D.A., Gupta, P., and Rodgers, J.R., 1980, Multihormone regulation of casein gene expression at the transcriptional and post-transcriptional levels in the mammary gland, *Recent Prog. Horm. Res.* **36:**157–193.
Rudland, P.S., Hallowes, R.C., Durbin, H., and Lewis, D., 1977, Mitogenic activity of pituitary hormones on cell cultures of normal and carcinogen-induced tumor epithelium from rat mammary glands, *J. Cell. Biol.* **73:**561–577.
Russell, D.H., and McVicker, T.A., 1972, Polyamine biogenesis in the rat mammary gland during pregnancy and lactation, *Biochem. J.* **130:**71–76.
Russell, J., Schneider, A.B., Katzhendler, J., Kowalski, K., and Sherwood, L.M., 1979, Modification of human placental lactogen with plasmin, *J. Biol. Chem.* **254:**2296–2301.
Sakai, S., Enami, J., Nandi, S., and Banerjee, M.R., 1978, Prolactin receptor on dissociated mammary epithelial cells at different stages of development, *Mol. Cell. Endocrinol.* **12:**285–298.
Sankaran, L., and Topper, Y.J., 1982, Effect of vitamin A deprivation on maintenance of

rat mammary tissue and on the potential of the epithelium for hormone-dependent milk protein synthesis, *Endocrinology* **111:**1061–1067.

Sankaran, L., and Topper, Y.J., 1983, Selective enhancement of the induction of α-lactalbumin activity in rat mammary explants by epidermal growth factor, *Biochem. Biophys. Res. Commun.* **117:**524–529.

Sankaran, L., and Topper, Y.J., 1984, Prolactin-induced α-lactalbumin activity in mammary explants from pregnant rabbits, *Biochem. J.* **217:**833–837.

Sapag-Hagar, M. and Greenbaum, A.L., 1974, Adenosine 3′,5′-monophosphate and hormone interrelationships in the mammary gland of the rat during pregnancy and lactation, *Eur. J. Biochem.* **47:**303–312.

Sapag-Hagar, M., Greensbaum, A.L., Lewis, D.J., and Hallowes, R.C., 1974, The effect of di-butyryl cAMP on enzymatic and metabolic changes in explants of rat mammary tissue, *Biochem. Biophys. Res. Commun.* **59:**261–268.

Sassin, J.F., Frantz, A.G., Weitzman, E.D., and Kapen, S., 1972, Human prolactin: 24 hr pattern with increased release during sleep, *Science* **177:**1205–1207.

Schams, D., Reinhardt, V., and Karg, H., 1972, Effects of 2-Br-α-ergokryptine on plasma prolactin level during parturition and onset of lactation in cows, *Experientia* **28:**697–699.

Schreiber, A.B., Libermann, T.A., Lax, I., Yarden, Y., and Schlessinger, J., 1983, Biological role of epidermal growth factor–receptor clustering, *J. Biol. Chem.* **258:**846–853.

Sheth, N.A., Tikekar, S.S., Ranadine, K.J., and Sheth, A.R., 1978, Influence of bromoergocryptine on estrogen-modulated prolactin receptors of mouse mammary gland, *Mol. Cell. Endocrinol.* **12:**167–176.

Shine, J., Seeburg, P.H., Martial, J.A., Baxter, J.D., and Goodman, H.M., 1977, Construction and analysis of recombinant DNA for human chorionic somatomammotropin, *Nature* **270:**494–499.

Shiu, R.P.C., 1980, Processing of prolactin by human breast cancer cells in long term tissue culture, *J. Biol. Chem.* **255:**4278–4281.

Shiu, R.P.C., and Friesen, H.G., 1974a, Solubilization and purification of a prolactin receptor from the rabbit mammary gland, *J. Biol. Chem.* **249:**7902–7911.

Shiu, R.P.C., and Friesen, H.G., 1974b, Properties of a prolactin receptor from the rabbit mammary gland, *Biochem. J.* **140:**301–311.

Shiu, R.P.C., and Friesen, H.G., 1976a, Studies on prolactin receptors, in: *Basic Applications and Clinical Uses of Hypothalamic Hormones* (A.L.C. Salgado, R. Fernandez-Durango, and J.C. Lopez-del-Campo, eds.), Excerpta Medica, American Elsevier, New York, pp. 71–75.

Shiu, R.P.C., and Friesen, H.G., 1976b, Blockade of prolactin action by an antiserum to its receptors, *Science* **192:**259–261.

Shiu, R.P.C., and Friesen, H.G., 1976c, Interaction of cell–membrane prolactin receptor with its antibody, *Biochem. J.* **157:**619–626.

Shiu, R.P.C., Kelly, P.A., and Friesen, H.G., 1973, Radioreceptor assay for prolactin and other lactogenic hormones, *Science* **180:**968–971.

Shiu, R.P.C., Elsholtz, H.P., Tanaka, T., Friesen, H.G., Gant, P.W., Beer, C.T., and Nobel, R.L., 1983, Receptor-mediated mitogenic action of prolactin in a rat lymphoma cell line, *Endocrinology* **113:**159–165.

Sideri, M., Virgilis, G., Guidobono, F., Borgese, N., Sereni, L.P., Nicolini, U., and Remotti, G., 1983, Immunologically undetectable human placental lactogen in a normal pregnancy. Case report, *Br. J. Obstet. Gynaecol.* **90:**771–773.

Sigel, M.B., Thorpe, N.A., Kobrin, M.S., Lewis, V.J., and Vanderlaan, W.P., 1981, Binding characteristics of a biologically active variant of human growth hormone (20K) to growth hormone and lactogen receptors, *Endocrinology* **108:**1600–1603.

Silberstein, G.B., Strickland, P., Trumpbour, V., Coleman, S., and Daniel, C.W., 1984, In vivo, cAMP stimulates growth and morphogenesis of mouse mammary ducts, *Proc. Natl. Acad. Sci. USA* **81:**4950–4954.

Silverstein, A.M., and Richards, J.F., 1979, Characterization of prolactin binding by membrane preparations from rat liver, *Biochem. J.* **178:**743–751.

Singh, D.V., and Bern, H.A., 1969, Interaction between prolactin and thyroxine in mouse mammary gland lobulo-alveolar development *in vitro, J. Endocrinol.* **45:**579–583.

Singh, R.N.P., Seavey, B.K., Rice, V.P., Lindsey, T.T., and Lewis, V.J., 1974, Modified forms of human growth hormone with increased biological activities, *Endocrinology* **94:**883–891.

Sinha, Y.N., and Baxter, S.R., 1979, Identification of a nonimmunoreactive but highly bioactive form of prolactin in the mouse pituitary by gel electrophoresis, *Biochem. Biophys. Res. Commun.* **86:**325–330.

Skarda, J., Urbanova, E., Houdebine, L.M., DeLouis, C., and Bilek, J., 1982a, Effects of insulin, cortisol, and prolactin on lipid, protein and casein syntheses in goat mammary tissue in organ culture, *Reprod. Nutr. Dev.* **22:**379–386.

Skarda, J., Urbanova, E., Houdebine, L.M., DeLouis, C., and Bilek, J., 1982b, Hormonal control of casein synthesis in mammary explants from pregnant goats, *Endocrinologie* **79:**301–307.

Smith, J.J., Capuco, A.V., Alston-Mills, B., and Vonderhaar, B.K., 1986, Isolation and purification of a prolactin binding protein from bovine mammary gland, Proceedings of the American Dairy Science Association Meeting, June 1986.

Smith, S., 1977, Structural and functional relationships of fatty acid synthetase from various tissues and species, in: *Immunochemistry of Enzymes and Their Antibodies* (M.R.H. Salton, ed.), Wiley, New York, pp. 125–146.

Smith, S., and Abraham, S., 1975, The composition and biosynthesis of milk fat, *Adv. Lipid Res.* **13:**195–239.

Smith, S., and Stern, A., 1981, Development of the capacity of mouse mammary glands for medium chain fatty acid synthesis during pregnancy and lactation, *Biochim. Biophys. Acta* **664:**611–615.

Smith, S., Pasco, D., Pawlak, J., Thompson, B.J., Stampfer, M., and Nandi, S., 1984, Thioesterase II, a new marker enzyme for human cells of breast epithelial origin, *J. Natl. Cancer Inst.* **73:**323–329.

Smith, V.G., Beck, T.W., Convey, E.M., and Tucker, H.A., 1974, Bovine serum prolactin, growth hormone, cortisol and milk yield after ergocryptine, *Neuroendocrinology* **15:**172–181.

Solari, R., and Kraehenbuhl, J.P., 1984, Biosynthesis of the IgA antibody receptor: A model for the transepithelial sorting of a membrane glycoprotein, *Cell* **36:**61–71.

Soltysiak, R.M., and Fellows, R.E., 1983, Prolactin receptor expression in monolayer cultures of rabbit mammary epithelial cells: Pre- and postpartum [^{125}I]-prolactin binding activity, *J. Cell. Biochem.* **22:**121–130.

Speake, B.K., Dils, R., and Mayer, R.J., 1975, Regulation of enzyme turnover during tissue differentiation: Studies on the effects of hormones on the turnover of fatty acid synthetase in rabbit mammary gland in organ culture, *Biochem. J.* **148:**309–320.

Strong, C.R., Carey, E.M., and Dils, R., 1973, The synthesis of medium-chain fatty acids by lactating rabbit mammary gland studied *in vitro, Biochem. J.* **132:**121–123.

Suard, Y.M., Kraehenbuhl, J.P., and Aubert, M.L., 1979, Dispersed mammary epithelial cells: Receptors of lactogenic hormones in virgin, pregnant, and lactating rabbits, *J. Biol. Chem.* **254:**10466–10475.

Suard, Y.M.L., Haeuptle, M.T., Farinon, E., and Kraehenbuhl, J.P., 1983, Cell proliferation and milk protein gene expression in rabbit mammary cell cultures, *J. Cell Biol.* **96:**1435–1442.

Subramanian, M.G., and Gala, R.R., 1986, Do prolactin levels measured by RIA reflect biologically active prolactin?, *J. Clin. Immunoassay* **9:**42–52.

Takemoto, T., Nagamatsu, Y., and Oka, T., 1980, Casein and α-lactalbumin mRNAs during the development of mouse mammary gland, *Dev. Biol.* **78:**247–257.

Taketani, Y., and Oka, T., 1983a, Biological action of epidermal growth factor and its functional receptors in normal mammary epithelial cells, *Proc. Natl. Acad. Sci. USA* **80:**2647–2650.

Taketani, Y., and Oka, T., 1983b, Possible physiological role of epidermal growth factor in the development of the mouse mammary gland during pregnancy, *FEBS Lett.* **152:**256–260.

Taketani, Y., and Oka, T., 1983c, Epidermal growth factor stimulates cell proliferation and inhibits functional differentiation of mouse mammary epithelial cells in culture, *Endocrinology* **113:**871–877.

Taketani, Y., and Oka, T., 1983d, Tumor promoter 12-*O*-tetradecanoyl phorbol 13-acetate, like epidermal growth factor, stimulates cell proliferation and inhibits differentiation of mouse mammary epithelial cells in culture, *Proc. Natl. Acad. Sci. USA* **80:**1646–1649.

Talamantes, F., Soares, M.J., Colosi, P., Haro, L., and Ogren, L., 1984, The biochemistry and physiology of mouse placental lactogen, in: *Prolactin Reproductive Hormone Action* (T.H. Hamilton, J.H. Clark, and W.A. Sadler eds.), Raven Press, New York, pp. 249–279.

Talwalker, P.K., and Meites, J., 1961, Mammary lobulo-alveolar growth induced by anterior pituitary hormones in adreno-ovariectomized and adreno-ovariectomized-hypophysectomized rats, *Proc. Soc. Exp. Biol. Med.* **107:**880–883.

Taylor, J.C., Peaker, M., and Linzell, J.L., 1975, Effects of prolactin on ion movements across the mammary epithelium of the rabbit, *J. Endocrinol.* **65:**26P.

Terada, N., and Oka, T., 1982, Selective stimulation of α-lactalbumin synthesis and its mRNA accumulation by thyroid hormone in the differentiation of the mouse mammary gland in vitro, *FEBS Lett.* **149:**101–104.

Terada, N., Ono, M., Nagamatsu, Y., and Oka, T., 1982, The reversal of cortisol-induced inhibition of α-lactalbumin production by prostaglandins in the mouse mammary gland in culture, *J. Biol. Chem.* **257:**11199–11202.

Terada, N., Leiderman, L.J., and Oka, T., 1983, The interaction of cortisol and prostaglandins on the phenotypic expression of the α-lactalbumin gene in the mouse mammary gland in culture, *Biochem. Biophys. Res. Commun.* **111:**1059–1065.

Terry, P.M., Banerjee, M.R., and Lui, R.M., 1977, Hormone-inducible casein messenger RNA in a serum-free organ culture of whole mammary gland, *Proc. Natl. Acad. Sci. USA* **74:**2441–2445.

Teyssot, B., and Houdebine, L.M., 1981, Induction of casein synthesis by prolactin and inhibition by progesterone in the pseudopregnant rabbit treated by colchicine without any simultaneous variations of casein and mRNA concentration, *Eur. J. Biochem.* **117:**563–568.

Topper, Y.J., and Freeman, C.S., 1980, Multiple hormone interactions in the developmental biology of the mammary gland, *Physiol. Rev.* **60:**1049–1106.

Topper, Y.J., Nicholas, K.R., Sankaran, L., and Kulski, J., 1984, Insulin as a developmental hormone, in: *Hormones and Cancer* (R.J. Soto, A. DeNicola, and J. Blaquier, eds.), Alan R. Liss, New York, pp. 63–77.

Tucker, H.A., 1979, Endocrinology of lactation, *Semin. Perinatol.* **3:**199–223.

Tucker, H.A., 1981, Physiological control of mammary growth, lactogenesis and lactation, *J. Dairy Sci.* **64:**1403–1421.

Turkington, R.W., and Topper, Y.J., 1966, Stimulation of casein synthesis and histological development of mammary gland by human placental lactogen *in vitro, Endocrinology* **79:**175–181.

Tyson, J.E., Hwang, P., Guyda, H., and Friesen, H.G., 1972, Studies of prolactin secretion in human pregnancy, *Am. J. Obstet. Gynecol.* **113:**14–20.

Tyson, J.E., Khojandi, M., Huth, J., and Andreasson, B., 1975, The influence of prolactin secretion on human lactation, *J. Clin. Endocrinol. Metab.* **40:**764–773.

Valverde, R.C., Chieffo, V., and Reichlin, S., 1972, Prolactin-releasing factor in porcine and rat hypothalamic tissue, *Endocrinology* **91:**982–993.

Vekemans, M., Delvove, R., L'Hermitte, M., and Robyn, C., 1972, Evolution des taux seriques de prolactine au cours du cycle menstruel, *C. R. Seances Acad. Sci. [D]* **275:**2247.

Vermouth, N.T., and Deis, R.P., 1975, Inhibitory effect of progesterone on the lactogenic and abortive action of prostaglandin $F_{2\alpha}$, *J. Endocrinol.* **66:**21–29.

Vonderhaar, B.K., 1975, A role of thyroid hormones in differentiation of mouse mammary gland *in vitro, Biochem. Biophys. Res. Commun.* **67:**1219–1225.

Vonderhaar, B.K., 1977, Studies on the mechanism by which thyroid hormones enhance α-lactalbumin activity in explants from mouse mammary glands, *Endocrinology* **100:**1423–1431.

Vonderhaar, B.K., 1984, Hormones and growth factors in mammary gland development, in: *Control of Cell Growth and Proliferation* (C.M. Veneziale, ed.), Van Nostrand-Reinhold, New York, pp. 11–33.

Vonderhaar, B.K., and Bhattacharjee, M., 1985, The mammary gland: A model for hormonal control of differentiation and preneoplasia, in: *Biological Responses in Cancer,* Vol. 4 (E. Mihich, ed.), Plenum Press, New York, pp. 125–159.

Vonderhaar, B.K., and Biswas, R., 1987, Prolactin effects and regulation of its receptors in human mammary tumor cells, in: *Cellular and Molecular Biology of Experimental Mammary Cancer* (D. Medina, W.R. Kidwell, G. Heppner, and E. Anderson, eds.), Plenum Press, New York, (in press).

Vonderhaar, B.K., and Nakhasi, H.L., 1986, Bifunctional activity of EGF on α- and κ-casein gene expression in rodent mammary glands *in vitro, Endocrinology* **119:**1178–1184.

Vonderhaar, B.K., and Smith, G.H., 1982, Dissociation of cytological and functional differentiation in virgin mouse mammary gland during DNA synthesis inhibition, *J. Cell Sci.* **53:**97–114.

Vonderhaar, B.K., and Topper, Y.J., 1974, Super-active forms of placental lactogen and prolactin, *Biochem. Biophys. Res. Commun.* **60:**1323–1330.

Vonderhaar, B.K., Owens, I.S., and Topper, Y.J., 1973, An early effect of prolactin on the formation of α-lactalbumin by mouse mammary epithelial cells, *J. Biol. Chem.* **248:**467–471.

Vonderhaar, B.K., Bhattacharya, A., Alhadi, T., Liscia, D.S., Andrew, E.M., Young, J.K., Ginsburg, E., Bhattacharjee, M., and Horn, T.M., 1985, Isolation, characterization, and regulation of the prolactin receptors, *J. Dairy Sci.* **68:**466–488.

von Werder, K., and Clemm, C., 1974, Evidence for "big" and "little" components of circulating immunoreactive prolactin in humans, *FEBS Lett.* **47:**181–184.

Vreeswijk, J.H.A., DePont, J.J.H.H.M., and Bonting, S.L., 1973, Studies on (Na^+-K^+)-activated ATPase. XXXII. Occurrence and properties of (Na^+-K^+)-ATPase in immature, lactating and involuted guinea pig mammary gland, *Biochim. Biophys. Acta* **330:**173–185.

Wallis, M., 1975, The molecular evolution of pituitary hormones, *Biol. Rev.* **50:**35–98.

Wallis, M., 1980, Growth hormone: Deletions in the protein and introns in the gene, *Nature* **284:**512.

Wallis, M., 1981, The molecular evolution of pituitary growth hormone, prolactin and placental lactogen: A protein family showing variable rates of evolution, *J. Mol. Evol.* **17:**10–18.

Wallis, M., 1984, The molecular evolution of prolactin and related hormones, in: *Prolactin Secretion: A Multidisciplinary Approach* (F. Mena and C. Valverde-R., eds.), Academic Press, New York, pp. 1–16.

Wallner, B.P., Mattaliano, R.J., Hission, C., Cate, R.L., Tizard, R., Sinclair, L.K., Foeller, C., Chow, E.P., Browning, J.L.. Ramachandran, K.L., and Pepinsky, R.B., 1986, Cloning and expression of human lipocortin, a phospholipase A_2 inhibitor with potential anti-inflammatory activity, *Nature* **320:**77–81.

Wang, D.Y., Hallowes, R.C., Bealing, J., Strong, C.R., and Dils, R., 1972, The effects of prolactin and growth hormone on fatty acid synthesis by pregnant mouse mammary gland in organ culture, *J. Endocrinol.* **53:**311–321.

Weisz-Carrington, P., Emancipator, S., and Lamm, M.E., 1984, Binding and uptake of immunoglobulins by mouse mammary gland epithelial cells in hormone-treated cultures, *J. Reprod. Immunol.* **6:**63–75.

Welsch, C.W., Dombroske, S.E., McManus, M.J., and Calaf, G., 1979a, Effect of human, bovine and ovine prolactin on DNA synthesis by organ culture of benign human breast tumors, *Br. J. Cancer* **40:**866–871.

Welsch, C.W., McManus, M.J., DeHoog, J.V., Goodman, G.T., and Tucker, H.A., 1979b, Hormone-induced growth and lactogenesis of grafts of bovine mammary gland maintained in the athymic "nude" mouse, *Cancer Res.* **39:**2046–2050.

Wicha, M.S., Liotta, L.A., and Kidwell, W.R., 1979, Effects of free fatty acids on the growth of normal and neoplastic rat mammary epithelial cells, *Cancer Res.* **39:**426–435.

Wicha, M.S., Laurie, G., Kohn, E., and Mahn, T., 1982, Extracellular matrix promotes mammary epithelial growth and differentiation *in vitro, Proc. Natl. Acad. Sci. USA* **79:**3213–3217.

Wilde, C.J., Hasan, H.R., and Mayer, R.J., 1984, Comparison of collagen gels and mammary extracellular matrix as substrata for study of terminal differentiation in rabbit mammary epithelial cells, *Exp. Cell Res.* **151:**519–532.

Wilson, G.D., Woods, K.L., Walker, R.A., and Howell, A., 1980, Effect of prolactin on lactalbumin production by normal and malignant human breast tissue in organ culture, *Cancer Res.* **40:**486–489.

Wood, B.G., Washburn, L.L., Mukherjee, A.S., and Banerjee, M.R., 1975, Hormonal regulation of lobulo-alveolar growth, functional differentiation and regression of whole mouse mammary gland in organ culture, *J. Endocrinol.* **65:**1–6.

Yadley, R.A., and Chrambach, A., 1973, Isohormones of human growth hormone. II. Plasmin-catalyzed transformation and increase in prolactin biological activity, *Endocrinology* **93:**858–865.

Yang, J., Richards, J., Guzman, R., Imagawa, W., and Nandi, S., 1980a, Sustained growth of primary culture of normal mammary epithelial cells embedded in collagen gels, *Proc. Natl. Acad. Sci. USA* **77:**2088–2092.

Yang, J., Guzman, R., Richards, J., Jentoft, V., DeVault, M.R., Wellings, S.R., and Nandi, S., 1980b, Primary culture of human mammary epithelial cells embedded in collagen gels, *J. Natl. Cancer Inst.* **65:**337–343.

Zick, Y., Kasuga, M., Kahn, C.R., and Roth, J., 1983, Characterization of insulin-mediated phosphorylation of the insulin receptor in a cell-free system, *J. Biol. Chem.* **258:**75–80.

13

Bovine Placental Lactogen

Structure and Function

Robert D. Bremel and Linda A. Schuler

1. Introduction

Mammary glands are organs of reproduction in mammals. Growth of the mammary gland is coordinated with gestation in such a way that the gland is developed and prepared to produce the nutrients required for survival of the young animal when it is born. It is obvious that there would have been very strong selective pressure against an animal that was incapable of producing sufficient food for the nourishment of its young. Over the years a great deal of research has been directed at determining the mechanisms that control the development of mammary glands. Thordarson and Talamantes, in Chapter 14 of this volume, compare the role of materials produced by the conceptus in a number of different species. Because of the obvious importance of the mammary gland to milk production, an understanding of the mechanisms controlling mammary growth and development are of special importance to the dairy industry. In this chapter, we focus on the work carried out in the bovine.

Reports from areas as diverse as endocrinology and population genetics have provided impetus for attempts to determine the factor(s) produced by the bovine fetoplacental unit that may contribute to the

Robert D. Bremel • Department of Dairy Science, College of Agricultural and Life Sciences, University of Wisconsin, Madison, Wisconsin 53706. ***Linda A. Schuler*** • Department of Comparative Biosciences, School of Veterinary Medicine, University of Wisconsin, Madison, Wisconsin 53706.

increases in maternal milk production. That the conceptus might play a role in the development of the mammary gland in cattle was first shown by Forsyth and her colleagues (Forsyth, 1973; Buttle and Forsyth, 1976) in the early 1970s. Using a coculture system of bovine placental tissue and midpregnant mouse mammary gland, they were able to demonstrate that placental tissue secreted a material that strongly stimulated the development of secretory activity by the mouse mammary tissue. A report by Skjervold and Fimland (1975) shortly thereafter showed that a statistically significant sire-of-fetus effect could be identified in randomly mated populations of cattle; namely, there was a genetic influence of the male on its mate's milk production in the subsequent lactation. Such an effect could be accounted for only by factors secreted by the conceptus altering maternal glandular development.

Work on placental lactogen in the bovine has been controversial from the outset because of the earlier notion that the placentas of all animals ought to be producing similar hormones and moreover that circulating levels of these hormones should also be similar. It has become clear that some animals do not have a placental lactogen at all. Here we review the evidence that the structural characteristics of bovine placental lactogen (bPL) and the levels at which it circulates in the cow are certainly very different from two of its close relatives, the sheep and the goat. If placental lactogen indeed plays a role in mammary development, then these observations raise questions about the validity of grouping ruminants together in dicussions of the role of the placenta in mammary development (Forsyth, 1986).

2. *Chemical Characterization of Bovine Placental Lactogen*

Following the identification of human placental lactogen in the 1960s, unsuccessful attempts were made to stain the syncytiotrophoblast of bovine placentas with antisera to human placental lactogen (PL). It was concluded therefore that the bovine did not produce a hormone equivalent to human PL. Subsequently, Buttle and Forsyth (1976) quite clearly showed that a factor(s) was produced by the fetal cotyledons of the bovine which stimulated the growth of mammary gland tissue from midpregnant mice. Shortly thereafter, Bolander and Fellows (1976) reported the isolation of two proteins from frozen bovine tissue which had the characteristics of placental lactogens: It bound to PRL and GH receptors in rabbit liver and stimulated mammary development in laboratory animals, but with activities only 0.13% that of bovine prolactin. Subsequent work from several other laboratories also produced apparently different proteins with the properties of placental lactogen (Beckers et al., 1980; Eakle et al., 1982; Murthy et al., 1982; Beckers, 1983; Arima and Bremel, 1983). When evaluated in radioreceptor assays with membrane receptors from rabbits, these proteins had activities essentially equivalent to that of bovine prolactin (bPRL) and bovine growth hormone (bGH). Thus, the activities of these preparations were about 1000 times higher than those reported by Bolander et al. (1976). To this time, the reason for this large discrepancy has not been determined. Perhaps a proteolytic fragment of bPL can be produced during certain isolation procedures that has only minute amounts of activity. Alternatively, the earlier workers may have isolated a totally different protein. Certainly a protein with such low activity would have been discarded during purification of a form 1000 times as potent.

The properties of what is now considered to be bovine placental lactogen (bPL) are clearly different from placental lactogens from all other species that have been characterized. These properties are summarized in Table I. All other placental lactogens that have been characterized have molecular weights similar to PRL and GH (i.e., approximately 22,000–23,000 M_r). The molecular weight of bPL, now corroborated independently in several laboratories, is considerably greater. In its denatured form, bPL has a molecular weight of about 32,000 M_r or 50% larger than PLs of other species. The mobility that it exhibits in gel filtration systems in salt solutions at neutral pH has always been anomalous. Under these conditions, its apparent molecular weight is in the range of 40,000–45,000 with one report as high as 60,000. The higher apparent molecular weight could be due to an inherent asymmetry in the molecule or due to molecular aggregation. Further physicochemical studies will be required to distinguish between these two possibilities.

A consistent pattern of the different purification protocols has been the low overall yield of hormone. In general, the final yields have been less than 5% of the starting activity, worrisome because the final product may not be truly representative of the starting material. The low yields have also greatly hampered efforts to obtain adequate amounts of material for the types of biological studies necessary to determine the effects of bPL. Obviously, this is a very acute problem when working with an animal the size of a cow. We have recently developed a technique by which bPL is isolated from a placental fraction enriched in secretory granules obtained by gentle homogenization of fetal cotyledons and centrifugation. These granules are then collected as a zone on a Percoll gradient, lysed, and the released protein subsequently purified in several simple chromatographic steps (Byatt et al., 1986). The overall yield of this process is much higher than that attained by other methods (25–

Table I. History of Detection and Characterization of Bovine Placental Lactogen

Method of characterization	Molecular weight	Method	p*I*	Reference
Existence (coculture)	N.D.	N.D.	N.D.	Buttle and Forsyth (1976)
Purification (41-fold)	60,000	SDS-PAGE	5.9	
	22,200	GFC (denatured)		Bolander and Fellows (1976)
Partial purification	60,000	GFC (salt)	N.D.	Roy et al. (1977)
Partial purification	45,000	GFC (salt)	5.3	Hayden and Forsyth (1979)
Purification (1500-fold)	N.D.	N.D.	N.D.	Beckers et al. (1980)
Partial purification	32,000	SDS-PAGE	N.D.	Eakle et al. (1982)
Purification (1200-fold)	32,000	SDS-PAGE	5.5	Murthy et al. (1982)
Purification (4200-fold)	32,000	SDS-PAGE	5.9, 5.5, 5.4	
	40,000	GFC (salt)		Arima and Bremel (1983)
Purification (1500-fold)	33,000	SDS-PAGE	5.2	Beckers (1983)

50% of starting activity is recovered) and has permitted the isolation of relatively large quantities of the hormone from small amounts of placental tissue. The protein obtained by this method is identical in all respects to that purified earlier in our laboratory from placental homogenates.

An explanation compatible with the larger size and multiple isoelectric forms is that bPL is glycosylated. When we realized that bPL had a much larger molecular weight than other PLs, we attempted to evaluate this possibility (Eakle et al., 1982). Our early attempts yielded negative results; some of ^{125}I-bPL bound to concanavalin A agarose but we were unable to displace it with α-methyl mannoside (the standard test for specificity of binding to this lectin). Subsequent attempts with more highly purified preparations of bPL and with other lectins have yielded virtually identical results. On the other hand, the cells in which we have localized bPL (see Section 3) by immunocytochemical procedures stain intensely with PAS, a characteristic that is typical of cells producing large amounts of glycoproteins. In addition, digestion of highly purified bPL with endoglycosidases suggests that at least 6 kDa of the bPL mass may be carbohydrate (K. Shimomura and R.D. Bremel, unpublished data).

Charge heterogeneity of bPL is seen clearly when techniques are used that separate proteins based on their isoelectric points (p*I* values) such as IEF/SDS-PAGE and chromatofocusing. Chromatofocusing, in which system proteins are eluted in the order of their isoelectric points, has greatly aided purification efforts. Using this technique, we have consistently shown multiple isoelectric forms of the protein. In our original studies, we could resolve three distinct peaks of activity in the chromatofocusing eluates (Arima and Bremel, 1983). The peaks eluted at pH values ranging from 4.8 to 5.5 (slightly lower than the protein's p*I*). A clearer picture of the heterogeneity of the protein preparations is seen in two-dimensional IEF/SDS-PAGE patterns (Fig. 1; Byatt et al., 1986). The higher resolving power of this system shows that there are perhaps as many as six different isoelectric forms of a protein that elutes as a single peak in HPRPC (high-performance reversed-phase chromatography). Two-dimensional electrophoretic analysis of various fractions eluting from the chromatofocusing column has confirmed the presence of multiple forms in each of the three peaks obtained from the column chromatographic procedure.

At present, we do not know whether all forms are secreted. It remains a possibility that by isolation of material from secretory granules, we have effectively obtained a "snapshot" of the posttranslational processing. We have attempted to address this issue by subjecting fetal calf serum to the same isolation protocol as the secretory granule lysates. The results from these experiments are intriguing. The forms of bPL

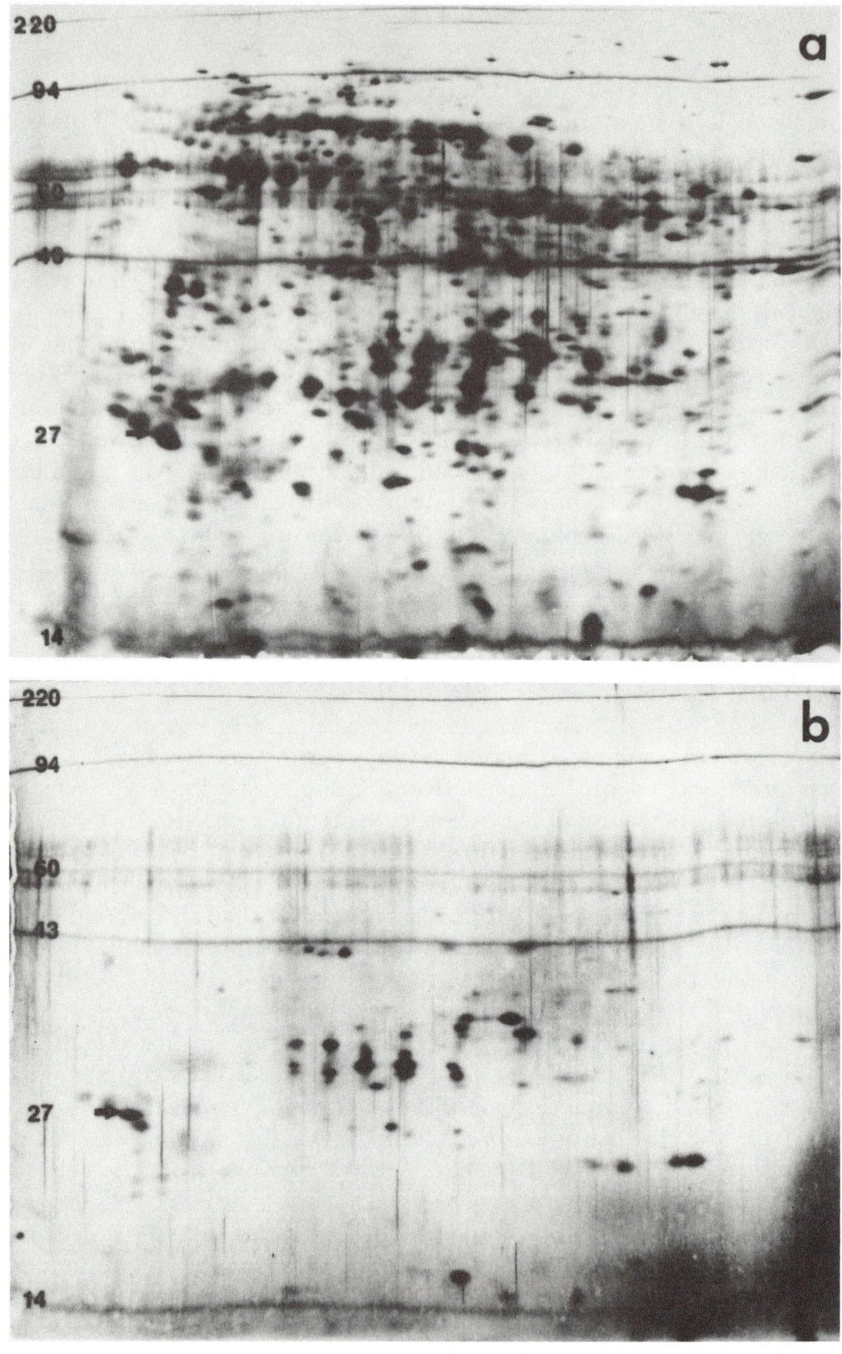

Figure 1. Two-dimensional IEF/SDS-PAGE patterns from (a) secretory granule lysates of the placenta, (b) Sephadex G-75 fractions containing the bPL activity, and (c) bPL eluted as a single peak from high-performance reversed-phase chromatography.

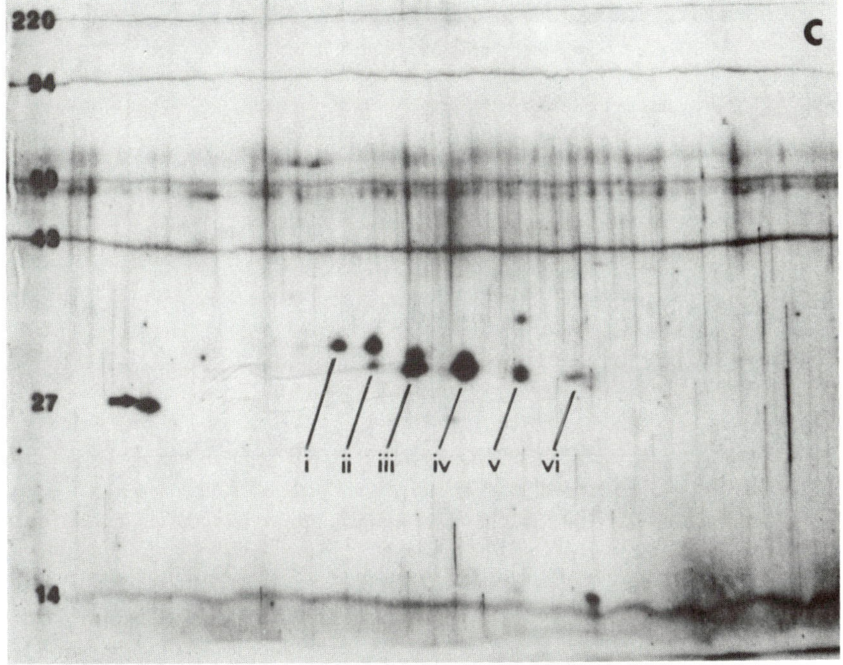

Figure 1. (*Continued*)

with the more basic p*I* values found in the preparations isolated from placental tissues, are not found in serum, but several quite acidic bPL forms, present in only very small (and variable) amounts in the placental granules, are found in relatively high concentrations in fetal calf serum (Fig. 2). Additional work is needed to determine whether the more acidic forms are more stable in serum or alternatively if only the more acidic forms are secreted.

3. Placental Cells Responsible for Secretion of Bovine Placental Lactogen

Placentas of cows, as well as those of sheep and goats, contain a population of highly granulated binucleate cells, thought to be a major secretory cell type in the placentas of these animals (Wooding, 1982). These cells stain intensely with PAS and phosphotungstic acid, both of

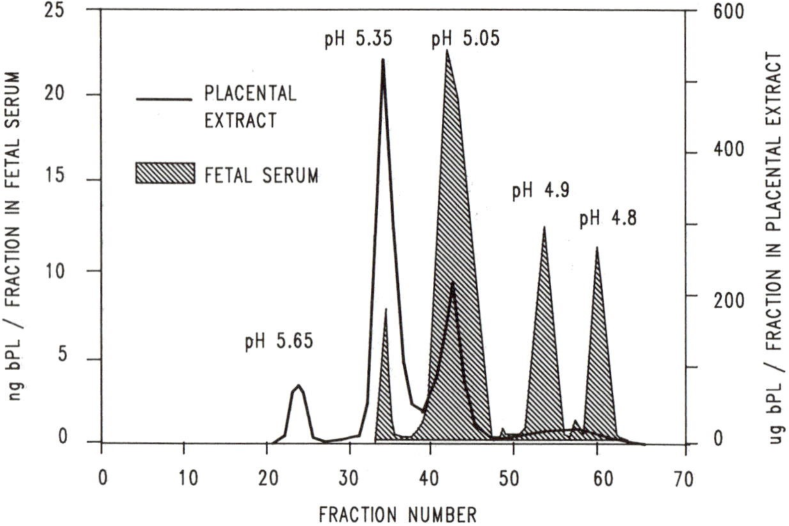

Figure 2. Comparison of the bPL activity (RIA) obtained from placental tissue and fetal calf serum and eluted from a chromatofocusing column.

these stains indicating the presence of glycoproteins. With the availability of specific antibodies for bPL, it has been possible to show by immunocytochemical techniques that these binucleate cells are the source of bPL (Fig. 3; Duello et al., 1986). The binucleate cells are found in the fetal epithelium and can be seen to change their appearance when they migrate and touch the maternal boundary. Since they are the only granulated cell type in the fetal placenta, it appears that the binucleate cells are the source granules from which we purify bPL. The granules certainly are the source of many other proteins as well, as is indicated by the two-dimensional gel electrophoresis patterns obtained from granule lysates (Byatt et al., 1986). bPL represents only a small fraction of the total proteins produced by these cells.

4. Bovine Placental Lactogen in Fetal and Maternal Serum

A minimal requirement for a proposed biological function is that the protein be present in the blood plasma in concentrations adequate to bind to receptors and thus to stimulate a hypothetical cellular response. Except for an initial report of concentrations in excess of 1 μg/ml by

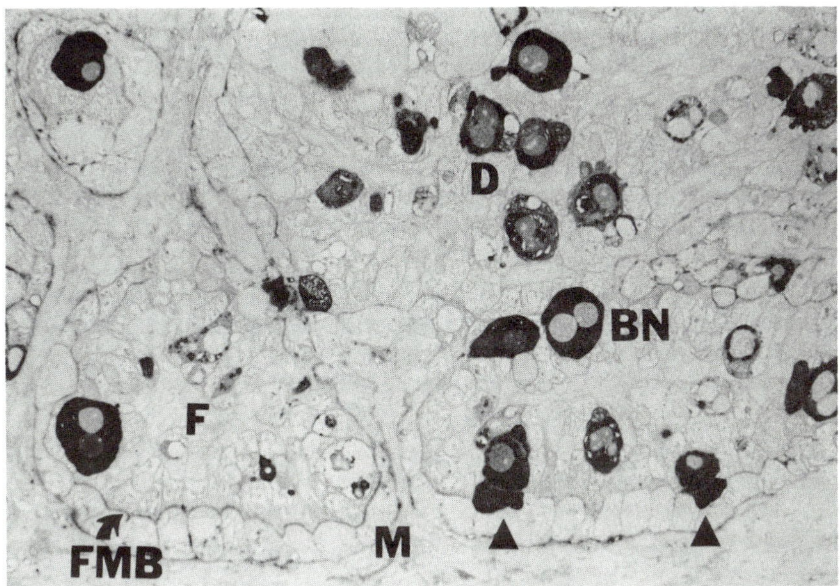

Figure 3. Immunocytochemical localization of bPL to binucleate (BN) cells of the bovine fetal placenta (Duello et al., 1986). The fetal–maternal boundary (FMB) can be seen separating the maternal uterine epithelium (M) from the fetal trophoblast (F). Staining was restricted to binucleate cells, some of which were sending processes (arrowhead) into the maternal epithelium. Some of the cells can be seen to be undergoing degenerative changes (D). Reprinted from *Endocrinology,* with permission.

Bolander et al. (1976), the levels found in bovine maternal serum in a number of laboratories by several independent methods have been uniformly low and in the range of 1 ng/ml. Using radioreceptor assays for PRL as well as GH, Kelly et al. (1976) found that bPL levels were much lower than PL levels in any of the other species tested. The levels they observed appeared to have been at the borderline of sensitivity of the assay and could be attributed to PRL in the serum samples. Buttle and Forsyth (1976) using a bioassay with a sensitivity of about 70 ng/ml were unable to detect bPL in cow serum other than that which could be attributed to PRL in the samples. Schellenberg and Friesen (1982) using the Nb2 lymphoma cell bioassay with a sensitivity of 1 ng/ml were unable to detect bPL from samples taken either during midpregnancy or near term. Again, all the activity could be attributable to PRL. Not until Beckers and colleagues (1982) used an RIA with a sensitivity of 5–10 pg was bPL consistently found in the sera of cows from day 100 to term; howev-

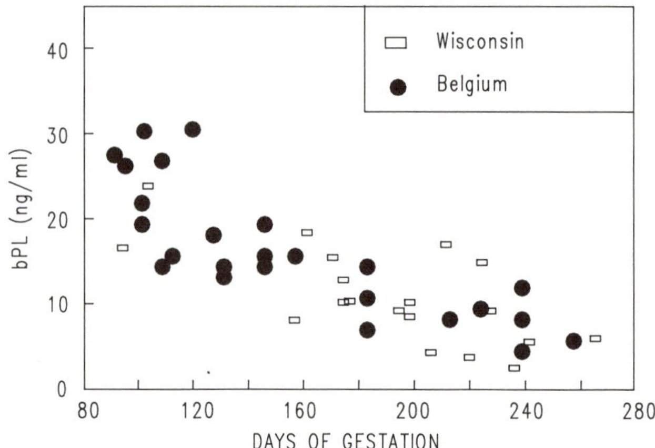

Figure 4. Levels of bPL in fetal calf serum determined independently in two laboratories. The Belgian data are from Beckers (1983).

er, the concentration never exceeded 2 ng/ml. In our laboratory, using a specific RIA with slightly lower sensitivity, we have not found samples to exceed 4 ng/ml (Byatt et al., 1986). Thus, when assays of sufficient sensitivity are used, bPL is clearly measurable in maternal serum samples albeit at concentrations 100–1000 times lower than those typically found in other species. Nevertheless, these concentrations are similar to plasma levels of a number of other protein hormones.

By contrast, the levels of bPL are relatively higher in fetal serum. The data obtained in our laboratory are superimposed on those of Beckers (1983) in Fig. 4. Beckers et al. (1982), using their RIA, reported a general decline from levels of 25–30 ng/ml at 90 days gestational age to 5–15 ng/ml toward term. Schellenberg and Friesen (1982) reported levels of 5–20 ng/ml at 180 days of gestation. Thus, similar results are obtained with independently purified proteins and independently developed assay procedures. These findings are particularly relevant to scientists examining the role of PRL and/or growth substances in cell culture systems where fetal calf serum is used.

5. Biological Activity of Bovine Placental Lactogen in Rabbit and Bovine Tissues

Placental lactogen in the maternal circulation of the bovine is certainly lower than that found in other species. But are the levels sufficient to evoke a biological response? Careful appraisal of the available data points out that the functions of bovine placental lactogen (and placental lactogen in all species for that matter) are largely hypothetical. There is no known biological indicator that is specific for a placental lactogen. All the assays used to assess the activity of PL are tests for PRL and/or GH activity and in general do not use tissue from the same species from which the hormone has been isolated. The results we have obtained in our attempts to evaluate the biological activity of bPL in *bovine* tissue

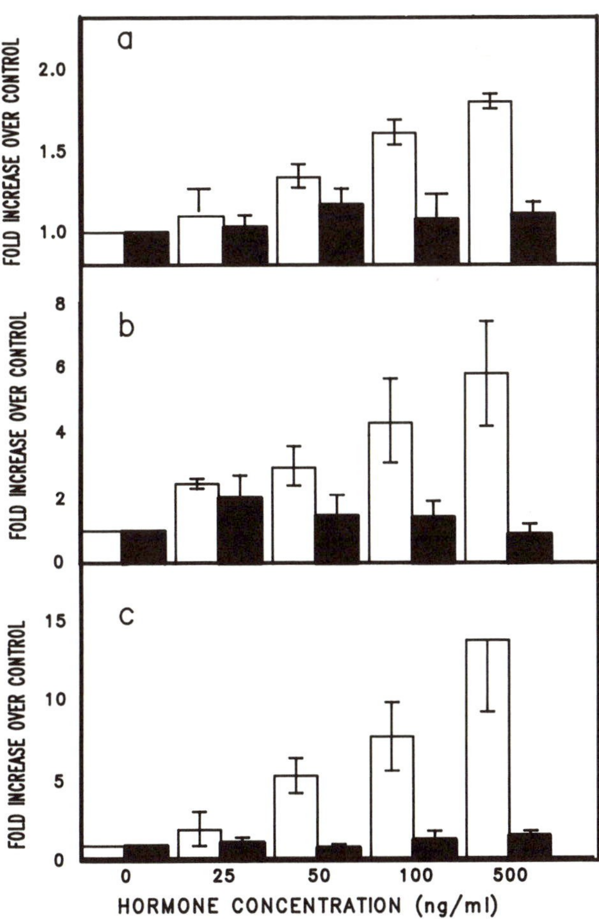

Figure 5. Comparison of the lactogenic activities of bPL (■) and bPRL (□) in bovine mammary tissue using several different indicators: (a) fatty acid synthesis; (b) casein synthesis; and (c) α-lactalbumin accumulation in the medium.

underscore the necessity to evaluate a supposed biological activity in the homologous species.

From its name, it is obvious that placental lactogen is thought to be lactogenic. A property that is characteristic of lactogenic hormones is their ability to stimulate the synthesis of milk constituents in mammary tissue from pregnant animals. Tissue from mice, rabbits, and rats is generally used. In our initial studies, we chose to use mammary tissue from a pregnant rabbit to test the biological activity of the preparations we had isolated. Two indicators were used: synthesis of milk fat and synthesis of casein (Byatt and Bremel, 1986). By both of these criteria, bPL had approximately the same potency as bPRL. We then evaluated the activity in tissue from midpregnant heifers using the same indicators and in addition with a specific RIA measured the secretion of α-lactalbumin. As in rabbit tissue, clear responses to increases in prolactin doses were seen with all indicators. However, bPL did not stimulate any of the lactogenic indicators (Fig. 5).

Two lines of evidence indicate that bovine placental lactogen binds to receptors in bovine mammary tissue. Beckers (1983) demonstrated high-affinity binding to bovine mammary tissue (Table II). He also showed high-affinity binding to membrane receptors from both corpus luteum and liver of pregnant cattle. When ^{125}I-bPL was used in competition assays with bPL, bPRL, and bGH, these receptors showed relatively low cross reactivities with either bPRL or bGH, indicating the presence of a receptor type in these tissues that was *specific* for bPL. Clearly, the presence of specific receptors along with the inability of these receptors to generate a typical PRL intracellular response indicates that the intracellular coupling mechanism is different from that of prolactin receptors. Moreover, to our surprise, we have found in some preliminary experiments that bPL is *antagonistic* to the action of PRL in bovine mammary tissue. Bovine placental lactogen totally blocked all PRL indicators when used in a concentration 10-fold in excess of that of PRL.

Table II. Characteristics of Receptors for Placental Lactogen in the Cow[a]

Tissue of origin	K_a (M^{-1})	Number of sites (fmol/mg)
Liver	6.7×10^9	8.5
Endometrium	9.3×10^9	13.3
Corpus luteum	8.4×10^9	3.1
Mammary	3.7×10^{10}	0.7
	1.0×10^9	15.6

[a]Data from Beckers (1983).

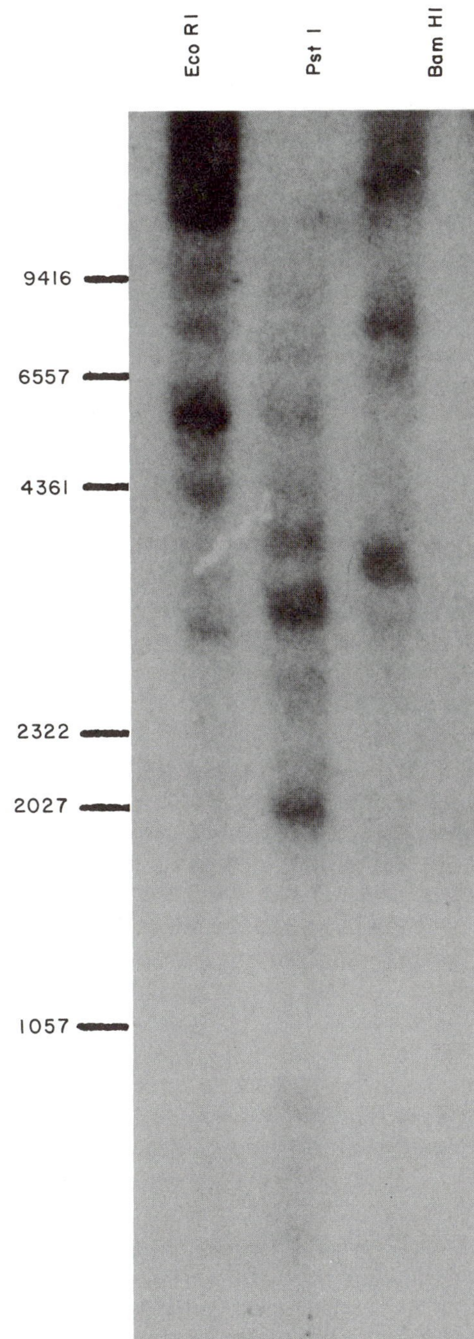

Figure 6. bPL related sequences in the bovine genome. Bovine pituitary DNA cut to completion, with the restriction endonucleases designated above, was fractionated by electrophoresis in 1% agarose, transferred to nitrocellulose, and hybridized to bPL582 (3 × SSC, 50-mm sodium phosphate, 5× Denhardt's, 0.1% SDS, 200 μg/ml herring sperm DNA at 65°C; washes 45 min each at 65°C, 2 × SSC, 0.2% SDS). Size markers in base pairs are noted on the left of the autoradiograph.

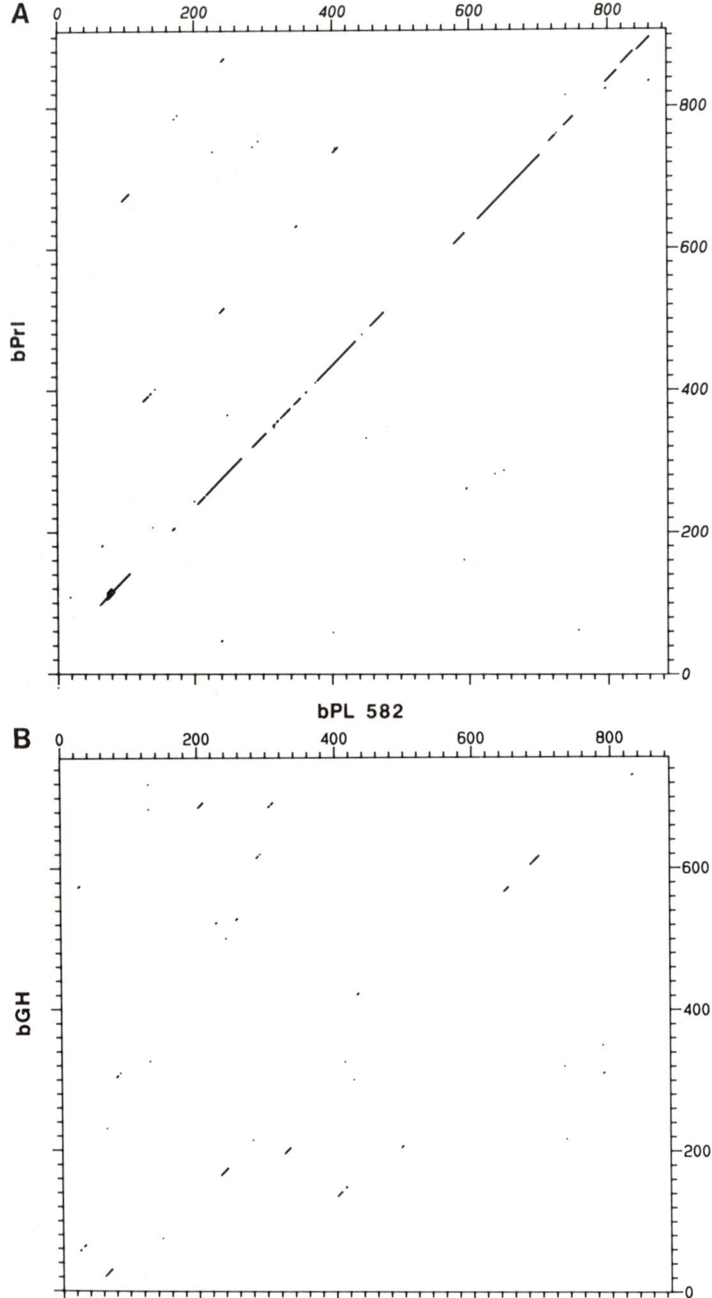
A
0
200
400
600
800
800
600
400
200
0
bPrl
bPL 582
B
0
200
400
600
800
600
400
200
0
bGH

6. Evidence for a Family of Related Genes Expressed in the Bovine Placenta

In our initial studies to identify the gene coding for bPL, we looked for a gene expressed by the placenta that was similar, but not identical, to prolactin and growth hormone. We were able to isolate a genomic clone from a bovine genomic library, a portion of which hybridized to bovine prolactin cDNA under conditions of low stringency. A restriction enzyme fragment from this clone was then used to screen a cDNA library made from bovine fetal cotyledon. This prolactin-related gene was expressed in bovine placenta, as shown by our isolation of a cDNA exemplified by bPL582. When this cDNA was hybridized to bovine genomic DNA cut with various restriction enzymes under conditions of moderate stringency, a complex pattern was seen (Fig. 6). This type of pattern is indicative of multiple related genes. Further screening of the cotyledonary cDNA library indicated that not only does the bovine genome contain more members of the growth hormone gene family than originally thought, but at least three of these genes are expressed in fetal placenta. We have identified three discrete, related cDNAs from our cotyledonary cDNA library which are members of this gene family. The mRNAs corresponding to these genes are present at moderately high levels, comprising 0.1–0.25% of the total RNA.

Each of the three cDNAs isolated from the bovine cotyledonary cDNA library is more similar to PRL than to GH (Fig. 7). Our three characterized cDNAs are about 70% homologous to bovine prolactin cDNA at the level of the nucleotide sequence and about 40% homologous at the level of predicted amino acid sequence. They are 75–90% similar to one another at the level of nucleotide sequence, and 50–75% homologous at the level of amino acid sequence. As expected, the predicted proteins have structural features that are more similar to prolactin than growth hormone. Six cysteine residues are positioned similarly to those of bPRL, suggesting three disulfide bonds, compared to two for GH. However, all three proteins contain more tryptophan residues than

---

Figure 7. Comparison of the nucleotide sequence of bPL582 (horizontal axes in base pairs) to (a) bovine prolactin cDNA and (b) bovine GH cDNA (vertical axes) (Sasavage et al., 1982; Woychik et al., 1982) using the Dotplot program of Devereux and Haeberli (1986). Dots are placed on the matrix in positions where the two sequences are homologous; if the sequences are identical, a solid line 45° to the ordinate would result. The relatively more continuous line resulting from the comparison of bovine prolactin cDNA to bPL582 indicates a higher level of homology of the placental hormone to prolactin than growth hormone.

other PRLs and GHs. These prolactin-related products from the placenta have three tryptophans, whereas mammalian prolactins generally have two, and growth hormones, a single residue. In addition, these cDNAs predict two to four potential sites for N-glycosylation (Asn-X-Ser or Asn-X-Thr), not found in bPRL. The conservation of these structural features suggests that they diverged from one another following the original gene duplication from prolactin, rather than having independently evolved from prolactin.

The bovine is not the only mammal where multiple prolactin-related genes are expressed by the placenta; similar findings have also been reported in the rat and mouse (Linzer and Nathans, 1984, 1985; Linzer et al., 1985; Peden et al., 1985; Duckworth et al., 1986). In primates, multiple placental lactogen genes also have been described. However, they code for proteins very similar to GH (reviewed by Moore et al., 1982; Miller and Eberhardt, 1983; Kidd et al., 1983). In contrast, our results, as well as work done with the rats and mice, indicate that these placental hormones in nonprimates may have a different evolutionary origin.

The relation of these cDNAs to the multiple isoelectric forms of the protein described above is not known at present. However, the demonstration, at both the protein and DNA levels, of unexpected complexity in these placental hormones suggests exciting possible roles for these hormones in a variety of actions, including those on mammary tissue during gestation.

7. Summary and Conclusions

Despite our biochemical understanding of these hormones in the bovine, little is known of their actions. Possible functions for what may be a family of hormones are as diverse as those reported for growth hormone and prolactin, including roles in both mother and fetus. In the mother, these hormones are good candidates for a prolactin-like role in the development of the mammary gland during pregnancy. A recent study by Schams et al. (1984) demonstrated that blockage of pituitary prolactin release in first-calf heifers during pregnancy did not affect development of mammary secretory apparatus. Mammary development that occurs during the first pregnancy is also an efficient predictor of the genetic merit of an animal and in addition may have a strong bearing on the lifetime production capability of an animal. Most available evidence now suggests that under normal conditions the amount of milk a cow will produce during a lactation is determined by events that take place prior to parturition (Forsyth, 1986). A mammogenic stimulus associated with placental lactogen remains a potential candidate for increasing the productivity of dairy cattle. Any positive effects on animal efficiency attained in this way would produce results that are additive with galactopoietic agents such as growth hormone.

Milk and dairy products made from milk are important components of the diets of many cultures around the world. Agricultural programs of many nations have concentrated on increasing the productive efficiency of their livestock populations. Milk production of different breeds of cattle varies considerably. Analysis of genetic information of dairy cattle populations indicates that a large number of genes are involved in the milk production trait. Although the heritability of milk production is relatively low, in the range of 0.2–0.3, the widespread application of population genetics to dairy cattle populations in Europe and North America has led to large increases in milk production. We are just now beginning to see the cumulative results of several generations of intensive selection and it is estimated that the current genetic trend in the United States is increasing milk production over 100 kg/year. Nevertheless, it is also apparent from the dramatic increases in milk production attained using bovine growth hormone produced by recombinant DNA technology that there exists a potential for major impacts on productive efficiency of dairy cows and other domestic species as well.

ACKNOWLEDGMENTS: This work was supported by the College of Agricultural and Life Sciences, Hatch Grant 5124, NSF Grant PCM 8416415, USDA 85-CRCR-1-1837, and USDA Cooperative Agreement 58-32U4-4-776.

References

Arima, Y., and Bremel, R.D., 1983, Purification and characterization of bovine placental lactogen, *Endocrinology* **113:**2186–2194.

Beckers, J.F., Fromont-Lienard, C., VanDerZwalmen, P., Wouters-Ballman, P., and Ectors, F., 1980, *Ann. Med. Vet.* **134:**585–595.

Beckers, J.F., De Coster, R., Wouters-Ballman, P., Fromont-Lienard, Ch., VanDer-Zwalmen, P., and Ectors, F., 1982, Dosage radioimmunologique de l'hormone placentaire somatotrope et memmotrope bovine, *Ann. Med. Vet.* **126:**9–21.

Beckers, J.F., 1983, L'Hormone placentaire somato-mammotrope bovine, Thesis, University of Liege, Belgium.

Bolander, F.F. Jr., and Fellows, R.E., 1976, Purification and characterization of bovine placental lactogen, *J. Biol. Chem.* **251:**2703–2708.

Bolander, F.F. Jr., Ulberg, L.C., and Fellows, R.E., 1976, Circulating placental lactogen levels in dairy and beef cattle, *J. Endocrinol.* **99:**1273–1278.

Byatt, J.D., Shimomura, K., Duello, R.D., and Bremel, R.D., 1986, Isolation and characterization of multiple forms of bovine placental lactogen from secretory granules of the fetal cotyledon, *Endocrinology* **119:**1343–1350.

Byatt, J.C., and Bremel, R.D., 1986, The lactogenic effect of bovine placental lactogen on pregnant rabbit but not pregnant heifer mammary gland explant, *J. Dairy Sci.* **69:**2066–2071.

Buttle, H.L., and Forsyth, I.A., 1976, Placental lactogen in the cow, *J. Endocrinol.* **68:**141–146.

Devereux, J., and Haeberli, P., 1986, Sequence analysis software package, University of Wisconsin Genetics Computer Group, Version 4, UW Biotechnology Center.

Duckworth, M.L., Peden, L., and Friesen, H.G., 1986, The characterization of two closely related prolactin-like cDNA clones from rat placenta, Sixty-eighth Annual Meeting of the Endocrine Society, Abstract 739.

Duello, T.M., Byatt, J.C., and Bremel, R.D., 1986, Immunocytochemical localization of placental lactogen in bovine placentomes, *Endocrinology* **119:**1351–1355.

Eakle, K.A., Arima, Y., Swanson, P., Grimek, H., and Bremel, R.D., 1982, A 32,000 molecular weight protein from bovine placenta with placental lactogen-like activity in radioreceptor assays, *Endocrinology* **110:**1758–1765.

Forsyth, I.A., 1973, Secretion of a prolactin-like hormone by the placenta in ruminants, in: *Le Corps Jaune (Colloque de la Société Nationale pour l'Étude de la Stérilité et de Fécondité)* (R. Denamur and A. Netter, eds.), Masson Press, Paris, pp. 239–255.

Forsyth, I.A., 1986, Variation among species in the endocrine control of mammary growth and function: The roles of prolactin, growth hormone and placental lactogen, *J. Dairy Sci.* **69:**886–903.

Hayden, T.J., Forsyth, I.A., 1979, Bovine placental lactogen: purification and characterization, *J. Endocrinol.* **80:**68p (Abstract).

Kelly, P.A., Tsushima, T., Shiu, R.P.C., and Friesen, H.G., 1976, Lactogenic and growth hormone-like activities in pregnancy determined by radioreceptor assays, *Endocrinology* **99:**765–774.

Kidd, V.M., Barrera-Saldana, H.A., and Saunders, G.F., 1983, The human growth hormone and placental lactogen gene complex, in: *Perspectives on Genes and the Molecular Biology of Cancer* (D.L. Robberson and G.F. Saunders, eds.), Raven Press, New York, pp. 143–181.

Linzer, D.I.H., and Nathans, D., 1984, Nucleotide sequence of a growth-related mRNA encoding a member of the prolactin-growth hormone family, *Proc. Natl. Acad. Sci. USA* **81:**4255–4259.

Linzer, D.I.H., and Nathans, D., 1985, A new member of the prolactin-growth hormone gene family expressed in mouse placenta, *EMBO J.* **4:**1419–1423.

Linzer, D.I.H., Lee, S.-J., Ogren, L., Talamantes, F., and Nathans, D., 1985, Identification of proliferin mRNA and protein in mouse placenta, *Proc. Natl. Acad. Sci. USA* **82:**4356–4359.

Miller, W.L., and Eberhardt, N.L., 1983, Structure and evolution of the growth hormone gene family, *Endocr. Rev.* **4:**97–130.

Moore, D.D., Conkling, M.A., and Goodman, H.M., 1982, Human growth hormone: A multigene family, *Cell* **29:**285–286.

Murthy, G.S., Schellenberg, C., and Friesen, H.G., 1982, Purification and characterization of bovine placental lactogen, *Endocrinology* **111:**2117–2124.

Peden, L., Duckworth, M.L., and Friesen, H.G., 1985, Characterization of a family of prolactin-like clones from rat placenta, Sixty-seventh Annual Meeting of the Endocrine Society, Baltimore, Abstract 526.

Roy, B.P., Grinwich, D.L., Murthy, G.S., and Friesen, H.G., 1977, Studies on bovine placental lactogen, Fifty-Ninth Annual Meeting of the Endocrine Society, Baltimore, Abstract 354.

Sasavage, N.L., Nilson, J.H., Horowitz, S., and Rottman, F.M., 1982, Nucleotide sequence of bovine prolactin messenger RNA, *J. Biol. Chem.* **257:**678–681.

Schams, D., Russe, I., Schallenberger, E., Prokopp, S., and Chan, J.S.D., 1984, The role of steroid hormones, prolactin and placental lactogen on mammary gland development in ewes and heifers, *J. Endocrinol.* **102:**121–130.

Schellenberger, C., and Freisen, H.G., 1982, The bioassay of bovine placental lactogen, *Endocrinology* **111:**2125–2128.

Skjervold, H., and Fimland, E., 1975, Evidence for a possible influence of the fetus on the milk yield of the dam, *Z. Tierzuchtung Zuchtungsbiol.* **92:**1313–1317.

Wooding, F.B.P., 1982, The role of the binucleate cell in ruminant placental structure, *J. Reprod. Fertil.* **76:**499–512.

Woychik, R.P., Camper, S.C., Lyons, R.L., Horowitz, S., Goodwin, E.C., and Rottman, F.M., 1982, Cloning and nucleotide sequencing of the bovine growth hormone gene, *Nucleic Acids Res.* **10:**7197–7211.

14

Role of the Placenta in Mammary Gland Development and Function

Gudmundur Thordarson and Frank Talamantes

1. Introduction

Successful mammary gland development and subsequent lactation are dependent on a complex interaction between a number of hormones. Using endocrinectomized (hypophysectomized, ovariectomized, and adrenalectomized) rats, Lyons et al. (1958) demonstrated the minimum hormonal requirements for mammary gland growth, differentiation, and milk secretion. They found that a combination of estrogen, growth hormone, and adrenal steroid was needed for duct growth. To obtain lobuloalveolar growth, two additional hormones were needed—progesterone and prolactin. For milk secretion, only prolactin and adrenal steroid were required. Similar hormonal requirements exist for mammary gland development and milk secretion in endocrinectomized mice (Nandi, 1958), It is not known to what extent these results apply to other species. Although these hormonal treatments may be sufficient to stimulate mammary development and milk secretion, the situation is normally much more complex. Insulin (Topper et al., 1984) and thyroid hormones (Bhattacharjee and Vonderhaar, 1984) affect mammary gland function directly, and hormones produced by the placenta undoubtedly make an important contribution to the development of the mammary gland.

Gudmundur Thordarson and Frank Talamantes • Department of Biology, Thimann Laboratories, University of California, Santa Cruz, California 95064.

The endocrine function of the placenta has been known since the turn of the century (see Allen, 1975, for references), and it is now well established that the placenta is the source of a variety of steroid and polypeptide hormones. The best-characterized placental polypeptide hormones are chorionic gonadotropin and placental lactogen. Chorionic gonadotropin has been purified and characterized from the human (Birken and Canfield, 1980) and horse (Papkoff et al., 1978) and identified in some other primate species (Hobson, 1983). Placental lactogen has been purified and partially characterized from three mammalian orders, Primata (Josimovich and MacLaren, 1962; Shome and Friesen, 1971; Josimovich et al., 1973), Rodentia (Robertson and Friesen, 1975; Colosi et al., 1982; Southard et al., 1986), and Artiodactyla (Chan et al., 1976; Murthy et al., 1982; Chapter 13 in this volume). Placental lactogen is structurally related to growth hormone and prolactin (Bewley et al., 1972; Bolander and Fellows, 1976; Hurley et al., 1977a,b; Shome and Parlow, 1977) and shows both growth hormone-like and prolactin-like activity in a variety of biological tests (Josimovich and MacLaren, 1962; Kaplan and Grumbach, 1964; Florini et al., 1966; Turtle and Kipnis, 1967; Forsyth and Folley, 1970; Chan et al., 1976; Hurley et al., 1977c; Butler et al., 1978; Colosi et al., 1982; Freemark and Handwerger, 1982, 1984; Southard et al., 1986; Thordarson et al., 1986). Relaxin, which may be important for mammary gland development (Wright and Anderson, 1982), has recently been detected in the human placenta (Yki-Järvinen and Wahlström, 1984; Koay et al., 1985) and has been purified from the rabbit placenta (Fields et al., 1982). The ability of the placenta to synthesize steroid hormones varies substantially even between related species. In the sheep, for example, the placenta secretes sufficient amounts of progesterone after days 50–60 to maintain pregnancy, but ovariectomy of goats causes abortion at any stage of pregnancy, since the corpus luteum remains the main source of progesterone throughout pregnancy (Thorburn et al., 1977).

In this chapter, we first briefly describe the mammary development that occurs during pregnancy in different species, and then we discuss the hormonal control provided by the placenta in the process. This chapter is limited to the effects of protein hormones of placental origin, as the effects of steroid hormones on mammary development are presented elsewhere in this book (see Chapter 15 in this volume). Similarly, as one of the chapters in this book is devoted to placental lactogen in the cow (see Chapter 13 in this volume), this species is not included in this presentation.

2. Mammary Gland Development during Pregnancy

2.1. General

The mammary gland consists of supportive adipose and connective tissue (stroma) and epithelial tissue (parenchyma). The growth of the mammary gland is slow from birth until puberty and does not exceed the growth rate of the rest of the body (isometric growth). At puberty or just before the onset of the ovarian cycle, mammary gland growth becomes allometric, growing at a faster rate than the rest of the body. Subsequently, this growth rate slows to isometric in unmated adult females (see reviews by Cowie and Tindal, 1971; Anderson, 1974). Mammary gland growth during the estrous cycle varies considerably between species, but formation of true alveolar tissue usually does not take place except during pseudopregnancy, when alveolar formation can be comparable to that seen in midpregnancy (Cowie et al., 1980). Further growth and differentiation of the mammary gland occur only during gestation. During pregnancy, the epithelial tissue grows and differentiates to form an active tissue capable of milk secretion, and by the time parturition occurs, stromal tissue has largely been replaced by secretory alveolar tissue.

Mammary gland development during pregnancy in mice, rats, hamsters, guinea pigs, goats, sheep, and humans is described briefly in the following sections. These species are specifically the subject of this chapter, since mammary development has been investigated in all of them to some extent and there is evidence to suggest that placental lactogenic hormones are involved in the mammary gland development of all these species. Mammary gland development under different physiological conditions has been reviewed previously by Cowie et al. (1980) and Topper and Freeman (1980).

2.2. Mouse

Using the total DNA content of the mammary gland to estimate growth, Brookreson and Turner (1959) found that about 30% of the total growth of the mammary gland during pregnancy and lactation took place between days 6 and 12 of gestation and about 47% occurred between day 12 of pregnancy and term. The remaining 20% of total mammary growth took place during the first 14 days of lactation. Similar results were obtained by Munford (1963, 1964). The proliferation rate of the epithelial cells in the mouse mammary gland has been estimated by radioautography after labeling with [^{3}H]-thymidine (Traurig, 1967). The highest rate of proliferation was found on day 4 of gestation with a second smaller peak on day 12. More recently, Zwierzchowski et al. (1984) observed a good correlation between DNA polymerase α activity and DNA synthesis during pregnancy with peaks again occurring on days 5 and 12.

The amount of RNA and the ratio of RNA to DNA have been used widely to assess protein synthesis in the mammary gland (see Munford, 1964, for review). In the mouse, the RNA content of the mammary gland increased steadily throughout pregnancy. The RNA : DNA ratio was less than one until just before parturition, when it exceeded unity (Yanai and Nagasawa, 1971). Banerjee et al. (1971) estimated the rate of RNA synthesis during pregnancy in mice by measuring [^{3}H]-uridine incorporation into the mammary gland. They found a sixfold increase in [^{3}H]-uridine incorporation on day 15 of pregnancy compared to tissue from virgin mice; a further increase was seen on day 5 of lactation. Characterization of the mammary gland RNA by sucrose density gradient centrifugation showed that rRNA is synthesized on day 12 of pregnancy and processing and migration of rRNA to the cytoplasm are similar during pregnancy and lactation. However, while the proportion of rRNA does not exceed 60% of the total RNA during pregnancy, rRNA constitutes about 85% of the total RNA in the lactating gland. Ribosomes in both virgin and midpregnant mice exist largely as monomers, as determined by sedimentation, but just before parturition, a peak of large ribosomal aggregates is found, indicative of augmented protein synthesis (Banerjee and Banerjee, 1973; Banerjee et al., 1977).

Measurements of specific milk constituents, in particular casein and α-lactalbumin, have also been used to assess mammary gland development. Casein is present in mammary tissue from midpregnant mice but the amount is small compared to the casein concentration just before parturition (Terry et al., 1975). Turkington et al. (1968) measured the concentrations of both components of lactose synthetase (galactosyltransferse and α-lactalbumin) in mammary tissue from pregnant and lactating mice. They found low concentrations of both proteins on day 10 of pregnancy. The concentration of galactosyltransferase rose rapidly during the second half of pregnancy to a near maximum before parturition, whereas the activity of α-lactalbumin remained relatively low until after parturition. Work in our own laboratory has yielded somewhat different results. We used a specific radioimmunoassay (RIA) (Thordarson et al., 1986) to measure the amount of mouse α-lactalbumin in mouse mammary homogenates during pregnancy. The total content and con-

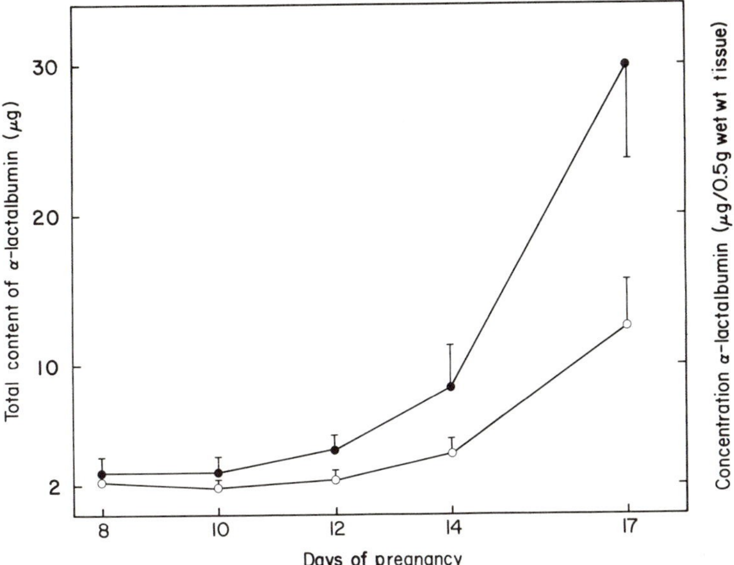

Figure 1. The total content (●) and concentration (○) of α-lactalbumin in the mammary glands obtained from mice at different stages of pregnancy. Each point represents the mean ± SEM (n = 12–14).

centration of α-lactalbumin remained low between days 8 and 14 of pregnancy but then rose sharply before parturition (Fig. 1; K. Bowens, G. Thordarson, and F. Talamantes, unpublished data). McKenzie et al. (1971) have also reported significant lactose synthetase activity in mouse mammary gland homogenates after day 15 of pregnancy.

Foster (1977) used cell volume to estimate the developmental changes in mouse mammary glands during pregnancy and lactation. On day 4 of pregnancy, he found a significant increase in cell volume over that of tissue from virgin mice, but the major enlargement in cell volume occurred between day 16 of gestation and parturition. An additional increase was observed during lactation.

2.3. Rat

The pattern of mammary gland growth and development in the rat is similar to that of the mouse (see Munford, 1964, for review). The total DNA content of the mammary gland shows an increase throughout pregnancy, which continues until day 10 or 12 of lactation (Munford, 1963; Tucker and Reece, 1963a,b). It has been estimated that only about

60% of the total mammary gland growth in the rat takes place during pregnancy (Griffith and Turner, 1961). The total RNA content of the rat mammary gland increases in parallel to the DNA content throughout pregnancy, and there is a gradual increase in the RNA : DNA ratio (Tucker and Reece, 1963a). A further increase in the RNA content occurs during the first 14 days of lactation and the RNA : DNA ratio triples during this period (Tucker and Reece, 1963b). Rosen et al. (1975) have assessed the casein mRNA activity of the developing rat mammary gland. They found an approximately 18-fold increase in the translation rate of casein mRNA between days 5 and 20 of pregnancy, whereas the total mRNA activity increased about 3.5-fold during the same period. Casein mRNA comprised about 5% of the total mammary gland mRNA on day 5 of pregnancy. This proportion increased to 25% at the end of gestation. Nakhasi and Qasba (1979) have measured the content of α-lactalbumin and three species of casein (42K, 29K, and 25K) as well as the activity and the content of the mRNA for these proteins in the rat mammary gland. Each of these parameters showed a substantial increase in the latter half of pregnancy. In contrast to these results, McKenzie et al. (1971) did not detect any lactose synthetase activity in rat mammary gland homogenates during pregnancy. These workers showed that the lack of lactose synthetase activity was due to the absence of α-lactalbumin. The discrepancy between these data has not been explained, but it may have been due to the use of different methods for measuring α-lactalbumin concentration.

2.4. Hamster

Mammary gland development in the hamster during pregnancy and lactation has been investigated by Sinha et al. (1970). In contrast to the mouse and rat, the growth of the mammary gland in the hamster is essentially complete at parturition as assessed by DNA content. The RNA content and the RNA : DNA ratio increase during pregnancy, with a further increase occurring at the beginning of lactation.

2.5. Guinea Pig

Nelson et al. (1962) investigated mammary development in guinea pigs throughout pregnancy and lactation. They found consistent but relatively slow increases in the total weight, nitrogen content, DNA content, and RNA : DNA ratio of the gland during pregnancy. A sharp increase in the same parameters was seen at parturition and this increase continued for the first 5 or 6 days of lactation. More recently, Anderson et al. (1982) used similar indices for assessing mammary gland development and found more substantial increases in mammary growth and development during pregnancy, especially during the latter half. An increase in mammary growth was also seen during the first days of lactation.

Guinea pig mammary tissue obtained in late pregnancy contained both α-lactalbumin mRNA and α-lactalbumin. The highest amounts of both were present at parturition. On the other hand, casein mRNA and casein synthesis were absent until after parturition (Burditt et al., 1981).

2.6. Goat and Sheep

Little mammary gland growth and development occurs during the first 80–90 days of gestation in the goat. By that time, an increase is found in udder volume (Fleet et al., 1975) and in DNA and lactose content as well as in the enzyme activity (Jones, 1979). Fleet and coworkers (1975) also found at days 80–90 of gestation that the fluid within the udder changes in composition from an extracellular fluid-like to a milk-like substance. They termed this onset of mammary gland secretory activity lactogenesis stage I. The commencement of copious milk secretion was designated lactogenesis stage II. After a spurt in mammary gland growth and differentiation at midgestation, DNA, lactose, and enzyme activity per unit mammary gland weight remained relatively constant until parturition (Jones, 1979). There was, on the other hand, a continuous increase in total DNA, mammary gland weight, and dry fat-free tissue (DFFT) throughout pregnancy, and both the total content of RNA and the RNA concentration increased. At days 90–100 of gestation, about 24% of the total mammary gland growth, estimated by the total DNA content, had occurred, and at parturition (days 148–150), mammary gland growth was 80% complete. The maximum DNA content was found on the fifth day of lactation. The RNA content of the mammary gland at parturition was only about half that found on day 5 of lactation (Anderson et al., 1981).

In the sheep, lactose synthesis begins between days 100 and 110 of gestation and coincides with the sharp increase in the total RNA and DNA contents of the mammary gland (Denamur, 1965). At parturition, mammary gland growth in the sheep is about 95–98% complete as estimated by DNA content (Denamur, 1965; Anderson, 1975b).

2.7. Human

Vorherr (1974) has summarized the histological changes that take place during pregnancy in the mammary gland in women. In the first trimester, there is an increase in terminal ductal sprouting, and lobuloalveolar formation begins during the third or fourth week of gestation. Toward the end of the third month of pregnancy, the alveolar epithelial cells change from being doublelayer to monolayer, indicating commencement of secretory activity. In the second trimester, there is enhancement of the branching of the ductal system and formation of lobular alveolar structures. Accumulation of secretory products within the alveolar lumen also begins during the second trimester. The third trimester is typified by the accumulation of abundant fat droplets in the secretory cells and further accumulation of secretory products in the alveolar lumen. During the third trimester, lobuloalveolar structure occupies most of the space in the gland, which before was occupied by fat and connective tissue.

The serum concentration of α-lactalbumin has been measured throughout pregnancy in women (Martin et al., 1980). There was a significant rise in α-lactalbumin concentration until the 26th week of gestation. After that, the α-lactalbumin concentration did not change significantly.

Kulski and Hartmann (1981) measured various constituents of the breast secretion in pregnant women beginning 110 days before parturition. Lactose and glucose are present 110 days before delivery and remain relatively constant throughout pregnancy, showing abrupt increases immediately after parturition.

In summary, mammary gland growth is generally slow before puberty when a spurt in cell proliferation takes place. Further development of the mammary gland only occurs during pregnancy or, to a lesser extent, in animals that undergo pseudopregnancy. The extent of mammary gland growth at parturition varies between species. In the sheep and hamster, for example, it is virtually complete by the end of pregnancy, but in other species growth of the mammary gland continues during early lactation. Rapid mammary gland differentiation and commencement of secretory activity usually occur at about midgestation, continue throughout pregnancy, and are completed during early lactation.

3. Lactogenic Hormones of Placental Origin

3.1. Early Studies in Rats and Mice

The term lactogenic hormone is used here to designate a group of protein hormones of pituitary and placental origin that are structurally similar to and/or show activity in radioreceptor assays for prolactin-like and/or GH-like hormones. All these hormones have been shown to possess lactogenic activity by bioassay.

The lactogenic activity of rat and mouse placentas has been known for several decades. Ray et al. (1955) demonstrated the prolactin-like activity of placental extract from 12-day pregnant rats in the pigeon crop sac assay. They also investigated the effect of placental extracts and placental implants from different stages of pregnancy on mammary gland development in hypophysectomized, ovariectomized rats that also received progesterone and estrogen injections. In these experiments, day-12 placentas (both injected extract and implants) were most active in inducing lobuloalveolar growth, but mammotropic activity was found in placentas from day 8 and in placentas obtained at later stages of pregnancy. Day-12 placental extract also induced milk secretion after cessation of progesterone and estrogen administration in the hypophysectomized, ovariectomized animals.

In addition to showing mammotropic activity, placental extract from 12-day pregnant rats also contained luteotropic activity. Subsequent studies confirmed the study of Ray and co-workers. Matthies (1965, 1967) and Cohen and Gala (1969) were able to correlate the appearance of the lactogenic and luteotropic factor(s) in the placenta with lactogenic and luteotropic activity in serum obtained from midpregnant rats. Furthermore, Matthies (1965) provided evidence for the placental origin of these factors by demonstrating their presence in the fetal component of the placenta and in the maternal serum from day-12 pregnant rats that had been hypophysectomized and ovariectomized on day 5 of gestation.

Mammary gland explant culture has widely been used to study mammary development and function. Using coculture of mouse mammary glands and mouse placentas, Kohmoto and Bern (1970) demonstrated the lactogenic activity of the mouse placenta by using histological criteria. They were able to detect lactogenic activity in placentas collected as early as day 6 of pregnancy and at any stage of pregnancy thereafter. Employing a similar technique, Talamantes (1975a,b) reported lactogenic activity in placentas from a number of species. He found high lactogenic activity in placentas from 12-day pregnant rats, but placentas obtained later in pregnancy also contained activity. Similar results were obtained for the mouse.

The development of a radioreceptor assay for lactogenic hormones (Shiu et al., 1973) enabled more accurate assessment of the lactogenic activity of the placenta. It was shown that two peaks of lactogenic activity were present in rat serum during pregnancy. The first one reached its highest value on day 12 of gestation and then declined, but on day 17 a second rise in activity, which continued until parturition, was seen. Only a small portion of this lactogenic activity was due to the presence of prolactin as assessed by a specific radioimmunoassay (RIA), and it was suggested that the remaining lactogenic activity originated in the placenta (Shiu et al., 1973). Subsequently, the radioreceptor assay was used to assess the lactogenic activity of serum and placental extract during pregnancy in a number of species. These studies confirmed that two peaks of lactogenic activity are present in rat serum during pregnancy, and they also revealed the presence of two molecular weight forms of lactogen in the placenta. Both forms were present on day 12 of pregnancy in serum and placental extract but only the smaller form was found in placentas and serum from late pregnant rats (Kelly et al., 1975, 1976). A very similar pattern of lactogenic activity was found in the serum from pregnant mice (Kelly et al., 1976). Kohmoto (1975) cultured placental explants from 12- to 14-day pregnant mice in the presence of [^{3}H]-leucine. He detected five radioactive protein bands after electrophoretic fractionation of the medium. Two of these protein bands showed lactogenic activity in the mouse mammary gland explant assay.

It has now been established that the placentas of both rats (Robertson and Friesen, 1981; Robertson et al., 1982) and mice (Soares et al., 1982, 1983; Talamantes et al., 1984a) secrete at least two lactogenic hormones during pregnancy. In rats, these lactogens have been designated placental lactogen I (the early, higher molecular weight form) and placental lactogen II (lower molecular weight form, present in the latter half of pregnancy; Robertson et al., 1982). In mice, the two lactogens are designated midpregnancy lactogen (the early, larger form; Soares et al., 1983) and placental lactogen (the smaller, later form; Colosi et al., 1982).*

3.2. Mouse Placental Lactogen

3.2.1. General

Mouse placental lactogen (mPL) has been purified from placentas obtained on days 14–18 of gestation (Colosi et al., 1982). The molecular weight of mPL is 21,812 daltons, as calculated from the amino acid

*Different nomenclatures have developed that describe the multiple lactogenic hormones produced by the mouse placenta. The 21,812-dalton protein, which is the predominant lactogen in the latter half of pregnancy, is designated mouse placental lactogen (mPL) in this chapter but has also been named mouse placental lactogen II (mPL II). Midpregnancy lactogen, also called mouse placental lactogen I (mPL I), refers to the higher molecular weight lactogen which reaches maximal concentration at midpregnancy.

sequence of the hormone (Jackson et al., 1986). This is identical to the molecular weight of mGH but less than that of mPRL (22,381 daltons; Linzer and Talamantes, 1985). The isoelectric point (p*I*) of mPL was estimated to be 7.1. A specific and sensitive RIA has been developed for mPL (Soares et al., 1982). Recently, Hall and Talamantes (1984) used antiserum to mPL and the avidin–biotin–peroxidase complex method to localize mPL in the placenta. They found heaviest staining in the basal zone of placentas from days 10, 12, 15, and 18 of gestation, most prominently in the cytoplasm of the giant cells and to a lesser extent in the cytoplasm of the basophilic cytotrophoblasts. Mouse PL was also localized to the giant cells of the decidua capsularis in 10-day placentas. No staining was observed in day 7 placentas.

The serum profile of mPL has been measured by RIA throughout pregnancy (Fig. 2a; see also Soares et al., 1982; Talamantes et al., 1984a). Mouse PL is first detected on day 9 of pregnancy and its concentration increases until day 14. After day 14, its concentration remains unchanged in C3H/HeN mice but continues to rise until term in BALB/c and Swiss Webster mice (Soares et al., 1982; Soares and Talamantes, 1983, 1985).

At the present time, little is known about the control of the synthesis and secretion of PL in mice. The genotype of the fetoplacental unit affects both the concentration and the secretion profile of mPL (Soares

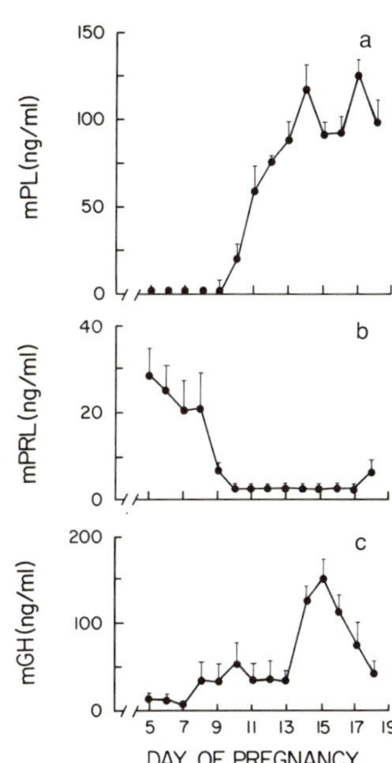

Figure 2. Serum profiles of mouse placental lactogen (a), mouse prolactin (b), and mouse growth hormone (c) on days 5–18 of pregnancy in C3H mice. Points represent the mean ± SEM (n = 7–8). From Talamantes et al. (1984a).

and Talamantes, 1983). The significance of this difference in the serum profile of mPL between mouse strains is not known. Hypophysectomy causes an increase in the circulating concentration of mPL (Day et al., 1986). It is not known what causes the rise in mPL after hypophysectomy. The effect may be direct through factor(s) released from the pituitary or indirect through organs influenced by the pituitary, possibly the ovaries or adrenals. The absence of the pituitary could also change the clearance rate of mPL from the circulation. Soares and Talamantes (1985) have shown that bilateral ovariectomy increases the serum concentration of mPL and that progesterone inhibits the release of mPL from placental explants in culture.

3.2.2. Lactogenic Activity of Mouse Placental Lactogen

Purified mPL shows prolactin-like activity in the pigeon crop sac assay and mPL is more effective than oPRL in displacing [^{125}I]-oPRL from rabbit mammary gland receptors (Colosi et al., 1982). The lactogenic activities of mPL, mGH, and mPRL have been compared in isolated mouse mammary epithelial cells grown on collagen; the release of α-lactalbumin was used to assess the lactogenic potency of the hormones (Thordarson et al., 1986). In this study, all three hormones showed lactogenic activity, but mPL was significantly more active than mPRL and mGH. Both mPL and mPRL caused dose-dependent increases in α-lactalbumin release while the enhancement in α-lactalbumin caused by mGH was not dependent on hormone dose (Fig. 3). It is of interest in this context that Markoff and Talamantes (1980) showed that although mGH is less potent than mPRL in inducing casein synthesis in mouse mammary explant culture, both hormones caused dose-related increases in casein synthesis. These findings suggest that the hormonal control of casein and α-lactalbumin synthesis differs in the mouse.

As shown in Fig. 2b, the serum concentration of mPRL is low in the mouse during the latter half of pregnancy, whereas the mPL concentration starts to rise on day 9 and reaches a high level by day 14. Although the serum concentration of mGH increases during the latter half of pregnancy (Fig. 2c), its elevation is not as pronounced as that of mPL. Mammary gland growth and differentiation will not proceed in the absence of mammotropic hormone(s); that is, PRL, GH, or PL (see Cowie and Tindal, 1971). It is therefore likely that mPL is the most important lactogen during the latter half of pregnancy in the mouse, since mPRL concentration is low at this time and mGH does not appear to be as potent a lactogen as either mPL or mPRL.

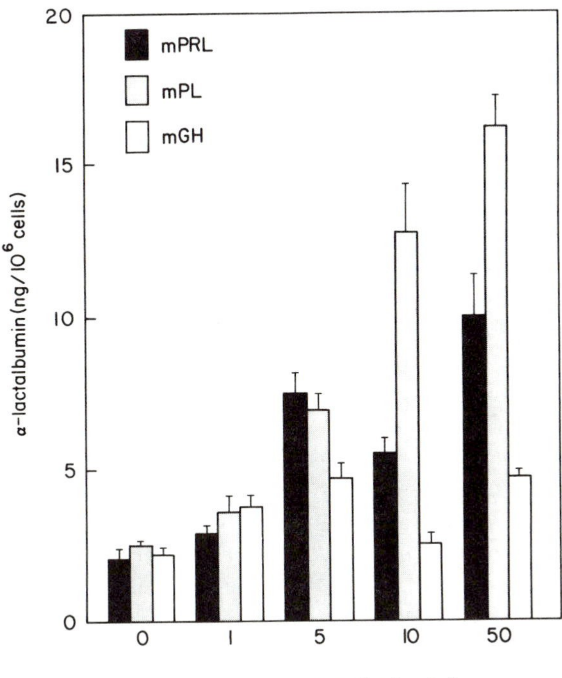

Figure 3. Concentration of α-lactalbumin in the medium from mouse mammary epithelial cells cultured on floating collagen gels in the presence of different concentrations of mouse placental lactogen, mouse prolactin, and mouse growth hormone. Each point represents the mean ± SEM (n = 4–8). From Thordarson et al. (1986).

There are also numerous indirect lines of evidence to support the notion that mPL is important for mouse mammary gland development. The appearance and rise of mPL in the circulation coincide with rapid changes in mammary gland growth and development (see Section 2.2 and Fig. 2a). It is known that the serum concentration of mPL is positively correlated with litter size (Markoff and Talamantes, 1981; Soares and Talamantes, 1983). Nagasawa and Yanai (1971) surgically adjusted the number of fetuses to 1–12 in C3H/He mice on day 8 of pregnancy. At the end of pregnancy (day 19) mammary gland development was estimated and correlated with the weight and number of placentas. All the indices used to assess mammary development (DNA, RNA, RNA : DNA, and lobuloalveolar development) were positively correlated with the weight and number of placentas, but no correlation was found between mammary development and the total contents or concentrations of PRL and GH in the anterior pituitary. Hemihysterectomy performed on day 8 of pregnancy as a means of reducing litter size caused a reduction in mammary development in late pregnancy (day 18) but was without effect on mammary development assessed on day 13 of pregnancy. By increasing the number of suckling pups postpartum, it was possible to compensate for the lack of mammary development during pregnancy (Knight and Peaker, 1982). Both studies provide circumstantial evidence for the importance of mPL in mammary gland development.

In mice, gestation is not disturbed after hypophysectomy if the ablation is performed during the latter half of pregnancy. Early studies showed that mice hypophysectomized after midpregnancy show transient milk secretion after parturition (Selye et al., 1934). Recent studies in our own laboratory have shown that substantial mammary gland development occurred after hypophysectomy on day 10 of pregnancy when mammary development was estimated on days 14 and 18 of gestation. When compared with intact and sham-operated control animals at the same stages of pregnancy, a significant reduction in the total DNA content of the mammary gland did not occur in the hypophysectomized mice on days 14 and 18 of pregnancy. Total RNA content and the RNA : DNA ratio were significantly reduced in the hypophysectomized mice on day 18. However, when compared with intact 10-day pregnant mice, significant increases in RNA and the RNA : DNA ratio had occurred in the hypophysectomized mice by day 18 of gestation (Table I; G. Thordarson, L. Ogren, J. Day, K. Bowens, P. Fielder, and F. Talamantes, unpublished data). As mentioned in Section 2.2, a sharp rise in both the total content and concentration of α-lactalbumin takes place on about day 16 of pregnancy in normal mice. After hypophysectomy, this increase in α-lactalbumin is greatly reduced (Fig. 4; G. Thordarson, L. Ogren, J. Day, K. Bowens, P. Fielder, and F. Talamantes, unpublished data). What prevents the usual rise in α-lactalbumin from occurring in late pregnant mice after hypophysectomy is not yet known. It is clear that although lactogenic hormones (PRL, PL, GH) are involved in regulating the synthesis of α-lactalbumin (Kleinberg et al., 1978; Akers et al., 1981; Goodman et al., 1983; Thordarson et al., 1986), synergistic effects of other hormone(s) are necessary for a normal rate of α-lactalbumin synthesis. There are a number of in vitro and in vivo studies that have shown the importance of adrenal steroids in mammary development and milk secretion (Lyons et al., 1958; Nandi, 1958; Turkington and Hill, 1969; Mills and Topper, 1970; Banerjee et al., 1971; Nagasawa and Yanai, 1973). In the mouse, there is a small increase in the circulating corticosterone concentration before day 10 of pregnancy, but there-

Table I. Nucleic Acid Content of Mammary Glands from Hypophysectomized, Sham-Operated, and Intact Pregnant Mice

			DNA		RNA		
Operation	Days of pregnancy	Number of animals	Total (mg) mean ± SEM	Concentration (mg/g tissue) mean ± SEM	Total (mg) mean ± SEM	Concentration (mg/g tissue) mean ± SEM	RNA : DNA mean ± SEM
Intact	10	9	1.81 ± 0.11	1.60 ± 0.13	0.79 ± 0.06	0.69 ± 0.05	0.44 ± 0.02
Intact	14	10	3.27 ± 0.25	1.80 ± 0.14	1.80 ± 0.19	0.98 ± 0.09	0.54 ± 0.03
Sham	14	11	3.06 ± 0.28	2.11 ± 0.14	1.69 ± 0.12	1.18 ± 0.06	0.58 ± 0.04
Hypox	14	14	3.03 ± 0.19	2.95 ± 0.16	1.20 ± 0.08	1.17 ± 0.06	0.40 ± 0.01
Intact	18	10	4.33 ± 0.24	1.65 ± 0.08	4.22 ± 0.25	1.62 ± 0.10	0.98 ± 0.04
Sham	18	13	4.10 ± 0.23	1.74 ± 0.09	4.08 ± 0.35	1.70 ± 0.11	0.99 ± 0.05
Hypox	18	15	3.86 ± 0.20	2.32 ± 0.15	3.03 ± 0.23	1.79 ± 0.13	0.77 ± 0.03

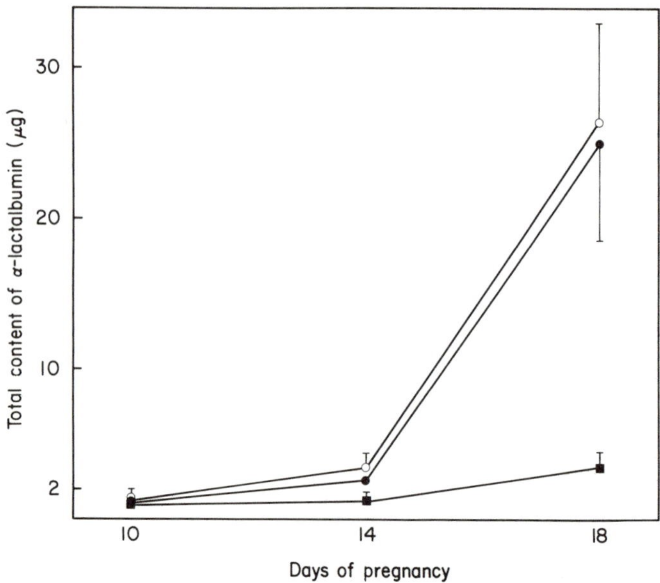

Figure 4. The total content of α-lactalbumin in the mammary glands of hypophysectomized (■), sham operated (○), and intact (●) pregnant mice. Each point represents the mean ± SEM (n = 9–15).

after a sharp increase in plasma concentration occurs, reaching the highest values at day 16 of gestation (Barlow et al., 1974). Thyroid hormones may also be important for normal mammary development and specifically for the synthesis and secretion of α-lactalbumin (Vonderhaar, 1975; Vonderhaar and Greco, 1979; Bhattacharjee and Vonderhaar, 1984). One may expect the concentration of both the adrenal steroids and the thyroid hormones to be reduced to low levels after the tropic effect of the pituitary on the adrenals and the thyroid has been removed. This may have prevented the rise of α-lactalbumin production in hypophysectomized animals.

3.3. Midpregnancy Lactogen

Midpregnancy lactogen has been purified recently and an RIA for the hormone has been developed (Colosi et al., 1987). The hormone is a glycoprotein that appears as several bands ranging in molecular weight from 29,000 to 42,000 on SDS polyacrylamide gels. The hormone is secreted by cells of the chorioallantoic and choriovitelline placenta (Soares et al., 1983). Midpregnancy lactogen is first detectable in maternal serum on day 6 of pregnancy and its concentration increases rapidly to reach a peak concentration of several micrograms per milliliter on day 10. Serum midpregnancy lactogen concentration then declines abruptly to barely detectable values on day 13 and remains low for the remainder of pregnancy (Colosi et al., 1986).

Little is known about the biological activity of midpregnancy lactogen. It stimulates secretory activity in mouse mammary explant culture (Soares et al., 1983) and α-lactalbumin synthesis in cultured mouse mammary epithelial cells (Colosi et al., 1987). The mouse conceptus contains luteotropic factor(s) at midpregnancy, and the luteotropic activity of mouse serum is enhanced at the same time (Critser et al., 1980, 1982). So far, these luteotropic factors have not been identified but it is interesting that the presence of the midpregnancy luteotropic activity of the placenta and serum coincides with the appearance of midpregnancy lactogen in the maternal circulation. It remains to be seen whether midpregnancy lactogen has luteotropic activity.

3.4. Proliferin and Proliferin-Related Protein

Identification of two new members of the prolactin–growth hormone family, as indicated by structural similarities to the pituitary hormones, has recently been reported. These two newly discovered proteins have been designated proliferin (PLF) and proliferin-related protein (PRP) (Linzer and Nathans, 1984, 1985). Both PLF mRNA and PRP mRNA have been found in mouse placental tissue, indicating that the placenta is the normal site of synthesis of these proteins (Linzer and Nathans, 1985; Linzer et al., 1985). The highest content of PLF mRNA was found in day 10 placentas, and day-14 placental explants secrete PLF. Immunologically, PLF is distinct from both mPL (Linzer et al., 1985) and midpregnancy lactogen (P. Colosi, personal communication). The highest content of PRP mRNA is found in day-12 placentas (Linzer and Nathans, 1985). As yet, nothing is known about the biological role of either of these proteins, but their structural similarity to prolactin may indicate an effect on the mammary gland, either direct or indirect via luteotropic activity.

In summary, the mouse placenta is the site of synthesis of at least four prolactin–growth hormone-related hormones: mPL, midpregnancy lactogen, PLF, and PRP. Mouse PL, which is highly lactogenic in a homologous system, is present in the circulation in high concentration during the latter half of pregnancy, when the concentration of other lactogenic hormones is low. It is suggested that mPL is the most important lactogen during this period. Midpregnancy lactogen is present in the serum in very high concentration at midgestation but the concentration remains low thereafter. It is lactogenic in a homologous system and it may also have a luteotropic effect. As yet, nothing is known about serum concentration or biological activity of PLF and PRP.

3.5. Rat Placental Lactogen I

Rat PL-I is first detectable in the circulation on day 8 of gestation, reaching maximal concentrations on day 12, and then its concentration declines rapidly and is barely detectable by day 15 (Robertson and Friesen, 1981). As yet, this protein has not been purified, but preliminary characterization of rPL-I has revealed that its molecular weight is about twice that of rPL-II and it has a p*I* of 4.5. Rat PL-I does not cross-react with antiserum to rPL-II. Rat PL-I is active in both the rabbit mammary gland radioreceptor assay and the Nb2 lymphoma bioassay (Robertson et al., 1982).

The rat placenta synthesizes luteotropic factors that show greatest activity at day 12 of gestation (Matthies, 1967; Linkie and Niswender, 1973; see also Section 3.1). At the present time, it is debatable whether this luteotropic activity is caused by rPL-I or whether the rat placenta also produces a chorionic gonadotropin (Blank et al., 1979; Tabarelli et al., 1982; Blank and Dufau, 1983; Tabarelli et al., 1983; Glaser et al., 1984, 1985). Therefore, rPL-I may be important for mammary gland development in at least two ways: (1) directly, by providing a mammotropic stimulus to the mammary gland, and (2) indirectly, by stimulating steroid production from the ovaries.

3.6. Rat Placental Lactogen II

3.6.1. General

Rat PL-II has been purified from placental tissue obtained from 17–19-day pregnant rats (Robertson and Friesen, 1975). The purified hormone has an apparent molecular weight of about 20,000, as estimated on SDS polyacrylamide gels and by chromatography on Sephadex G-100, and it has a p*I* of 6.0–6.4 (Robertson et al., 1982). The serum concentration of rPL-II has been measured throughout pregnancy with a specific RIA. The concentration is low on day 10 of gestation and shows a relatively small peak between days 12 and 13 of pregnancy. After day 14, the rPL-II concentration of the serum increases continuously, reaching a maximum value of about 1000 ng/ml before parturition (Robertson and Friesen, 1981).

It has been shown that PL-II cross-reacts with antiserum to pituitary prolactin (Robertson and Friesen, 1981; Robertson et al., 1982). Tabarelli et al. (1983) found immunoactivity to rat prolactin antiserum in trophoblast giant cells of 15- and 17-day rat placentas and in the endometrium and adjacent decidual cells. More recently, Soares et al. (1985) demonstrated that rPL-II is synthesized and secreted from cultured rat trophoblast cells.

The lactogenic activity of serum from 21-day pregnant rats (presumably mostly rPL-II) is positively correlated with the number of conceptuses (Robertson and Friesen, 1981). Hypophysectomy on day 14 of pregnancy increases the serum lactogenic activity by day 16 (Daughaday et al., 1979). More recently, Robertson et al. (1984a) showed that hypophysectomy at midpregnancy causes a significant increase in rPL-II in late pregnancy. Ovarian factor(s) seems to inhibit and fetal factor(s) appears to enhance rPL-II secretion since ovariectomy increases and fetectomy decreases circulating levels of rPL-II. Adrenalectomy augments the elevation of rPL-II obtained after ovariectomy although adrenalectomy alone is without effect (Robertson et al., 1984a,b).

3.6.2. Lactogenic Activity of Rat Placental Lactogen II

Direct evidence for the mammotropic activity of rPL-II is scarce, but there are a number of studies that indicate the importance of the placenta for normal mammary development in rats. A purified preparation of rPL-II is about 41% as effective as oPRL in a radioreceptor assay using receptors from rabbit mammary glands and [^{125}I]-oPRL as the radioligand (Robertson and Friesen, 1975). As in the mouse, the latter half of pregnancy in the rat is a time of rapid mammary development (see Section 2.3), which coincides with high serum concentrations of rPL-II (Robertson and Friesen, 1981). On the other hand, the serum concentration of rPRL is low after day 10 of pregnancy (Smith and Neill, 1976) until just before parturition (Amenomori et al., 1970). The blood concentration of GH does not appear to be elevated during pregnancy in rats (Schalch and Reichlin, 1966). Normal pseudopregnancy, which lasts approximately 12 days in rats, will result in mammary development. However, the extent of this mammary development is less than that of 12-day pregnant rats. If pseudopregnancy is prolonged to 18 or 21 days either by hysterectomy or by inducing deciduomata, no further increase in mammary gland development beyond that of normal pseudopregnancy occurs (Anderson and Turner, 1968; Desjardins et al., 1968). These results show that the fetoplacental unit is needed for normal mammary gland development during pregnancy. It was also shown that removal of the fetus and the fetal placenta on days 12 and 16 of pregnancy prevented normal mammary growth when assessed on day 21 of gestation. Fetectomy alone did not retard mammary development if performed after day 16 (Desjardins et al., 1968).

Lactose synthesis (Bussmann et al., 1983) and γ-glutamyltransferase activity (Bussmann and Deis, 1984) were enhanced in late pregnant rats after the withdrawal of progesterone regardless of serum PRL concentrations, provided that the conceptuses remain intact. If a reduction in PRL concentration (by bromocriptine treatment) was accompanied by hysterectomy, thereby eliminating placental hormones from the circulation, no increase in lactose synthesis or γ-glutamyltransferase activity over controls was observed.

Early studies demonstrated that rats hypophysectomized at midpregnancy show milk secretion for a few hours after parturition (Collip et al., 1933; Selye et al., 1934). Anderson (1975a) showed that hypophysectomy at midgestation does not reduce mammary development (as estimated by DNA and RNA content) when compared with sham-operated animals on day 20 of pregnancy. Furthermore, mammary development in hypophysectomized pregnant rats was dependent on the number of conceptuses. At least three conceptuses were needed for full mammary development.

In summary, the rat placenta secretes at least two lactogenic hormones, rPL-I and rPL-II. Indirect evidence indicates that both hormones may be important for mammary development during pregnancy.

3.7. Hamster Placental Lactogen

The lactogenic activity of the hamster placenta was demonstrated by coculture of hamster placentas and mouse mammary tissue and by treating mouse mammary explant cultures with hamster placental extract (Talamantes, 1975a,b). Later studies used a radioreceptor assay to confirm the presence of lactogenic activity in the hamster placenta (Kelly et al., 1976; Soares and Talamantes, 1982).

A lactogenic hormone designated hamster placental lactogen (haPL) has recently been purified from the hamster placenta (Southard et al., 1986). The apparent molecular weight of this hormone, as estimated on SDS polyacrylamide gels, is 25,200. Isoelectric focusing of haPL revealed three distinct bands with p*I* values from 8.3 to 8.8.

Hamster PL displaces [^{125}I]-oPRL from rabbit mammary gland receptors with about 42% of the efficiency of oPRL, and purified haPL stimulates the secretion of α-lactalbumin by cultured mouse mammary epithelial cells.

The lactogenic activity present in serum obtained from pregnant hamsters has been measured by radioreceptor assay (Kelly et al., 1976; Soares and Talamantes, 1982). It was found that the lactogenic activity is low during early pregnancy but a rapid increase occurs at about midgestation. The concentration remains high throughout pregnancy and increases further just before parturition (Soares and Talamantes, 1982). It is likely that most of the activity measured by the radioreceptor assay is of placental origin, as circulating concentrations of pituitary prolactin are reduced in late-pregnant hamsters (Bast and Greenwald, 1974; Talamantes et al., 1984b) and purified hamster PRL shows low activity in the rabbit mammary gland radioreceptor assay using oPRL as the radioligand (Colosi et al., 1981). Mammotropic activity may be of particular importance during pregnancy in the hamster because the gestation period lasts only 16 days, and because virtually no mammary growth occurs after parturition (Sinha et al., 1970; see also Section 2.4). It is not known to what extent mammary gland development during pregnancy is dependent on haPL, but milk secretion occurred at parturition in hamsters that had been hypophysectomized on day 12 of gestation (Greenwald, 1967).

3.8. Guinea Pig Placental Lactogen

Placental extract from 40- and 50-day pregnant guinea pigs stimulates secretion in cultured mouse mammary explants (Talamantes, 1975a), and lactogenic activity has been detected by radioreceptor assay in placental extracts and plasma samples obtained from pregnant guinea pigs (Kelly et al., 1976). The lactogenic activity in plasma is low until about midgestation. Shortly after midterm, lactogenic activity increases sharply and then gradually declines toward parturition (Kelly et al., 1976; Thordarson and Forsyth, 1982). Milk yield in guinea pigs increases with the number of fetuses carried, the litter size ranging from one to five (Davis et al., 1979). Interestingly, it was not possible to compensate for low milk yield caused by a small number of fetuses carried during pregnancy by increasing the number of young suckling postpartum.

Thordarson and Forsyth (1982) have shown that mammary gland development (DNA, RNA content and lactose synthetase and glucose-6-P-dehydrogenase activity) at parturition is correlated with total lactogenic activity during pregnancy as measured by radioreceptor assay and also with the weight of the litter at birth. Both studies provide circumstantial evidence for the importance of guinea pig placental lactogen in mammary gland development. Furthermore, some milk secretion occurred after parturition in guinea pigs that were hypophysectomized on day 40 of pregnancy (Pencharz and Lyons, 1934).

3.9. Placental Lactogen in Sheep and Goats

3.9.1. General

Using rabbit mammary gland organ culture, Buttle et al. (1972) demonstrated lactogenic activity that was immunologically distinct from goat PRL in the plasma of pregnant goats. It was subsequently shown that this lactogenic activity was of placental origin (Forsyth, 1973). As yet, only partial purification of caprine PL (cPL) has been reported with an estimated molecular weight of 20,000–24,000 and estimated p*I* of 8.8 (Becka et al., 1977; Currie et al., 1977).

In the sheep, Kelly et al. (1974) first measured high concentrations of ovine placental lactogen (oPL) by radioreceptor assay. This activity was immunologically distinct from oPRL. Ovine PL was subsequently purified and characterized by several groups of workers (Martal and Djiane, 1975; Chan et al., 1976; Hurley et al., 1977a; Reddy and Watkins, 1978a). The estimation of the molecular weight of various preparations of oPL ranges from 20,000 to 24,000 using either size exclusion chromatography (Chan et al., 1976; Reddy and Watkins, 1978a) or SDS–polyacrylamide gel electrophoresis (Martal and Djiane, 1975; Hurley et al., 1977a). The estimation of p*I* for oPL also differs between laboratories and ranges from 6.8 to 8.8 (Martal and Djiane, 1975; Chan et al., 1976; Hurley et al., 1977a; Reddy and Watkins, 1978a). Limited information about the structural relation between oPL and bovine PL (bPL) and their homologous growth hormones and prolactins indicates that the PL of both these species is structurally intermediate between GH and PRL (Bolander and Fellows, 1976; Hurley et al., 1977a,b)

Using coculture of goat placental tissue and mouse mammary explants, Forsyth (1973) found that the lactogenic activity of the goat placenta was restricted to the cotyledonary tissue. The author also found that the fetal part of the placentome stimulated mouse mammary tissue more consistently than did the maternal tissue and suggested that the fetal trophoblast was the site of cPL synthesis. In the sheep, PL has been localized in mono- and binucleate cells in the epithelium of the chorionic villi by immunofluorescence techniques (Martal et al., 1977; Reddy and Watkins, 1978b) and in mononucleate cells of the maternal epithelial syncytium and binucleate cells of the chorionic membrane (Watkins and Reddy, 1980). Using a technique of higher resolution (electron microscope immunocytochemistry), Wooding (1981) localized oPL exclusively within granules and in the Golgi region of the binucleate cells of the fetal epithelium of the chorionic villi and in granules of similar size and shape that were scattered throughout the maternal syncytial epithelium of the placentome.

Kelly et al. (1974) measured the PL concentration of plasma samples obtained from pregnant ewes using a radioreceptor assay. They found activity from day 60 of gestation that increased and reached a peak of 1000–2000 ng/ml between days 95 and 114 of gestation. The concentration declined toward the end of gestation and was about 500–700 ng/ml 12 h before parturition (days 148–150).

More recently, an RIA was used to measure PL concentrations in sheep. Handwerger et al. (1977) detected oPL in the maternal circulation at days 41–50 of gestation. The concentration of the hormone gradually increased and reached a peak of about 2500 ng/ml between days 121 and 130 of pregnancy in singleton gestations. Ewes carrying twins tended to have higher PL concentrations than those carrying single fetuses. Other investigators have found similar patterns of oPL secretion but somewhat lower concentrations (Chan et al., 1978a; Gluckman et al., 1979). Gluckman et al. (1979) also found a significantly higher plasma concentration of oPL in twin than in singleton pregnancies.

In the goat, the blood concentration of PL has been measured during pregnancy by radioreceptor assay. Currie et al. (1977) first detected activity on about day 60 of pregnancy. The concentration was less than 100 ng/ml (oPRL and GH equivalents) and then gradually increased and reached a peak of 400–600 ng/ml between days 100 and 130 of gestation. The activity decreased during the last 15 days of gestation. Hayden et al. (1980) reported similar patterns and concentrations of cPL and also found higher PL concentrations in goats carrying twins and triplets than in goats carrying single fetuses. The plasma concentration of cPL was found to fluctuate markedly in hourly samples taken during 24-h periods during weeks 10, 14, and 20 of gestation.

3.9.2. *Lactogenic Activity of Ovine and Caprine Placental Lactogen*

Purified oPL is as effective as oPRL in displacing [^{125}I]-oPRL from rabbit mammary gland receptors (Chan et al., 1976; Reddy and Watkins, 1978a). The hormone is also active in stimulating casein synthesis in rabbit mammary gland explant culture (Chan et al., 1976) and secretory activity in the rabbit mammary gland when administered intraductally (Reddy and Watkins, 1978a). Recently it has been shown that oPL stimulates the synthesis of α-lactalbumin in mammary explants obtained from late-pregnant sheep although the potency of oPL was somewhat less than that of oPRL (I. Forsyth, J. Byatt, G. Thordarson, and S. Iley, unpublished results).

The appearance and rise of PL in the circulation of both sheep and goats (Gluckman et al., 1979; Hayden et al., 1980) coincide with a rapid increase in mammary gland growth and development during pregnancy (see Section 2.6). On the other hand, plasma concentrations of PRL are low during pregnancy in both sheep (Kelly et al., 1974) and goats (Buttle et al., 1972; Hayden et al., 1980), except for a rise just before parturition. Growth hormone concentration is also low during pregnancy in goats (Thordarson, 1984) and sheep, although some increase occurs during the month before lambing (Blom et al., 1976).

In the goat, the presence of a lactogenic protein hormone is essential for mammary gland development. Cowie et al. (1966) showed that the mammary gland of ovariectomized, nonpregnant goats will respond to estrogen and progesterone administration, provided that the pituitary is intact. A combination of estrogen, progesterone, PRL, GH, and adrenocorticotropic hormone (ACTH) administered to ovariectomized, hypophysectomized, nonpregnant goats also caused significant lobuloalveolar growth. The importance of the pituitary hormones in mammary gland development in goats was further confirmed by the fact that the regular milking stimulus will cause mammary growth and lactation in the absence of ovarian steroids in ovariectomized nulliparous goats. Surgical transection of the pituitary stalk completely prevented the response, indicating the pituitary origin of the mammotropic stimulus (Cowie et al., 1968). It was later shown that PRL is probably the most important of the pituitary hormones in mammogenesis in the goat (Hart, 1976).

It has been postulated that PL may play an important role in mammogenesis during pregnancy in goats and sheep when circulating levels of both PRL and GH are low (Cowie et al., 1980). Supporting the role of PL in mammogenesis is the finding that the total lactogenic activity of plasma during pregnancy in goats (mostly PL) is positively correlated with milk yield postpartum (Hayden et al., 1979). Furthermore, in sheep, the PL concentration of the plasma is correlated with litter size, and milk production is also directly related to the number of offspring (Butler et al., 1981).

Further evidence for lactogenic activity of PL in goats and sheep has been derived from experiments in which PRL was removed or suppressed during pregnancy, either by hypophysectomy or by treatment with the dopamine agonist bromocriptine. Buttle et al. (1979) found a fivefold increase in the weight of the lobuloalveolar mammary tissue in hypophysectomized or bromocriptine-treated goats between days 60 and 120 of gestation as compared with a 10-fold increase in intact goats. They also found that mammary tissue maintained the ability to synthesize lactose and showed normal structure, examined histologically, in both hypophysectomized and bromocriptine-treated animals. Pregnant sheep show mammary gland development after hypophysectomy (Denamur and Martinet, 1961). Schams et al. (1984) found comparable stages of mammogenesis at the end of gestation in normal sheep and in those treated with bromocriptine from day 60 of pregnancy. Forsyth et al. (1985) examined mammary development during pregnancy and milk yield postpartum in goats that had been treated with bromocriptine (5 mg/day) between weeks 8 and 20 of gestation. They found that the accumulation of precolostrum in the udder was not affected by the bromocriptine treatment in goats carrying twin fetuses but in singleton gestation it was delayed about 4–6 weeks, that is, to week 17 of pregnancy. Secretion was unobtainable from the udder and the α-lactalbumin concentration of the plasma remained low. Although udder volume was significantly reduced during weeks 15–16 in bromocriptine-treated goats, a reduction was not found during weeks 20–21 of pregnancy nor did bromocriptine treatment affect milk yield after 50 or 203 days of lactation. Placental lactogen concentrations in late pregnancy were correlated with milk yield postpartum and this correlation was more prominent on day 50 of lactation than on day 203, indicating that prepartum factors are more influential in early lactation than later on. In spite of these results, which strongly support the lactogenic activity of PL in both goats and sheep, Chan et al. (1978b) found very low specific binding of [^{125}I]-oPL to ovine mammary tissue and Servely et al. (1983) showed that oPL has only about 1–10% of the activity of oPRL in inducing casein mRNA accumulation in sheep mammary explants.

In summary, both the sheep and the goat secrete placental lactogens. There is a good correlation between the plasma concentrations of oPL and cPL and the rapid increase in mammary development during the latter half of pregnancy, indicating the involvement of these hormones in mammogenesis.

3.10. Primate Placental Lactogen

3.10.1. General

Ito and Higashi (1961) detected a prolactin-like substance in human placental extract and Josimovich and MacLaren (1962) were the first to purify and characterize this prolactin-like placental substance, which they designated placental lactogen. A structural comparison of human placental lactogen (hPL) and human GH (hGH) has revealed a substantial similarity between these two hormones with amino acid sequence identity of 85% (Bewley et al., 1972). There is, on the other hand, only 13% amino acid sequence identity between hPL and human PRL (hPRL) (Shome and Parlow, 1977).

Human PL has been located in the syncytiotrophoblast of the chorionic villi using immunocytochemical techniques (Sciarra et al., 1963; Ikonicoff and Cedard, 1973). In addition to locating hPL in the syncytiotrophoblastic layer, Dujardin et al. (1977) found the hormone in multinucleated giant cells of the basal plate and in several non-Langhansian cytotrophoblastic cells. More recently, Hoshina et al. (1982) used in situ hybridization to localize hPL mRNA. They found hPL mRNA exclusively in the syncytial layer and suggested that the synthesis of hPL does not commence until after formation of fully differentiated syncytiotrophoblast.

In women, PL can first be detected in plasma at about days 30–40 of pregnancy and its concentration rises gradually toward term, with a tendency to plateau or decrease during the last 20–30 days of gestation. The maximum plasma concentration may be as high as 5–10 μg/ml (Samaan et al., 1966; Grumbach et al., 1968; Lindberg and Nilsson, 1973; Gaspard and Franchimont, 1974).

In addition to the human, PL has been purified from two other primate species, rhesus monkey and baboon. Shome and Friesen (1971) isolated two forms of PL from full-term rhesus monkey placentas, and Josimovich et al. (1973) reported purification of a PL from the baboon. This protein was immunologically similar to hPL. Belanger et al. (1971) used an RIA to estimate the PL concentration in the plasma of rhesus monkeys. They found a gradual rise in the plasma concentration during pregnancy, reaching 4–8 μg/ml at term.

3.10.2. Lactogenic Activity of Placental Lactogen in Primates

There are a number of studies that have shown lactogenic activity of hPL in a variety of bioassays for lactogenic hormones. These include activity in the pigeon crop sac assay (Ito and Higashi, 1961; Josimovich and MacLaren, 1962; Forsyth, 1967), stimulation of mammary gland secretory activity in pseudopregnant rabbits after intraductal administration (Josimovich and MacLaren, 1962; Forsyth, 1967) and in pregnant rabbits after subcutaneous administration (Friesen, 1966), stimulation of casein synthesis (Turkington and Topper, 1966; Sherwood et al., 1971; Ways et al., 1979), and secretory activity (Forsyth, 1967; Talamantes, 1975b) in mouse mammary gland explants. When hPL alone was administered to nonpregnant, nonlactating rhesus monkeys, it did not affect the morphology of the mammary glands, but it facilitated mammary development when given in combination with 17β-estradiol and progesterone (Beck, 1972). Human PL had no effect on milk production when administered to lactating monkeys (Beck, 1972).

DNA synthesis in benign breast tumors was enhanced after administration of hPL both in organ culture (Welsch and McManus, 1977) and when the benign tissue was transplanted into athymic "nude" mice (McManus et al., 1978). Prop (1969) cultured human breast tissue obtained from a lactating woman after mastectomy. He administered hPL or oPRL to the culture medium in the presence and absence of progesterone and hydrocortisone. Human PL maintained the alveolar structure of the mammary tissue and caused substantial epithelial ductal growth independent of the presence of the steroid hormones but it did not stimulate secretory activity. Ovine PRL, on the other hand, stimulated secretory activity of the cultured mammary tissue.

There is no direct evidence for the lactogenic activity of hPL in humans in vivo but circumstantial evidence indicates mammotropic activity during pregnancy. Mammary development and transient lactation have been reported in a woman after hypophysectomy during pregnancy (Kaplan, 1961). However, it is not known whether some PRL secretion continued after the operation as no assessment of plasma PRL in the patient was reported. In another case, the serum concentration of PRL was measured during pregnancy in a woman who previously had a pituitary tumor removed. The PRL concentration remained low throughout pregnancy, at about 15 ng/ml (Franks et al., 1977). Normally, a continuous rise in PRL occurs during pregnancy in women, with concentrations reaching 100 ng/ml before parturition (Rigg et al., 1977). This low prolactin concentration did not seem to affect mammary development and adequate lactation took place postpartum.

In summary, human PL enhances growth of human mammary tissue in vitro, although it does not stimulate secretory activity. Mammary development does occur in women when circulating concentrations of PRL are abnormally low or even absent, indicating the mammotropic activity of hPL in vivo. On the other hand, it is known that normal mammary development can occur in women who have very low or no circulating PL during pregnancy because of partial or complete deletion of the hPL genes (Gaede et al., 1978; Nielsen et al., 1979; Wurzel et al., 1982; Parks et al., 1985).

At the present time, no information is available about the lactogenic activity of purified preparations of PLs in rhesus monkeys and baboons, but it is known that rhesus monkeys that are hypophysectomized during pregnancy show mammary development and temporary milk secretion after parturition (Agate, 1952; P. E. Smith, 1954).

3.11. Relaxin

Although the corpus luteum appears to be the primary site of synthesis of relaxin in most species (Anderson, 1982), it is now apparent that the ovaries are not the only source of this hormone (Bryant-Greenwood, 1981; Fields et al., 1981). Relaxin has now been localized by immunocytochemical techniques to the human placenta (Fields and Larkin, 1981; Yki-Järvinen and Wahlström, 1984; Koay et al., 1985) and a partially purified preparation of relaxin has been obtained from the human term placenta (Fields and Larkin, 1981). Relaxin has also been purified from the rabbit placenta (Fields et al., 1982).

The primary physiological role of relaxin has long been considered to be the softening of the cervix and relaxation of the pelvic ligaments to facilitate delivery. It has also been suggested that relaxin may enhance mammary development (Hamolsky and Sparrow, 1945; T. C. Smith, 1954; Wada and Turner, 1959). More recently, relaxin was shown to increase the lengthening of mammary ducts and to synergize with other mammotropic hormones in mammary gland differentiation in hypophysectomized rats (Wright and Anderson, 1982). Relaxin also enhanced ductal growth and the differentiation of myoepithelial cells in mice when administered in combination with ovarian steroids (Bani and Bigazzi, 1984; Bani et al., 1985).

4. Conclusions

The contribution of placental polypeptide hormones to mammary development during pregnancy is discussed in this chapter. There are species differences with respect to polypeptide hormones synthesized by the placenta. So far, PL has been detected in three orders of mammals, Primata, Rodentia, and Artiodactyla, but attempts to detect placental lactogenic activity using radioreceptor assays and bioassays have been unsuccessful in several other mammalian orders (Talamantes et al., 1980; Forsyth, 1986). Lactogenic hormones (PRL, PL, GH) are necessary for mammary development in rats, mice, and goats (Lyons et al., 1958; Nandi, 1958; Cowie et al., 1966, 1968; Cowie and Tindal, 1971). It is not known to what extent this applies to other species, with the exception that lactogenic hormones do not seem to be essential for mammary development in rabbits (A. Norgren, 1966, 1968, cited by Cowie and Tindal, 1971). In those species having a PL, the importance of the hormone for mammary development may vary considerably. In mice and rats, PL (the smaller molecular weight form that is present during the latter half of pregnancy) is probably the most important lactogen in the latter half of pregnancy when PRL concentration is low. Similarly, PRL and GH remain low during pregnancy in sheep and goats, whereas PL is present in the circulation in high concentrations in the latter half of pregnancy in both these species. In the human, on the other hand, PRL shows a continuous rise throughout pregnancy. However, mammary development also takes place when the PRL concentration is low or absent during pregnancy and normal mammary development occurs in the absence of PL, indicating that these hormones can be replaced by each other to some extent.

There is very limited knowledge about the mechanism of action of PL. Binding to receptors on the plasma membrane is the first step in the action of polypeptide hormones. So far, specific PL receptors have only been reported in ovine fetal liver (Freemark and Handwerger, 1986) but it is not known whether specific receptors for PL exist in the mammary gland or whether PL acts exclusively through receptors that also bind other lactogens. Similarly, it is not known whether one lactogenic hormone (PRL, PL, GH) can completely replace another or whether they synergize in their action on the mammary gland. It is interesting to note in this context that artificial induction of lactation in goats and cows by hormonal treatments has, at best, only approached the milk yield obtained after parturition, but usually the milk yield is considerably less (see Cowie et al., 1980, for references). The lack of success in inducing lactation by hormonal treatment may be caused by the absence of appropriate hormonal stimulation from the placenta.

The establishment of a mammary epithelial cell culture has provided an opportunity for many kinds of studies on the hormonal control of the mammary gland. Synergistic effects of the lactogens and the receptor specificity of each of these hormones are two areas that are important to investigate to understand further the role of each of the lactogenic hormones in mammogenesis. Moreover, it is now feasible to extend the studies of the mammary gland to the molecular level by using molecular probes to examine the hormonal control of the expression of genes that code for specific milk proteins.

ACKNOWLEDGMENTS: We gratefully acknowledge the valuable assistance and advice of Karol Bowens, Dr. Peter Colosi, Paula Folger, Gulla Gisladottir, Dr. Luis Haro, Dr. Linda Ogren, and Dr. Jonathan Southard. This work was supported by NIH Grants HD14966 and RR08132 and NSF Grant PCM-8217382 to Dr. F. Talamantes.

References

Agate, F.J., 1952, The growth and secretory activity of the mammary glands of the pregnant rhesus monkey (*Macaca mulatta*) following hypophysectomy, *Am. J. Anat.* **90:**257–283.

Akers, R.M., Bauman, D.E., Capuco, A.V., Goodman, G.T., and Tucker, H.A., 1981, Prolactin regulation of milk secretion and biochemical differentiation of mammary epithelial cells in periparturient cows, *Endocrinology* **109:**23–30.

Allen, W.R., 1975, Endocrine function of the placenta, in: *Comparative Plancentation* (D.H. Steven, ed.), Academic Press, London, pp. 214–267.

Amenomori, Y., Chen, C.L., and Meites, J., 1970, Serum prolactin levels in rats during different reproductive states, *Endocrinology* **86:**506–510.

Anderson, L.L., 1982, Relaxin localization in porcine and bovine ovaries by assay and morphologic techniques, in: *Advances in Experimental Medicine and Biology,* Vol. 143, *Relaxin* (R.R. Anderson ed.), Plenum Press, New York, pp. 1–67.

Anderson, R.R., 1974, Endocrinological control, in: *Lactation,* Vol. I (B.L. Larson and V.R. Smith, eds.), Academic Press, New York, pp. 97–140.

Anderson, R.R., 1975a, Mammary gland growth in the hypophysectomized pregnant rat, *Proc. Soc. Exp. Biol. Med.* **148:**283–287.

Anderson, R.R., 1975b, Mammary gland growth in sheep, *J. Anim. Sci.* **41:**118–123.

Anderson, R.R., and Turner, C.W., 1968, Mammary gland growth during pseudopregnancy and pregnancy in the rat, *Proc. Soc. Exp. Biol. Med.* **128:**210–214.

Anderson, R.R., Harness, J.R., Snead, A.F., and Salah, M.S., 1981, Mammary growth pattern in goats during pregnancy and lactation, *J. Dairy Sci.* **64:**427–432.

Anderson, R.R., Salah, M.S., Harness, J.R., and Snead, A.F., 1982, Mammary growth patterns in guinea pigs during puberty, pregnancy and lactation, *Biol. Reprod.* **26:**620–627.

Banerjee, D.N., and Banerjee, M.R., 1973, Rapidly-labelled RNA in the mouse mammary gland before and during lactation, *J. Endocrinol.* **56:**145–152.

Banerjee, M.R., Rogers, F.M., and Banerjee, D.N., 1971, Hormonal regulation of RNA and protein synthesis in the mouse mammary gland before and during lactation, *J. Endocrinol.* **50:**281–291.

Banerjee, M.R., Terry, P.M., Sakai, S., and Lin, F.K., 1977, Regulation of messenger RNA and specific milk protein in mammary gland, *J. Toxicol. Environ. Health* **3:**281–308.

Bani, G., and Bigazzi, M., 1984, Morphological changes induced in mouse mammary gland by porcine and human relaxin, *Acta Anat.* **119:**149–154.

Bani, G., Bigazzi, M., and Bani, D., 1985, Effects of relaxin on the mouse mammary gland. 1. The myoepithelial cells, *J. Endocrinol. Invest.* **8:**207–215.

Barlow, S.M., Morrison, P.J., and Sullivan, F.M., 1974, Plasma corticosterone levels during pregnancy in the mouse: The relative contributions of the adrenal glands and foeto-placental units, *J. Endocrinol.* **60:**473–483.

Bast, J.D., and Greenwald, G.S., 1974, Daily concentrations of gonadotrophins and prolactin in the serum of pregnant and lactating hamsters, *J. Endocrinol.* **63:**527–532.

Beck, P., 1972, Lactogenic activity of human chorionic somatomammotropin in rhesus monkeys, *Proc. Soc. Exp. Biol. Med.* **140:**183–187.

Becka, S., Bilek, J., Slaba, J., Skarda, J., and Mikulas, I., 1977, Some properties of the goat placental lactogen, *Separatum Experientie* **33:**771–772.

Belanger, C., Shome, B., Friesen, H., and Myers, R.E., 1971, Studies of the secretion of monkey placental lactogen, *J. Clin. Invest.* **50:**2660–2667.

Bewley, T.A., Dixon, J.S., and Li, C.H., 1972, Sequence comparison of human pituitary growth hormone, human chorionic somatomammotropin, and ovine pituitary growth and lactogenic hormones, *Int. J. Pept. Protein Res.* **4:**281–287.

Bhattacharjee, M., and Vonderhaar, B.K., 1984, Thyroid hormones enhance the synthesis and secretion of α-lactalbumin by mouse mammary tissue *in vitro, Endocrinology* **115:**1070–1077.

Birken, S., and Canfield, R.E., 1980, Chemistry and immunochemistry of human chorionic gonadotropin, in *Chorionic Gonadotropin* (S.J. Segal, ed.), Plenum Press, New York, pp. 65–88.

Blank, M.S., and Dufau, M.L., 1983, Rat chorionic gonadotropin: Augmentation of bioactivity in the absence of the pituitary, *Endocrinology* **112:**2200–2202.

Blank, M.S., Dufau, M.L., and Friesen, H.G., 1979, Demonstration of potent gonadotropin-like biological activity in the serum of rats during midpregnancy, *Life Sci.* **25:**1023–1028.

Blom, A.K., Hove, K., and Nedkvitne, J.J., 1976, Plasma insulin and growth hormone concentrations in pregnant sheep. II: Post-absorptive levels in mid- and late-pregnancy, *Acta Endocrinol.* **82:**553–560.

Bolander, F.F., and Fellows, R.E., 1976, Purification and characterization of bovine placental lactogen, *J. Biol. Chem.* **251:**2703–2708.

Brookreson, A.D., and Turner, C.W., 1959, Normal growth of mammary gland in pregnant and lactating mice, *Proc. Soc. Exp. Biol. Med.* **102:**744–745.

Bryant-Greenwood, G.D., 1981, Relaxin from non-corpus luteum sources, in: *Relaxin, Proceedings of a Workshop on the Chemistry and Biology of Relaxin* (G.D. Bryant-Greenwood, H.D. Niall, and F.C. Greenwood, eds.), Elsevier North Holland, New York, pp. 171–173.

Burditt, L.J., Parker, D., Craig, R.K., Getova, T., and Campbell, P.N., 1981, Differential expression of α-lactalbumin and casein genes during the onset of lactation in the guinea-pig mammary gland, *Biochem. J.* **194:**999–1006.

Bussmann, L.E., and Deis, R.P., 1984, γ-Glutamyltransferase activity in mammary gland of pregnant rats and its regulation by ovarian hormones, prolactin and placental lactogen, *Biochem. J.* **223:**275–277.

Bussmann, L.E., Koninckx, A., and Deis, R.P., 1983, Effect of estrogen and placental lactogen on lactogenesis in pregnant rats, *Biol. Reprod.* **29:**535–541.

Butler, S.R., Hurley, T.W., Schanberg, S.M., and Handwerger, S., 1978, Ovine placental lactogen stimulation of ornithine decarboxylase activity in brain and liver of neonatal rats, *Life Sci.* **22:**2073–2078.

Butler, W.R., Fullenkamp, S.M., Cappiello, L.A., and Handwerger, S., 1981, The relationship between breed and litter size in sheep and maternal serum concentrations of placental lactogen, estradiol and progesterone, *J. Anim. Sci.* **53:**1077–1081.

Buttle, H.L., Forsyth, I.A., and Knaggs, G.S., 1972, Plasma prolactin measured by radioimmunoassay and bioassay in pregnant and lactating goats and the occurrence of a placental lactogen, *J. Endocrinol.* **53:**483–491.

Buttle, H.L., Cowie, A.T., Jones, E.A., and Turvey, A., 1979, Mammary growth during pregnancy in hypophysectomized or bromocryptine-treated goats, *J. Endocrinol.* **80:**343–351.

Chan, J.S.D., Robertson, H.A., and Friesen, H.G., 1976, The purification and characterization of ovine placental lactogen, *Endocrinology* **98:**65–76.

Chan, J.S.D., Robertson, H.A., and Friesen, H.G., 1978a, Maternal and fetal concentrations of ovine placental lactogen measured by radioimmunoassay, *Endocrinology* **102:**1606–1613.

Chan, J.S.D., Robertson, H.A., and Friesen, H.G., 1978b, Distribution of binding sites for ovine placental lactogen in the sheep, *Endocrinology* **102:**632–640.

Cohen, R.M., and Gala, R.R., 1969, Detection of luteotropic and mammotropic activity in the serum of rats at midpregnancy, *Proc. Soc. Exp. Biol. Med.* **132:**683–685.

Collip, J.B., Selye, H., and Thomson, D.L., 1933, Further observations on the effect of hypophysectomy on lactation, *Proc. Soc. Exp. Biol. Med.* **30:**913.

Colosi, P., Markoff, E., Levy, A., Ogren, L., Shine, N., and Talamantes, F., 1981, Isolation and partial characterization of secreted hamster pituitary prolactin, *Endocrinology* **108:**850–854.

Colosi, P., Marr, G., Lopez, J., Haro, L., Ogren, L., and Talamantes, F., 1982, Isolation, purification, and characterization of mouse placental lactogen, *Proc. Natl. Acad. Sci. USA* **79:**771–775.

Colosi, P., Ogren, L., and Talamantes, F., 1986, RIA and gestational serum profile of mouse midpregnancy lactogen, *Endocrinology* **118** (suppl.)**:** 79.

Colosi, P., Ogren, L., Thordarson, G., and Talamantes, F., 1987, Purification and partial characterization of two prolactin-like glycoprotein hormone complexes from the midpregnant mouse conceptus, *Endocrinology* **120:** 2500–2511.

Cowie, A.T., and Tindal, J.S., 1971, *The Physiology of Lactation,* Edward Arnold Ltd., London.

Cowie, A.T., Tindal, J.S., and Yokoyama, A., 1966, The induction of mammary growth in the hypophysectomized goat, *J. Endocrinol.* **34:**185–195.

Cowie, A.T., Knaggs, G.S., Tindal, J.S., and Turvey, A., 1968, The milking stimulus and mammary growth in the goat, *J. Endocrinol.* **40:**243–252.

Cowie, A.T., Forsyth, I.A., and Hart, I.C., 1980, *Monographs on Endocrinology,* Vol. 15, *Hormonal Control of Lactation* (F. Gross, M.M. Grumbach, A. Labhart, M.B. Lipsett, T. Mann, L.T. Samuels, and J. Zander, eds.), Springer-Verlag, Berlin.

Critser, E.S., Rutledge, J.J., and French, L.R., 1980, Role of the uterus and the conceptus in regulating luteal lifespan in the mouse, *Biol. Reprod.* **23:**558–563.

Critser, E.S., Savage, P.J., Rutledge, J.J., and French, L.R., 1982, Control of luteal function during pregnancy: Antiluteolytic and luteotropic properties of the developing mouse conceptus, *Biol. Reprod.* **27:**1042–1048.

Currie, W.B., Kelly, P.A., Friesen, H.G., and Thorburn, G.D., 1977, Caprine placental lactogen: Levels of prolactin-like and growth hormone-like activities in the circulation of pregnant goats determined by radioreceptor assays, *J. Endocrinol.* **73:**215–226.

Daughaday, W.H., Trivedi, B., and Kapadia, M., 1979, The effect of hypophysectomy on rat chorionic somatomammotropin as measured by prolactin and growth hormone radioreceptor assays: Possible significance in maintenance of somatomedin generation, *Endocrinology* **105:**210–214.

Davis, S.R., Mepham, T.B., and Lock, K.J., 1979, Relative importance of pre-partum and post-partum factors in the control of milk yield in the guinea-pig, *J. Dairy Res.* **46:**613–621.

Day, J.R., Ogren, L.M., and Talamantes, F., 1986, The effect of hypophysectomy on serum placental lactogen and progesterone in the mouse, *Endocrinology* **119:**898–903.

Denamur, R., 1965, Les acides nucleiques et les nucleotides libres de la glande mammaire pendant la lactogenese et la galactopoiese, *Excerpta Med. Int. Congr. Ser.,* 83, *Part* **1:**434–462.

Denamur, R., and Martinet, J., 1961, Effets de l'hypophysectomie et de la section de la tige pituitaire sur la gestation de la brebis, *Ann. Endocrinol.* **22:**755–759.

Desjardins, C., Paape, M.J., and Tucker, H.A., 1968, Contribution of pregnancy, fetuses, fetal placentas and desiduomas to mammary gland and uterine development, *Endocrinology* **83:**907–910.

Dujardin, M., Robyn, C., and Wilkin, P., 1977, Mise en evidence immunohistoenzymologique de l'hormone chorionique somatomammotrope (HCS). Au niveau des divers constituants cellulaires du placenta humain normal, *Biol. Cell.* **30:**151–154.

Fields, P.A., and Larkin, L.H., 1981, Purification and immunohistochemical localization of relaxin in the human term placenta, *J. Clin. Endocrinol. Metab.* **52:**79–85.

Fields, P.A., Pardo, R., and Larkin, L.H., 1981, Non-ovarian sources of relaxin, in: *Relaxin,*

Proceedings of a Workshop on the Chemistry and Biology of Relaxin (G.D. Bryant-Greenwood, H.D. Niall, and F.C. Greenwood, eds.), Elsevier North Holland, New York, pp. 179–182.

Fields, P.A., Larkin, L.H., and Pardo, R.J., 1982, Purification of relaxin from the placenta of the rabbit, *Ann. N.Y. Acad. Sci.* **380:**75–86.

Fleet, I.R., Goode, J.A., Hamon, M.H., Laurie, M.S., Linzell, J.L., and Peaker, M., 1975, Secretory activity of goat mammary glands during pregnancy and the onset of lactation, *J. Physiol.* **251:**763–773.

Florini, J.R., Tonelli, G., Breuer, C.B., Coppola, J., Ringler, I., and Bell, P.H., 1966, Characterization and biological effects of purified placental protein (human), *Endocrinology* **79:**692–708.

Forsyth, I.A., 1967, Lactogenic and pigeon crop-stimulating activities of a human placental lactogen preparation, *J. Endocrinol.* **37:**35–37.

Forsyth, I.A., 1973, Secretion of a prolactin-like hormone by the placenta in ruminants, in: *Le corps jaune* (R. Denamur and A. Netter, eds.), Masson, Paris, pp. 239–255.

Forsyth, I.A., 1986, Variation between species in the endocrine control of mammary growth and function: The roles of prolactin, growth hormone and placental lactogen, *J. Dairy Sci.* **69:**886–903.

Forsyth, I.A., and Folley, S.J., 1970, Prolactin and growth hormone in man and other mammals, in: *Ovo-implantation. Human Gonadotropins and Prolactins* (P.O. Hubinont, F. Leroy, C. Robyn, and P. Leleux, eds.), Karger, Basel, pp. 266–278.

Forsyth, I.A., Byatt, J.C., and Iley, S., 1985, Hormone concentrations, mammary development and milk yield in goats given long-term bromocriptine treatment in pregnancy, *J. Endocrinol.* **104:**77–85.

Foster, R.C., 1977, Changes in mouse mammary epithelial cell size during mammary gland development, *Cell Differ.* **6:**1–8.

Franks, S., Kiwi, R., and Nabarro, J.D.N., 1977, Pregnancy and lactation after pituitary surgery, *Br. Med. J.* **1:**882.

Freemark, M., and Handwerger, S., 1982, Ovine placental lactogen stimulates amino acid transport in rat diaphragm, *Endocrinology* **110:**2201–2203.

Freemark, M., and Handwerger, S., 1984, Ovine placental lactogen stimulates glycogen synthesis in fetal rat hepatocytes, *Am. J. Physiol.* **246:**E21–E24.

Freemark, M., and Handwerger, S., 1986, The glycogenic effects of placental lactogen and growth hormone in ovine fetal liver are mediated through binding to specific fetal ovine placental lactogen receptors, *Endocrinology* **118:**613–618.

Friesen, H.G., 1966, Lactation induced by human placental lactogen and cortisone acetate in rabbits, *Endocrinology* **104:**1828–1833.

Gaede, P., Trolle, D., and Pedersen, H., 1978, Extremely low placental lactogen hormone (hPL) values in an otherwise uneventful pregnancy preceding delivering of a normal baby, *Acta Obstet. Gynecol. Scand.* **57:**203–209.

Gaspard, U., and Franchimont, P., 1974, HCS, HCG and HCG subunit serum levels during multiple pregnancies, *Acta Genet. Med. Gemellol.* **22:**195–199. (Supplement, P. Parisi, ed., Proceedings of an International Symposium, Multiple Pregnancy and Twin Care.)

Glaser, L.A., Kelly, P.A., and Gibori, G., 1984, Differential action and secretion of rat placental lactogens, *Endocrinology* **115:**969–976.

Glaser, L.A., Khan, I., Pepe, G.J., Kelly, P.A., and Gibori, G., 1985, Further studies on rat placental lactogens, in: *Prolactin. Basic and Clinical Correlates,* Vol. I (R.M. MacLeod, M.O. Thorner, and U. Scapagnini, eds.), Liviana Press, Padova, pp. 495–499.

Gluckman, P.D., Kaplan, S.L., Rudolph, A.M., and Grumbach, M.M., 1979, Hormone ontogeny in the ovine fetus. II. Ovine chorionic somatomammotropin in mid- and late gestation in the fetal and maternal circulations, *Endocrinology* **104:**1828–1833.

Goodman, G.T., Akers, R.M., Friderici, K.H., and Tucker, H.A., 1983, Hormonal regulation of α-lactalbumin secretion from bovine mammary tissue cultured *in vitro, Endocrinology* **112:**1324–1330.

Greenwald, G.S., 1967, Luteotropic complex of the hamster, *Endocrinology* **80:**118–130.

Griffith, D.R., and Turner, C.W., 1961, Normal growth of rat mammary glands during pregnancy and early lactation, *Proc. Soc. Exp. Biol. Med.* **106:**448–450.

Grumbach, M.M., Kaplan, S.L., Sciarra, J.J., and Burr, I.M., 1968, Chorionic growth hormone-prolactin (CGP): Secretion, disposition, biological activity in man, and postulated function as the "growth hormone" of the second half of pregnancy, *Ann. N.Y. Acad. Sci.* **148:**501–531.

Hall, J., and Talamantes, F., 1984, Immunocytochemical localization of mouse placental lactogen in the mouse placenta, *J. Histochem. Cytochem.* **32:**379–382.

Hamolsky, M., and Sparrow, R.C., 1945, Influence of relaxin on mammary development in sexually immature female rats, *Proc. Soc. Exp. Biol. Med.* **60:**8–9.

Handwerger, S., Crenshew, C., Maurer, W.F., Barrett, J., Hurley, T.W., Golander, A., and Fellows, R.E., 1977, Studies on ovine placental lactogen secretion by homologous radioimmunoassay, *J. Endocrinol.* **72:**27–34.

Hart, I.C., 1976, Prolactin growth hormone, insulin and thyroxine: Their possible roles in steroid-induced mammary growth and lactation in the goat, *J. Endocrinol.* **71:**41P–42P.

Hayden, T.J., Thomas, C.R., and Forsyth, I.A., 1979, Effect of number of young born (litter size) on milk yield of goats: Role for placental lactogen, *J. Diary Sci.* **62:**53–57.

Hayden, T.J., Thomas, C.R., Smith, S.V., and Forsyth, I.A., 1980, Placental lactogen in the goat in relation to stage of gestation, number of fetuses, metabolites, progesterone and time of day, *J. Endocrinol.* **86:**279–290.

Hobson, B.M., 1983, An appraisal of the mouse uterine weight assay for the bioassay of chorionic gonadotrophin in the macaque term placenta, *J. Reprod. Fertil.* **68:**457–463.

Hoshina, M., Boothby, M., and Boime, I., 1982, Cytological localization of chorionic gonadotropin α and placental lactogen mRNAs during development of the human placenta, *J. Cell Biol.* **93:**190–198.

Hurley, T.W., Handwerger, S., and Fellows, R.E., 1977a, Isolation and structural characterization of ovine placental lactogen, *Biochemistry* **16:**5598–5604.

Hurley, T.W., Grissom, F.E., Handwerger, S., and Fellows, R.E., 1977b, Purification and partial characterization of the cyanogen bromide fragments of ovine placental lactogen, *Biochemistry* **16:**5605–5609.

Hurley, T.W., D'Ercole, A.J., Handwerger, S., Underwood, L.E., Furlanetto, R.W., and Fellows, R.E., 1977c, Ovine placental lactogen induces somatomedin: A possible role in fetal growth, *Endocrinology* **101:**1635–1638.

Ikonicoff, L.K. de, and Cedard, L., 1973, Localization of human chorionic gonadotropic and somatomammotropic hormones by the peroxidase immunohistoenzymologic method in villi and amniotic epithelium of human placentas (from six weeks to term), *Am. J. Obstet. Gynecol.* **116:**1124–1132.

Ito, Y., and Higashi, K., 1961, Studies of the prolactin-like substance in human placenta, *Endocrinol. Jap.* **8:**279–287.

Jackson, L.L., Colosi, P., Talamantes, F., and Linzer, D.I.H., 1986, Molecular cloning of mouse placental lactogen cDNA, *Proc. Natl. Acad. Sci. USA,* **83:**8496–8500.

Jones, E.A., 1979, Changes in the activity of lactose synthetase in the goat udder during pregnancy, *J. Dairy Res.* **46:**35–40.

Josimovich, J.B., and MacLaren, J.A., 1962, Presence in the human placenta and term serum of a highly lactogenic substance immunologically related to pituitary growth hormone, *Endocrinology* **71:**209–220.

Josimovich, J.B., Levitt, M.J., and Stevens, V.C., 1973, Comparison of baboon and human placental lactogens, *Endocrinology* **93:**242–244.

Kaplan, N.M., 1961, Successful pregnancy following hypophysectomy during the twelfth week of gestation, *J. Clin. Endocrinol. Metab.* **21:**1139–1145.

Kaplan, S.L., and Grumbach, M.M., 1964, Studies of a human and simian placental hormone with growth hormone-like and prolactin-like activities, *J. Clin. Endocrinol. Metab.* **24:**80–100.

Kelly, P.A., Robertson, H.A., and Friesen, H.G., 1974, Temporal pattern of placental lactogen and progesterone secretion in sheep, *Nature* **248:**435–437.

Kelly, P.A., Shiu, R.P.C., Robertson, M.C., and Friesen, H.G., 1975, Characterization of rat chorionic mammotropin, *Endocrinology* **96:**1187–1195.

Kelly, P.A., Tsushima, T., Shiu, R.P.C., and Friesen, H.G., 1976, Lactogenic and growth hormone-like activities in pregnancy determined by radioreceptor assays, *Endocrinology* **99:**765–774.

Kleinberg, D.L., Todd, J., and Niemann, W., 1978, Prolactin stimulation of α-lactalbumin in normal primate mammary gland, *J. Clin. Endocrinol. Metab.* **47:**435–441.

Knight, C.H., and Peaker, M., 1982, Mammary development in mice: Effects of hemi-hysterectomy in pregnancy and of litter size *post partum*, *J. Physiol.* **327:**17–27.

Koay, E.S.C., Bagnell, C.A., Bryant-Greenwood, G.D., Lord, S.B., Cruz, A.C., and Larkin, L.H., 1985, Immunocytochemical localization of relaxin in human decidua and placenta, *J. Clin. Endocrinol. Metab.* **60:**859–863.

Kohmoto, K., 1975, Synthesis of two lactogenic proteins by the mouse placenta *in vitro*, *Endocrinol. Jap.* **22:**275–278.

Kohmoto, K., and Bern, H.A., 1970, Demonstration of mammotrophic activity of the mouse placenta in organ culture and by transplantation, *J. Endocrinol.* **48:**99–107.

Kulski, J.K., and Hartmann, P.E., 1981, Changes in human milk composition during the initiation of lactation, *Aust. J. Exp. Biol. Med. Sci.* **59:**101–114.

Lindberg, B.S., and Nilsson, B.A., 1973, Variations in maternal plasma levels of human placental lactogen (HPL) in normal pregnancy and labor, *J. Obstet. Gynaecol. Br. Commonw.* **80:**619–626.

Linkie, D.M., and Niswender, G.D., 1973, Characterization of rat placental luteotropin physiological and physicochemical properties, *Biol. Reprod.* **8:**48–57.

Linzer, D.I.H., and Nathans, D., 1984, Nucleotide sequence of a growth-related mRNA encoding a member of the prolactin-growth hormone family, *Proc. Natl. Acad. Sci. USA* **81:**4255–4259.

Linzer, D.I., and Nathans, D., 1985, A new member of the prolactin-growth hormone gene family expressed in mouse placenta, *EMBO J.* **4:**1419–1423.

Linzer, D.I.H., and Talamantes, F., 1985, Nucleotide sequence of mouse prolactin and growth hormone mRNAs and expression of these mRNAs during pregnancy, *J. Biol. Chem.* **260:**9574–9579.

Linzer, D.I.H., Lee, S.-J., Ogren, L., Talamantes, F., and Nathans, D., 1985, Identification of proliferin mRNA and protein in mouse placenta, *Proc. Natl. Acad. Sci. USA* **82:**4356–4359.

Lyons, W.R., Li, C.H., and Johnson, R.E., 1958, The hormonal control of mammary growth and lactation, *Recent Prog. Horm. Res.* **14:**219–254.

Markoff, E., and Talamantes, F., 1980, The lactogenic response of mouse mammary explants to mouse prolactin and growth hormone, *Endocr. Res. Commun.* **7:**269–278.

Markoff, E., and Talamantes, F., 1981, Serum placental lactogen in mice in relation to day of gestation and number of conceptuses, *Biol. Reprod.* **24:**846–851.

Martal, J., and Djiane, J., 1975, Purification of a lactogenic hormone in sheep placenta, *Biochem. Biophys. Res. Commun.* **65:**770–778.

Martal, J., Djiane, J., and Dubois, M.P., 1977, Immunofluorescent localization of ovine placental lactogen, *Cell Tissue Res.* **184:**427–433.

Martin, R.H., Glass, M.R., Chapman, C., Wilson, G.D., and Woods, K.L., 1980, Human α-lactalbumin and hormonal factors in pregnancy and lactation, *Clin. Endocrinol.* **13:**223–230.

Matthies, D.L., 1965, Evidence for the synthesis of a protein mammotropin by the mid-pregnancy rat placenta, *Anat. Rec.* **151:**383.

Matthies, D.L., 1967, Studies of the luteotropic and mammotropic factor found in trophoblast and maternal peripheral blood of the rat at mid-pregnancy, *Anat. Rec.* **159:**55–61.

McKenzie, L., Fitzgerald, D.K., and Ebner, K.E., 1971, Lactose synthetase activities in rat and mouse mammary glands, *Biochim. Biophys. Acta* **230:**526–530.

McManus, M.J., Dembroske, S.E., Pienkowski, M.M., Anderson, T.J., Mann, L.C., Schuster, J.S., Vollwiler, L.L., and Welsch, C.W., 1978, Successful transplantation of human benign breast tumors into the athymic nude mouse and demonstration of enhanced DNA synthesis by human placental lactogen, *Cancer Res.* **38:**2343–2348.

Mills, E.S., and Topper, Y.J., 1970, Some ultrastructural effects of insulin, hydrocortisone, and prolactin on mammary gland explants, *J. Cell. Biol.* **44:**310–328.

Munford, R.E., 1963, Changes in the mammary glands of rats and mice during pregnancy, lactation and involution, *J. Endocrinol.* **28:**17–34.

Munford, R.E., 1964, A review of anatomical and biochemical changes in the mammary gland with particular reference to quantitative methods of assessing mammary development, *Dairy Sci. Abstr.* **26:**293–304.

Murthy, G.S., Schellenberg, C., and Friesen, H.G., 1982, Purification and characterization of bovine placental lactogen, *Endocrinology* **111:**2117–2124.

Nagasawa, H., and Yanai, R., 1971, Quantitative participation of placental mammotropic hormones in mammary development during pregnancy of mice, *Endocrinol. Jap.* **18:**507–510.

Nagasawa, H., and Yanai, R., 1973, Effects of adrenalectomy and/or deficiency of pituitary prolactin secretion on initiation and maintenance of lactation in mice, *J. Endocrinol.* **58:**67–73.

Nakhasi, H.L. and Qasba, P.K., 1979, Quantitation of milk proteins and their mRNAs in rat mammary gland at various stages of gestation and lactation, *J. Biol. Chem.* **154:**6016–6025.

Nandi, S., 1958, Endocrine control of mammary-gland development and function in the C3H/He Crgl mouse, *J. Natl. Cancer Inst.* **21:**1039–1063.

Nelson, W.L., Heytler, P.G., and Ciaccio, E.I., 1962, Guinea pig mammary gland growth changes in weight, nitrogen and nucleic acids, *Proc. Soc. Exp. Biol. Med.* **109:**373–375.

Nielsen, P.V., Pedersen, H., and Kampmann, E.M., 1979, Absence of human placental lactogen in an otherwise uneventful pregnancy, *Am. J. Obstet. Gynecol.* **135:**322–326.

Papkoff, H., Bewley, T.A., and Ramachandran, J., 1978, Physicochemical and biological characterizations of pregnant mare serum gonadotropin and its subunits, *Biochim. Biophys. Acta* **532:**185–194.

Parks, J.S., Nielsen, P.V., Sexton, L.A., and Jorgensen, E.H., 1985, An effect of gene dosage on production of human chorionic somatomammotropin, *J. Clin. Endocrinol. Metab.* **60:**994–997.

Pencharz, R.I., and Lyons, W.R., 1934, Hypophysectomy in the pregnant guinea-pig, *Proc. Soc. Exp. Biol. Med.* **31:**1131–1132.

Prop, F.J.A., 1969, Action of prolactin and human placental lactogen (HPL) on human mammary gland *in vitro,* in: *Protein and Polypeptide Hormones,* Part 2, Proceedings of an

International Symposium (M. Margoulies, ed.), Excerpta Medica Foundation, Amsterdam, pp. 508–510.

Ray, E.W., Averill, S.C., Lyons, W.M.R., and Johnson, R.E., 1955, Rat placental hormonal activities corresponding to those of pituitary mammotropin, *Endocrinology* **56:**359–373.

Reddy, S., and Watkins, W.B., 1978a, Purification and some properties of ovine placental lactogen, *J. Endocrinol.* **78:**59–69.

Reddy, S., and Watkins, W.B., 1978b, Immunofluorescence localization of ovine placental lactogen, *J. Reprod. Fertil.* **52:**173–174.

Rigg, L.A., Lein, A., and Yen, S.S.C., 1977, Pattern of increase in circulating prolactin levels during human gestation, *Am. J. Obstet. Gynecol.* **129:**454–456.

Robertson, M.C., and Friesen, H.G., 1975, The purification and characterization of rat placental lactogen, *Endocrinology* **97:**621–629.

Robertson, M.C., and Friesen, H.G., 1981, Two forms of rat placental lactogen revealed by radioimmunoassay, *Endocrinology* **108:**2388–2390.

Robertson, M.C., Gillespie, B., and Friesen, H.G., 1982, Characterization of the two forms of rat placental lactogen (rPL): rPL-I and rPL-II, *Endocrinology* **111:**1862–1866.

Robertson, M.C., Owens, R.E., Klindt, J., and Friesen, H.G., 1984a, Ovariectomy leads to a rapid increase in rat placental lactogen secretion, *Endocrinology* **114:**1805–1811.

Robertson, M.C., Owens, R.E., McCoshen, A., and Friesen, H.G., 1984b, Ovarian factors inhibit and fetal factors stimulate the secretion of rat placental lactogen, *Endocrinology* **114:**22–30.

Rosen, J.M., Woo, S.L.C., and Comstock, J.P., 1975, Regulation of casein messenger RNA during the development of the rat mammary gland, *Biochemistry* **14:**2895–2903.

Samaan, N., Yen, S.C.C., Friesen, H., and Pearson, O.H., 1966, Serum placental lactogen levels during pregnancy and in trophoblastic disease, *J. Clin. Endocrinol. Metab.* **26:**1303–1308.

Schalch, D.S., and Reichlin, S., 1966, Plasma growth hormone concentration in the rat determined by radioimmunoassay: Influence of sex, pregnancy, lactation, anesthesia, hypophysectomy and extrasellar pituitary transplants, *Endocrinology* **79:**275–280.

Schams, D., Rüsse, I., Schallenberger, E., Prokopp, S., and Chan, J.S.D., 1984, The role of steroid hormones, prolactin and placental lactogen on mammary gland development in ewes and heifers, *J. Endocrinol.* **102:**121–130.

Sciarra, J.J., Kaplan, S.L., and Grumbach, M.M., 1963, Localization of anti-human growth hormone serum within the human placenta: Evidence for a human chorionic growth hormone-prolactin, *Nature* **199:**1005–1006.

Selye, H., Collip, J.B., and Thomson, D.L., 1934, Effect of hypophysectomy upon pregnancy and lactation in mice, *Proc. Soc. Exp. Biol. Med.* **31:**82–83.

Servely, J.-L., Emane, M.N., Houdebine, L.-M., Djiane, J., Delouis, C., and Kelly, P.A., 1983, Comparative measurement of the lactogenic activity of ovine placental lactogen in rabbit and ewe mammary gland, *Gen. Comp. Endocrinol.* **51:**255–262.

Sherwood, L.M., Handwerger, S., McLaurin, W.D., and Pang, E.C., 1971, Comparison of the structure and function of human placental lactogen and human growth hormone, *Excerpta Med. Int. Congr. Ser.* **244:**209–223.

Shiu, R.P.C., Kelly, P.A., and Friesen, H.G., 1973, Radioreceptor assay for prolactin and other lactogenic hormones, *Science* **180:**968–971.

Shome, B., and Friesen, G.H., 1971, Purification and characterization of monkey placental lactogen, *Endocrinology* **89:**631–641.

Shome, B., and Parlow, A.F., 1977, Human pituitary prolactin (hPRL): The entire linear amino acid sequence, *J. Clin. Endocrinol. Metab.* **45:**1112–1115.

Sinha, K.N., Anderson, R.R., and Turner, C.W., 1970, Growth of the mammary glands of the golden hamster, *Mesocricetus auratus, Biol. Reprod.* **2:**185–188.

Smith, M.S., and Neill, J.D., 1976, Termination at midpregnancy of the two daily surges of plasma prolactin initiated by mating in the rat, *Endocrinology* **98:**696–701.

Smith, P.E., 1954, Continuation of pregnancy in rhesus monkeys (*Macaca mulatta*) following hypophysectomy, *Endocrinology* **55:**655–664.

Smith, T.C., 1954, The action of relaxin on mammary gland growth in the rat, *Endocrinology* **54:**59–70.

Soares, M.J., and Talamantes, F., 1982, Placental and serum hormone changes during the second half of pregnancy in the hamster, *Biol. Reprod.* **27:**523–529.

Soares, M.J., and Talamantes, F., 1983, Genetic and litter size effects on serum placental lactogen in the mouse, *Biol. Reprod.* **29:**165–171.

Soares, M.J., and Talamantes, F., 1985, Placental lactogen secretion in the mouse: *In vitro* responses and ovarian and hormonal influences, *J. Exp. Zool.* **234:**97–104.

Soares, M.J., Colosi, P., and Talamantes, F., 1982, The development and characterization of a homologous radioimmunoassay for mouse placental lactogen, *Endocrinology* **110:**668–670.

Soares, M.J., Colosi, P., Ogren, L., and Talamantes, F., 1983, Identification and partial characterization of a lactogen from the midpregnant mouse conceptus, *Endocrinology* **112:**1313–1317.

Soares, M.J., Julian, J.A., and Glasser, S.R., 1985, Trophoblast giant cell release of placental lactogens: Temporal and regional characteristics, *Dev. Biol.* **107:**520–526.

Southard, J.N., Thordarson, G., and Talamantes, F., 1986, Purification and characterization of hamster placental lactogen, *Endocrinology* **119:**508–514.

Tabarelli, M., Kofler, R., Schwarz, S., and Wick, G., 1982, Rat placental hormones: Attempts for identification of rat chorionic gonadotropin and rat placental lactogen by *in vivo* experiments, *Acta Endocrinol.* **99:**288–294.

Tabarelli, M., Kofler, R., and Wick, G., 1983, Placental hormones: I. Immunofluorescence studies of the localization of chorionic gonadotrophin, placental lactogen and prolactin in human and rat placenta and in the endometrium of pregnant rats, *Placenta* **4:**379–388.

Talamantes, F., 1975a, Comparative study of the occurrence of placental prolactin among mammals, *Gen. Comp. Endocrinol.* **27:**115–121.

Talamantes, F., 1975b, *In vitro* demonstration of lactogenic activity in the mammalian placenta, *Am. Zool.* **15:**279–284.

Talamantes, F., Ogren, L., Markoff, E., Woodard, S., and Madrid, J., 1980, Phylogenetic distribution, regulation of secretion, and prolactin-like effects of placental lactogens, *Fed. Proc.* **39:**2582–2587.

Talamantes, F., Soares, M.J., Colosi, P., Haro, L., and Ogren, L., 1984a, The biochemistry and physiology of mouse placental lactogen, in: *Prolactin Secretion: A Multidisciplinary Approach* (F. Mena and C.M. Valverde-R., eds.), Academic Press, New York, pp. 31–41.

Talamantes, F., Marr, G., DiPinto, M.N., and Stetson, M.H., 1984b, Prolactin profiles during estrous cycle and pregnancy in hamster as measured by homologous RIA, *Am. J. Physiol.* **247:**E126–E129.

Terry, P.M., Ball, E.M., Ganguly, R., and Banerjee, M.R., 1975, An indirect radioimmunoassay for mouse casein using ^{125}I-labeled antigen, *J. Immunol. Methods* **9:**123–124.

Thorburn, G.D., Challis, J.R.C., and Currie, W.B., 1977, Control of parturition in domestic animals, *Biol. Reprod.* **16:**18–27.

Thordarson, G., 1984, Ph.D. Thesis, University of Reading, Reading, England.

Thordarson, G., and Forsyth, I.A., 1982, Plasma lactogenic activity and mammary development in guinea-pigs, *Programme of Winter Meeting of the Society for the Study of Fertility*, Abstract 34.

Thordarson, G., Villalobos, R., Colosi, P., Southard, J., Ogren, L., and Talamantes, F., 1986, Lactogenic response of cultured mouse mammary epithelial cells to mouse placental lactogen, *J. Endocrinol.* **109:**263–274.

Topper, Y.J., and Freeman, C.S., 1980, Multiple hormone interactions in the developmental biology of the mammary gland, *Physiol. Rev.* **60:**1049–1106.

Topper, Y.J., Nicholas, K.R., Sankaran, L., and Kulski, J.K., 1984, Insulin biology from the perspective of studies on mammary gland development, in: *Biochemical Actions of Hormones,* Vol. XI (G. Litwack, ed.), Academic Press, Orlando, FL, pp. 163–186.

Traurig, H.H., 1967, A radioautographic study of cell proliferation in the mammary gland of the pregnant mouse, *Anat. Rec.* **159:**239–247.

Tucker, H.A., and Reece, R.P., 1963a, Nucleic acid content of mammary glands of pregnant rats, *Proc. Soc. Exp. Biol. Med.* **112:**370–372.

Tucker, H.A., and Reece, R.P., 1963b, Nucleic acid content of mammary glands of lactating rats, *Proc. Soc. Exp. Biol. Med.* **112:**409–412.

Turkington, R.W., and Hill, R.L., 1969, Lactose synthetase: Progesterone inhibition of the induction of α-lactalbumin, *Science* **163:**1458–1460.

Turkington, R.W., and Topper, Y.J., 1966, Stimulation of casein synthesis and histological development of mammary gland by human placental lactogen *in vitro, Endocrinology* **79:**175–181.

Turkington, R.W., Brew, K., Vanaman, T.C., and Hill, R.L., 1968, The hormonal control of lactose synthetase in the developing mouse mammary gland, *J. Biol. Chem.* **243:**3382–3387.

Turtle, J.R., and Kipnis, D.M., 1967, The lipolytic action of human placental lactogen on isolated fat cells, *Biochim. Biophys. Acta* **144:**583–593.

Vonderhaar, B.K., 1975, A role of thyroid hormones in differentiation of mouse mammary gland *in vitro, Biochem. Biophys. Res. Commun.* **67:**1219–1225.

Vonderhaar, B.K., and Greco, A.E., 1979, Lobulo-alveolar development of mouse mammary glands is regulated by thyroid hormones, *Endocrinology* **104:**409–418.

Vorherr, H., 1974, *The Breast, Morphology, Physiology and Lactation,* Academic Press, New York.

Wada, H., and Turner, C.W., 1959, Effect of relaxin on mammary gland growth in female mice, *Proc. Soc. Exp. Biol. Med.* **101:**707–709.

Watkins, W.B., and Reddy, S., 1980, Ovine placental lactogen in the cotyledonary and intercotyledonary placenta of the ewe, *J. Reprod. Fertil.* **58:**411–414.

Ways, J., Markoff, E., Ogren, L., and Talamantes, F., 1979, Lactogenic response of mouse mammary explants from different days of pregnancy to placental lactogen and pituitary prolactin, *In Vitro* **15:**891–894.

Welsch, C.W., and McManus, M.J., 1977, Stimulation of DNA synthesis by human placenlactogen or insulin in organ cultures of benign human breast tumors, *Cancer Res.* **37:**2257–2261.

Wooding, F.B.P., 1981, Localization of ovine placental lactogen in sheep placentomes by electron microscope immunocytochemistry, *J. Reprod. Fertil.* **62:**15–19.

Wright, L.C., and Anderson, R.R., 1982, Effect of relaxin on mammary growth in the hypophysectomized rat, in: *Advances in Experimental Medicine and Biology,* Vol. 143, *Relaxin* (R.R. Anderson, ed.), Plenum Press, New York, pp. 341–355.

Wurzel, J.M., Parks, J.S., Herd, J.E., and Nielsen, P.V., 1982, A gene deletion is responsible for absence of human chorionic somatomammotropin, *DNA* **1**:251–257.

Yanai, R., and Nagasawa, H., 1971, Mammary growth and placental mammotropin during pregnancy in mice with high or low lactational performance, *J. Dairy Sci.* **54**:906–910.

Yki-Järvinen, H., and Wahlström, T., 1984, Immunohistochemical demonstration of relaxin in the placenta after removal of the corpus luteum, *Acta Endocrinol.* **106**:544–547.

Zwierzchowski, L., Kleczkowska, D., Niedbalski, W., and Grochowska, I., 1984, Variation of DNA polymerase activities and DNA synthesis in mouse mammary gland during pregnancy and early lactation, *Differentiation* **28**:179–185.

15

Role of Sex Steroid Hormones in Normal Mammary Gland Function

Sandra Z. Haslam

1. Introduction

The mammary gland is composed of epithelial, adipose, and fibrous connective tissues; the relative proportion of each tissue type varies with the species of origin and/or the developmental state of the gland. In the nonpregnant nulliparous animal, the epithelial component of the gland is organized into a branching ductal system. The epithelial cells lining the ducts are invested with a basal layer of myoepithelial cells and a continuous basement membrane encloses the whole epithelial system. Fibrous connective tissue surrounds the ducts and separates them from the subadjacent adipose stroma.

Mammary growth from birth to the approach of puberty is isometric. With the onset of puberty and ovarian cycles in females, growth in all tissues of the mammary gland accelerates (Cowie, 1949; Silver, 1953). The duct system proliferates within the adipose stroma, and with each successive ovarian cycle further ductal growth may occur. Postovulatory phases may be characterized by varying degrees of ductal or alveolar development (Purnell and Saggers, 1974).

During pregnancy, further ductal elongation and branching occur along with extensive lobuloalveolar development and organization of the epithelium such that it fills in the stroma between the ducts. Epithelial cell proliferation continues through pregnancy and into early

Sandra Z. Haslam • Department of Anatomy, Michigan State University, East Lansing, Michigan 48824.

lactation with a concomitant depletion of the adipose stroma during pregnancy and lactation (Elias et al., 1973). When lactation ceases, the mammary gland involutes and there is degeneration and loss of the secretory epithelium (Munford, 1963). The adipose stroma is restored and the epithelial component resumes the form of a branching ductal system. In most species, regression is not complete and some residual alveolar buds remain. With each ensuing pregnancy, the pattern described above is repeated.

The ovarian steroid hormones, estrogen and progesterone, are critically involved in the stimulation of mammary growth at puberty and during pregnancy (Lyons et al., 1958; Nandi, 1958). Estrogens promote ductal elongation and also regulate progesterone receptor concentration. Progestins stimulate ductal branching and lobuloalveolar development; they also inhibit lactogenesis during pregnancy (Assairi et al., 1974). Once established, lactation can proceed in the absence of the ovaries; thus, neither estrogen nor progesterone appear to be required for the maintenance of lactation (Simpson et al., 1973).

The effects of estrogen and/or progesterone cannot be demonstrated in hypophysectomized animals (Lyons et al., 1958; Nandi, 1958), indicating a relation between the pituitary and ovarian hormones. However, because mammary cells contain specific receptors for estrogen and progesterone (Shyamala and Haslam, 1980), a direct effect of these hormones is also implied. In this context, it is important to note that the existence and extent of direct versus indirect effects of ovarian hormones on mammary tissue is still unresolved.

1.1. Mechanism of Steroid Hormone Action

Steroid hormones are believed to produce their biological effects in target cells through a receptor-mediated mechanism. The two-step model for the mechanism of steroid hormone action states that the hormone enters the target cells and binds to a specific, high-affinity, macromolecular cytoplasmic receptor (Gorski et al., 1968; Jensen et al., 1968). The hormone receptor complex undergoes an *activation process* that is both hormone and temperature dependent and results in binding to acceptor sites on the nuclear chromatin. A variety of metabolic processes are then activated, resulting ultimately in the induction of new proteins. How induction of macromolecular synthesis results in tissue growth is still largely unknown.

Over the years, the validity of a cytoplasmic receptor and the two-step model has been questioned (Sheridan, 1975). Recent evidence has lent support to the proposal that in their native state steroid hormone receptors reside only in the nuclear compartment of target cells (King and Green, 1984; Welshons et al., 1984). The demonstration of cytoplasmic receptors is now considered by some to be an artifact resulting from leaching of the receptor from the nucleus during tissue homogenization. Until this controversy is resolved, the bulk of the evidence for estrogen and progesterone action can still be examined in the context of the two-step model, since the receptors still appear to exist in two different states, activated and nonactivated.

The prevailing methodological approach used to study steroid hormone receptors and hormone action employs tissue homogenization with subsequent receptor analysis under cell-free conditions. This approach has been criticized because it fails to consider target organ cellular heterogeneity and receptor distribution. There is good evidence in a number of organs, including mammary gland, that steroid hormone receptors are present in more than one cell type (Haslam and Shyamala, 1981; Cunha et al., 1983). There is further evidence to suggest that certain steroid hormones do not act directly on epithelial cells but rather stimulate the secretion of hormone-induced growth factors or inductors in neighboring stromal cells (Cunha et al., 1983) or alternatively in organs or tissues elsewhere in the body (Sirbasku, 1980).

The purpose of this chapter is to summarize recent advances in our understanding of the role(s) and mechanism(s) of action of estrogen and progesterone in normal mammary gland function. Hormonal effects are analyzed in relation to regulation and function of steroid hormone receptors. In the studies to be reviewed, receptor concentration was determined by ligand binding and does not refer in most cases to independent measurement of the receptor molecule itself. Mammary gland cellular heterogeneity and the possibility that epithelial–stromal interactions have a role in mediating hormonal effects are examined. Furthermore, evidence for direct versus indirect effects of estrogen and/or progesterone are considered. Because rodent mammary gland has been studied most extensively in this regard, studies in mice and rats provide the main focus for this chapter.

2. Estrogen Action in the Mammary Gland

2.1. Estrogen Effects in Vivo

Many studies have shown that estrogen plays a key role in mammary growth in vivo (for review see Leung, 1982). Two particularly prominent effects are (1) stimulation of ductal growth and (2) an increase in progesterone receptor concentration. This latter effect may be the basis for the observed synergistic action of estrogen and progesterone on lobuloalveolar development (Nandi, 1958).

The effect of estrogen on mammary ductal growth in vivo was carefully investigated by Bresciani (1968). Using the technique of DNA historadiography, he showed that estrogen injection in ovariectomized adult mice caused stimulation of DNA synthesis in the duct end epithelium but not in the epithelium of the duct proper. Much later, Shyamala and Ferenczy (1984) found that estrogen also stimulated stromal DNA synthesis, preceding epithelial DNA synthesis by 24 h, thus raising the possibility that the effects of estrogen are initiated in the mammary stroma.

The effect of estrogen in vivo on noncancerous human mammary biopsy tissue has been studied indirectly using subcutaneous implants in athymic nude mice. In this preparation, McManus and Welsch (1981, 1984) observed that estrogen, administered systemically, stimulated DNA synthesis in the ductal epithelium.

Progesterone receptor concentration varies with the developmental state of the mammary gland; progesterone receptors are abundant in the mammary glands of virgin mice but they are reduced during pregnancy and undetectable during lactation (Haslam and Shyamala, 1980). A similar decrease in mammary progesterone receptor concentration during pregnancy and lactation has been reported in the rat (Wiehle and

Table I. Relationship between Mammary Gland Developmental Site and Progesterone Receptor Responsiveness to Estrogen Regulation

	Progesterone receptor specific ^{3}H-R5020$_a$ binding (fmol/mg DNA)	
Developmental state	Saline control	17β-estradiol
Virgin[b]	487 ± 54[c]	993 ± 53
Pregnant	100 ± 25	1500 ± 175
Postpartum (days)		
7–10, nipple intact	0	0
7–10, thelectomized	180 ± 20	320 ± 25
28, nipple intact	249 ± 10	480 ± 27
35, nipple intact	331 ± 67	675 ± 16

[a]R5020, 17,21-dimethyl-19-nor-4,9-pregnadiene-3,20-dione.
[b]In all cases, mice were ovariectomized or ovariectomized and hysterectomized (pregnant mice) 5–7 days prior to injection with 1–3 μg 17β-estradiol or saline, I.P. Specific ^{3}H-R5020 binding was assayed 24 h after injection as described in Haslam and Shyamala (1980).
[c]Mean ± SEM.

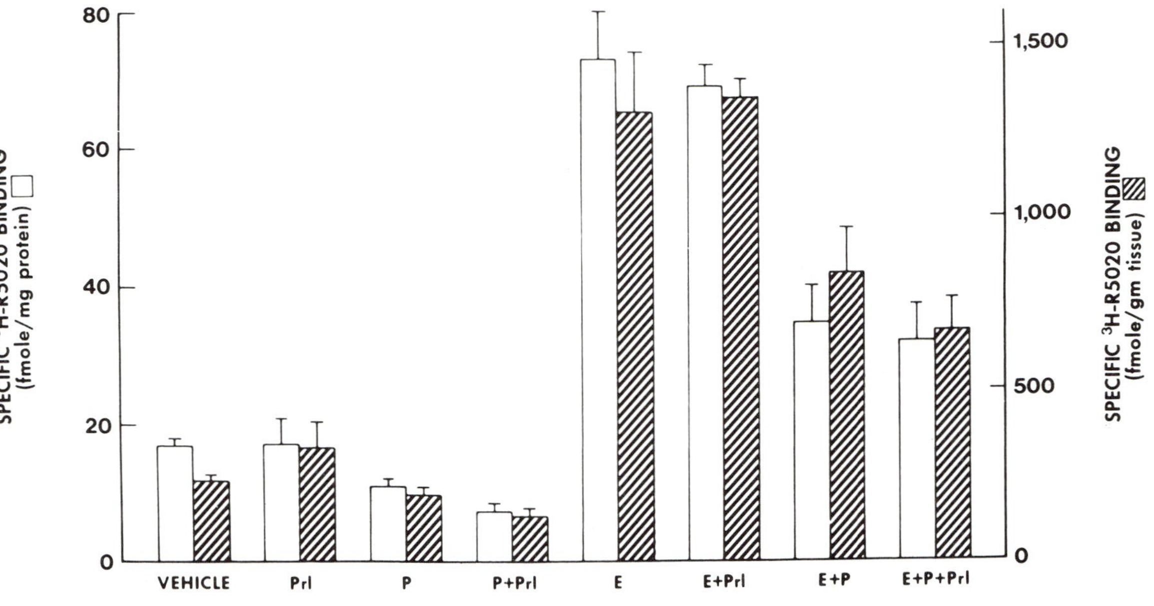

Figure 1. The effects of estrogen, progesterone, and prolactin on mammary progesterone receptor concentration after 14–16 days of pregnancy. Ovariectomized and hysterectomized mice received five daily injections of vehicle, or estrogen (E, 1 μg), or progesterone (P, 1 mg), or prolactin (Prl, 1 μg) alone or in combination as indicated. 24 h after the last injection, cytoplasmic extracts were assayed for specific ^{3}H-R5020 binding. Each value represents the mean ± SEM of three to four experiments.

Wittliff, 1983), the rabbit (Kelly et al., 1983), and the cow (Capuco et al., 1982). Progesterone receptors in mammary glands of virgin and pregnant mice are regulated by estrogen (Table I); thus, these two stages of mammary gland development represent estrogen-responsive states. By contrast, progesterone receptors cannot be restored by estrogen treatment during lactation. The refractoriness of the lactating mammary gland to estrogen is intrinsic to the mammary gland since another estrogen target tissue, the uterus, is not refractory to estrogen in lactating mice (Haslam and Shyamala, 1979).

The relation between secretory activity on the one hand and mammary gland progesterone receptor concentration and responsiveness to estrogen on the other hand have been investigated in the mouse (Haslam and Shyamala, 1980). Absence of progesterone receptors and loss of responsiveness to estrogen occur after parturition upon the acquisition of secretory function. If the nipples are removed on one side of the animal prior to parturition (unilateral thelectomy), that half of the mammary glands remain nonsecretory; the other, nipple-intact, glands are fully secretory. Using this treatment (Table I), we observed that the thelectomized, nonsecretory glands maintained both basal progesterone receptor levels and responsiveness to estrogen. Estrogen stimulation of DNA synthesis paralleled these findings (Shyamala and Ferenczy, 1982). In contrast, the nipple-intact, secretory glands lacked progesterone receptor and were refractory to estrogen. These results indicate that refractoriness to estrogen during lactation is not due to the hormonal milieu but is related to the secretory state of the mammary gland. The condition is reversible as shown by the progressive restoration of progesterone receptor concentration to prepregnancy levels at 35 days postpartum on completion of involution (Table I). The estrogen response is restored in parallel.

Prolactin is a potential mediator of certain estrogenic effects since estrogen stimulates the release of pituitary prolactin and the pituitary is required for estrogen stimulation of mammary growth. It is of interest, however, that an in vivo effect of prolactin on mammary progesterone receptor concentration has not been observed (Fig. 1).

To delineate potential direct versus indirect effects of estrogen on the mammary gland and its component cell populations, studies in vitro in both organ and cell culture systems are reviewed next.

2.2. Estrogen Effects in Vitro

2.2.1. Organ Culture

Organ culture studies undertaken to identify the potential direct effect(s) of estrogen fall into two categories: cultures using (1) serum-supplemented medium and (2) chemically defined medium without serum.

Mammary glands of the 10–15 day fetal mouse (Lasfargues and Murray, 1959) or the 17-day fetal rat (Ceriani, 1970) could be maintained and grew slowly for up to 9 days in defined medium without hormones. However, fetal rudiments grew better in serum-containing medium (Kratochwil, 1969). Exposure of fetal mouse tissues to estrogen in defined medium inhibited growth of the epithelium and at the same time favored the development of adipose tissue (Lasfargues and Murray, 1959). The lack of stimulation of epithelial proliferation by estrogen could be due to an inability to respond to estrogen. However, 16-day fetal mouse mammary gland exhibited epithelial cell proliferation and fully differentiated morphology 9 days after transplantation to the mammary fat pad of a pregnant animal (Hoshino, 1983). These results argue against a lack of capacity to respond to estrogen but instead suggest that the hormone may not act directly on the epithelium.

Estrogen did not promote growth in organ cultures of mammary glands from 3–4 week-old mice in defined medium (Ichinose and Nandi, 1966; Tonelli and Sorof, 1980). However, if the mice were pretreated in vivo with estrogen plus progesterone (E + P) for 9 days, the combination of insulin, prolactin, aldosterone, and hydrocortisone (I,P,A,H) effected subsequent lobuloalveolar development in vitro (Ichinose and Nandi, 1966). The requisite 9-day pretreatment time prior to organ culture was shortened to 6 days when epidermal growth factor (EGF) was included in the culture medium (Vonderhaar, 1984). The E + P in vivo pretreatment also caused a 15–20-fold increase in mammary epithelium EGF receptors and led to increased in vivo EGF concentration in submaxillary glands. Furthermore, extracts of E + P pretreated mammary glands contain an EGF-like mammary growth factor that is much more potent than EGF in facilitating mammary differentiation in organ culture (Vonderhaar, 1984). These results support the estromedin hypothesis (Sirbasku, 1978, 1980), which states that estrogen does not have a direct growth-promoting effect on mammary epithelium but acts indirectly through specifically induced polypeptide, EGF-like growth factors called estromedins.

In contrast to experiments performed in *defined* medium, in studies where adult rat mammary tissue has been subjected to organ culture in the presence of serum, growth-promoting effects of estrogen have been demonstrated (Koyama et al., 1972). The difference in response to estrogen in the presence or absence of serum is not likely mediated by prolactin since prolactin cannot substitute for serum (Koyama et al., 1972). These results suggest that effects of estrogen on adult mammary tissue may be synergistic with growth factors in serum.

Although lactation can proceed in the absence of ovaries, recent studies suggest that estrogen can influence secretory function. In organ cultures of primate mammary tissue, prolactin-induced α-lactalbumin synthesis was specifically inhibited by physiological levels of estrogen (Kleinberg et al., 1982, 1983). In contrast, estrogen stimulated lactose synthetase activity and casein synthesis in organ cultures of midpregnant mouse mammary gland (Bolander and Topper, 1979).

2.2.2. Cell Culture

Primary cell cultures enriched for normal mammary epithelial cells grown on plastic or on the surface of or within collagen gels have failed to demonstrate a cell proliferative response to estrogen in the majority of cases. This was the case for mammary epithelium from virgin or midpregnant mice and rats (Nandi et al., 1981; Kidwell et al., 1984; Haslam, 1986) as well as noncancerous human biopsy specimens (Yang et al., 1981). Two exceptions were cultured mouse and rat mammary end buds (Richards et al., 1982, 1983). When cultured within a collagen–gel matrix, a growth response was obtained with a medium containing prolactin, estrogen, progesterone, and hydrocortisone; however, the specific effects of individual hormones were not determined. End buds are developmentally unique mammary structures (Silberstein and Daniel, 1982; Williams and Daniel, 1983) and it is possible that they exhibit hormone responsiveness not shared by adult tissue. In another instance, noncancerous human mammary epithelium showed a specific response to estrogen characterized by morphological changes such as an increase in the number and length of microvilli and dispersal of condensed chromatin (Chambon et al., 1984). The relation between these morphological responses to estrogen and cell proliferation has not been established.

In contrast to normal cells, several epithelial cell lines derived from human mammary carcinomas have been shown to contain estrogen receptors and to exhibit an estrogen-specific increase in cell proliferation (Lippman et al., 1976; Drabre et al., 1983). Furthermore, the production of several specific proteins such as progesterone receptor (Horwitz and McGuire, 1977a), an undefined 52,000-dalton secretory glycoprotein (Westley and Rochefort, 1980), a plasminogen activator (Butler et al., 1979), and a major 24,000-dalton intracellular protein (Edwards et al., 1981) have been shown to be stimulated in a specific manner by estrogen. The absence of similar effects in cultured normal cells is paradoxical and raises important questions. Possible explanations for the discrepancy include: (1) loss or inactivation of estrogen receptor in normal cells as a consequence of cell culture; (2) lack of a direct effect of estrogen on epithelial cells when other cells or "factors" required for an estrogen effect are lacking; or (3) cancerous cells respond to estrogen in an abnormal manner.

We have explored the first possibility and have shown that both estrogen and progesterone receptors are present in normal mouse mammary epithelial cells for up to 7 days of culture on plastic (Haslam and Levely, 1985). Similar results have been obtained for both rat and mouse mammary epithelial cells cultured within collagen gels (Edery et al., 1984a,b). Therefore, the lack of response does not appear to be due to the absence of estrogen receptor.

The possibility that stromal cells are required for an estrogen effect in mammary epithelial cells has also been explored. McGrath (1983) observed estrogen-specific stimulation of DNA synthesis and mitosis in mouse mammary epithelial cells cultured in direct contact with mammary stromal fibroblasts. In a similar vein, we have shown that estrogen stimulation of progesterone receptor in normal mouse mammary epithelial cultures is facilitated by the presence of mammary fibroblasts (Haslam and Levely, 1985). The estrogen effect appeared to be specific for the epithelial cell population in these mixed cultures, since fibroblasts cultured alone did not contain progesterone receptors even when treated with estrogen.

Recently, we investigated further the mammary stromal fibroblast influence on normal mouse mammary epithelial cell responses to estrogen in cell culture (Haslam, 1986). Estrogen responsiveness in these cells was assayed by either measuring progesterone receptors or DNA synthesis. Our results suggested that mammary fibroblasts affect estrogen-specific responses in vitro both by stimulating extracellular matrix production and through a direct, metabolism-dependent mechanism. Stimulation of progesterone receptor number by estrogen was seen in the presence of both live, metabolically active fibroblasts and glutaraldehyde-killed fibroblasts. Pretreating the culture surface with type I collagen was also effective. This suggests that fibroblasts may promote the progesterone receptor response via an extracellular matrix or substratum effect on the epithelial cells. Normal rat and mouse mammary epithelial cells grown inside a collagen–gel matrix have been shown to possess estrogen receptors and to exhibit an estrogen-dependent increase in progesterone receptors (Edery et al., 1984a,b). The use of more complex mammary-specific extracellular matrix material has also been reported to promote estrogen-specific stimulation of rat mammary epithelial cell DNA synthesis in primary culture (Wicha, 1982). Epithelial cell shape, production of basal laminae, and acquisition of polarity are all influenced by collagenous substrata (Emerman et al, 1979). The exact mechanism(s) by which the collagen substratum or other potential extracellular matrix components promote mammary epithelial cell response to estrogen and other hormones remains to be elucidated. Further discussion of this problem may be found in Chapter 4 in this volume.

In contrast to their effect on progesterone receptor response, mammary fibroblasts apparently need to be metabolically active and either in close contact with epithelial cells or present in sufficient numbers to promote estrogen-dependent stimulation of epithelial cell DNA synthesis (Haslam, 1986). It is of interest that, under the same conditions, mammary epithelial cells promote estrogen-dependent increase in fibroblast DNA synthesis. These results indicate that some form of interaction between the two cell types occurs; it does not indicate, however, whether only one or both cell types are targets for estrogen action. Fibroblast-conditioned medium was not effective in stimulating epithelial cell DNA synthesis, suggesting that a readily diffusible extracellular factor(s) is not involved. However, the results do not exclude the possibility that a diffusible factor(s) acts only over a short distance or that an effective concentration is reached only when fibroblasts are present in high numbers. Another possibility is that communication occurs by direct transfer of informational molecules across cell membranes by specialized channels, such as gap junctions (Lowenstein, 1981).

In vivo, the mammary epithelium exists within a complex stromal environment. The data obtained in cell culture suggest that the nature of epithelial–fibroblast interactions can determine and modulate epithelial cell responses to estrogen and may reflect in vivo regulatory processes.

The results obtained to date in cell culture studies with normal and neoplastic epithelial cells support the hypothesis that estrogen acts directly on mammary epithelial cells to regulate progesterone receptor concentration. In contrast, the question of whether the mitogenic effects of estrogen on epithelial cells are direct or indirect has not been resolved. Both normal and neoplastic mammary epithelial cells respond to EGF and EGF-like growth factors in vitro (Osborne et al., 1980; Yang et al., 1981; Imai et al., 1982; Kidwell et al., 1982). Recently, it has been shown that mammary tumor cells can secrete growth factors in culture (Solomon et al., 1984) and the synthesis/secretion of such growth factors can be regulated specifically by estrogen (Dickson et al., 1985; Vignon et al., 1986). All in vitro evidence tends to support the hypothesis that estrogen is an indirect mitogen for mammary epithelial cells. The extent to which mitogenic effects of estrogen are mediated by other mammary cell types, such as stromal fibroblasts or adipocytes, or by autocrine factors produced in the epithelial cell itself remains to be determined.

2.3. Analysis of Estrogen Receptor in Relation to Estrogen-Mediated Effects

2.3.1. Ontogeny and Cellular Distribution of Estrogen Receptor

Direct effects of estrogen are believed to be mediated via specific receptor molecules in the cells comprising target tissues. The acquisition of responsiveness of the mammary gland to estrogen therefore would be expected to be related to the acquisition of cellular estrogen receptors. Steroid autoradiography has shown that in the 16-day fetal mammary gland, the earliest stage yet examined, cells that possess estrogen receptors are restricted to the mesenchyme directly surrounding the epithelial rudiment and are not present in the epithelium or extraprimordial mesenchymal cells (Narbaitz et al., 1980). Since injection of estrogens in the neonatal period can result in numerous epithelial malformations (Raynaud and Raynaud, 1954), mammary mesenchyme, the stromal percursor, appears to be an estrogen target tissue capable of estrogenic responses that affect the epithelium.

In another study, estrogen receptor concentrations were measured in mammary gland homogenates from mice of different ages (Muldoon, 1979). By this methodology, no estrogen receptors were detected prior to 2 weeks of age and were maximal in the 4-week-old animal. Neither the specific age at which estrogen receptors are acquired by mammary epithelial cells nor the fate of the mesenchymal estrogen receptors observed in fetal mammary gland has been determined.

To assess the relative distribution of estrogen receptor in the epithelial and stromal compartments of the adult mammary gland, estrogen receptors have been quantified either in intact mammary gland or in mammary stroma from which the epithelium has been removed surgically. The data are presented in Table II. In the adult virgin, the epithelium-devoid mammary stroma contained approximately 50% of the total estrogen receptor present in the intact organ. During pregnancy, the total estrogen receptor decreased significantly. Since the estrogen receptor concentration in the stroma is the same as that of the virgin gland, this indicates that the decrease in estrogen receptor concentration occurs in the epithelium. Estrogen receptor concentration in the lactating mammary gland decreases by 53% in both intact mammary gland

Table II. Distribution of Estrogen Receptors between Stromal and Epithelial Components of Adult Mammary Gland at Different States of Development

Developmental state[a]	Intact mammary gland specific ^{3}H-E$_2$ binding (fmol/mg DNA)	Epithelium-devoid stroma specific ^{3}H-E$_2$ binding (fmol/mg DNA)
Virgin (2–5 months)	1733 ± 277[b]	923 ± 138
Pregnancy (14 days)	1023 ± 153	920 ± 120
Lactation (7–10 days)	787 ± 118	430 ± 56

[a]In all cases, mice were ovariectomized or ovariectomized and hysterectomized (pregnant mice) 5–7 days prior to assay to remove endogenous estrogens. Thus, measured = total cytoplasmic estrogen receptor. Estrogen receptor concentration was determined by Scatchard analysis. For methods see Haslam and Shyamala (1981).
[b]Mean ± SEM.

and stroma and is most likely due to a decrease in stromal estrogen receptor. Thus, modulations of estrogen receptor concentration occur in both epithelial and stromal cells at different stages of mammary gland development.

Steroid autoradiographic analysis of estrogen receptor distribution among mammary cell types of ovariectomized pregnant or lactating rats (Sar and Stumpf, 1975) revealed weak ^{3}H-estradiol nuclear labeling in some ductal and alveolar cells, while no labeling was seen in others. In the lactating mammary gland, nuclear labeling was also seen in unspecified cells of the surrounding connective tissue; myoepithelial cells and adipocytes were not labeled.

Mammary tissues of the dog, calf, and rabbit also have been shown to contain estrogen receptor (for a review see Leung, 1982). Although mammary neoplasms of human breast have been shown to possess estrogen receptors (for a review see Leung, 1982), it has been difficult to demonstrate estrogen receptors in normal human mammary tissue (Hahnel et al., 1971; Rosen et al., 1975; Seshadri et al., 1979). Most likely, either low epithelial content or endogenous saturation of estrogen receptors is responsible for the difficulty since no exchange assays were employed. Recently, benign human mammary lesions were examined by steriod autoradiography after incubation with ^{3}H-estradiol in vitro (Buell and Tremblay, 1984). These conditions favor exchange of endogenously bound estrogens; nuclear labeling was found in some epithelial cells while stromal cells and myoepithelial cells were uniformly negative. The absence of stromal cell label observed with human tissue may be due to a species difference or alternatively to estrogen receptor levels too low to be detected by this method.

2.3.2. Factors Influencing Estrogen Receptor Concentration

In view of the proliferative response to estrogen during pregnancy and the contrasting lack of response during lactation, it is of interest to compare estrogen receptor concentrations at these two developmental states. In studies using mice depleted of endogenous estrogen, the highest concentration of estrogen receptor per cell is present in mammary glands of virgin mice (Table II). Significant decreases were observed during pregnancy and lactation. Others have reported either no differences in estrogen receptor concentration (Shyamala and Nandi, 1972; Auricchio et al., 1976) or an increase during lactation (Hseuh et al., 1973; Leung et al., 1976) in mice and rats. It should be noted, however, that in most of these studies ovary-intact animals were used without using exchange assays; thus, endogenously bound estrogens could preclude an accurate estrogen receptor measurement. Variations in estrogen receptor concentration in mammary glands from virgin, pregnant, and lactating mammary glands of rat and rabbit have also been reported (Kelly et al., 1983; Wiehle and Wittliff, 1983).

Estrogen receptor concentration may also be subject to hormonal regulation. Prolactin has been reported to increase rat mammary estrogen receptor in vitro (Edery et al., 1984a) and to increase mouse mammary estrogen receptor concentration in vivo (Muldoon, 1981).

Genetic factors also appear to have a significant influence on estrogen receptor concentration in mammary tissues of mice (Richards et al., 1974). The values obtained for BALB/c, C57BL, and C3H mouse strains were similar to each other ($\sim 45 \times 10^{-17}$ mol/g DNA), whereas the I, RIII, and GR strains had a value of $\sim 120 \times 10^{-17}$ mol/g DNA. The C57BL × I F_1 hybrid had an intermediate value ($\sim 90 \times 10^{-17}$ mol/g DNA). Similarly, strain differences in mammary estrogen receptor concentrations have been reported for the rat (Wiehle and Wittliff, 1983).

The influence of the mouse mammary tumor virus (MMTV) on mammary gland estrogen receptor concentration has also been investigated. In the C3H mouse strain, the presence or absence of MMTV did not influence estrogen receptor concentration (Bondy and Okey, 1978). In another study, however, it was reported that in the BR6 strain the presence of MMTV reduced mammary gland DNA synthesis response to estrogen (Lee, 1983).

During lactation, no causal relation between estrogen receptor concentration and lack of estrogen responsiveness has been demonstrated. Since estrogen receptors are present in both epithelial and stromal compartments, a more detailed analysis of modulations in receptor concentrations among the various mammary cell types is required before meaningful conclusions can be drawn about receptor concentration and cellular response. On the other hand, those effects of estrogen that may be mediated indirectly might be expected to be independent of mammary tissue estrogen receptor concentration.

2.3.3. Physicochemical Analysis of Cytoplasmic Estrogen Receptor

Elucidation of the molecular mechanism(s) of estrogen action has centered around analyses of the physicochemical properties of the receptor and receptor hormone complex. In early studies on rodent mammary gland, the cytoplasmic receptor was investigated in lactating animals (Shyamala and Nandi, 1972; Wittliff et al., 1972; Hsueh et al., 1973) and identified a macromolecular, metalloprotein (MW ~ 93,000 daltons) that binds to estrogen with low capacity (~5000–6000 sites/cell), high-affinity (K_D = 0.5 nM), and specificity for estrogenic compounds (Shyamala and Nandi, 1972; Shyamala and Yeh, 1977).

Since virgin mouse mammary gland is responsive to estrogen and lactating mouse mammary gland is not, differences in physical properties and function of cytoplasmic estrogen receptor were examined. Analysis of molecular size on low ionic strength sucrose density gradients showed the cytoplasmic estrogen receptor hormone complex of both virgin and lactating mice sediments as an 8S moiety (Shyamala and Nandi, 1972; Wittliff et al., 1972; Auricchio et al., 1976). A high-affinity 4S binder observed in virgin tissue (Muldoon, 1981) is now believed to represent artifactual degradation of the native 9S cytoplasmic estrogen receptor (Gaubert et al., 1982).

Activation is considered to be an essential event in estrogen action, and studies using weak estrogens and estrogen antagonists (Weichman and Notides, 1980) provide evidence that the activation process underlies the biological regulatory function of estrogen receptors. In uterine tissue as a result of temperature-induced activation, the cytoplasmic estrogen receptor complex (1) undergoes a 4S to 5S change in sedimentation coefficient in a high salt medium (Jensen et al., 1969; Shyamala and Gorski, 1969), (2) displays a decrease in dissociation rate of the hormone from the receptor (Weichman and Notides, 1977), and (3) acquires an enhanced ability to bind to DNA and nuclei (DeSombre et al., 1972).

In one study, Shyamala and Yeh (1977), using normal lactating mammary gland estrogen receptor, were unable to show the 4S to 5S change in sedimentation coefficient after temperature-induced activation (Shyamala and Yeh, 1977). We have examined this problem further by measuring ^{3}H-estradiol–receptor dissociation kinetics and sedimentation coefficients on high salt gradients (Haslam et al., 1984). The kinetic and gradient data revealed: (1) a fast dissociating 4S form that appeared to be the nonactivated receptor and (2) a slow dissociating 5S form that appeared to be the activated receptor. In vitro cell-free conditions, such as heating, high salt concentration, dilution, and ammonium sulfate fractionation, which promote activation of estrogen receptors in other systems and activation of other steroid hormone receptors, were effective in promoting activation of mammary gland estrogen receptor. Sodium molybdate, an effective inhibitor of activation of other steroid hormone receptors (Leach et al., 1979; Nishigori and Toft, 1980), also inhibited mammary gland estrogen receptor activation. In summary, no significant differences were observed between cytoplasmic estrogen receptor from virgin and lactating mammary gland animals. However, since we used whole organ homogenates and biochemical methods to investigate receptor function, we cannot assess the possibility that receptor function could be altered in certain cell populations within the mammary gland and was not detected by the methods used.

2.3.4. Nuclear Estrogen Receptor

Interaction of the steroid–hormone receptor complex with target cell nuclei is required for an estrogenic response. However, the nature of the nuclear interaction and the molecular events related to biological response have not been clearly identified.

^{3}H-estradiol injected in vivo is localized mainly to the nuclei of mammary cells. This was originally demonstrated in lactating mouse (Shyamala and Nandi, 1972) and rat mammary gland (Hseuh et al., 1973). We have compared dissociation kinetics and sedimentation behavior on high salt sucrose density gradients of nuclear estrogen receptor from virgin and lactating mouse mammary gland (Haslam et al, 1984). We found that for both virgin and lactating mammary glands the nuclear estrogen receptor is predominantly represented by the slow dissociating form, indistinguishable from the activated cytoplasmic estrogen receptor; it sediments as a 5S moiety under appropriate experimental conditions.

The kinetics of nuclear estrogen receptor binding and the length of retention in the nucleus have also been proposed to be associated with induction of estrogenic responses (Clark and Peck, 1976). Our evidence indicates that there are significant differences in the kinetics of estrogen receptor interactions in the nucleus between ovariectomized virgin and lactating mice (Table III). One hour after injection, there was depletion of ^{3}H-estradiol bound cytoplasmic estrogen receptor and translocation

Table III. Relative Distribution of Cytoplasmic and Nuclear Estrogen Receptors in Virgin and Lactating Mouse Mammary Glands

Time after injection (h)	Estrogen receptor (fmol/g tissue)			
	Virgin		Lactator	
	Cytoplasmic[a]	Nuclear[b]	Cytoplasmic[a]	Nuclear[b]
0	416 ± 30[c]	—	611 ± 70	—
1	348 ± 29	100 ± 15	429 ± 35	284 ± 30
4	387 ± 30	52 ± 10	1673 ± 100	107 ± 15
24	291 ± 30	6 ± 1	1551 ± 130	32 ± 5

[a]Cytoplasmic estrogen receptor measured both unfilled and endogenously filled receptor sites.
[b]Nuclear estrogen receptors measured only unfilled estrogen receptors.
[c]Mean ± SEM.

to the nuclear compartment, 22 and 40% for virgin and lactating mouse mammary glands, respectively. In both cases, there was an approximate 50% decrease in nuclear estrogen receptors by 4 h, with a further decrease observed at 24 h. Interestingly, in lactating mouse mammary glands, concomitant with the decrease in nuclear estrogen receptors there was a replenishment and approximately a twofold increase in cytoplasmic estrogen receptors. This replenishment was already evident at 4 h. In distinct contrast, cytoplasmic estrogen receptors in virgin mouse mammary glands were not replenished. In fact, at 24 h only ~50% of preinjection cytoplasmic estrogen receptors were detectable. These results suggest that differences exist in nuclear retention, processing, and/or cytoplasmic replenishment of estrogen receptor between virgin and lactating mouse mammary glands. Nuclear retention (Clark and Peck, 1976) and nuclear processing (Horwitz and McGuire, 1978) have been proposed to be required for biological responses.

Differences in the ability to bind to DNA have been reported for virgin versus lactating mouse mammary gland estrogen receptor (Gaubert et al., 1986). Only 20% of total estrogen receptor from lactating mouse mammary glands binds to calf thymus DNA as compared with 60–80% of virgin mouse mammary gland estrogen receptor. A putative low molecular weight factor(s) is proposed to be the inhibitor of DNA binding in lactating mouse mammary gland. The data in Table III, however, do not show significant differences in the proportion of estrogen receptor associated with the nucleus after in vivo injection of ^{3}H-estradiol to virgin or lactating mice. In fact, in both cases very similar proportions of total estrogen receptor are associated with the nuclear compartment.

The cellular heterogeneity of intact mammary gland and our previous observation that mammary stroma also contains estrogen receptor make it difficult to interpret the nuclear estrogen receptor results. At present, it is not possible to discriminate between nuclear estrogen receptor events occurring in epithelium versus stroma. A meaningful analysis of estrogen action in normal mammary gland may require a separate analysis of estrogen receptor and estrogenic effects in epithelial cells versus stromal cells.

3. Progesterone Action in the Mammary Gland

3.1. Progesterone Effects in Vivo

Although there are significant gaps in our understanding of estrogen action in normal mammary gland, there is an even greater deficit in our knowledge about progesterone action in normal mammary tissues. Proliferation of mammary epithelium and lobuloalveolar morphogenesis during pregnancy clearly require progesterone (Nandi, 1958; Bresciani, 1968). While progesterone does not appear to be required for ductal elongation, the development of alveoli is dependent on progesterone in the mouse (Freeman and Topper, 1978). In the rat, prolactin rather than progesterone appears to play a key role in alveolar development (Lyons et al., 1958). Bresciani (1968) reported that in ovariectomized adult virgin mice progesterone stimulated DNA synthesis in the epithelium of the duct proper as well as in the duct ends. Because only basal levels of progesterone receptor would be present in these ovariectomized animals (Haslam and Shyamla, 1979), these observations suggest that progesterone can have effects that are independent of estrogen. Enhancement of DNA synthesis, however, was observed when estrogen and progesterone were administered together, possibly because of estrogen stimulation of progesterone receptor number.

Some information is available in humans. Biopsy specimens of human breast tissue obtained from patients in the luteal phase of the menstrual cycle exhibited higher DNA synthesis in ductal epithelium than did specimens obtained from women in the follicular phase (Masters et al., 1977; Meyer, 1977). Increased DNA synthesis appeared to correspond to elevated estrogen and progesterone blood levels during the luteal phase (Brown, 1981). In contrast to these observations, no stimulation of DNA synthesis by progesterone was observed in the ductal epithelium of normal human mammary tissue transplanted into athymic nude mice; this was the case with or without added estrogen (McManus and Welsch, 1984). Why progesterone promotes cell proliferation in human mammary tissue in situ but not in the athymic nude mouse is not known.

A second major effect of progesterone in vivo is the inhibition of lactogenesis (for a review see Kuhn, 1977). It is believed that the high plasma levels of progesterone present during gestation prevent premature lactation; milk secretion can be initiated experimentally by reducing plasma progesterone levels (Kuhn, 1969). There is evidence that progesterone acts indirectly, blocking casein gene expression by antagonizing glucocorticoid action (Rosen et al., 1978). This antagonistic effect of progesterone appears to be due to the ability of progesterone to bind to the glucocorticoid receptor (for a review see Shyamala, 1982).

3.2. Progesterone Effects in Vitro

3.2.1. Organ Culture

Using 10–15-day embryonic mouse tissue and defined medium, Lasfargues and Murray (1959) reported that progesterone at a physiological concentration caused no stimulation of the epithelial rudiment and in fact caused histolysis of the collagenous connective tissue. When combined with estrogen, progesterone caused an unfolding of the epithelial bud; however, this process did not involve cell proliferation but rather was believed to be due to cell rearrangement. It was hypothesized that progesterone contributed to this process by loosening the connective tissue. Ceriani (1970), using defined medium, reported that progesterone either alone or with estrogen produced no effect on the mammary epithelium of embryonic rat tissue. However, progesterone in combination with insulin and prolactin did enhance ductal proliferation.

The effect of progesterone in combination with estrogen has also been tested in immature 3–4-week-old mouse mammary gland using defined medium; no effect on cell proliferation was observed (Ichinose and Nandi, 1966). Using older mice (5–7 weeks) and serum-supplemented media, Prop (1966) reported that progesterone alone promoted some alveolar development and inhibited secretory activity induced by hydrocortisone.

Mammary glands of adult 50- to 60-day-old rats have also been studied for progesterone responses in organ culture (Koyama et al., 1972). Using serum-supplemented media, Koyama and co-workers showed that progesterone plus insulin induced significant lobuloalveolar development at 6–9 days with significant increases in both epithelial labeling and mitotic indexes. Addition of prolactin caused further lobuloalveolar development. When insulin, estrogen, progesterone, and prolactin were used in combination, maximal stimulation was observed. Other hormone combinations were not effective. The results of the above studies suggest that serum factors and/or prolactin are important for promoting progesterone-dependent cell proliferation.

3.2.2. Cell Culture

The in vitro effects of progesterone have also been investigated in cell culture. When cultured on plastic, adult virgin or perphenazine pretreated rat mammary epithelial cells did not proliferate in response to progesterone (Hallowes et al., 1977). To date, the only increase in cell proliferation due to progesterone has been observed when normal rat mammary epithelial organoids were cultured within a collagen–gel matrix (Edery et al., 1984b). Cells from virgin rats responded to neither progesterone nor prolactin alone; however, a three- to fourfold increase in cell number was observed with prolactin plus progesterone. It is of interest to note that in the same culture system progesterone receptors were increased by estrogen; however, estrogen had no effect on cell proliferation, either alone or in combination with progesterone. In similar studies using mouse epithelial cells, Imagawa et al. (1985) reported a synergistic effect of prolactin and progesterone on cell proliferation. Cells from midpregnant mice were less responsive than those from virgin mice; estrogen again did not potentiate the effect of progesterone.

Although there is abundant evidence in vivo demonstrating the requirement of progesterone for cell proliferation, very little is known about its mechanism of action. To date, most studies have been carried out in vitro using human mammary carcinoma cell lines such as T47D, which contains high levels of progesterone receptor and no estrogen receptor (Horwitz et al., 1982), and the MCF-7 cell line, which contains both estrogen receptor and progesterone receptor (Horwitz and McGuire, 1978). In both cell lines, progesterone apparently triggers a decrease in cell proliferation (Horwitz and Freidenberg, 1985). Recently, however, progestins have also been shown to increase EGF receptors in T47D cells (Murphy et al., 1986) and a 48,000-dalton protein has been reported to be induced specifically by progestins in T47D cells (Rochefort and Chalbos, 1984). All these progestin-specific effects appear to be mediated via progesterone receptor. The biological significance of these protein and growth factor promoting or inhibiting activities of progesterone in mammary cells is not known.

The inhibition of cell proliferation in neoplastic human mammary cells by progesterone in vitro is in distinct contrast to its growth-promoting effects on normal rodent mammary cells both in vivo and in vitro. It is difficult to explain such opposite effects of progesterone on the basis of species differences, since in vivo progesterone action in humans is consistent with promotion of mammary epithelial cell proliferation (Masters et al., 1977; Meyer, 1977).

3.3. Analysis of Progesterone Receptor in Relation to Progesterone-Mediated Effects

3.3.1. Ontogeny and Cellular Distribution of Progesterone Receptor

Virtually nothing is known about the detailed ontogeny of progesterone receptor in normal mammary gland. Progesterone receptors are known to be present in mammary glands of adult virgin mice (Haslam and Shyamala, 1979), rats (Yu and Leung, 1982; Wiehle and Whittliff, 1983), rabbits (Kelly et al., 1983), and cows (Capuco et al., 1982). In the human female, progesterone receptors were detected in four of 10 individuals 13–25 years of age and eight of eight individuals 27–50 years of age (Seshadri et al., 1979). However, the specific age when progesterone receptors are first detectable in mammary tissue of any species is not known.

The distribution of progesterone receptors between the epithelial and stromal components of the mammary gland has been investigated in cell-free homogenate preparations of mouse tissue (Haslam and Shyamala, 1981). About 20% of the progesterone receptors present in intact mammary gland were associated with the stroma (Fig. 2). Stromal progesterone receptor concentration in epithelium-devoid fat pads was quite stable during various developmental states and appeared to be constitutive; that is, estrogen independent. Progesterone receptors in intact glands, on the other hand, were regulated by estrogen and were the class of progesterone receptor lost during lactation. This class of progesterone receptor appears to be associated with the epithelium. Stromal progesterone receptors may be present but not detectable during lactation in intact glands as a result of their dilution by the increased number of receptor-negative epithelial cells.

Steroid autoradiographic analysis of progesterone receptor cellular distribution has been carried out in only one species, the mature female of the prosimian primate, galago (Warembourg, 1983). In this study, estrogen-stimulated progesterone receptors appeared to be localized in the ductal epithelium. No selective labeling of connective tissue or

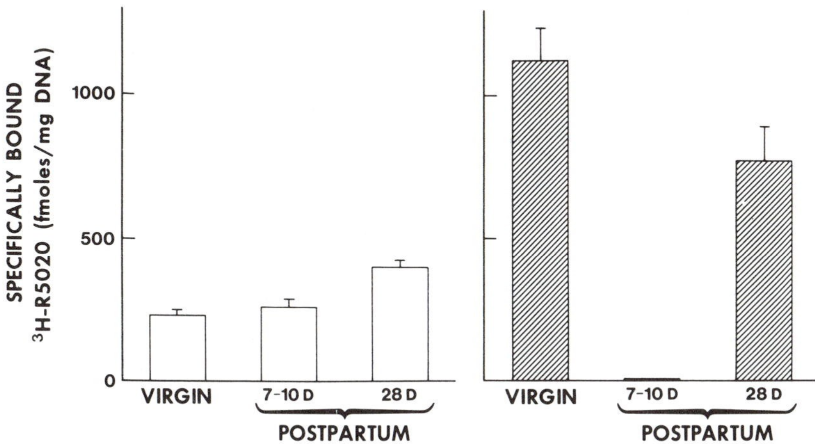

Figure 2. Comparison of the progesterone receptor concentration in epithelium-devoid mammary stroma and intact mammary glands of virgin and postpartum mice. Cytoplasmic extracts of mammary stroma (▨) and intact glands (□) were assayed for specific ^{3}H-R5020 binding as described in Haslam and Shyamala (1981). Each value represents the mean ± SEM of three to five experiments.

adipose tissue was noted. Cell culture studies using normal mouse mammary cells also substantiate the observations that the major concentration of progesterone receptor is in the epithelial component of the mammary gland (Haslam and Levely, 1985). However, the relative distribution of progesterone receptor in adipocytes, ductal versus alveolar epithelial cells, or other topographically or developmentally distinct mammary gland structures such as endbuds is unknown.

3.3.2. Factors Influencing Progesterone Receptor Concentration

In the mature mouse (Haslam and Shyamala, 1979), rat (Yu and Leung, 1982; Wiehle and Whittliff, 1983), rabbit (Kelly et al., 1983), and bovine (Capuco et al., 1982), mammary gland progesterone receptor concentration changes with the developmental state of the gland. In all cases, progesterone receptors are highest in concentration in mammary tissues of virgin or nonpregnant, nonlactating animals. With the onset of pregnancy, progesterone receptors decrease and are generally undetectable or absent during lactation. The basis for this observed modulation has been investigated in detail in the mouse as described earlier in this chapter (Haslam and Shyamala, 1979, 1980).

The presence of mouse mammary tumor virus is reported to be

related to increased responsiveness of mammary tissue to cell proliferative effects of progestins in nonpregnant, nonlactating animals (Lee, 1983). The biological basis for viral-enhanced progestin effects is not known.

The observed modulations in progesterone receptor concentration appear to be compatible with progesterone's role in mammary gland function. Progesterone acts on virgin mammary gland to produce lobuloalveolar morphogenesis and thus the high concentration of progesterone receptor observed in the virgin gland is consistent with the high degree of responsiveness of this tissue to progesterone. During late pregnancy, another role of progesterone, the inhibition of lactation, comes into play. This effect of progestin is believed to be mediated indirectly via the glucocorticoid receptor. Established lactation does not require the presence of progesterone; therefore, the absence of progesterone receptor is compatible with secretory function.

In one study of premenopausal women, mammary progesterone receptor concentration varied with the menstrual cycle, being highest at the time of ovulation, indicating a positive influence of estrogens on progesterone receptor in human tissue (Pollow et al., 1977).

The only effect of progestins studied in detail in organ culture has been the inhibition of lactogenesis (for a review see Banerjee et al., 1982). No detailed studies of progestin effects on cell proliferation have been carried out; furthermore, there is no information about maintenance or regulation of progesterone receptors in organ culture.

Progesterone receptors have been identified and quantitated in primary culture of mouse mammary epithelial cells grown on plastic (Haslam and Levely, 1985) and in mouse and rat epithelial cells cultured within collagen gels (Edery et al., 1984a,b). When mouse epithelial cells are cultured on plastic, only basal levels of progesterone receptors are detectable and estrogenic regulation of progesterone receptor is not observed. However, if epithelial cells are grown in combination with mammary stromal fibroblasts, the ability of estrogen to regulate progesterone receptor is maintained in a manner similar to that observed in vivo.

As discussed earlier, analysis of the fibroblast influence has revealed that these cells most likely are providing an appropriate substratum. In the absence of stromal cells, collagen gels were also effective in maintaining epithelial cell progesterone receptors and their regulation by estrogen (Edery et al., 1984a,b). Under the latter condition, in contrast to the in vivo situation, both prolactin and progesterone together caused a maximal increase in progesterone receptor. Progesterone plus prolactin also stimulated cell proliferation; similar observations have been made using rat cells. There appears to be a positive correlation between progesterone receptor concentration and progestin effects in cell culture, suggesting that progesterone may act directly as a mitogen for mammary epithelial cells via a receptor-mediated mechanism.

Although progesterone receptors have been identified in mammary stroma in vivo, they do not appear to be associated with or maintained in vitro in stromal fibroblasts. It is possible that progesterone receptor may be present in adipocytes in vivo and cannot be detected in vitro since adipocytes are not maintained during the procedures used for cell dissociation.

3.3.3. *Multiple Pathways of Progesterone Action*

Analysis of the mechanism(s) of progesterone action in mammary tissues is complicated by the potential multiple pathways available for progestin-induced effects. First, target cells for progestins contain specific receptors and certain progestin effects are believed to be mediated via these receptors. At least four progesterone receptor-mediated responses have been identified in human mammary carcinoma cell lines: (1) a decrease in cell proliferation (Horwitz and Freidenberg, 1985), (2) regulation (increase) of a progestin-specific 48,000-dalton protein (Rochefort and Chalbos, 1984), (3) an increase in EGF receptors (Murphy et al., 1986), and (4) a decrease in an estrogen-induced 52,000-dalton protein (Vignon et al., 1983). Similar progesterone receptor-mediated effects in normal mammary cells have not been reported.

Second, progestins at high concentrations can bind to glucocorticoid and androgen receptors having agonist/antagonist effects (Rochefort and Chalbos, 1984). Normal mammary tissue may contain both progesterone and glucocorticoid receptors and progestins can bind to both receptors (Shyamala, 1973; Wittliff, 1975). The demonstration that exclusion of sulfhydryl reducing agents during tissue homogenization results in the selective loss of glucocorticoid receptor but not progesterone receptor (Haslam et al., 1982) may be useful in distinguishing these effects.

Finally, since progesterone is subject to extensive metabolism in mammary cells, the possibility that progestin effects are mediated by metabolites must be considered (Verma et al., 1978; Lloyd, 1979; Horwitz et al., 1983). Normal tissues have low levels of 5-α-reductase, 20-α-hydroxysteroid dehydrogenase, and 3-α-hydroxysteroid dehydrogenase activities. Fibrocystic disease-derived tissues as well as carcinomas had increased 5-α-reductase activity, apparently associated with increased epithelial content (Lloyd, 1979). Mammary adipocytes also possess all three enzyme activities and 5-α-reductase activity is present in fibroblasts. Of the metabolites produced, 5-α-dihydroprogesterone was shown to be an effective competitor of progesterone binding to progesterone receptor. The biological significance and role of these metabolites have not been determined.

In the T47D cell line, the major metabolite has been tentatively identified as an 11-hydroxypregnanolone (Horwitz et al., 1983). In T47D cells, the rapid metabolism of progesterone permits the replenishment of cytoplasmic receptors and ensures maintenance of a progestin-responsive state. Thus, steroid metabolism can have a major effect on intracellular receptor levels and distribution and can thereby play a major role in the regulation of biological response.

3.3.4. Physicochemical Analysis of Cytoplasmic Progesterone Receptor

The equilibrium constant (K_D) for mammary cytosolic progesterone receptor ranges from 0.15 to 5.8 n*M* and is similar in all species tested. Analysis of steroid binding specificity also demonstrates that compounds with the highest binding affinity have the greatest progestin biological potency (Haslam and Shyamala, 1979).

Sucrose density gradient analysis has been used to investigate the molecular size of progesterone receptor in mammary tissues. A "7–8S" and/or a "4–5S" species have been observed on low ionic strength sucrose gradients. Based on studies with uterine progesterone receptor, it has been proposed that the nonactivated form of progesterone receptor exists as an oligomer composed of either identical or dissimilar subunits. This form of the receptor–hormone complex sediments at 7–8S. After activation, the receptor–hormone complex sediments at 4–5S, thought to be due to enzymatic or conformational changes.

As can be seen from Table IV, there is considerable variation in the distribution of the 7–8S and 4–5S forms of the receptor among the various mammary tissue sources of progesterone receptor. Atger et al. (1974) proposed that the predominant occurrence of progesterone receptor in a 4–5S form in other tissues may be due to low cellular progesterone receptor concentration. In our own studies, mouse mammary gland obtained from ovary-intact virgin mice yielded only 4.5S progesterone receptor (Fig. 3A). In contrast, progesterone receptors from ovariectomized virgin mice injected with estradiol, sediment as the 7S form (Fig. 3B). In this case, the difference is not due to differences in progesterone receptor concentration since equivalent amounts of receptor were detected under both conditions.

Although a number of factors and/or conditions are known to pro-

Table IV. Progesterone Receptor Sedimentation on Low Salt Sucrose Gradients

Animal	Tissue	PgR sedimentation coefficients		Reference
Mouse				
Ovary-intact virgin	Whole gland	4.5S	—	Haslam and Shyamala (1979)
OVX virgin + E_2	Whole gland	4.5S	7.5S	Haslam, this chapter
Virgin	MXT mammary tumor	4.3S	7.5S	Watson et al. (1979)
Rat	DMBA mammary tumors	4.3S	—	Horwitz and McGuire (1977b)
Rabbit, virgin	Whole gland	—	7–8S	Kelly et al. (1983)
Human				
Tissue biopsies	Noncancerous	4S	7S	Pollow et al. (1977)
	Cancerous	4S	7S	Verma et al. (1978)
		4S	—	Lloyd (1979)
Cultured cancerous cell lines	MCF-7	—	8S	Horwitz and McGuire (1978)
	T47D	—	8S	Horwitz et al. (1982)

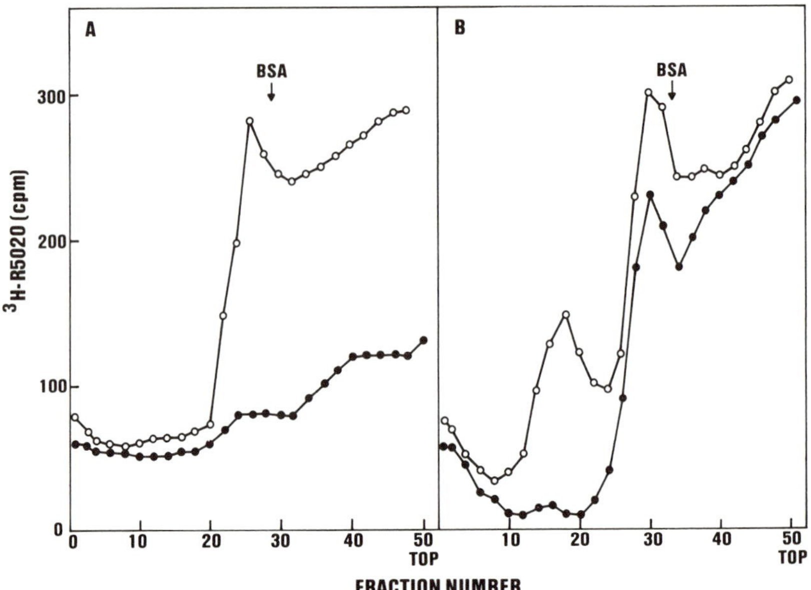

Figure 3. Sucrose density gradient profiles of ^{3}H-R5020 labeled cytoplasmic extracts of virgin mouse mammary glands. Aliquots of extracts from (A) intact, untreated virgin or (B) ovariectomized virgin mice injected for 7 days with 1 μg 17β-estradiol daily were incubated with 5 n*M* ^{3}H-R5020 plus 500 n*M* unlabeled dexamethasone (○) or with 5 n*M* ^{3}H-R5020 plus 500 n*M* unlabeled R5020 (●). For detailed methods see Haslam and Shyamala (1979). Specific ^{3}H-R5020 binding layered on gradients: A = 17,092 cpm; B = 16,505 cpm.

mote progesterone receptor activation in vitro (for a review see Moudgil, 1983), little is known about the process of in vivo activation. One possible explanation for the presence of 7.5S progesterone receptor in mammary tissue of estrogen-treated mice is that the newly synthesized progesterone receptors have not yet been exposed to in vivo activating conditions. The actual significance of 7–8S versus 4–5S extracted progesterone receptor forms in relation to tissue responsiveness of normal mammary gland remains to be established.

3.3.5. Nuclear Progesterone Receptor

The only mammary cells in which nuclear progesterone receptor related events have been investigated is the T47D human mammary carcinoma cell line (Horwitz et al., 1983; Mockus and Horwitz, 1983). Studies on T47D have shown that exposure to progesterone results in nuclear localization of 70–90% of progesterone receptor within 5 min. The nuclear receptor could be recovered quantitatively only in the first 5 min; afterward, 50–80% of the nuclear receptor was lost or "processed" to a form that no longer bound marker hormones. The authors postulated that this receptor processing step, similar to estrogen receptor processing, may involve interaction of the receptors with DNA. Replenishment of progesterone receptor to the cytoplasm after progesterone removal occurred 16–20 h later and appeared to be dependent on an early protein synthesis step, since in the first 4 h exposure to cycloheximide inhibited replenishment. Chronic exposure to progesterone or nonmetabolizable progestins inhibits receptor replenishment and subsequent hormone receptor binding, thereby attenuating continued hormonal effects.

T47D cells have also provided information about the molecular structure of the human mammary progesterone receptor. In general, receptors for each of the different steroid hormones are believed to be oligomers composed of identical subunits with one hormone binding site per polypeptide chain. The nonactivated receptors are multimers of this protein. An exception to this is chick oviduct progesterone receptor, which is composed of oligomers of dissimilar subunits (for a review see Moudgil, 1983). The progesterone receptor of human uterus has only one molecular weight species and thereby conforms to the identical subunit structure (Smith et al., 1981). However, recent studies using T47D human mammary carcinoma cells have demonstrated dissimilar subunits comparable to chick oviducts progesterone receptor (Lessey et al., 1983). The same subunits are present in the nucleus after translocation (Horwitz and Alexander, 1983), and this observation suggests that acquisition of nuclear binding capacity does not involve subunit proteolysis or other major modification of the receptor.

4. Summary and Conclusions

Estrogen and progesterone are clearly required for the promotion of mammary growth in vivo. In the case of estrogen, specific cellular hormone receptors are present in both the epithelial and stromal components of the gland. The ability of estrogen to regulate progesterone receptors appears to be due to a direct effect of the hormone on the epithelial cells. The mitogenic effects of estrogen, on the other hand, are elicited in both the epithelium and the stroma. Most recent evidence indicates that the mitogenic effects of estrogen are indirect, elicited via the induction of paracrine or autocrine growth factors. Furthermore, there is evidence that epithelial–stromal interactions play a role in modulating tissue responsiveness to estrogen. Analyses of estrogen receptor function in relation to biological responses indicate that the nature of hormone receptor interactions with target cell nuclei may be the most critical factor determining biological responsiveness.

The nature and mechanism(s) of progesterone effects on normal mammary gland are less well understood. Progesterone receptors that are regulated by estrogen are predominantly localized in the mammary epithelium; however, there appears to be a subpopulation of estrogen-independent progesterone receptors associated with mammary stroma. Progesterone clearly stimulates cell proliferation in rodent mammary tissue both in vivo and in vitro. Prolactin and/or serum factors may mediate or modulate this progestin effect. In the case of human mammary tissue, the evidence indicates that progesterone also stimulates cell proliferation in vivo. However, in vitro studies with human cancerous mammary cells indicate that progestins inhibit cell proliferation. The basis of this discrepancy in progestin effects with human tissue remains unresolved. To date, most studies of progesterone receptor function in relation to biological response have been carried out using cancerous cells in vitro. At present, very little is known about progesterone receptor function in normal mammary tissue.

ACKNOWLEDGMENTS: This chapter is dedicated to the memory of a dear colleague and friend, Dr. Robert Echt. The author thanks Ms. K. Gale, M. Levely and S. Dachtler for their expert technical assistance, Ms. J. Bullis and B. Holmer-Heckman for typing the manuscript. This work was supported by NIH grants CA31774 and CA40104.

References

Assairi, L., Delouis, C., Houdebine, L.M., Ollivier-Bousquet, M., and Denamur, R., 1974, Inhibition by progesterone of the lactogenic effect of prolactin in the pseudopregnant rabbit, *Biochem. J.* **144:**245–252.

Atger, M., Baulieu, E.-E., and Milgrom, E., 1974, An investigation of progesterone receptors in guinea pig vagina, uterine cervix, mammary glands, pituitary and hypothalamus, *Endocrinology* **94:**161–166.

Auricchio, F., Rotondi, A., and Bresciani, F., 1976, Oestrogen receptor in mammary gland cytosol of virgin, pregnant and lactating mice, *Mol. Cell. Endocrinol.* **4:**55–60.

Auricchio, F., Rotondi, A., Schiavone, E., and Bresciani, F., 1978, Oestrogen receptor of mammary gland. Inhibition of aggregation and characterization of receptor from lactating gland in the presence of sodium bromide, *Biochem. J.* **169:**481–488.

Banerjee, M.R., Ganguly, R., Mehta, N.M., and Ganguly, N., 1982, Hormone regulation of casein gene expression in normal and neoplastic cells in murine mammary glands, in: *Hormonal Regulation of Mammary Tumor,* Vol. II (B.S. Leung, ed.), Eden Press, Vermont, pp. 229–283.

Bolander, F.F., Jr., and Topper, Y.J., 1979, Stimulation of lactose synthetase activity and casein synthesis in mouse mammary explants by estradiol, *Endocrinology* **106:**490–495.

Bondy, G.P., and Okey, A.B., 1978, Estrogen binding in mammary tissue of C3H mice with or without the mouse mammary tumor virus, *Oncology* **35:**127–131.

Bresciani, F., 1968, Topography of DNA synthesis in the mammary gland of the C3H mouse and its control by ovarian hormones: An autoradiographic study, *Cell Tissue Kinet.* **1:**51–63.

Brown, J.B., 1981, Hormone profiles in young women at risk of breast cancer, in: *Hormones and Breast Cancer, Banbury Report #8* (M.C. Pike, P.K. Siiteri, and C.W. Welsch, eds.) Cold Spring Harbor Laboratory, Cold Spring Harbor, NY, pp. 33–56.

Buell, R.H., and Tremblay, G., 1984, Autoradiographic demonstration of ^{3}H-estradiol incorporation in benign human mammary lesions, *Am. J. Clin. Pathol.* **81:**30–34.

Butler, W.B., Kirkland, W.L., and Jorgensen, T.L., 1979, Induction of plasminogen activator by estrogen in a human breast cancer cell line (MCF-7), *Biochem. Biophys. Res. Commun.* **90:**1328–1334.

Capuco, A.V., Feldhoff, P.A., Akers, R.M., Whittliff, J.L., and Tucker, H.A., 1982, Progestin binding in mammary tissue of prepartum, nonlactating cows, *Steroids* **40:**502–517.

Ceriani, R.L., 1970, Fetal mammary gland differentiation *in vitro* in response to hormones. I. Morphological findings, *Dev. Biol.* **21:**506–529.

Chambon, M., Cavalie-Barthez, G., Vieth, F., Vignon, F., Hallowes, R., and Rochefort, H., 1984, Effect of estradiol on nonmalignant human mammary cells in primary culture, *Cancer Res.* **44:**5733–5743.

Clark, J.H., and Peck, E.J. Jr., 1976, Nuclear retention of receptor–estrogen complex and nuclear acceptor sites, *Nature* **260:**635–637.

Cowie, A.T., 1949, The relative growth of the mammary gland in normal gonadectomized and adrenalectomized rats, *J. Endocrinol.* **6:**145–157.

Cunha, G.R., Chung, L.W.K., Shannon, J.M., Taguehi, O., and Fujii, H., 1983, Hormone induced morphogenesis and growth: Role of mesenchymal–epithelial interactions, *Recent Prog. Horm. Res.* **39:**559–595.

Darbre, P., Yates, J., Curtis, S., and King, R.J.B., 1983, Effect of estradiol on human breast cancer cells in culture, *Cancer Res.* **43:**349.

DeSombre, E.R., Mohla, S., and Jensen, E.V., 1972, Estrogen-independent activation of the receptor protein of calf uterine cytosol, *Biochem. Biophys. Res. Commun.* **48:**1601–1606.

Dickson, R.B., Huff, K.K., Spencer, E.M., and Lippman, M.E., 1985, Induction of EGF-related polypeptides by 17β-estradiol in MCF-7 human breast cancer cells, *Endocrinology* **118:**138–142.

Edery, M., Imagawa, W., Larson, L., and Nandi, S., 1984a, Regulation of estrogen and progesterone receptor levels in mouse mammary epithelial cells grown in serum-free collagen gel cultures, *Endocrinology* **116:**105–112.

Edery, M., McGrath, M., Larson, L., and Nandi, S., 1984b, Correlation between *in vitro* growth and regulation of estrogen and progesterone receptors in rat mammary epithelial cells, *Endocrinology* **115:**1691–1697.

Edwards, D.P., Adams, D.J., and McGruire, W.L., 1981, Estradiol stimulates synthesis of a major intracellular protein in MCF-7 human breast cancer cell line, *Breast Cancer Res. Treat.* **1:**209–223.

Elias, J.J., Pitelka, D.R., and Armstrong, R.C., 1973, Changes in fat cell morphology during lactation in the mouse, *Anat. Res.* **177:**533–548.

Emerman, J.T., Burwen, S.J., and Pitelka, D.R., 1979, Substrate properties influencing ultrastructural differentiation of mammary epithelial cells in culture, *Tissue Cell* **11:**109–119.

Flaxman, B.A., and Lasfargues, E.Y., 1973, Hormone-independent DNA synthesis by epithelial cells of adult human mammary gland in organ culture, *Proc. Soc. Exp. Biol. Med.* **143:**371–374.

Freeman, C.S., and Topper, Y.J., 1978, Progesterone is not essential to the differentiative potential of mammary epithelium in the male mouse, *Endocrinology* **103:**186–192.

Gaubert, C.-M., Biancucci, S., and Shyamala, G., 1982, A comparison of the cytoplasmic estrogen receptors of mammary gland from virgin and lactating mice, *Endocrinology* **110:**683–685.

Gaubert, C.-M., Carriero, R., and Shyamala, G., 1986, Relationships between mammary estrogen receptor and estrogenic sensitivity. Molecular properties of cytoplasmic receptor and its binding to DNA, *Endocrinology* **118:**1504–1512.

Gorski, J., Toft, D., Shyamala, G., Smith, D., and Notides, A.C., 1968, Hormone receptors: Studies on the interaction of estrogen with the uterus, *Recent Prog. Horm. Res.* **24:**45–80.

Hahnel, R., Twaddle, E., and Vivian, A.B., 1971, Estrogen receptors in human breast cancer. 2. *In vitro* binding of estradiol by benign and malignant tumors, *Steroids* **18:**681–708.

Hallowes, R.C., Rudland, P.S., Hawkins, R.A., Lewis, D.J., Bennett, D., and Durbin, H., 1977, Comparison of the effects of hormones on DNA synthesis in cell cultures of nonneoplastic and neoplastic mammary epithelium from rats, *Cancer Res.* **37:**2492–2504.

Haslam, S.Z., 1986, Mammary fibroblast influence on normal mouse mammary epithelial cell responses to estrogen *in vitro, Cancer Res.* **45:**310–316.

Haslam, S.Z., and Levely, M.L., 1985, Estrogen responsiveness of normal mouse mammary cells in primary cell culture: Association of mammary fibroblasts with estrogenic regulation of PgR, *Endocrinology* **116:**1835–1844.

Haslam, S.Z., and Shyamala, G., 1979, Effect of oestradiol on progesterone receptors in normal mammary glands and its relationship to lactation, *Biochem. J.* **182:**127–131.

Haslam, S.Z., and Shyamala, G., 1980, Progesterone receptors in normal mammary gland: Receptor modulations in relation to differentiation, *J. Cell. Biol.* **86:**730–737.

Haslam, S.Z., and Shyamala, G., 1981, Relative distribution of estrogen and progesterone receptors among epithelial, adipose and connective tissues of normal mammary gland, *Endocrinology* **108:**825–830.

Haslam, S.Z., McBlain, W.A., and Shyamala, G., 1982, An empirical basis for the competition by dexamethasone to progesterone receptors as estimated with the synthetic progestin R5020, *J. Receptor Res.* **2:**435–451.

Haslam, S.Z., Gale, K.J., and Dachtler, S.L., 1984, Estrogen receptor activation in normal mammary gland, *Endocrinology* **114:**1163–1172.

Horwitz, K.B., and Alexander, P.S., 1983, *In situ* photo linked nuclear progesterone receptors of human breast cancer cells: Subunit molecular weights after transformation and translocation, *Endocrinology* **113:**2195–2201.

Horwitz, K.B., and Freidenberg, G.R., 1985, Growth inhibition and increase of insulin receptors in antiestrogen-resistant $T47d_{co}$ human breast cancer cells by progestins: Implications for endocrine therapies, *Cancer Res.* **45:**167–173.

Horwitz, K.B., and McGuire, W.L., 1977a, Estrogen control of progesterone receptor in human breast cancer, *J. Biol. Chem.* **253:**2223–2228.

Horwitz, K.B., and McGuire, W.L., 1977b, Progesterone and progesterone receptors in experimental breast cancer, *Cancer Res.* **37:**1733–1738.

Horwitz, K.B., and McGuire, W.L., 1978, Estrogen control of progesterone receptors in human breast cancer: Correlation with nuclear processing of estrogen receptors, *J. Biol. Chem.* **253:**8185–8191.

Horwitz, K.B., Mockus, M.B., and Lessey, B.A., 1982, Variant T47D human breast cancer cells with high progesterone-receptor levels despite estrogen and anti-estrogen resistance, *Cell* **28:**633–642.

Horwitz, K.B., Mockus, M.B., Pike, A.W., Tennessey, P.V., and Sheridan, R.L., 1983, Progesterone receptor replenishment in T47D human breast cancer cells, *J. Biol. Chem.* **258:**7603–7610.

Hoshino, K., 1983, *In vivo* induction of lactation in mammary glands isografted from neonates to pregnant mice, *J. Endocrinol.* **99:**245–250.

Hseuh, A.J.W., Peck, E.J., Jr., and Clark, J.H., 1973, Oestrogen receptors in the mammary gland of the lactating rat, *J. Endocrinol.* **58:**503–511.

Ichinose, R.R., and Nandi, S., 1966, Influence of hormones on lobuloalveolar differentiation of mouse mammary glands *in vitro, J. Endorcrinol.* **35:**331–340.

Imagawa, W., Tomooka, Y., Hamamoto, S., and Nandi, S., 1985, Stimulation of mammary epithelial cell growth *in vitro:* Interaction of epidermal growth factor and mammogenic hormones, *Endocrinology* **116:**1514–1524.

Imai, Y., Leung, C.K.H., Friesen, H.G., and Shui, R.P.C., 1982, Epidermal growth factor receptors and effect of epidermal growth factor on growth of human breast cancer cells in long-term tissue culture, *Cancer Res.* **42:**4394–4398.

Jensen, E.V., Suzuki, T., Numata, M., Smith, S., and DeSombre, E.R., 1969, Estrogen-binding substances of target tissues, *Steroids* **13:**417–421.

Jensen, E.V., Suzuki, T., Kawashima, T., Stumpf, W.E., Jungblut, P.W., and DeSombre, E.R., 1968, A two-step mechanism for the interaction of estradiol with rat uterus, *Proc. Natl. Acad. Sci. USA* **59:**632–638.

Kelly, P.A., Dijane, J., and Malancon, R., 1983, Characterization of estrogen, progesterone and glucocorticoid receptors in rabbit mammary glands and their measurement during pregnancy and lactation, *J. Steroid Biochem.* **18:**215–221.

Kidwell, W.R., Salomon, D.S., Liotta, L.A., Zweibel, J.A., and Bano, M., 1982, Effect of growth factors on mammary epithelial cell proliferation and basement membrane synthesis, in: *Growth of Cells in Hormonally Defined Media* (G.H. Sato, A.B. Pardee, and D.A. Sirbasku, eds.), Cold Spring Harbor Conferences on Cell Proliferation, Vol. 9, Cold Spring Harbor Laboratory, Cold Spring Harbor, NY, pp. 807–818.

Kidwell, W.R., Bano, M., and Salomon, D.S., 1984, Growth of normal mammary epithelium on collagen in serum-free medium, in: *Cell Culture Methods for Molecular and Cell Biology,* Vol. 2, *Methods for Serum-Free Culture of Cells of the Endocrine System* (D.W. Barnes, D.A. Sirbasku, and G.H. Sato, eds.), Alan R. Liss, New York, pp. 105–126.

King, W.J., and Greene, G.L., 1984, Monoclonal antibodies localize oestrogen receptor in the nuclei of target cells, *Nature* **307:**745–747.

Kleinberg, D.L., Todd, J., Babitsky, G., and Greising, J., 1982, Estradiol inhibits prolactin induced α-lactalbumin production in normal primate mammary tissue *in vitro, Endocrinology* **110:**279–281.

Kleinberg, D.L., Todd, J., and Babitsky, G., 1983, Inhibition of the lactogenic effect of prolactin in primate mammary tissue: Reversal by antiestrogens LY156758 and tamoxifen, *Proc. Natl. Acad. Sci. USA* **80:**4144–4148.

Koyama, H., Sinha, D., and Dao, T.L., 1972, Effects of hormones and 7,12-dimethylbenz-[a]anthracene on rat mammary tissue grown in organ culture, *J. Natl. Cancer Inst.* **48:**1671–1680.

Kratochwil, K., 1969, Organ specificity in mesenchymal induction demonstrated in the embryonic development of the mammary gland of mouse, *Dev. Biol.* **20:**46–71.

Kuhn, N.J., 1969, Progesterone withdrawal as the lactogenic trigger in the rat, *J. Endocrinol.* **44:**39–54.

Kuhn, N.J., 1977, Lactogenesis: The search for trigger mechanisms in different species, in: *Comparative Aspects of Lactation* (M. Peaker, ed.), Academic Press, New York, pp. 165–192.

Lasfargues, E.Y., and Murray, M.R., 1959, Hormonal influences on the differentiation and growth of embryonic mouse mammary glands in organ culture, *Dev. Biol.* **1:**413–435.

Leach, K.L., Dahmer, M.K., Hammond, N.D., Sando, J.J., and Pratt, W.B., 1979, Molybdate inhibition of glucocorticoid receptor inactivation and transformation, *J. Biol. Chem.* **254:**11884–11890.

Lee, A.E., 1983, Proliferative response of mouse mammary glands to 17β-estradiol and progesterone and modification by mouse mammary tumor virus, *J. Natl. Cancer Inst.* **71:**1265–1269.

Lessey, B.A., Alexander, P.S., and Horwitz, K.B., 1983, The subunit structure of human breast cancer progesterone receptors: Characterization by chromatography and photoaffinity labeling, *Endocrinology* **112:**1267–1274.

Leung, B.S., 1982, Estrogen receptor in normal and neoplastic mammary tissues, in: *Hormonal Regulation of Mammary Tumors* Vol. 1 (B.S. Leung, ed.), Eden Press, Vermont, pp. 118–154.

Leung, B.S., Wenche, J.M., and Reiney, C.G., 1976, Estrogen receptor in mammary glands and uterus of rats during pregnancy, lactation and involution, *J Steroid Biochem.* **7:**88–95.

Lippman, M., Bolan, G., and Huff, K., 1976, The effect of estrogens and antiestrogens on hormone responsive breast cancer in long-term culture, *Cancer Res.* **36:**4595.

Lloyd, R.V., 1979, Studies on the progesterone receptor content and steroid metabolism in normal and pathological human breast tissues, *J. Clin. Endocrinol. Metab.* **48:**585–593.

Lowenstein, W.R., 1981, Junctional intercellular communication: The cell-to-cell membrane chanel, *Physiol. Rev.* **61:**829–913.

Lyons, W.R., Li, C.H., and Johnson, R.E., 1958, The hormonal control of mammary growth and lactation, *Recent Prog. Horm. Res.* **14:**219–254.

Masters, J.R.W., Drife, J.O., and Scarisbreck, J.J., 1977, Cyclic variation of DNA synthesis in human breast epithelium, *J. Natl. Cancer Inst.* **58:**1263–1265.

McGrath, C.M., 1983, Augmentation of response of normal mammary epithelial cells to estradiol by mammary stroma, *Cancer Res.* **43:**1355–1360.

McManus, J.M., and Welsch, C.W., 1981, Hormone-induced ductal DNA synthesis of human breast tissues maintained in the athymic nude mouse, *Cancer Res.* **41:**3300–3305.

McManus, J.M., and Welsch, C.W., 1984, The effect of estrogen progesterone, thyroxine, and human placental lactogen on DNA synthesis of human breast ductal epithelium maintained in athymic nude mice, *Cancer Res.* **54:**1920–1927.

Meyer, J.S., 1977, Cell proliferation in normal human breast ducts, fibroadenomas and other ductal hyperplasias measured by nuclear labeling with tritiated thymidine, *Human Pathol.* **8:**67–81.

Mockus, M.B., and Horwitz, K.B., 1983, Progesterone receptors in human breast cancer, *J. Biol. Chem.* **258:**4778–4783.

Moudgil, V.K., 1983, Progesterone receptor, in: *Principles of Receptorology* (M.K. Agarwal, ed.), Walter de Gruyter, Berlin, pp. 273–379.

Muldoon, T.G., 1979, Mouse mammary tissue estrogen receptors: Ontogeny and molecular heterogeneity, in: *Ontogeny of Receptors and Reproductive Hormone Action* (T.H. Hamilton, J.H. Clark, and W.A. Sadler, eds.), Raven Press, New York, pp. 225–247.

Muldoon, T.G., 1981, Interplay between estradiol and prolactin in the regulation of steroid hormone receptor levels, nature and functionality in normal mouse mammary tissue, *Endocrinology* **109:**1339–1346.

Munford, R.E., 1963, Changes in mammary glands of rats and mice during pregnancy, lactation and involution, *J. Endocrinol.* **28:**1–15.

Murphy, L.J., Sutherland, R.L., Slead, B., Murphy, L.C., and Lazarus, L., 1986, Progestin regulation of epidermal growth factor receptor in human mammary carcinoma cells, *Cancer Res.* **46:**728–734.

Nandi, S., 1958, Endocrine control of mammary gland development and function in the C3HHe Crgl mouse, *J. Natl. Cancer Inst.* **21:**1039–1063.

Nandi, S., Yang, J., Richards, J., and Guzman, R., 1981, Role of hormones in mammogenesis and carcinogenesis, in: *Hormones and Breast Cancer, Banbury Report #8* (M.C. Pike, P.K. Siiteri, and C.W. Welsch, eds.), Cold Spring Harbor Laboratory, Cold Spring Harbor, NY, pp. 445–456.

Narbaitz, R., Stumpf, W.E., and Sar, M., 1980, Estrogen receptors in mammary gland primordia of fetal mouse, *Anat. Embryol.* **158:**161–166.

Nishigori, H., and Toft, D.O., 1980, Inhibition of progesterone receptor activation by sodium molybdate, *Biochemistry* **19:**77–83.

Osborne, C.K., Hamilton, B., Titus, G., and Livingston, R.B., 1980, Epidermal growth factor stimulation of human breast cancer cells in culture, *Cancer Res.* **40:**2361–2366.

Pollow, K., Sinnecker, R., Schmidt-Gollwitzer, M., Boquoi, E., and Pollow, B., 1977, Binding of [^{3}H]-progesterone to normal and neoplastic tissue samples from tumor bearing breasts, *J. Mol. Med.* **2:**69–82.

Prop, F.J.A., 1966, Effect of donor age on hormone reactivity of mouse mammary gland organ cultures, *Exp. Cell Res.* **42:**386–388.

Purnell, D.M., and Saggers, G.C., 1974, Topologic assessment by use of whole-mounts of mitotic activity in hamster mammary gland during the estrous cycle, *J. Natl. Cancer Inst.* **53:**825–828.

Raynaud, A., and Raynaud, J., 1954, Les diverses malformations mammaires produites chez les foetus de souris par l'action des hormones sexuelles, *C.R. Soc. Biol. Paris* **148:**963–968.

Richards, J., Guzman, R., Konrad, M., Yang, J., and Nandi, S., 1982, Growth of mouse mammary gland end buds cultured in a collagen gel matrix, *Exp. Cell Res.* **141:**433–443.

Richards, J., Hamamoto, S., Smith, S., Pasco, D., Guzman, R., and Nandi, S., 1983, Response of end bud cells from immature rat mammary gland to hormones when cultured in collagen gel, *Exp. Cell Res.* **147:**95–109.

Richards, J.E., Shyamala, G., and Nandi, S., 1974, Estrogen receptor in normal and neoplastic mouse mammary tissues, *Cancer Res.* **34:**2764–2772.

Rochefort, H., and Chalbos, D., 1984, Progestin-specific markers in human cell lines: Biological and pharmacological applications, *Mol. Cell. Endocrinol.* **36:**3–10.

Rosen, J.M., O'Neal, D.L., McHugh, J.E., and Comstock, J.P., 1978, Progesterone-mediated inhibition of casein mRNA and polysomal casein synthesis in the rat mammary gland during pregnancy, *Biochemistry* **17:**290–297.

Rosen, P.P., Mendez-Botet, C.J., Nisselbaum, J.S., Urban, J.A., Mike, V., Fracchea, A., and Schwartz, M.K., 1975, Pathological review of breast lesions analyzed for estrogen receptor protein, *Cancer Res.* **35:**3187–3194.

Salomon, D.S., Zwiebel, J.A., Bano, M., Losonczy, A., Fehne, P., and Kidwell, W.R., 1984,

Presence of transforming growth factors in human breast cancer cells, *Cancer Res.* **44:**4069–4077.

Sar, M., and Stumpf, W.E., 1975, Autoradiography of mammary glands and uteri of mice and rats after injection with [^{3}H]-estradiol, *J. Steroid Biochem.* **7:**391–394.

Seshadri, R., Shah, P.N., and Shindi, S.R., 1979, Presence of sex steroid receptors in normal breast of human females, *Endokrinologie* **13:**353–355.

Sheridan, P.J., 1975, Is there an alternative to the cytoplasmic receptor model for the mechanism of action of steroids?, *Life Sci.* **17:**497–502.

Shyamala, G., 1973, Specific cytoplasmic glucocorticoid hormone receptors in lactating mammary gland, *Biochemistry* **12:**3085–3090.

Shyamala, G., 1982, Glucocorticoid receptors: Mode of action in normal and neoplastic mammary tissues in: *Hormonal Regulation of Mammary Tumors,* Vol. 1 (B.S. Leung, ed.), Eden Press, Vermont, pp. 245–286.

Shyamala, G., and Ferenczy, A., 1982, The nonresponsiveness of lactating mammary gland to estradiol, *Endocrinology* **110:**1249–1256.

Shyamala, G., and Ferenczy, A., 1984, Mammary fat pad may be a potential site for initiation of estrogen action in normal mouse mammary glands, *Endocrinology* **115:**1078–1081.

Shyamala, G., and Gorski, J., 1969, Estrogen receptors in the rat uterus. Studies on the interaction of cytosol and nuclear binding sites, *J. Biol. Chem.* **244:**1097–1022.

Shyamala, G., and Haslam, S.Z., 1980, Estrogen and progesterone receptors in normal mammary gland during different functional states, in: *Perspectives in Steroid Receptor Research* (F. Bresciani, ed.), Raven Press, New York, pp. 193–216.

Shyamala, G., and Nandi, S., 1972, Interactions of 6,7-^{3}H-17β-estradiol with the mouse lactating mammary tissue *in vivo* and *in vitro, Endocrinology* **91:**861–867.

Shyamala, G., and Yeh, Y.-F., 1977, Estrogen receptors of mammary glands: A molecular analysis of the cytoplasmic estrogen binding proteins, in: *Multiple Molecular Forms of Steroid Hormone Receptors* (M.K. Agarwal, ed.), Elsevier/North Holland Biomedical Press, New York, pp. 129–147.

Silberstein, G.B., and Daniel, C.W., 1982, Glycosaminoglycans in the basal lamina and extracellular matrix of the developing mouse mammary duct, *Dev. Biol.* **90:**215–222.

Silver, M., 1953, The onset of allometric mammary growth in the female hooded Norway rat, *J. Endocrinol.* **10:**35–45.

Simpson, A.A., Simpson, M.H.W., and Kulharni, D.N., 1973, Prolactin production and lactogenesis in rats after ovariectomy in late pregnancy, *J. Endocrinol.* **57:**425–429.

Sirbasku, D.A., 1978, Estrogen induction of growth factors specific for hormone-responsive mammary, pituitary and kidney tumor cells, *Proc. Natl. Acad. Sci. USA* **75:**3786–3790.

Sirbasku, D.A., 1980, Estromedins. Uterine derived growth factors for estrogen responsive tumor cells, in: *Control Mechanisms in Animal Cells: Specific Growth Factors* (L.J. DeAsua, ed.), Raven Press, New York, pp. 293, 315.

Smith, R.G., dIstria, M., and Van, N.T., 1981, Purification of a human progesterone receptor, *Biochemistry* **20:**5557–5564.

Strum, J.M., and Hillman, E.A., 1981, Human breast epithelium in organ culture: Effect of hormones on growth and morphology, *In Vitro* **17:**33–43.

Tonelli, Q.J., and Sorof, S., 1980, Epidermal growth factor requirement for development of cultured mammary gland, *Nature* **285:**250–252.

Verma, V., Kapur, M.M., and Laumas, K.R., 1978, Characterization of progesterone receptors and metabolism of progesterone in the normal and cancerous human mammary gland, *J. Steroid Biochem.* **9:**569–577.

Vignon, F., Bardon, S., Chalbos, D., and Rochefort, H., 1983, *J. Clin. Endocrinol. Metab.* **56:**1124–1129.

Vignon, F., Capony, F., Chambon, M., Freiss, G., Garcia, M., and Rochefort, H., 1986, Autocrine growth stimulation of MCF-7 breast cancer cells by the estrogen-regulated 52K protein, *Endocrinology* **118:**1537–1545.

Vonderhaar, B.K., 1984, Hormones and growth factors in mammary gland development, in: *Control of Cell Growth and Proliferation* (C.M. Veneziale, ed.), Van Nostrand Reinhold, New York, pp. 11–33.

Warembourg, M., 1983, Progestagen-concentrating cells in the brain, uterus, vagina and mammary glands of the galago (*Galago senegalensis*), *J. Reprod. Fertil.* **68:**189–193.

Watson, C.S., Medina, D., and Clark, J.H., 1979, Characterization and estrogen stimulation of cytoplasmic progesterone receptor in the ovarian-dependent MXT-3590 mammary tumor line, *Cancer Res.* **39:**4098–4104.

Weichman, B.M., and Notides, A.C., 1977, Estradiol-binding kinetics of the activated and non-activated estrogen receptor, *J. Biol. Chem.* **252:**8856–8862.

Weichman, B.M., and Notides, A.C., 1980, Estrogen receptor activation and the dissociation kinetics of estradiol, estriol and estrone, *Endocrinology* **106:**435–439.

Welshons, W.V., Lieberman, M.E., and Gorski, J., 1984, Nuclear localization of unoccupied oestrogen receptors, *Nature* **307:**747–749.

Westley, B., and Rochefort, H., 1980, A secreted glycoprotein induced by estrogen in human breast cancer cell lines, *Cell* **20:**353–362.

Wicha, M.S., 1982, Growth and differentiation of rat mammary epithelium on mammary gland extracellular matrix in: *Extracellular Matrix* (S. Hawk, ed.), Academic Press, New York, pp. 309–314.

Wiehle, R.D., and Wittliff, J.L., 1983, Alterations in sex-steroid hormone receptors during mammary gland differentiation in the rat, *Comp. Biochem. Physiol.* **76B:**409–417.

Williams, J.M., and Daniel, C.W., 1983, Mammary ductal elongation: Differentiation of myoepithelium and basal lamina during branching morphogenesis, *Dev. Biol.* **97:**214–290.

Wittliff, J.L., 1975, Steroid binding proteins in normal and neoplastic mammary cells, *Methods Cancer Res.* **11:**293–354.

Wittliff, J.L., Gardner, D.G., Battema, W.L., and Gilbert, P.J., 1972, Specific estrogen-receptors in the neoplastic and lactating mammary gland of the rat, *Biochem. Biophys. Res. Commun.* **48:**119–125.

Yang, J., Elias, J.J., Petrakis, N.L., Wellings, S.R., and Nandi, S., 1981, Effects of hormones and growth factors on human mammary epithelial cells in collagen gel culture, *Cancer Res.* **41:**1021–1027.

Yang, J., Guzman, R., Richards J., Imagawa, W., McCormick, K., and Nandi, S., 1980, Growth factor- and cyclic nucleotide-induced proliferation of normal and malignant mammary epithelial cells in primary culture, *Endocrinology* **107:**35–41.

Yu, W.C.Y., and Leung, B.S., 1982, Variation of cytoplasmic content of estrogen and progesterone receptors in the mammary gland and uterus of rats at time of parturition, *Biol. Reprod.* **27:**658–664.

16

Regulation of Mammary Glucose Metabolism in Lactation

Anne Faulkner and Malcolm Peaker

The importance of glucose to the lactating mammary gland was demonstrated many years ago when, using the isolated perfused udder of a goat, Hardwick et al. (1961) showed conclusively that omission of glucose from the perfusion medium stopped milk lactose and water secretion completely. Secretion was reestablished on reintroduction of glucose into the perfusate. Earlier, Foa (cited by Linzell, 1974) had demonstrated that lactose could only be detected in milk from a perfused sheep's udder when glucose was present in the perfusate and Kleiber et al. (1955), using radioactive glucose injections into the jugular vein, had shown that about 80% of milk lactose was derived from the plasma glucose pool in the cow in vivo. These classic experiments highlighted the unique and essential role of glucose in the synthesis of lactose and hence in the maintenance of milk production in the lactating mammary gland.

In this chapter, we provide a brief review of the biochemical foundation for our studies, following with a discussion of the relation between glucose availability and milk synthesis and then reviewing mechanisms other than glucose availability that may be involved in the regulation of glucose metabolism in the mammary gland.

Anne Faulkner and Malcolm Peaker • Hannah Research Institute, Ayr KA6 5HL, Scotland.

1. Pathways of Glucose Metabolism in the Mammary Gland

1.1. Lactose Biosynthesis

Lactose is the predominant carbohydrate in the milk from most mammalian species; its concentration varies from being almost undetectable in some aquatic mammals to 200 m*M* (7 g/dl) in the human (Jenness and Sloan, 1970). Within most species, the concentration of lactose is quite constant and maintains the osmolarity of milk (Jenness, 1974). Because glucose is the sole precursor of lactose, it plays an important role in the function of the mammary gland. In ruminants, up to 70% of the glucose taken up by the mammary gland appears as lactose in milk; most of the rest is oxidized. Mammary uptake can be 60–85% of the total glucose entering the circulation (Annison and Linzell, 1964; Chaiyabutr et al., 1980).

The final step in the synthesis of lactose is catalyzed by the enzyme, galactosyltransferase, according to the reaction

$$\text{UDP-galactose} + \text{glucose} \rightarrow \text{lactose} + \text{UDP}$$

Galactosyltransferases are found in many tissues where they are involved in the biosynthesis of glycoproteins, glycolipids, polysaccharides, and mucin (Roseman, 1970). The galactosyltransferases are characteristically associated with the membrane fractions of cells, being bound to the inner membrane of the Golgi vesicle. In other tissues, the acceptors of the galactose moiety are *N*-acetylglucosamine residues. Only in the mammary gland is free glucose the acceptor. This change of specificity of galactosyltransferase is achieved by the interaction of the enzyme with a second protein, α-lactalbumin, which increases the affinity of galactosyltransferase for glucose. Because the mammary gland is incapable of synthesizing free glucose from other precursors because of the absence of the enzyme glucose 6-phosphatase (Threadgold and Kuhn, 1979), glucose for the synthesis of lactose can be obtained only from the blood supply.

UDP-Galactose, the second precursor of lactose, is also derived principally from glucose by a series of enzymatic reactions within the cytosol of the mammary gland. These are

$$\text{glucose} + \text{ATP} \xrightarrow{①} \text{glucose 6-phosphate} \xrightarrow{②} \text{glucose 1-phosphate}$$

$$\text{glucose-1-phosphate} + \text{UTP} \xrightarrow{③} \text{UDP-glucose} \xrightarrow{④} \text{UDP-galactose}$$

The enzymes involved in the synthesis are: (1) hexokinase, (2) phosphoglucomutase, (3) uridine 5′-diphosphoglucose pyrophosphorylase, and (4) uridine 5′-diphosphoglucose 4-epimerase. Enzymes (2), (3), and (4) are thought to catalyze equilibrium reactions; hexokinase catalyzes an irreversible reaction. In theory, L-lactate could also be a precursor of the UDP-galactose used for lactose synthesis since the enzymes required to catalyze the formation of glucose 6-phosphate from lactate are all known to be present in the mammary gland (Baird, 1969). In practice, it is unlikely that substantial quantities of UDP-galactose are formed in this way, since radioactivity from L-lactate does not appear in lactose. On the other hand, isotopic studies in cows and goats have indicated that up to 20% of the glucose 6-phosphate used for UDP-galactose formation may be derived from triose phosphates that arise from pentose phosphate metabolism (Wood et al., 1965; Chaiyabutr et al., 1980), thus making maximum use of the glucose available to the mammary gland.

Further details of the mechanism and regulation of the lactose synthase reaction can be found in several reviews (Brew, 1970; Ebner and Schanbacher, 1974; Kuhn, 1983).

1.2. Pentose Phosphate Pathway

The pentose phosphate pathway provides a mechanism for the generation of NADPH by the oxidative decarboxylation of glucose 6-phosphate to ribulose 5-phosphate. Subsequent reactions of carbon transfer can then regenerate glucose 6-phosphate from pentose phosphate such as ribose 5-phosphate (Fig. 1) so that the overall reaction may be written:

$$12\ \text{NADP} + 6\ \text{glucose 6-phosphate} \rightarrow 5\ \text{glucose 6-phosphate} + 6\ \text{CO}_2 + 12\ \text{NADPH}$$

The lactating mammary gland, a tissue with a high rate of fatty acid synthesis (see Chapter 17 in this volume), has a considerable requirement for reducing equivalents in the form of NADPH. This requirement can be fulfilled in several ways (Gumaa et al., 1973; Bauman and Davis, 1974). However, the importance of the pentose phosphate pathway in lactation in most species is suggested by the high activities of the enzymes involved (Bauman and Davis, 1974) and by the large increases in the activities of these enzymes, which are seen at the onset of lactation (Gumaa et al., 1971, 1973). These statements imply further that the pathway might be more important in nonruminant species where glucose is more available. However, experiments in vivo in goats using 3-[^{3}H]-glucose infusions showed that in this species 20% of the glucose

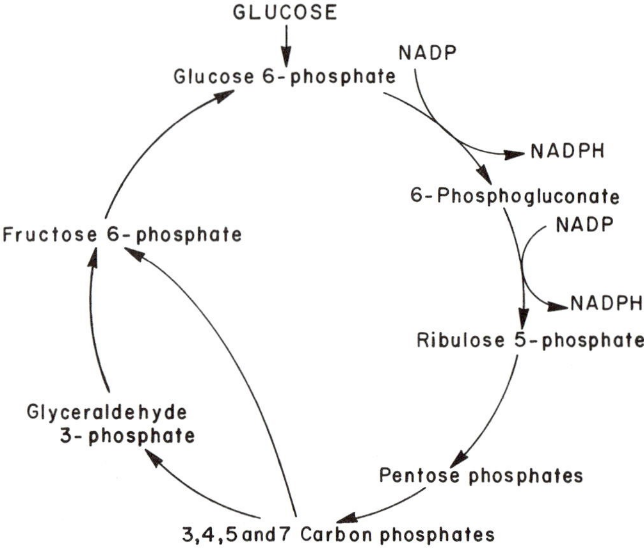

Figure 1. Glucose metabolism via the pentose phosphate pathway.

taken up by the mammary gland was metabolized via the pentose phosphate pathway, providing about 25% of the total NADPH required for de novo fatty acid synthesis in the mammary gland of the fed animal (Chaiyabutr et al., 1980). In studies in vitro using acini prepared from lactating rat mammary gland, metabolism via the pentose phosphate pathway accounted for 25–50% of the glucose taken up by the acini and provided 70–100% of the NADPH required for fatty acid synthesis (Katz et al., 1974; Robinson and Williamson, 1977b).

1.3. Fatty Acid and Triglyceride Biosynthesis

Major differences between species occur in the utilization of glucose for fatty acid synthesis. In nonruminant species, a considerable proportion of the glucose taken up by the mammary gland is used for fat synthesis de novo (Katz et al., 1974; Robinson and Williamson, 1977a). In ruminant species, essentially no glucose is used for this purpose; rather, acetate is the major fatty acid precursor (Hardwick et al., 1963; McCarthy and Smith, 1972). However, all species require glucose as a precursor for the glycerol 3-phosphate needed for the esterification of fatty acids to triglycerides.

In both ruminant and nonruminant species, glucose for fatty acid esterification must first be converted to glyceraldehyde 3-phosphate either via glycolysis or the pentose phosphate pathway (Fig. 2). Metabolism via the pentose phosphate pathway also has the advantage of generating the NADPH required for fatty acid synthesis. The available evidence suggests that, in the ruminant, triose phosphate is formed almost exclusively via the pentose phosphate pathway (Chaiyabutr et al., 1980; Smith, 1971). In nonruminants, formation via glycolysis also occurs; here, isotope studies indicate that 35–50% is provided by the pentose phosphate pathway (Katz et al., 1974; Robinson and Williamson, 1977b).

Synthesis of fatty acids from glucose involves further metabolism of glyceraldehyde 3-phosphate to produce pyruvate in the cytosol, followed by oxidative decarboxylation to acetyl-CoA, a reaction catalyzed by the enzyme pyruvate dehydrogenase, which is located in the mito-

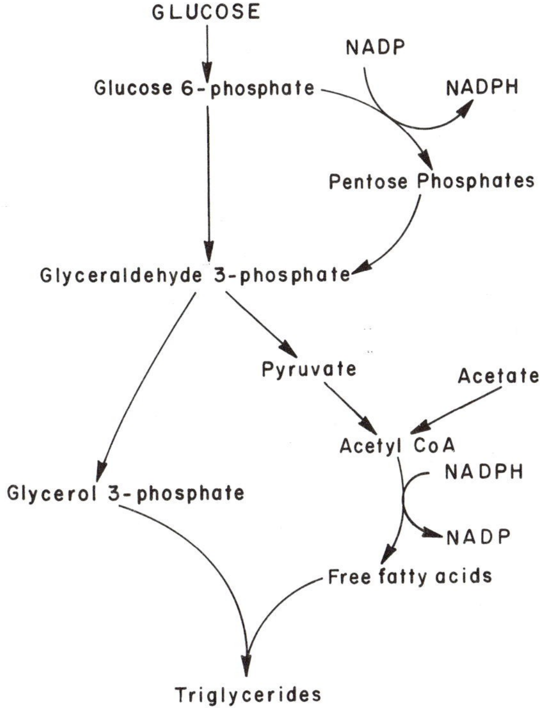

Figure 2. Glucose metabolism and the biosynthesis of lipid.

chondrial compartment (Bauman and Davis, 1974). The acetyl-CoA generated within the mitochondria is then translocated to the cytosol, where lipogenesis takes place. These reactions and their regulation mainly by phosphorylation–dephosphorylation reactions are discussed extensively by Munday and Hardie (Chapter 17 in this volume).

In nonruminants, utilization of glucose for fatty acid synthesis de novo accounts for a substantial proportion of the glucose taken up by the mammary gland. In the mammary tissue of ruminants, the activity of one of the enzymes linking glucose metabolism to fatty acid synthesis, ATP–citrate lyase, is very low (Hanson and Ballard, 1967). Pyruvate dehydrogenase activity (both total and active state) is also relatively lower than in nonruminant species (Read et al., 1977; R.G. Vernon, unpublished data). These low enzyme activities probably account for the very low contribution of glucose to de novo fatty acid synthesis in the mammary tissue of ruminants.

1.4. Glycolysis and the Tricarboxylic Acid Cycle

In addition to producing triose phosphate and pyruvate (and subsequently acetyl-CoA) for lipid biosynthesis, glucose may be metabolized to produce energy for the mammary gland, resulting in the production of lactate as the end product of glycolysis or carbon dioxide if complete oxidation occurs in the tricarboxylic acid cycle. (See Fig. 1 of Chapter 17 in this volume). The evidence available for most species suggests that the use of glucose solely for energy production is minimal in the mammary gland of the normal, fed, lactating animal. In fact, studies of arteriovenous differences indicate that lactate is taken up in vivo in both the rat (Robinson and Williamson, 1977a) and goat (Chaiyabutr, 1980) rather than being produced. Under conditions where rates of milk secretion fall (e.g., starvation), and glucose requirements are decreased, rates of glycolysis and lactate production may increase substantially (Robinson and Williamson, 1977a; Williamson et al., 1979; Chaiyabutr et al., 1980).

The complete oxidation of acetyl-CoA produced from glucose in the tricarboxylic acid cycle appears to be low in the mammary glands of most species. Thus, in the cow and goat, the CO_2 produced by the lactating udder from radioactively labeled glucose can be accounted for almost entirely by the oxidation of glucose in the pentose phosphate pathway (Wood et al., 1965; Smith, 1971; Chaiyabutr et al., 1980). In lactating rat mammary tissue in vitro, CO_2 produced in the tricarboxylic acid cycle accounts for only about 10% of the total CO_2 produced from glucose (Katz et al., 1974; Robinson and Williamson, 1977a).

2. Glucose Availability and Milk Synthesis

2.1. Effects of Blood Flow and Arterial Glucose Concentrations on Glucose Availability

Availability of glucose to the mammary gland is a major factor in the maintenance of milk secretion. When no glucose is presented to the gland, lactose synthesis is arrested and milk secretion ceases (Hardwick et al., 1961, 1963). The availability of glucose to the mammary gland is dependent on two factors: (1) blood flow to the organ and (2) concentration of glucose in the blood.

Mammary blood flow increases greatly at the onset of lactation in all species in which it has been measured (Reynolds, 1970; Hanwell and Linzell, 1973; Burd et al., 1978; Ota and Peaker, 1979). However, during established lactation, the variations in mammary blood flow are small in undisturbed animals and milk secretion is also stable. Mild stresses (e.g., starvation or cold exposure), however, do result in a fall in mammary blood flow and the rate of the milk secretion (Annison et al., 1968; Treacher et al., 1976; Chaiyabutr et al., 1980; Faulkner et al., 1980). In both the cow and goat, there is a good correlation between changes in mammary blood flow and milk yield (Linzell, 1974), but the control mechanisms involved in regulating mammary blood flow in lactating animals are still unknown.

In general, the arterial concentration of glucose is held within narrow limits and is under the control of circulating hormones. However, arterial concentrations may be lowered by treatment with insulin, or elevated by infusing glucose or treatment with anti-insulin serum. In addition, in ruminants, arterial glucose concentrations can be lowered some 10–20% by short-term starvation (Annison et al., 1968; Chaiyabutr et al., 1980) or elevated by cold-exposure (Faulkner et al., 1980). As arterial glucose concentrations fall, milk yields fall, but they recover when glucose is infused into hypoglycemic animals (Linzell, 1967; Hove, 1978a,b). Euglycemic animals infused with glucose show either a small or no response in their milk yields (Linzell, 1967; Treacher et al., 1976; Chaiyabutr, 1980). In hypoglycemic or euglycemic goats, about 30% of the glucose presented to the mammary gland is extracted. In hyperglycemic animals, the glucose extraction ratio falls and the increased availability of glucose (defined as arterial concentration × blood flow) does not result in higher rates of glucose uptake by the mammary gland. Thus, when glucose is infused into fed and starved goats, glucose availability increases from 1107 to 1622 μmol/min in fed and 317 to 862

Table I. Mean Concentrations of Glucose in Milk and Plasma and Glucose Uptake in Goats

Treatment		Milk (μmol/ml)	Plasma (μmol/ml)	Glucose uptake (μmol/min)
Colchicine—treated gland	Day 0	0.135	3.37	453
	Day 1	0.290	3.71	244
—untreated gland	Day 0	0.170	3.37	—
	Day 1	0.287	3.71	—
	Day 2	0.334	3.48	—
Starved goat	Day 0	0.150	3.06	363
	Day 1	0.080	2.85	—
	Day 2	0.039	2.92	92
Starved goat infused	Day 0	0.182	4.15	354
with glucose	Day 2	0.096	5.25	106

μmol/min in starved animals, but glucose uptake and milk glucose concentrations are unchanged (Table I); milk yields increase only in starved animals and do not increase in proportion to the increased glucose availability (Chaiyabutr, 1980). There appears to be no simple relation between glucose uptake and arterial glucose concentrations, as there is for mammary blood flow and glucose uptake.

2.2. Intracellular Glucose Concentrations

Of crucial importance is the intracellular concentration of glucose because it determines substrate availability for, and at low levels regulates the activity of, enzymes of glucose metabolism. Evaluation of the intracellular concentration of glucose in any tissue is difficult because of the high concentrations of glucose present in plasma occupying intercellular spaces. In the mammary gland, there is the additional complication of the extracellular milk space. Isolated cells or acini, which can be separated rapidly from surrounding medium, have been used for the measurement of the glucose content of rat mammary tissue after incubation in vitro and yield values for intracellular glucose concentrations of 0.3–0.5 m*M* (Wilde and Kuhn, 1981)—very much lower than the concentrations present in plasma (about 5 m*M*).

The realization that the aqueous phase of milk is derived from the fluid contained in the Golgi vesicles of the epithelial secretory cells (see Linzell and Peaker, 1971) led to the speculation that the concentration of glucose in the aqueous phase of milk may be equal to its intracellular concentration (Kuhn and White, 1975). In support of this concept, milk from several species has been shown to have a glucose concentration of about 0.2–0.3 m*M*, similar to that found in isolated mammary cells (Faulkner et al., 1981). Furthermore, it has been demonstrated that glucose readily crosses the apical membrane of the mammary epithelial cell in both directions (Faulkner et al., 1985a). When udder milk was diluted by infusion of an iso-osmotic solution of sucrose into the udder, the glucose concentration in the lumen of the mammary gland fell initially then increased steadily to reach a plateau at the preinfusion levels about 90 min following the infusion; when udder milk was diluted by infusion of an iso-osmotic solution containing glucose into the udder, the glucose concentration in the lumen initially increased then fell steadily to the preinfusion levels about 4 h following the infusion. These findings indicated the establishment of an equilibrium between intracellular and milk glucose concentrations (Faulkner et al., 1985a). These two pieces of data—(1) the similarity of milk glucose concentrations to those found in isolated mammary cells and (2) the ability of glucose to cross the apical membrane freely in both directions—provide strong evidence that the glucose concentration in milk can be equated with intracellular glucose levels and that both change in parallel.

Various physiological and pharmacological treatments produce changes in the concentration of glucose in milk that can be interpreted in terms of changing intracellular glucose concentrations. For example, withdrawal of food from lactating goats resulted in a rapid decrease in milk yield (up to 75%), which was accompanied by a fall in the concentration of glucose in milk of a similar magnitude (Fig. 3A). There are many physiological adaptations occurring during short-term starvation

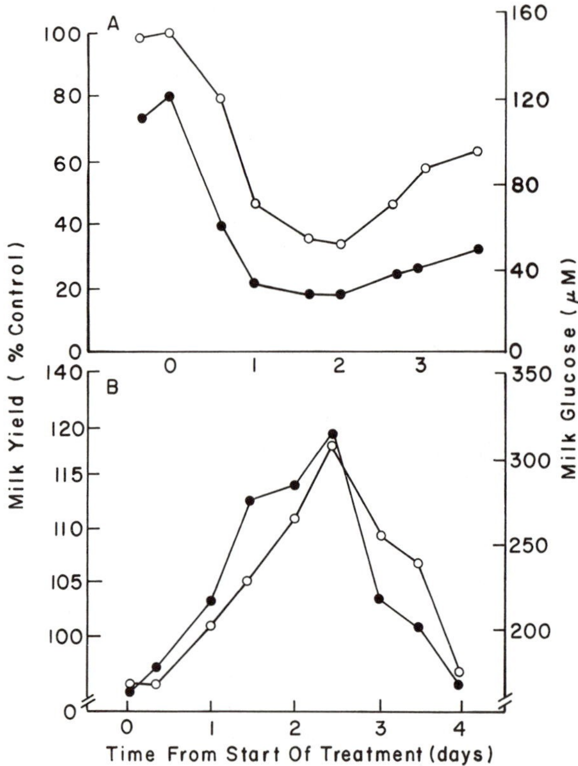

Figure 3. Changes in the concentration of glucose in milk (●) and milk yield (○) (A) during 48-h starvation and (B) in the untreated gland during inhibition of milk secretion in the treated gland by colchicine. Control values are those obtained on day 0 before treatment started. Feed was withdrawn from starved animals after afternoon milking on day 0 and offered again after afternoon milking on day 2. A single dose of colchicine (5 mg) was infused aseptically via the teat canal into one side of the udder on day 0 and day 1. Data are means of six animals for both experiments.

in the goat. The blood flow to the mammary gland falls rapidly to about 30% of fed values and glucose uptake also falls by the same amount. Extraction of glucose by the gland is unchanged and plasma glucose concentrations are maintained or fall by no more than 20% (Annison et al., 1968; Chaiyabutr et al., 1980). The reduced availability of glucose to the mammary gland caused by the reduced blood flow is probably the major contributor to the decrease in glucose uptake and milk glucose concentrations, but other factors may also operate (see Section 2.1). At the present time, we do not know what controls mammary blood flow or glucose uptake during starvation, but we have shown that changes in the rates of lactose synthesis (calculated from lactose concentrations in milk and milk yields) correlate well with the changes in concentrations of glucose in milk ($r = 0.91$; $p < 0.01$), suggesting that during starvation, reduced availability of glucose limits lactose synthesis and hence milk secretion (Faulkner et al., 1981). The converse also appears to be true; when milk yields increase, concentrations of glucose in milk rise. This was observed during the compensatory increase in milk yield in the untreated gland of lactating goats following inhibition of milk secretion in the other gland by treatment with colchicine (Henderson and Peaker, 1980). In this experiment, a 25% increase in milk yield was accompanied by a 100% increase in the concentration of glucose in milk (Faulkner et al., 1984) (Fig. 3B). With both the starvation and compensatory increase experiments, large changes in milk glucose concentrations were observed in the absence of major changes in arterial plasma glucose concentrations.

On the other hand, there are situations where the concentration of glucose in milk does not correlate well with milk secretion. Thus, when milk secretion is inhibited with alkaloids like colchicine or vincristine there is a large but transient increase in milk glucose in the treated gland at the onset of inhibition (Fig. 4A; Faulkner et al., 1984). At parturition, a similar transient increase in milk glucose is consistently observed before the onset of copious milk production (Fig. 4B; Faulkner et al., 1982). These transient accumulations of glucose in milk are suggestive of a buildup of precursor immediately following a block in lactose synthesis or, at around parturition, before lactogenesis.

The large changes in the concentration of glucose in milk (Figs. 3 and 4) are independent of plasma glucose concentration (Table I). If these changes can be interpreted to reflect changes in cytosolic glucose, they must be attributed to increased rates of entry of glucose into the cells or decreased rates of glucose utilization. The effects of alkaloids are particularly interesting in this regard. The increased concentrations of glucose observed following inhibition of milk secretion in the treated

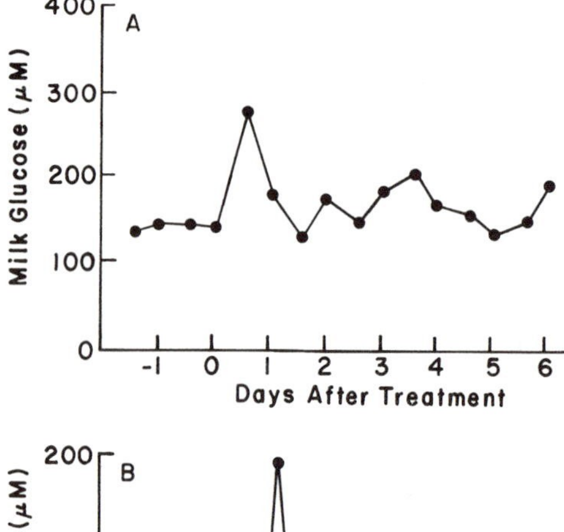

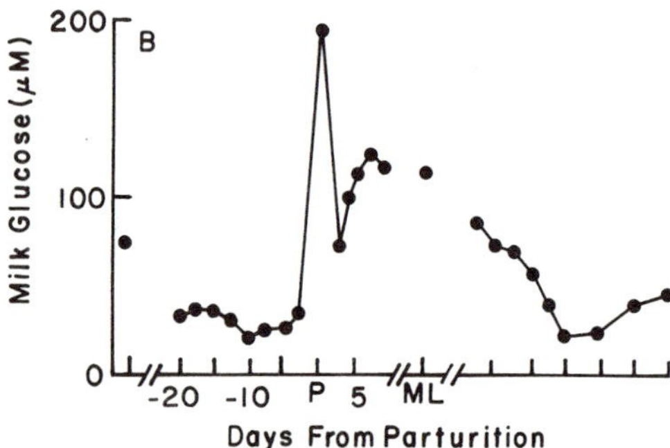

Figure 4. Changes in the concentration of glucose in milk (A) during colchicine treatment of the mammary gland and (B) through pregnancy and lactation. P — parturition; ML — midlactation. Colchicine treatment is as in Fig. 4. Fluid was removed aseptically from the udders of pregnant goats. Data are from six animals.

gland (Fig. 4A) are indicative of decreased utilization (i.e., reduced milk secretion); however, the increased concentration of glucose in the untreated gland (Fig. 3B) must be due to enhanced glucose entry since milk secretion is actually increasing at this time. The lack of correlation between arterial glucose concentration and milk glucose concentrations (Table I) indicates some form of control of glucose entry into the mammary epithelial cell. Experiments in vitro using mammary acini from lactating rats have provided evidence for a glucose transport system on the membrane of the mammary epithelial cell in this species (Threadgold et al., 1982). Using nonmetabolizable analogs of glucose, these workers showed inhibition of glucose uptake by glucose transport inhibitors and described a specific saturable process for glucose uptake and phosphorylation with an apparent K_m within the physiological range as well as a nonspecific process. They concluded that transport of glucose into the mammary epithelial cell was rate-limiting in the overall metabolism of glucose in the rat.

The hormonal control of glucose entry in most tissues that use large amounts of glucose is closely associated with plasma levels of insulin.

However, in the mammary gland, unlike muscle or adipose tissue, there is little evidence to suggest that insulin actually controls the entry of glucose into the mammary epithelial cell (Hove, 1978a,b; Robinson et al., 1978; Jones et al., 1984). Furthermore, infusion of insulin into lactating goats had no effect on the concentration of glucose in milk (A. Faulkner, unpublished data). In the ruminant in vivo, changes in plasma insulin concentration in either direction have no effect on milk yield or composition (Hove, 1978a,b); insulin effects are observed only when there are associated changes in plasma glucose concentrations; these can then be attributed to the effects of substrate availability rather than direct effects of insulin on the tissue. In the rat, responses to insulin have been observed but these appear to be associated almost exclusively with the metabolism of glucose to fatty acids (see Chapter 17 in this volume). There is also some evidence that insulin activates the glycolytic pathway (Jones et al., 1984), increasing the flux of glucose to pyruvate.

2.3. Intra-Golgi Glucose Concentrations

The rate of lactose synthesis is dependent not on cytosolic but on intra-Golgi glucose concentrations. Experiments in vitro using isolated Golgi vesicles from rat mammary gland suggested that there is very little restriction on glucose entry into these vesicles. Purified Golgi vesicles were penetrated by glucose, mannose, fructose, sorbitol, mannitol, and 3-*O*-methyl glucose but not by sucrose or lactose (White et al., 1981). Thus, carbohydrate entry into Golgi vesicles from rat mammary tissue appeared to be governed mainly by size, and a simple water-filled pore or channel was proposed as the mode of glucose entry. Such a system would impose few restrictions of glucose availability for lactose synthesis and leads to the prediction that glucose in the Golgi vesicles readily equilibrates with the cytosol. However, it is possible that the Golgi vesicular membrane is modified in some way by the techniques involved in isolation and that this may result in some loss of specificity of the hexose transporter. Similar size-discriminating pores in Golgi membranes have been produced by detergent action (Wallace and Kuhn, 1986).

A lack of specificity of metabolite entry into Golgi vesicles of mammary cells can also be implied from experiments performed on goats in vivo. Thus, milk has been shown to contain a wide variety of metabolites (Faulkner, 1980), including intermediates of glycolysis such as glucose 6-phosphate, phosphoenolpyruvate, fructose 6-phosphate, and glycerate 3-phosphate, which are present normally in the cytosol of the cell, as well as carboxylic acids such as 2-oxoglutarate, L-malate, and isocitrate; their concentrations in milk are similar to those within the cytosol (Table II;

Table II. Metabolite Concentrations in Milk and Mammary Tissue in the Goat[a]

Metabolite	Milk (μmol/ml)	Mammary gland (μmol/g)
Glucose 6-phosphate	0.12	0.095
UDP-glucose	0.167	0.127
UDP-galactose	0.334	0.074
2-Oxoglutarate	0.14	0.156
Isocitrate	0.065	0.121
Glycerate 3-phosphate	0.074	0.131
Phosphoenolpyruvate	0.052	0.049
Fructose 6-phosphate	0.035	0.031
L-Malate	0.064	0.193

[a]From Faulkner (1980).

Faulkner, 1980). These substances have been shown to be secreted into milk, along with lactose, via the secretory vesicles (Faulkner et al., 1985a). The presence of these metabolites at cytosolic concentrations, and their secretion via the secretory vesicles in the goat, points to entry of hexose, triose phosphates, and carboxylic acids into Golgi vesicles but gives no information on their rate of entry. Studies performed on the transport of hexoses across the apical membrane of the mammary epithelial cell of the goat in vivo, however, do suggest the presence of specific transport mechanisms as discussed next.

2.4. Glucose Transport across the Apical Membrane of the Mammary Epithelial Cell

The apical membrane of the mammary epithelial cell is in a state of constant change during lactation. Sections of the membrane are lost when the milk fat globule is secreted by a membranous envelope and new membrane is added when secretory vesicles fuse with the apical membrane, discharging their contents of protein and lactose (Linzell and Peaker, 1971; Mather and Keenan, 1983; Chapter 7 in this volume). The apical membrane may therefore be an amalgam of plasma and secretory vesicular membrane. If the membrane of the secretory vesicle is retained intact in the apical membrane after fusion, the apical membrane should exhibit some of the transport properties of the secretory vesicle. Therefore, studies on transport across the apical membrane in vivo may provide more meaningful information on the transport sys-

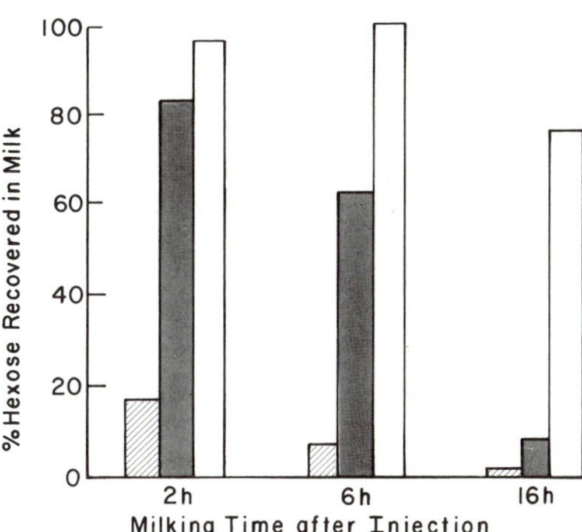

Figure 5. Retention of hexoses in the lumen of the mammary gland of goats. Solutions containing glucose (▨), galactose (■), and fructose (□) were infused aseptically via the teat canal into one-half of the udder. Animals were then milked at 2, 6, and 16 h after infusion and the recovery of glucose, galactose, and fructose calculated from their concentrations in milk and the milk volume. Data are means from experiments on four goats.

tems of the vesicles than studies performed on isolated vesicles, which may display artifacts due to isolation procedures.

The apical membrane is accessible to investigation of hexose transport via the teat canal and lumen of the gland in vivo (i.e., studying transport in the direction of lumen to cytosol). The results of such studies in the goat show that glucose crosses the apical membrane readily, but other hexoses are slower to cross. Galactose is lost from the lumen of the gland at less than half the rate of glucose, and fructose is almost entirely retained within the lumen (Faulkner et al., 1985b; Fig. 5). This specificity for glucose in hexose transport across the apical membrane is strong evidence for the presence of a specific glucose transporter whose properties are similar to those described for the plasma membrane of the mammary epithelial cell of the rat (Threadgold and Kuhn, 1984); this transporter would differ considerably from that described for the Golgi vesicular membrane of the rat in vitro (White et al., 1981). Such a specific transport system could be a point of regulation of glucose availability for lactose synthesis, but given the rapid rate of transport of glucose across the apical membrane, it is unlikely that it would be rate-limiting for milk synthesis.

2.5. Effects of Glucose Concentrations on Enzyme Activities

Intracellular glucose concentrations affect most directly the rate of the reactions utilizing free glucose, that is, hexokinase and lactose synthetase.

The hexokinases of mammary tissue of the rat are mainly types I and II, which have reported K_m values for glucose of 4.5×10^{-5} *M* and 2.3×10^{-4} *M*, respectively (Grossbard and Schimke, 1966; Walters and McLean, 1967). The activity of the type II hexokinase increases at the onset of lactation and is the predominant form in fully lactating mammary tissue. Thus, at the levels of glucose (about 200 μ*M*) that appear to be present in the cytosol of the mammary epithelial cell, type II hexokinase would not be expected to be saturated with substrate and low intracellular glucose concentrations may decrease glucose phosphorylation.

Lactose synthetase, the second enzyme that uses free glucose, apparently has a very much higher K_m for glucose than hexokinase. In the presence of optimum concentrations of α-lactalbumin, K_m values of around 3 m*M* have been reported for the bovine (Schanbacker and Ebner, 1970), human (Morrison and Ebner, 1971), and rat enzymes (Murphy et al., 1973). On the other hand, recent data on the rate of lactose synthesis determined in vivo in the mammary gland of the goat suggest that in vivo the K_m for glucose may be much lower. Thus, when the rate of lactose secretion is plotted as a function of the concentration of glucose in milk under a variety of experimental conditions, a hyperbolic plot is obtained, characteristic of an enzyme exhibiting normal Michaelis–Menten type kinetics. The corresponding double-reciprocal plot is a straight line and a K_m value for glucose of 160 μ*M* can be

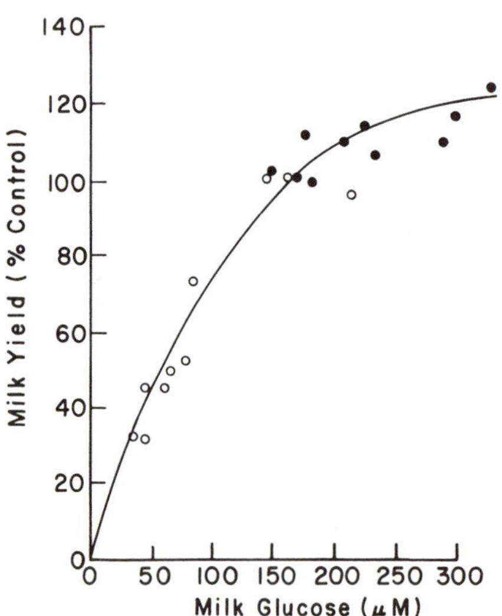

Figure 6. Relation between the concentration of glucose in milk and the rate of lactose production. Lactose production is expressed as milk yield since the lactose content of milk varied little during treatment. Treatment is as in Fig. 4 for starved goats (○) and goats treated with colchicine (●).

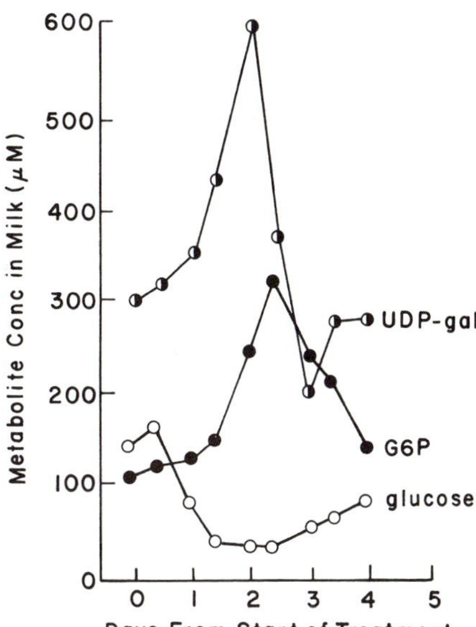

Figure 7. Changes in the concentrations of glucose 6-phosphate (●), UDP-galactose (◑), and glucose (○) in milk from starved goats. Feed was withdrawn from animals on day 0 and reoffered on day 2. Data are means from experiments on six goats.

obtained from it (Faulkner, 1985) (Fig. 6). If this is a true estimate of the K_m for glucose of the lactose synthetase system in its natural environment, the K_m value is very similar to the proposed cytosolic concentration of glucose (see Section 2.2).

The estimated K_m values for glucose for both type II hexokinase and lactose synthetase suggest that both compete on nearly equal terms for the available intracellular glucose. However, experiments in the goat in vivo suggest that at low intracellular glucose concentrations the activity of lactose synthetase decreases to a greater extent than that of hexokinase. During short-term starvation, lactose secretion falls as does the concentration of glucose in milk, but the concentration of UDP-galactose, the second substrate for the lactose synthetase reaction, increases twofold in milk and that of glucose 6-phosphate increases threefold (Fig. 7; Faulkner et al., 1981). If these changes in metabolite concentrations mirror changes occurring in the Golgi vesicles and/or cytosol of the cell, the accumulation of glucose 6-phosphate and UDP-galactose suggests that the rate of glucose phosphorylation is greater than that of lactose synthesis. This could imply that the relative rates of reaction of these enzymes are regulated by factors other than glucose availability under these conditions.

3. Regulation of Glucose Metabolism by Mechanisms Other Than Glucose Concentrations

3.1. Lactose Synthesis

The most investigated of the factors that regulate galactosyl transferase is its interaction with the second protein, α-lactalbumin (for reviews see Ebner and Schanbacher, 1974; Kuhn, 1983). To summarize, α-lactalbumin is a soluble protein that binds to the galactosyltransferase present on the inner membrane of the Golgi vesicle to form lactose synthetase. The presence of α-lactalbumin increases the affinity of lactose synthetase for glucose, reducing the K_m for glucose from 1.4 *M* to about 5 m*M* in vitro (Schanbacher and Ebner, 1970). Because α-lactalbumin is secreted continuously into milk, constant synthesis of this protein is required to maintain lactose biosynthesis. The lactose and α-lactalbumin contents of milks from various species appear to be correlated, supporting the hypothesis of regulation of lactose synthesis by α-lactalbumin (Brew, 1970; Schmidt et al., 1971). In addition, the lactose and α-lactalbumin content of rats' milk are proportional for the first 20 days of lactation (Nicholas et al., 1981). However, this proportionality is lost completely during weaning and other restricting factors must then operate.

The concentration of the second precursor of lactose, UDP-galactose, might also be expected to affect the rate of lactose synthesis. The K_m for UDP-galactose is about 60 μ*M* (Kuhn et al., 1980). The concentration of UDP-galactose in milk is 350 μ*M* (Faulkner, 1980). UDP-Galactose has been shown to be secreted via the secretory vesicles, so that the concentration in milk could be similar to that in the Golgi vesicle at the site of lactose synthesis (Faulkner et al., 1985a). Changes that result in decreases in the concentration of UDP-galactose may therefore alter the rate of lactose synthesis. Changes in the concentration of UDP-galactose could arise for several reasons. The availability of glucose could limit UDP-galactose synthesis in the cytosol of the mammary epithelial cell; but the evidence in Fig. 7 suggests that in the starved animal UDP-galactose is synthesized even when cytosolic glucose levels are reduced (Faulkner et al., 1981). Regulation of UDP-galactose synthesis by the enzymes involved in its biosynthetic pathway also is unlikely except possibly at the onset of lactation. Before parturition, the activities of these enzymes increase slightly (Kuhn and Lowenstein, 1967); subsequently, they appear to operate at equilibrium as their activities are in excess of that of galactosyltransferase.

The permeability of the Golgi vesicular membrane also may be a factor in regulating the concentration of UDP-galactose available for lactose synthesis. Although small molecules such as glucose appear to cross the membrane of the Golgi vesicle readily, larger molecules such as lactose are not transported (White et al., 1981). Evidence has been presented for a specific transporter for UDP-galactose into the Golgi vesicle (Kuhn and White, 1976) and this may be rate-limiting. The high ratio of UDP-galactose to UDP-glucose in goats' milk compared to that in mammary tissue (Table II) supports the theory of specific entry of UDP-galactose into the Golgi vesicles (Faulkner, 1980).

The permeability of the Golgi membrane to the products of the lactose synthetase reaction may also regulate its activity. Neither lactose nor UDP can cross the Golgi vesicular membrane (Kuhn and White, 1977). Whereas high concentrations of lactose do not appear to be inhibitory, UDP has been shown to be a powerful inhibitor of the reaction (Khatra et al., 1974). The accumulation of UDP in the vesicles is prevented by the presence of a nucleoside diphosphatase on the inner Golgi membrane, which hydrolyzes it to UMP and inorganic phosphate (Kuhn and White, 1977), both of which can cross the Golgi vesicular membrane to reenter the cytosol. Although the additional reaction imposes a higher energy cost on lactose synthesis (2 molecules of ATP are required to regenerate UTP), it allows an additional means of regulating the system. Accumulation of nucleoside diphosphate in goats' milk has been observed during times of decreased milk production such as in starvation (Chaiyabutr et al., 1981), inhibition of milk secretion by colchicine (A. Faulkner, unpublished data), and during the drying off period (Faulkner et al., 1982). Thus, an increase in the nucleoside diphosphate concentrations inside the Golgi vesicles could play a part in limiting lactose synthesis at these times; why UDP concentration increases under these conditions is a matter for further research.

3.2. Hexokinase

The activity of hexokinase in the lactating mammary gland is not high compared with that of other enzymes (Gumaa et al., 1971) and it is likely that the enzyme is working at near maximum capacity. The predominant form of hexokinase present in mammary tissue is type II (Walters and McLean, 1967), which is inhibited noncompetitively by physiological concentrations ($K_i = 1.6 \times 10^{-4}$ *M*) of glucose 6-phosphate (Grossbard and Schimke, 1966). In milk from the starved lactating goat, the concentration of glucose 6-phosphate increased two- to threefold within the range that could inhibit hexokinase activity (Fig. 7; Chaiyabutr et al., 1981; see Section 2.5). An increased glucose 6-phosphate content in mammary tissue from the starved compared to the fed or refed rat (Williamson et al., 1985) supports the concept that changes in milk concentrations of this metabolite mirror changes within the cytosol and that these changes are of a magnitude to regulate hexokinase activity.

3.3. Pentose Phosphate Pathway

As we have described earlier, the role of glucose metabolized via the pentose phosphate pathway is to provide NADPH for fatty acid synthesis. Metabolism by this pathway must therefore be closely linked to fatty acid synthesis de novo in the mammary gland. The activity of the initial enzymes involved in the pathway is inhibited by NADPH (Glock and McLean, 1953; Glaser and Brown, 1955). Thus, when the rates of fatty acid synthesis are rapid, NADPH is used and the pentose phosphate pathway is active, but when the rates of fatty acid synthesis decrease, NADPH accumulates and the pentose phosphate pathway is inhibited (Fig. 2).

In the ruminant, NADPH for fatty acid synthesis is produced not only by the pentose phosphate pathway (Fig. 2) but also by the isocitrate dehydrogenase reaction (see Fig. 1 in Chapter 17 of this volume) in the cytosol (Bauman and Davis, 1974). The reactants of the isocitrate dehydrogenase reaction, isocitrate and 2-oxoglutarate, are present in milk and their concentrations change in a way that could mirror changes occurring in the cytosol as evinced by the correlation (r = 0.768; $p <$ 0.001) between the ratio of the concentration of 2-oxoglutarate to isoci-

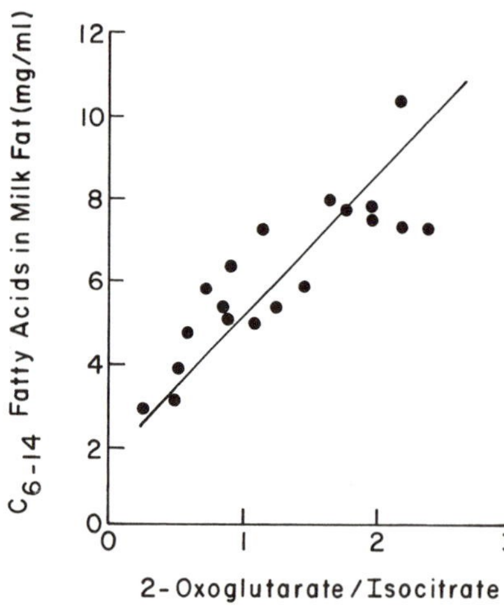

Figure 8. Relation between the 2-oxoglutarate : isocitrate ratio in milk and fatty acid synthesis de novo in the mammary gland of the cow. Fatty acid synthesis de novo was calculated from the content of short- and medium-chain fatty acids in milk triglycerides. Diets contained silage and concentrates with various amounts of added fat. Data are from five cows.

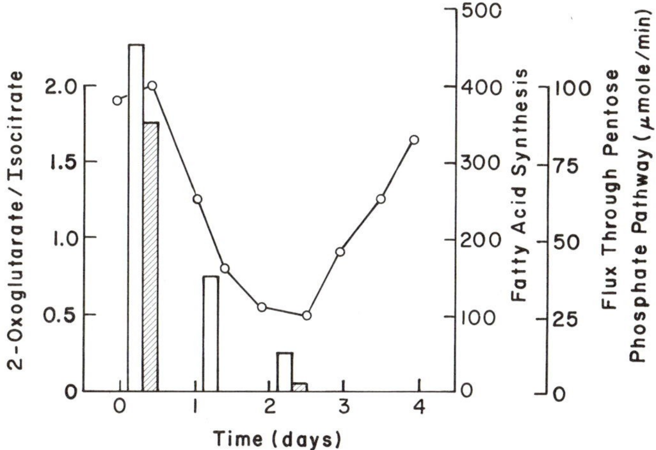

Figure 9. Changes in the ratio of the concentrations of isocitrate to 2-oxoglutarate in milk (○), fatty acid synthesis de novo in the mammary gland (□), and flux through the pentose phosphate pathway (▨) in goats during food withdrawal. Fatty acid synthesis in the mammary gland was calculated from the content of short- and medium-chain fatty acids in milk triglycerides and from the yield of milk fat. Flux through the pentose phosphate pathway was calculated from the incorporation of tritium into milk fat following a 4-h infusion of 3-[^{3}H]-glucose into the jugular vein of the goat.

trate and the short- and medium-chain fatty acids in milk fat (Fig. 8; Faulkner and Clapperton, 1981). Since the isocitrate dehydrogenase reaction is thought to be at equilibrium, changes in the NADP : NADPH ratio should correlate with changes in the 2-oxoglutarate : isocitrate ratio in the cytosol (and hence in milk). Thus, changes in the NADP : NADPH can be followed by measuring changes in [2-oxoglutarate] : [isocitrate].

Flux through the pentose phosphate pathway has been followed in vivo in the goat by measuring the incorporation of tritium from 3-[^{3}H]-glucose into milk fat. Hydrogen from the 3-position of glucose is transferred to NADP at the glucose 6-phosphate dehydrogenase reaction and then incorporated into fatty acids (Fig. 2) (Chaiyabutr et al., 1980). Incorporation falls during starvation as does the [2-oxoglutarate] : [isocitrate] ratio (Fig. 9). This correlation indicated that flux through the pentose phosphate pathway is correlated with the NADP : NADPH ratio in vivo.

It is also interesting to note that the concentration of glucose 6-phosphate (the substrate for the pentose phosphate pathway) in milk rises during starvation, while that of the triose phosphates (the product of the pentose phosphate pathway) falls (Chaiyabutr et al., 1981). This also suggests pentose phosphate pathway inhibition during starvation.

Similar decreases in triose phosphate are observed in milk from glands treated with alkaloids to inhibit milk secretion, but, in this case, glucose 6-phosphate concentrations also decrease and the changes appear to be connected more with variations in the rate of glycolysis than with the pentose phosphate pathway (Faulkner et al., 1984).

3.4. Glycolysis

In the mammary gland of the normal ruminant, metabolism of glucose via glycolysis appears to be minimal, with the flux through the pentose phosphate pathways being sufficient to account for the CO_2 and glycerol 3-phosphate produced from glucose (Smith, 1971; Chaiyabutr et al., 1980). However, in the nonruminant, substantial quantities of glucose are metabolized via glycolysis and ultimately this provides the acetyl-CoA required for the high rates of lipogenesis from glucose in the lactating mammary gland (Katz et al., 1974; Robinson and Williamson, 1977b). The rates of glycolysis observed do not appear to be in excess of the requirement for acetyl-CoA production as there is no net production of L-lactate by the mammary gland of the normal fed lactating rat in vivo (Robinson and Williamson, 1977b). On the other hand, in vivo lactate metabolism changes from a net uptake by the mammary gland in the fed animal to a net output in the 24-h starved animal (Robinson and Williamson, 1977b). This difference is maintained in acini prepared from mammary glands of fed and starved lactating rats. It is likely that the reduced rates of fatty acid biosynthesis are responsible in part for the net lactate production with the active form of pyruvate dehydrogenase decreasing during starvation (Baxter and Coore, 1973; Munday and Williamson, 1981, 1982).

The effect of starvation on lactate metabolism in the ruminant is not as dramatic as in the rat, but lactate uptake is reduced (Chaiyabutr, 1980). However, under other conditions, glycolysis can be activated in the mammary gland of the ruminant. Thus, when milk secretion is inhibited by colchicine or vincristine, the concentrations of lactate and pyruvate in milk increase two- to threefold, suggesting large increases in their cytosolic concentrations (Fig. 10). These large increases occur at a time when glucose uptake by the gland is unaffected by the treatment although lactose synthesis is decreased. When rates of milk secretion recover, the lactate and pyruvate concentrations in milk fall to pretreatment levels (Faulkner et al., 1984).

A similar switch to increased rates of glycolysis and lactate production is seen when mammary tissue is incubated in vitro. Slices of rat mammary gland show a relatively high rate of lactate and pyruvate production (Williamson et al., 1975) and isolated acini from mammary

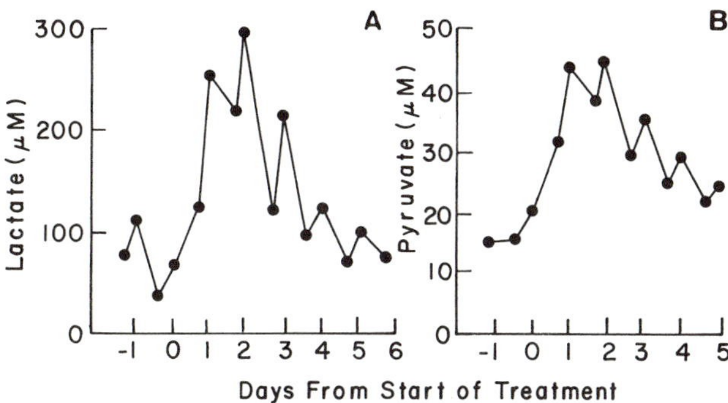

Figure 10. Changes in the concentration of (A) L-lactate and (B) pyruvate in milk from colchicine-treated glands of the goat. Treatment is same as in Fig. 4.

glands of normal fed rats also show a net lactate production although rates are lower than with slices; in vivo there is a net uptake of lactate by the mammary gland in these animals (Robinson and Williamson, 1977b). A similar large production of lactate from glucose has also been observed in slices from mammary glands of ruminants (A. Faulkner, unpublished data).

4. Conclusions

Although the pathways of glucose metabolism in the mammary gland are now understood, much remains to be known of the regulation and integration of these pathways. The observation that many intracellular metabolites are found in milk at levels similar to those in the tissue (Table II), and that their concentrations change under different experimental conditions, opens up a new approach to the investigation of mammary metabolism. For glucose, there is good evidence that the concentrations in milk can be equated with intracellular concentrations. The evidence for this is (1) the similarity in concentrations present in milk and in isolated mammary cells or acini (Faulkner et al., 1981), (2) the ability of glucose to cross the apical membrane in both directions (Faulkner et al., 1985a), and (3) the changes that occur in milk glucose concentrations can be interpreted in terms of the biochemical changes occurring in the mammary gland (Faulkner et al., 1981; 1984). For other metabolites such as hexose or triose phosphate and carboxylic acid, there is less evidence that the changes in concentrations in milk mirror cytosolic changes. These metabolites appear to be secreted into milk via the secretory vesicles (Faulkner et al., 1985a) and there is much to be learned of the way in which they enter these vesicles and to what extent, if any, entry is regulated. However, the content of these metabolites in milk is very similar to that in mammary tissue (Table II) (Faulkner, 1980) and many of the changes in their concentrations correlate with metabolic changes in the mammary gland (e.g., [2-oxoglutarate] : [isocitrate] and de novo fatty acid synthesis, Fig. 8; Faulkner and Clapperton, 1980; Chaiyabutr et al., 1981; Faulkner et al., 1984). In addition, where changes in the content of a metabolite in mammary tissue have been measured, as with glucose 6-phosphate during starvation in the rat (Williamson et al., 1985), the changes in tissue content are similar to the changes observed in goats' milk (Chaiyabutr et al., 1981). Thus, from this circumstantial evidence, it is likely that many of the changes in concentrations described for the metabolites in milk reflect similar changes occurring within the cytosol or Golgi vesicle of the mammary epithelial cell. Therefore, we could now have a simple and noninvasive method of following metabolic changes as they occur within the mammary gland.

Assuming that changes in the concentration of metabolites in milk can be equated with, or mirror, changes occurring in the cytosol, our studies enable us to make some deductions about glucose metabolism in the mammary gland. First, intracellular glucose concentrations show large variations; and these are not related to changes in plasma glucose concentations. It is therefore possible that there is some control of glucose entry into the mammary epithelial cell and that this could regulate lactose synthesis. Rates of lactose synthesis show strong positive correlations with glucose concentrations and the activity of lactose synthetase appears to be controlled by glucose availability to a much greater extent than is the activity of hexokinase. Glucose metabolism via the pentose phosphate pathway in vivo is regulated by NADP : NADPH in the cytosol, which is in turn regulated by the rate of fatty acid synthesis. In ruminants, very little glucose is metabolized via glycolysis but in nonruminants, glucose metabolism via glycolysis is important in generating acetyl-CoA for fatty acid synthesis. When rates of lactose synthesis are decreased, relative rates of glucose metabolism via glycolysis may increase with the production of lactate and pyruvate in both ruminants and nonruminants.

References

Annison, E.F., and Linzell, J.L., 1964, The oxidation and utilization of glucose and acetate by the mammary gland of the goat in relation to their over-all metabolism and to milk formation, *J. Physiol.* **175:**372–385.

Annison, E.F., Linzell, J.L., and West, C.E., 1968, Mammary and whole animal metabolism of glucose and fatty acids in fasting lactating goats, *J. Physiol.* **197:**445–459.

Baird, G.D., 1969, Fructose-1,6-diphosphatase and phosphopyruvate carboxykinase in bovine lactating mammary gland, *Biochim. Biophys. Acta* **177:**343–345.

Bauman, D.E., and Davis, C.L., 1974, Biosynthesis of milk fat, in: *Lactation: A Comprehensive Treatise,* Vol. II (B.L. Larson and V.R., Smith, eds.), Academic Press, New York, pp. 31–75.

Baxter, M.A., and Coore, H.G., 1978, The mode of regulation of pyruvate dehydrogenase of lactating rat mammary gland, *Biochem. J.* **174:**553–561.

Brew, K., 1970, Lactose synthetase: Evolutionary origins, structure and control, *Essays Biochem.* **6:**93–118.

Burd, L.I., Ascherman, G., Dowers, S., Scommegna, A., and Auletta, F.J., 1978, The effect of 2-Br-α-ergocryptine on mammary blood flow and endocrine changes at the time of parturition in the ewe, *Endocrinology* **102:**1223–1229.

Chaiyabutr, N., 1980, Control of mammary function during pregnancy and lactation in the goat: Effects of starvation, Ph.D. Thesis, University of Glasgow.

Chaiyabutr, N., Faulkner, A., and Peaker, M., 1980, The utilization of glucose for the synthesis of milk components in the fed and starved lactating goat *in vivo, Biochem. J.* **186:**301–308.

Chaiyabutr, N., Faulkner, A., and Peaker, M., 1981, Changes in the concentrations of the minor constituents of goat's milk during starvation and on refeeding of the lactating animal and their relationship to mammary gland metabolism, *Br. J. Nutr.* **45:**149–157.

Ebner, K.E., and Schanbacher, F.L., 1974, Biochemistry of lactose and related carbohydrates, in: *Lactation: A Comprehensive Treatise,* Vol. II (B.L. Larson and V.R. Smith, eds.), Academic Press, London, pp. 77–113.

Faulkner, A., 1980, The presence of cellular metabolites in milk, *Biochim. Biophys. Acta* **630:**141–145.

Faulkner, A., 1985, Glucose availability and lactose synthesis in the goat, *Biochem. Soc. Trans.* **13:**496.

Faulkner, A., and Clapperton, J.L., 1981, Changes in the concentration of some minor constituents of milk from cows fed low- or high-fat diets, *Comp. Biochem. Physiol.* **68A:**281–283.

Faulkner, A., Thomson, E.M., Bassett, J.M., and Thompson, G.E., 1980, Cold exposure and mammary glucose metabolism in the lactating goat, *Br. J. Nutr.* **43:**163–170.

Faulkner, A., Chaiyabutr, N., Peaker, M., Carrick, D.T., and Kuhn, N.J., 1981, Metabolic significance of milk glucose, *J. Dairy Res.* **48:**51–56.

Faulkner, A., Blatchford, D.R., White, J.M., and Peaker, M., 1982, Changes in the concentrations of metabolites in milk at the onset and cessation of lactation in the goat, *J. Dairy Res.* **49:**399–405.

Faulkner, A., Henderson, A.J., and Peaker, M., 1984, The effects of colchicine and vincristine on the concentrations of glucose and related metabolites in goat's milk, *Biochim. Biophys. Acta* **802:**335–339.

Faulkner, A., Henderson, A.J. and Blatchford, D.R., 1985a, The transport of metabolites into goats' milk, *Biochem. Soc. Trans.* **13:**495.

Faulkner, A., Blatchford, D.R., and Pollock, H.T., 1985b, The transport of hexoses across the apical membrane of the mammary gland of the goat, *Biochem. Soc. Trans.* **13:**689–690.

Glaser, L., and Brown, D.H., 1955, Purification and properties of D-glucose 6-phosphate dehydrogenase, *J. Biol. Chem.* **216:**67–79.

Glock, G.E., and McLean, P., 1953, Further studies on the properties and assay of glucose

6-phosphate dehydrogenase and 6-phospho-gluconate dehydrogenase of rat liver, *Biochem. J.* **55:**400–408.

Grossbard, L., and Schimke, R.T., 1966, Multiple hexokinases of rat tissues. Purification and comparison of soluble forms, *J. Biol. Chem.* **241:**3546–3560.

Gumaa, K.A., Greenbaum, A.L., and McLean, P., 1971, The control of pathways of carbohydrate metabolism in mammary gland, in: *Lactation* (I.R. Falconer, ed.), Butterworths, London, pp. 197–238.

Gumaa, K.A., Greenbaum, A.L., and McLean, P., 1973, Adaptive changes in satellite systems related to lipogenesis in rat and sheep mammary gland and in adipose tissue, *Eur. J. Biochem.* **34:**188–198.

Hanson, R.W., and Ballard, F.J., 1967, The relative significance of acetate and glucose as precursors for lipid synthesis in liver and adipose tissue from ruminants, *Biochem. J.* **105:**529–536.

Hanwell, A., and Linzell, J.L., 1973, The time course of cardiovascular changes in lactation in the rat, *J. Physiol.* **233:**93–109.

Hardwick, D.C., Linzell, J.L., and Price, S.M., 1961, The effect of glucose and acetate on milk secretion by the perfused goat udder, *Biochem. J.* **80:**37–45.

Hardwick, D.C., Linzell, J.L., and Mepham, T.B., 1963, Metabolism of acetate and glucose by the isolated perfused udder. The contribution of acetate and glucose to carbon dioxide and milk constituents, *Biochem. J.* **88:**213–220.

Henderson, A.J., and Peaker, M., 1980, The effects of colchicine on milk secretion, mammary metabolism and blood flow in the goat, *Q. J. Exp. Physiol.* **65:**367–378.

Hove, K., 1978a, Maintenance of lactose secretion during acute insulin deficiency in lactating goats, *Acta Physiol. Scand.* **103:**173–179.

Hove, K., 1978b, Effects of hyperinsulinemia on lactose secretion and glucose uptake by the goat mammary gland, *Acta Physiol. Scand.* **104:**422–430.

Jenness, R., 1974, The composition of milk, in: *Lactation: A Comprehensive Treatise,* Vol. III (B.L. Larson and V.R. Smith, eds.), Academic Press, New York, pp. 3–107.

Jenness, R., and Sloan, R.E., 1970, The composition of milks of various species: A review, *Dairy Sci. Abstr.* **32:**599–612.

Jones, R.G., Ilic, V., and Williamson, D.H., 1984, Regulation of lactating rat mammary gland lipogenesis by insulin and glucagon *in vivo, Biochem. J.* **223:**345–351.

Katz, J., Wals, P.A., and Van de Velde, R.L., 1974, Lipogenesis by acini from mammary gland of lactating rats, *J. Biol. Chem.* **249:**7348–7357.

Khatra, B.S., Herries, D.G., and Brew, K., 1974, Some kinetic properties of human milk galactosyltransferase, *Eur. J. Biochem.* **44:**537–560.

Kleiber, M., Black, A.L., Brown, M.A., Baxter, C.F., Luick, J.R., and Stadtman, F.H., 1955, Glucose as a precursor of milk constituents in the intact dairy cow, *Biochim. Biophys. Acta* **17:**252–260.

Kuhn, N.J., 1983, The biosynthesis of lactose, in: *Biochemistry of Lactation* (T.B. Mepham, ed.), Elsevier, Amsterdam, pp. 159–176.

Kuhn, N.J., and Lowenstein, J.M., 1967, Lactogenesis in the rat. Changes in metabolic parameters at parturition, *Biochem. J.* **105:**995–1002.

Kuhn, N.J., and White, A., 1975, Milk glucose as an index of the intracellular glucose concentration of rat mammary gland, *Biochem. J.* **152:**153–155.

Kuhn, N.J., and White, A., 1976, Evidence for a specific transport of uridine diphosphate galactose across the Golgi membrane of rat mammary gland, *Biochem. J.* **154:**243–244.

Kuhn, N.J., and White, A., 1977, The role of nucleoside diphosphatase in a uridine nucleotide cycle associated with lactose synthesis in rat mammary gland Golgi apparatus, *Biochem. J.* **168:**423–433.

Kuhn, N.J., Wooding, F.B.P., and White, A., 1980, Properties of galactosyltransferase-enriched vesicles of Golgi membranes for lactating-rat mammary gland, *Eur. J. Biochem.* **103:**377–385.

Linzell, J.L., 1967, The effects of infusions of glucose, acetate and amino acids on hourly milk yields, *J. Physiol.* **190:**347–357.

Linzell, J.L., 1974, Mammary blood flow and methods of identifying and measuring precursors of milk, in: *Lactation: A Comprehensive Treatise,* Vol. I (B.L. Larson and V.R. Smith, eds.), Academic Press, New York, pp. 143–225.

Linzell, J.L., and Peaker, M., 1971, Mechanisms of milk secretion, *Physiol. Rev.* **51:**564–597.

Mather, I.H., and Keenan, T.W., 1983, Function of endomembranes and the cell surface in the secretion of organic milk constituents, in: *Biochemistry of Lactation* (T.B. Mepham, ed.), Elsevier, Amsterdam, pp. 231–283.

McCarthy, S., and Smith, G.H., 1972, Synthesis of milk fat from β-hydroxybutyrate and acetate by ruminant mammary tissue *in vitro, Biochim. Biophys. Acta* **260:**185–196.

Morrison, J.F., and Ebner, K.E., 1971, Studies on galactosyltransferase. Kinetic effects of α-lactalbumin and N-acetylglucosamine and glucose as galactosyl group acceptors, *J. Biol. Chem.* **246:**3992–3998.

Munday, M.R., and Williamson, D.H., 1981, Role of pyruvate dehydrogenase and insulin in the regulation of lipogenesis in the lactating mammary gland of the rat during the starved-refed transition, *Biochem. J.* **196:**831–837.

Munday, M.R., and Williamson, D.H., 1982, Effects of starvation, insulin or prolactin deficiency on the activity of acetyl CoA carboxylase in mammary gland and liver of lactating rats, *FEBS Lett.* **138:**285–288.

Murphy, G., Ariyanayagam, A.D., and Kuhn, N.J., 1973, Progesterone and the metabolic control of the lactose biosynthetic pathway during lactogenesis in the rat, *Biochem. J.* **136:**1105–1116.

Nicholas, K.R., Hartman, P.E., and McDonald, B.L., 1981, α-Lactalbumin and lactose concentrations in rat milk during lactation, *Biochem. J.* **194:**149–154.

Ota, K., and Peaker, M., 1979, Lactation in the rabbit: Mammary blood flow and cardiac output, *Q. J. Exp. Physiol.* **64:**225–238.

Read, G., Crabtree, B., and Smith, G.H., 1977, The activities of 2-oxoglutarate dehydrogenase and pyruvate dehydrogenase in hearts and mammary glands from ruminants and non-ruminants, *Biochem. J.* **164:**349–355.

Reynolds, M., 1970, Proportion of cardiac output and of total body oxygen consumption which is used by the mammary glands, *Physiologist* **13:**292–293.

Robinson, A.M., and Williamson, D.H., 1977a, Comparison of glucose metabolism in the lactating mammary gland of the rat *in vivo* and *in vitro.* Effects of starvation, prolactin or insulin deficiency, *Biochem. J.* **164:**153–159.

Robinson, A.M., and Williamson, D.H., 1977b, Control of glucose metabolism in isolated acini of the lactating mammary gland of the rat. The ability of glycerol to mimic some of the effects of insulin, *Biochem. J.* **168:**465–474.

Robinson, A.M., Girard, J.R., and Williamson, D.H., 1978, Evidence for a role of insulin in the regulation of lipogenesis in lactating rat mammary gland, *Biochem. J.* **176:**343–346.

Roseman, S., 1970, The synthesis of complex carbohydrates by multiglycosyltransferase systems and their potential function in intercellular adhesion, *Chem. Phys. Lipids* **5:**270–297.

Schanbacker, F.L., and Ebner, K.E., 1970, Galactosyltransferase acceptor specificity of the lactose synthetase A protein, *J. Biol. Chem.* **245:**5057–5061.

Schmidt, D.V., Walker, L.E., and Ebner, K.E., 1971, Lactose synthetase activity in northern fur seal milk, *Biochim. Biophys. Acta* **252:**439–442.

Smith, G.H., 1971, Glucose metabolism in the ruminant, *Proc. Nutr. Soc.* **30:**265–272.

Threadgold, L.C., and Kuhn, N.J., 1979, Glucose 6-phosphate hydrolysis by lactating rat mammary gland, *Int. J. Biochem.* **10:**683–685.

Threadgold, L.C., and Kuhn, N.J., 1984, Monosaccharide transport in the mammary gland of the intact lactating rat, *Biochem. J.* **218:**213–219.

Threadgold, L.C., Coore, H.G., and Kuhn, N.J., 1982, Monosaccharide transport into lactating rat, mammary acini, *Biochem. J.* **204:**493–501.

Treacher, R.J., Baird, G.D., and Young, J.L., 1976, Anti-ketogenic effect of glucose in the lactating cow deprived of food, *Biochem. J.* **158:**127–134.

Wallace, A.V., and Kuhn, N.J., 1986, Incorporation into phospholipid vesicles of pore-like properties from Golgi vesicles of lactating-rat mammary gland, *Biochem. J.* **236:**91–96.

Walters, E., and McLean, P., 1967, Multiple forms of glucose-adenosine triphosphate phosphotransferase in rat mammary gland, *Biochem. J.* **104:**778–783.

White, M.D., Kuhn, N.J., and Ward, S., 1981, Mannitol and glucose movement across the Golgi membrane of lactating-rat mammary gland, *Biochem. J.* **194:**173–177.

Wilde, C.J., and Kuhn, N.J., 1981, Lactose synthesis and the utilization of glucose by rat mammary acini, *Int. J. Biochem.* **13:**311–316.

Williamson, D.H., McKeown, S.R., and Ilic, V., 1975, Metabolic interactions of glucose, acetoacetate, and insulin in mammary gland slices of lactating rats, *Biochem. J.* **150:**145–152.

Williamson, D.H., Stewart, H.J., and Robinson, A.M., 1979, Effects of progesterone on glucose metabolism in isolated acini from mammary glands of lactating rats, *Arch. Biochem. Biophys.* **198:**462–469.

Williamson, D.H., Ilic, V., and Jones, R.G., 1985, Evidence that the stimulation of lipogenesis in the mammary gland of starved lactating rats refed with a chow diet is dependent on continued hepatic gluconeogenesis during the absorption period, *Biochem. J.* **228:**727–733.

Wood, H.G., Peeters, G.J., Verbeke, R., Laurssens, M., and Jacobson, B., 1965, Estimation of the pentose cycle in the perfused cow's udder, *Biochem. J.* **96:**605–615.

17

Role of Protein Phosphorylation in the Regulation of Fatty Acid Synthesis in the Mammary Gland of the Lactating Rat

Michael R. Munday and D. Grahame Hardie

1. Fatty Acid Synthesis in the Lactating Mammary Gland in Vivo

Glucose utilization and fatty acid synthesis in rat liver and white adipose tissue are known to be regulated hormonally by the phosphorylation and dephosphorylation of certain key regulatory enzymes (Denton et al., 1981; Hardie et al., 1984). In recent years, it has become increasingly evident that such mechanisms are also important in controlling the biosynthesis of lipid, a major component of milk, in the mammary gland of the rat during lactation. The aim of this chapter is to review the evidence that supports a role for protein phosphorylation in regulating fatty acid synthesis in the mammary gland of the lactating rat.

Compared with other species, rat milk has a relatively high fat content (cf. rat milk w/v 8.4% protein, 2.6% lactose, 10.3% fat; human milk w/v 1% protein, 7.0% lactose, 3.8% fat; Williamson et al., 1984). With a daily milk yield of some 40 ml at peak lactation, this produces a considerable demand on the lactating rat mammary gland for triacylglycerol production. Half of this demand is met from circulating lipoproteins of both dietary and hepatic origin (Hawkins and Williamson, 1972), mam-

Michael R. Munday • Department of Pharmaceutical Chemistry, The School of Pharmacy, University of London, London WC1N 1AS, United Kingdom. ***D. Grahame Hardie*** • M.R.C. Protein Phosphorylation Group, Department of Biochemistry, University of Dundee, Dundee DD1 4HN, Scotland.

mary gland having a very active lipoprotein lipase (Otaway and Robinson, 1968; Hamosh et al., 1970). The remaining half is synthesized de novo within the gland predominantly as medium-chain fatty acids, which are products of fatty acid synthase and a mammary gland-specific medium-chain thioesterase (Libertini and Smith, 1978, 1979). The exact physiological role of the medium-chain fatty acids is unclear, but they may be important in the maintenance of milk fluidity. There is an induction of fatty acid synthesis in the mammary gland during lactation in parallel with increased milk production (Wilde and Kuhn, 1979; Martyn and Hansen, 1980) so that at peak lactation (12–14 days postpartum) the rate of mammary gland lipogenesis is some 15-fold higher than that in virgin rats of a similar age (Agius et al., 1979). Expressed per gram wet weight of tissue, the rate of fatty acid synthesis in the mammary gland at peak lactation is higher than that observed in any other tissue in either lactating or nonlactating rats. This high rate of lipogenesis in the mammary gland produces a very large demand for substrate, supplied predominantly by blood glucose. It has been calculated that at peak lactation, glucose uptake by the rat mammary gland over 24 h is equivalent to the whole body glucose turnover of a male rat of similar age and weight. This substantial glucose uptake for fatty acid (and lactose) synthesis is met both by a higher dietary intake and a decreased utilization of this substrate by other tissues such as white adipose tissue (Williamson, 1980). However, fatty acid biosynthesis in the lactating mammary gland must be able to respond rapidly to changes in the availability of glucose in the circulation to maintain maternal carbohydrate balance. Hence, the rate of mammary gland lipogenesis is stringently regulated according to the dietary status of the rat and is sensitive both to the amount of food eaten and the composition of the diet.

1.1. Fatty Acid Synthesis and the Availability of Food

During lactation, rats eat fairly continuously throughout the 24-h cycle, consuming 35% of their daily food intake during the light period compared with 14% consumed by virgin controls. However, there is still a pronounced diurnal variation in the food intake of lactating rats, resembling that of nonlactating animals. This diurnal variation is paralleled by a similar diurnal pattern of mammary gland lipogenesis underlining the close relation between the two (Munday and Williamson, 1983). The relation between lipogenic rate and dietary status is further illustrated by dietary and physiological manipulations of lactating rats in vivo (Table I). Withdrawal of food for 24 h results in a 98% inhibition of mammary gland lipogenesis, which is rapidly reversed by refeeding chow for 2 h. These changes correlate with changes in circulating insulin concentrations (Robinson et al., 1978) and the induction of short-term insulin deficiency by administration of streptozotocin to lactating rats results in a substantial inhibition of lipogenesis (Table I). Evidence that insulin is the hormonal signal responsible for the activation of mammary gland lipogenesis is provided by the administration of streptozotocin to 24-h-starved rats prior to refeeding with chow. The resulting insulin deficiency totally abolishes the reactivation of lipogenesis by refeeding (Table I). Furthermore, administration of insulin and glucose to a 24-h-starved rat partially reactivates mammary gland lipogenesis, mimicking the refeeding effect (Table I). The response of mammary gland lipogenesis to food withdrawal is obviously rapid since a period of only 6-h starvation also produces a dramatic (88%) inhibition of lipogenesis. Refeeding 6-h-starved rats, or infusion of physiological concentrations of

Table I. Rates of Lipogenesis in Lactating Rat Mammary Gland in Vivo[a]

Rats killed at 10.00 h		
1. Chow fed	128 ± 17	(9)
2. 24-h Starved	2.3 ± 0.23	(10)
3. 24-h Starved/2-h refed	152 ± 7.9	(10)
4. 24-h Starved/2-h Streptozotocin/2-h refed	3.2 ± 0.92	(3)
5. 24-h Starved/oral glucose (8 mmol) + insulin (10 U) 2.5 h	76 ± 4.1	(4)
6. Chow fed/2-h streptozotocin	17 ± 5.5	(4)
7. Chow + high-fat biscuit diet (20% fat)	63 ± 19	(6)
8. 20% Peanut oil (82% C_{18})	33 ± 7.3	(6)
9. 20% Coconut oil (50% C_{12})	68 ± 16	(6)
10. Chow fed + oral load long-chain triacylglycerol 2 h	9.9 ± 1.6	(7)
11. Chow fed + oral load medium-chain triacylglycerol 2 h	16.8 ± 1.3	(8)
Rats killed at 14.30 h		
12. Chow fed	73 ± 19	(8)
13. Chow fed/insulin infusion 1.5 h (120 mU/kg body wt/h)	146 ± 22	(5)
14. 6-h Starved	8.0 ± 1.5	(8)
15. 6-h Starved/insulin infusion 1.5 h (120 mU/kg body wt/h)	54 ± 11	(8)
16. 6-h Starved/refed 2 h	73 ± 9.0	(5)

[a]Values are means ± SEM for the number of experiments shown in parentheses and are expressed as μmol ^3H_2O incorporated into fatty acids/h/g wet wt tissue. Results are taken from: 1,7—Munday and Williamson (1987); 2,3,5—Munday and Williamson (1981); 4,6—Robinson et al. (1978); 8,9—Grigor & Warren (1980); 10,11—Agius and Williamson (1980); 12–15—Jones et al. (1984a); 16—Jones and Williamson (1984).

insulin (Jones et al., 1984a), restores rates of lipogenesis to those of chow-fed controls measured at the same time of day (i.e., 14.30 h; Table I). Table I illustrates the previously mentioned diurnal variation in lipogenesis, in that the rates measured at 14.30 h are significantly less than at 10.00 h. Thus, infusion of insulin into fed rats at 14.30 h produces a significant increase in the lipogenic rate.

It is clear that in response to starvation, the lactating rat shuts down both mammary gland lipogenesis (Table I) and milk production (Brosnan et al., 1982; Sampson and Jansen, 1985). This mechanism favors the survival of the mother rather than the litter, which is a sensible choice given the rat's high fertility.

1.2. Fatty Acid Synthesis and Dietary Composition

Unlike starvation, increasing the fat composition of the diet from parturition onward has relatively little effect on milk yield, nor does it change the percentage of fat in the milk (Grigor and Warren, 1980). However, the fatty acid composition of the milk fat does alter to resemble that of the dietary lipid (Garton, 1963; Coniglio and Bridges, 1966; Grigor and Warren, 1980). This implies that the lactating rat switches from synthesizing fatty acids de novo to utilizing those of dietary origin in its provision of milk lipid. Hence, a high-fat diet given throughout lactation considerably decreases the rate of lipogenesis in rat mammary glands (Agius et al., 1980; Grigor and Warren, 1980; Munday and Williamson, 1987). Table I shows that feeding rats a diet containing 20% coconut oil or 20% peanut oil inhibited lipogenesis by approximately 50 and 70%, respectively. In these experiments, triacylglycerols with long-chain fatty acids were more effective in producing inhibition of mammary gland lipogenesis than those with predominantly medium-chain fatty acids. Intragastric loading of both long-chain and medium-chain triacylglycerols produced a rapid and dramatic reduction in the rate of mammary lipogenesis, and again, long-chain triacylglycerols produced the greater effect (Table I).

Feeding rats a palatable diet of standard laboratory chow together with high-fat cheese biscuits (McVities "Cheddars," London, U.K.) increases the proportion of fat consumed from 2 to 20% of the total weight of food eaten and inhibits (50%) the rate of mammary gland lipogenesis measured in vivo (Agius et al., 1980; Gibbons et al., 1983; Munday and Williamson, 1987; Table I). This lipogenic inhibition persists through the isolation of mammary acini and can be completely reversed by incubation of these cells in vitro with insulin (Agius et al., 1980; Munday and Williamson, 1987; Table III). This is in agreement with the observations that administration of insulin to rats in vivo can partially reverse the inhibition of mammary gland lipogenesis brought about by high-fat feeding (Agius et al., 1981) or by intragastric triacylglycerol loading (Agius and Williamson, 1980).

1.3. Hormonal Regulation of Mammary Gland Lipogenesis

The lactating rat mammary gland is rich in insulin receptors (Flint, 1982) and is a highly insulin-sensitive and insulin-responsive tissue (Burnol et al., 1983; Jones et al., 1984a,b). Insulin stimulates fatty acid synthesis in this tissue, as demonstrated by its reactivation of lipogenesis in mammary glands of lactating rats that have been starved (Table I) or have increased their consumption of dietary fat (Agius et al., 1980; Agius and Williamson, 1980). However, signals that are counter-regulatory to insulin in the lactating mammary gland are not so easily identified. In the major lipogenic tissues of nonlactating rats (i.e., liver and white adipose tissue) glucagon and glucagon and adrenaline, respectively, are antagonistic to the stimulation of lipogenesis by insulin. These hormones raise cAMP concentrations in these tissues and activate cAMP-dependent protein kinase. This in turn phosphorylates and inactivates acetyl-CoA carboxylase, a key regulatory enzyme in the synthesis of fatty acids (for a review see Hardie et al., 1984). In white adipose tissue, these hormones, acting through cAMP, also antagonize the insulin stimulation of glucose transport (Green, 1983; Smith et al., 1984). The role of cAMP in mediating hormonal effects on mammary gland metabolism is less well defined. In keeping with the changes in lipogenic rate, rat mammary cAMP levels decrease with the onset of lactation and increase at weaning (Sapag-Hagar and Greenbaum, 1973; Louis and Baldwin, 1975a). The induction of acute insulin deficiency results in elevated cAMP concentrations in this tissue (Louis and Baldwin, 1975b). However, fatty acid synthesis in the lactating rat mammary gland appears to be insensitive to hormones that act via increased cAMP concentrations. Thus, lipogenesis is not inhibited by adrenaline or glucagon in the rat mammary gland in vivo (Bussman et al., 1984; Jones et al., 1984a) or in isolated mammary acini in vitro (Williamson et al., 1983; Robson et al., 1984). Furthermore, the stimulation of fatty acid synthesis by insulin in vitro in acini from high-fat fed rats is not antagonized by adrenaline or the addition of dibutyryl cAMP (Munday and Williamson, 1987). If anything, adrenaline tends to stimulate the rate of fatty acid synthesis in rat mammary acini in vitro (Plucinski and Baldwin, 1982; Munday and Williamson, 1987).

While there is evidence that mammary acinar cells lack receptors for glucagon (Robson et al., 1984), there is no doubt that they possess competent β-adrenergic receptors (Lavandero et al., 1985), which have been characterized as the β_2-subtype (Clegg and Mullaney, 1985). These are functionally coupled to adenylate cyclase in the plasma membrane (Bar, 1973) and the remaining elements in this signaling system have also been identified in the lactating mammary gland: cAMP (Sapag-Hagar and Greenbaum, 1974; Plucinski and Baldwin, 1982; Clegg and Mullaney, 1985), cAMP-dependent protein kinase (Burchell et al., 1978; Munday and Hardie, 1984), and phosphodiesterase (Mullaney and Clegg, 1984). In the presence of β_2-adrenergic agonists and phosphodiesterase inhibitors, it is possible to raise the basal cAMP content of mammary acini by 20-fold (Clegg and Mullaney, 1985). However, such increases in cAMP concentration have no effect on the rates of fatty acid synthesis in these acini (Clegg et al., 1986) or on the activity or phosphorylation state of acetyl-CoA carboxylase (Clegg et al., 1987). This insensitivity of lactating rat mammary gland to glucagon or to changes in cAMP concentration compared with white adipose tissue has led to the hypothesis that the increased glucagon : insulin ratio observed in lactation is part of the reintegration of tissue metabolism that directs substrates toward the mammary gland and away from other tissues (Robinson et al., 1978; Robson et al., 1984).

The role of prolactin in enzyme regulation in the lactating mammary gland is not altogether clear, although it appears to be concerned with the longer-term control of lipogenic enzyme concentrations (Field and Coore, 1976; McNeillie and Zammit, 1982). Consequently, insulin is the only hormone that is known to exert short-term control over the rates of lipogenesis in this tissue. The changes in lipogenic rate shown in Table I correlate well with changes in the arterial plasma insulin concentration (Robinson et al., 1978; Jones et al., 1984a) with the notable exception of high-fat fed rats. Preliminary results (M.R. Munday and D.H. Williamson, unpublished data) suggest that arterial plasma insulin concentrations are not significantly different between lactating rats fed chow or the high-fat biscuit diet. This observation might suggest that increased consumption of dietary fat reduces the insulin sensitivity of the lactating mammary gland as has been reported for white adipose tissue in nonlactating rats (Ip et al., 1976; Sun et al., 1977; Lavau et al., 1979). An alternate mechanism is that increased tissue concentrations of fatty acids from increased hydrolysis of lipoprotein triglyceride may act as feedback inhibitors of fatty acid synthesis, particularly as long-chain fatty acyl-CoA is known to be a potent inhibitor of acetyl-CoA carboxylase in the mammary gland (Miller and Levy, 1969; Miller et al., 1970). This hypothesis is supported by the observation that exogenously added fatty acids inhibit the in vitro incorporation of [^{14}C]-glucose into lipid, in mammary gland slices from lactating mice (Rao and Abraham, 1975), and in mammary acini from lactating rats (Robinson and Williamson,

1978a). Whatever the signals responsible for the changes in mammary gland fatty acid synthesis observed in vivo, they must act by altering the catalytic capability of one or more of the regulatory steps in this pathway.

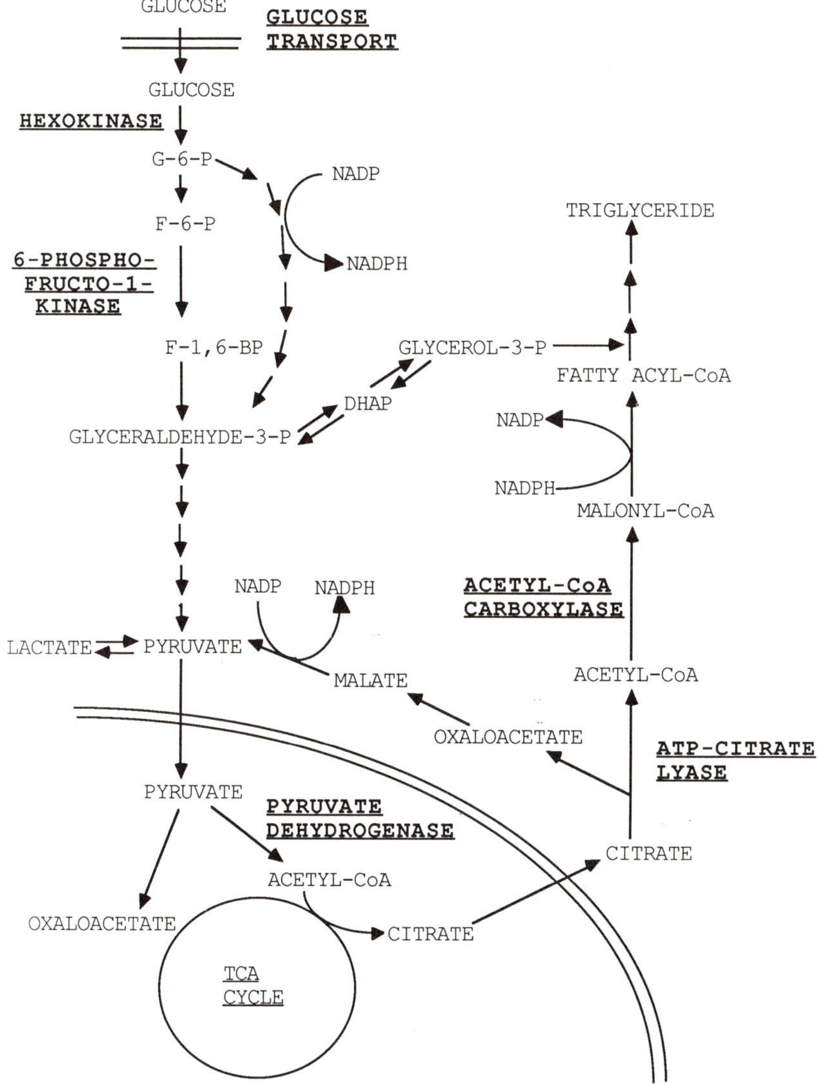

Figure 1. The pathway of fatty acid synthesis from glucose in the lactating mammary gland of the rat.

1.4. Potential Regulatory Enzymes of Fatty Acid Synthesis

Since fatty acids are synthesized predominantly from glucose in the lactating rat mammary gland, there are a number of potential rate-limiting steps in the pathway from glucose to fatty acid (Fig. 1). One method of identifying regulatory steps is to compare the activities of the enzymes of the pathway with the rate of flux of substrate through this pathway. In a normal chow-fed lactating rat, the rate of glucose utilization by the mammary gland is close to the relative enzyme activities of hexokinase, 6-phosphofructo-1-kinase, pyruvate dehydrogenase, and acetyl-CoA carboxylase (Gumaa et al., 1971; Williamson, 1980) and to the rate of glucose transport across the plasma membrane (Threadgold et al., 1982; Threadgold and Kuhn, 1984). Each of these steps has been implicated as a site of metabolic regulation in other tissues (Newsholme and Start, 1981) and each has the potential to be regulated hormonally via phosphorylation–dephosphorylation mechanisms. The extent to which this is applicable in the lactating rat mammary gland will be discussed for each of these steps individually.

2. Glucose Transport

Kuhn and co-workers have established that the secretory cells of the lactating rat mammary gland possess a sugar transport system similar to that found in the mammalian erythrocyte (Jung, 1975) and the white adipocyte (Livingstone and Lockwood, 1974; Czech, 1976; Vinten et al., 1976). The measured rate of 2-deoxy-D-glucose transport into isolated mammary acini was very close to the rate of glucose uptake by these cells, suggesting that under these conditions, transport controls the overall rate of glucose utilization by this tissue (Threadgold et al., 1982). This is in accordance with a substantial concentration gradient of glucose across the plasma membrane of the lactating rat mammary gland, which decreases from 5–6 m*M* extracellularly to less than 0.5 m*M* intracellularly (Kuhn and White, 1975; Wilde and Kuhn, 1981). Some elegant measurements of 3-*O*-methylglucose and 2-deoxyglucose uptake by the lactating rat mammary gland in vivo appear to confirm the rate-limiting nature of glucose transport in this tissue (Threadgold and Kuhn, 1984). Furthermore, these experiments showed that, in parallel with the changes in lipogenic rate shown in Table I, the rate of glucose transport is inhibited by 90–95% following prolonged starvation (16 h); the inhibition was completely reversed by refeeding the rat with chow for 2 h. The administration of insulin to starved rats mimics the effect of refeeding and restores the rate of glucose transport close to the value measured in mammary glands of fed lactating rats (Threadgold and Kuhn, 1984). These effects were ascribed to changes in the V_{max} of transport rather than the apparent affinity (K_m) of the transporter for glucose, mainly by analogy with the effects of insulin on glucose transport in white adipose tissue.

The hormonal regulation of glucose transport in muscle and white adipose tissue has been the subject of much investigation (for a review see Simpson and Cushman, 1986). Insulin appears to increase the V_{max} of glucose transport in adipocytes principally by stimulating the recruitment of functional transporters from an intracellular pool to the plasma membrane (Cushman and Wardzala, 1980; Karnieli et al., 1981). This effect is readily reversible upon withdrawal of insulin. However, the nature of the signal that elicits this response to insulin is still unknown despite intense investigation (for a review see Czech, 1985; Kahn, 1985). The translocation of the glucose transporters to the plasma membrane actually precedes the onset of glucose transport activation by approximately 1.5 min (Karnieli et al., 1981). This raises the possibility that some further modification of the glucose transporter molecule itself is required for full activation of transport (Pilch et al., 1980). The insulin stimulation of glucose transport in adipocytes is antagonized by agents that increase cAMP concentrations, that is, glucagon (Green, 1983) and β-agonists (Smith et al., 1984), and potentiated by adenosine, which decreases cAMP concentrations (Smith et al., 1984; Kuroda et al., 1985), but these changes are not accompanied by any corresponding changes in the number of glucose transporters in the plasma membrane (Joost et al., 1986; Simpson and Cushman, 1986). There is thus good evidence that the regulation of glucose transport may be achieved at least in part via changes in the intrinsic activity of those glucose transporters present in the plasma membrane. An obvious candidate for such regulation is a covalent modification of glucose transporters. In the past, changes in disulfide bonding (Czech, 1977) or in phosphorylation state (Forn and Greengard, 1976) have been proposed. The effects of glucagon and β-agonists described above can be mimicked by dibutyryl cAMP exogenously added to the adipocyte (Taylor and Halperin, 1979; Smith et al., 1984) and this has suggested a possible role for cAMP-dependent protein kinase. However, partially purified human erythrocyte transporters could not be phosphorylated in vitro by cAMP-dependent protein kinase, casein kinase 1, or casein kinase 2, but they were phosphorylated on serine residues by partially purified rat brain protein kinase C (Witters et al., 1985). This is consistent with an increase in the basal level of phosphorylation of transporters in intact human red blood cells in response to phorbol esters (Witters et al., 1985). These experiments did not report any corresponding changes in glucose transport activity, although phorbol esters have been shown to stimulate glucose transport in mouse fibroblasts in a Ca^{2+}-dependent manner (Yamanishi et al., 1983).

For the reasons described in Section 1.2, it seems unlikely that cAMP is involved in regulating glucose transport in the lactating rat mammary gland, but there is good evidence that glucose transport is under the control of insulin (Threadgold and Kuhn, 1984). Evidence to support this has been gained from refeeding starved lactating rats, where the recovery of glucose uptake by the mammary gland in vivo is closely coupled to the rise in plasma insulin and precedes the stimulation of glucose incorporation into either fatty acids or lactose (Bussman et al., 1984; Page and Kuhn, 1986; Mercer and Williamson, 1986). The mechanism of glucose transport regulation by insulin, via transporter recruitment and/or modification of transporter activity that occurs in white adipose tissue, could equally well operate in the lactating rat mammary gland. There is a potential role for protein phosphorylation in mediating the signal for translocation or the changes in intrinsic activity of the transporter molecule, but this will require much further investigation.

3. Hexokinase and 6-Phosphofructo-1-kinase

Changes in glucose and glucose-6-phosphate in the lactating rat mammary gland in response to starvation suggest regulation of steps early in the pathway from glucose to fatty acid (Jones et al., 1984a). The percentage of glucose accumulating as glucose-6-phosphate decreases from 40% in fed rats to 21 and 10% in 6- and 24-h-starved rats, respectively, suggesting that hexokinase is inhibited (Jones et al., 1984a). Williamson and co-workers have also reported a significant inverse correlation between the short-term changes in the concentration of glucose-6-phosphate and lipogenic rate in the lactating mammary gland in vivo (Jones et al., 1984a; Williamson et al., 1985), indicating that a point beyond glucose-6-phosphate is inhibited when glucose utilization is decreased. Increases in glucose-6-phosphate concentration in the mammary gland in response to lipogenic inhibition are accompanied by decreases in fructose 1,6-bisphosphate concentration. Thus, classic crossover analysis pinpoints 6-phosphofructo-1-kinase (PFK-1), as the primary site responsible for inhibition of glycolytic flux under these conditions (Jones et al., 1984a).

A possible regulatory role for PFK-1 in the lactating rat mammary gland was earlier suggested from work on tissue slices (Williamson et al., 1975) and in diabetic rats (Martin and Baldwin, 1971). The mammary enzyme is inhibited by citrate (Zammit, 1979), the K_i (0.2 mM) being very similar to physiological concentrations of citrate in this tissue under normal conditions (Williamson et al., 1975; Robinson and Williamson, 1977b). Thus, regulation of PFK-1 in mammary gland may well be linked to ketone body metabolism, via changes in citrate concentration, as described for other tissues (Randle et al., 1964). Ketone bodies inhibit the utilization of glucose by the lactating mammary gland in vivo (Robinson and Williamson, 1977b) and in vitro (Williamson et al., 1975; Robinson and Williamson, 1977c) and this correlates with a significant increase in the tissue concentration of citrate (Williamson et al., 1975; Robinson and Williamson, 1977b). Starvation also increases both circulating ketone body concentrations and mammary gland citrate concentrations in the lactating rat (Robinson and Williamson, 1977a; Jones et al., 1984a). The activity of acetyl-CoA carboxylase plays an important part in determining the cytosolic concentration of citrate. In the lactating rat mammary gland, this enzyme is known to be phosphorylated and inactivated in response to prolonged starvation (Munday and Hardie, 1986; Section 6.2.2a). This is therefore likely to augment the rise in citrate concentration that would result from an increased uptake of ketone bodies during starvation. In mammary acini in vitro, insulin reverses the inhibition of glucose utilization by ketone bodies (Robinson and Williamson, 1977c). This occurs with a concomitant decrease in citrate concentrations, relieving inhibition of PFK-1, and has been ascribed to an activation of acetyl-CoA carboxylase by insulin in these cells. It is important to note that regulation of fatty acid synthesis by this mechanism could be supplemented by regulation of pyruvate dehydrogenase. This enzyme would be inhibited by the increased acetyl-CoA : CoA ratio resulting from increased ketone body uptake by mammary gland (see Section 4.1).

PFK-1 purified from rabbit muscle (Foe and Kemp, 1982) or from rat liver (Sakakibara and Uyeda, 1983) can be phosphorylated by cAMP-dependent protein kinase in vitro. While this does not affect the V_{max} of the enzyme, it does appear to affect its allosteric properties such that the phosphorylated form of PFK-1 is much more sensitive to inhibition by citrate (Foe and Kemp, 1982; Sakakibara and Uyeda, 1983). Although there is no evidence at present for phosphorylation of PFK-1 in the lactating mammary gland, this would be an attractive control mechanism to superimpose on the citrate sensitivity of PFK-1 in this tissue.

Recent studies on rat hepatic PFK-1 resulted in the discovery of fructose 2,6-bisphosphate (F 2,6-BP) which activates PFK-1 and inhibits fructose 1,6-bisphosphatase (F 1,6-BPase) and plays a prominent role in the hormonal regulation of hepatic glycolysis and gluconeogenesis (Hers and Van Schaftingen, 1982; Pilkis et al., 1982). This unique sugar diphosphate is synthesized and degraded in the cytosol by 6-phosphofructo-2-kinase (PFK-2) and fructose 2,6-bisphosphatase (F 2,6-BPase), respectively. These enzyme activities, from rat or bovine liver, copurify and appear to be present within the same polypeptide chain. A comprehensive review of this bifunctional enzyme and its regulation is given by Pilkis et al. (1984). Purified PFK-2/F 2,6-BPase is phosphorylated stoichiometrically (1 mole phosphate/mole enzyme subunit) on a single serine residue, by cAMP-dependent protein kinase in vitro. The effect of this phosphorylation is to inhibit the phosphotransferase activity of PFK-2 (decreased V_{max}, increased K_m for fructose-6-phosphate) and activate the phosphohydrolase activity of F 2,6-BPase (increased V_{max}, decreased K_m for F 2,6-BP) (El-Maghrabi et al., 1981, 1982; Van Schaftingen et al., 1981, 1982). Consequently, hormones that have been shown to modulate intracellular cAMP concentrations in the liver (e.g., glucagon, adrenaline, insulin) can regulate the level of F 2,6-BP via changes in the phosphorylation state of the bifunctional enzyme. Additions of glucagon or cAMP to hepatocytes results in a dose-dependent decrease in the intracellular concentration of F 2,6-BP. At glucagon concentrations less than 0.7 n*M*, insulin (10 n*M*) progressively antagonizes this effect and increases the concentration of cAMP necessary to produce a half-maximal decrease in F 2,6-BP concentration, from 12 to 36 μ*M* (Pilkis et al., 1983). These changes are the result of parallel changes in the activity ratio of PFK-2 : F 2,6-BPase, where glucagon (0.2 n*M*) decreases the activity ratio by 95% and insulin (10 n*M*) opposes the effect of glucagon, restoring the ratio to 30% of control values (Pilkis et al., 1983). Thus, hormonally induced phosphorylation–dephosphorylation of the bifunctional enzyme by cAMP-dependent protein kinase and an as yet unidentified protein phosphatase controls the concentration of F 2,6-BP, which in turn allosterically regulates PFK-1, imposing hormonal regulation on glycolytic flux.

F 2,6-BP has been identified in a number of other tissues including the rat mammary gland. The content of F 2,6-BP in this tissue is threefold higher at peak lactation compared with a 20-day pregnancy, which correlates with a fourfold increase in the activity of PFK-1 (Sochor et al., 1984). The decreases in citrate concentration and the increases in ATP concentration in the mammary gland during lactation (Sochor et al., 1984) would allosterically activate not only PFK-1 but also PFK-2 (Hers et al., 1982) and are therefore probably, at least in part, responsible for the rise in F 2,6-BP concentration. In addition, there is also a large and significant decrease in the concentration of cAMP in the mammary gland over this period (Sapag-Hagar and Greenbaum, 1974; Sochor et al., 1984); it can be speculated that if the bifunctional PFK-2/F 2,6-BPase were a substrate for cAMP-dependent protein kinase in this tissue, then decreased cAMP might also contribute to the increase in F 2,6-BP concentration. As discussed in Section 1.3, changes in cAMP concentration and phosphorylation by cAMP-dependent protein kinase appear to play little part in the short-term regulation of fatty acid synthesis in the lactating rat mammary gland. However, this tissue does contain a cyclic nucleotide-independent protein kinase, termed acetyl-CoA carboxylase kinase-2 (ACCK-2) (Munday and Hardie, 1984), which phosphorylates the same serine residues in the same sequences of amino acids recognized by cAMP-dependent protein kinase (Section 6.3), that is, basic amino acid-(X)-serine(P) (Cohen, 1985). The sequence surrounding the phosphorylated residue on PFK-2/F 2,6-BPase from rat liver is VAL-LEU-GLN-ARG-ARG-ARG-GLY-SER(P)-SER-ILE-PRO-GLN (Murray et al., 1984). This contains the recognition site and could therefore be a substrate for ACCK-2 in the lactating rat mammary gland, providing a potential mechanism for regulation via phosphorylation in this tissue.

In contrast to the hepatic regulation of PFK-2/F 2,6-BPase, it has been noted that PFK-2 activity in crude preparations from rat muscle and heart is not inactivated upon incubation with ATP and cAMP-dependent protein kinase (Rider et al., 1985). The reason appears to be that there are separate isoenzymes of PFK-2/F 2,6-BPase in liver and muscle (Van Schaftingen and Hers, 1986). The enzyme from pigeon muscle (M_r 53,000) is smaller than that from chicken liver (M_r 54,000) and presumably lacks the phosphorylation site, because it cannot be phosphorylated, and is entirely unresponsive to regulation by cAMP-dependent protein kinase. It is therefore important when considering the potential of PFK-2/F 2,6-BPase in the regulation of lipogenesis to know which of these isoenzymes exists in the lactating mammary gland.

A further level of regulation involving F 2,6-BP can be achieved via phosphorylation of PFK-1. It has been reported that phosphorylation of PFK-1 from rabbit muscle and rat liver by cAMP-dependent protein kinase, not only makes it more sensitive to citrate, but also makes it less sensitive to activation by F 2,6-BP (Foe and Kemp, 1982; Sakakibara and Uyeda, 1983). PFK-1 from brown or white adipose tissue is phosphorylated to a low stoichiometry in vitro by cAMP-dependent protein kinase and in isolated cells in response to isoprenaline treatment. In contrast to the enzyme in liver and muscle, phosphorylation of PFK-1 in adipose tissue appears to activate the enzyme making it more sensitive to F 2,6-BP and less sensitive to inhibition by ATP (Sale and Denton, 1985a,b). There is as yet no evidence that either PFK-2/F 2,6-BPase or PFK-1 are regulated by phosphorylation in the lactating rat mammary gland. Nevertheless, comparison with the regulatory mechanism in liver and the existence of cyclic nucleotide-independent kinases like ACCK-2 (Munday and Hardie, 1984) in the mammary gland make this an exciting possibility.

Small but significant changes in F 2,6-BP concentration in the lactating rat mammary gland have already been reported in response to starvation and refeeding (Ward and Kuhn, 1985). These authors confirmed that the activity of PFK-1, measured at *physiological* concentrations of effectors, is very likely to limit the rate of glycolytic flux in the mammary gland. However, while the enzyme has an absolute requirement for F 2,6-BP, the physiological intracellular concentrations of F 2,6-BP that were measured approached saturation of the enzyme (Ward and Kuhn, 1985). There is thus some doubt that the changes in concentration of this effector alone, in response to starvation (40% decrease) and refeeding (130% increase), are sufficient to cause a great enough change in PFK-1 activity to account for the changes in glycolytic flux (Ward and Kuhn, 1985). But considering the synergism of AMP, citrate, F 2,6-BP, and phosphorylation state in determining PFK-1 activity, it is clear that further investigation is required before we fully understand the role of this enzyme, and its potential for regulation by phosphorylation mechanisms, in the control of mammary gland fatty acid synthesis.

4. Pyruvate Dehydrogenase

In the oxidative catabolism of glucose, pyruvate dehydrogenase (PDH) plays an important role in ATP synthesis, but in rat liver, adipose tissue, and lactating mammary gland it is also an important enzyme in the synthesis of fatty acids. In keeping with the increased lipogenic capacity of the rat mammary gland from late pregnancy to peak lactation, there is a sevenfold induction of *total* pyruvate dehydrogenase activity (Gumaa et al., 1973; Coore and Field, 1974). The oxidative decarboxylation of pyruvate to acetyl-CoA, which is catalyzed by PDH in the mitochondria, is essentially an irreversible step:

$$CH_3{\cdot}CO{\cdot}COO^- + CoA + NAD^+ \rightarrow CH_3{\cdot}CO{\cdot}CoA + CO_2 + NADH$$

$$(\Delta G^\circ = -39.5 \text{ kJ/mol}, K_{eq} = 8.4 \times 10^6, \text{pH } 7)$$

Animals lack the means of synthesizing glucose from acetyl-CoA, so that this reaction represents a net loss of carbohydrate from the body. In the mammary gland of the lactating rat, the rate of glucose utilization is very high (Williamson, 1980). Therefore, the regulation of this step according to the availability of food would seem essential in maintaining a balanced carbohydrate metabolism, particularly since the end products of mammary gland glycolysis, pyruvate and lactate, are readily reconverted into glucose via hepatic gluconeogenesis.

Arteriovenous differences across the mammary glands of lactating rats show that whereas there is a net uptake of lactate in chow-fed animals, this changes to a net lactate output of equal magnitude following 24-h starvation (Robinson and Williamson, 1977a). Lactate uptake by the mammary gland is restored again when the 24-h-starved rat is refed chow for 2.5 h (Robinson and Williamson, 1978b). These changes indicate a decrease in mammary gland PDH activity in response to starvation, which increases again in response to refeeding. Williamson and coworkers have consistently taken the accumulation of pyruvate and lac-

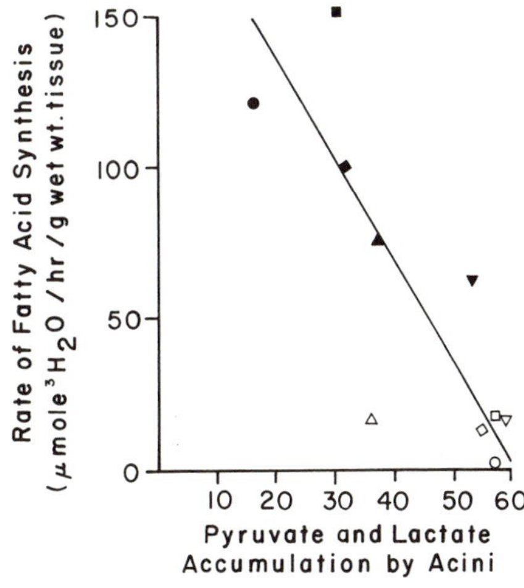

Figure 2. Correlation between rates of lipogenesis in the lactating rat mammary gland in vivo and the activity of pyruvate dehydrogenase as indicated by the accumulation of lactate and pyruvate in mammary acini in vitro. Lipogenesis was measured in the lactating rat mammary gland in vivo as described by Robinson et al. (1978). Acini were prepared and incubated with glucose and the rate of glucose uptake and lactate and pyruvate accumulation were measured as described by Robinson and Williamson (1977a). The rate of pyruvate and lactate accumulation is expressed as a percentage of the rate of glucose uptake by the acini. The physiological status of each rat was as follows. For rats killed at 10.00 h: ●, chow fed; ○, 24-h starved; ■, 24-h starved/2.5-h refed; □, 24-h starved + oral glucose (8 mmol) 2.5 h; ▲, 24-h starved + oral glucose (8 mmol) + insulin (10 U) 2.5 h; ▼, chow fed + streptozotocin 2 h; △, chow fed + bromocryptine 24 h; ▽, 24-h starved + insulin (1 U) 2h. For rats killed at 14.30 h: ◆, chow fed; ◇, 6-h starved. Results were taken from Robinson and Williamson (1977a); Robinson et al. (1978); Munday and Williamson (1981); and Williamson et al. (1983). The coefficient of correlation is $r = -0.81$; $p < 0.0025$.

tate in isolated mammary acini in vitro as a reliable indicator of the activity of PDH in the mammary gland in vivo prior to isolation of the cells (Robinson and Williamson, 1977a, 1978b; Munday and Williamson, 1981). This is supported by a remarkable inverse correlation ($r = -0.81$; $p < 0.0025$) between the percentage of the glucose taken up by the acini in vitro that accumulates as pyruvate and lactate and the rate of lipogenesis measured in the mammary gland in vivo (Fig. 2). It is clear than in response to starvation, or insulin deficiency, inhibition of lipogenesis in vivo is accompanied by an increased accumulation of pyruvate and lactate in isolated acini in vitro, indicative of an inhibition of PDH (Fig. 2). Reactivation of lipogenesis by refeeding, or by administration of insulin with glucose, is accompanied by a reactivation of PDH, which is reflected in decreased accumulation of pyruvate and lactate in the mammary cells in vitro (Fig. 2). The mechanisms by which these changes in PDH activity in the lactating rat mammary gland are achieved are discussed in the next section.

4.1. Regulation Mechanism of Pyruvate Dehydrogenase

Pyruvate dehydrogenase (PDH) is a large multienzyme complex (M_r > 7,000,000 daltons) located in mitochondria. Its structure and regulation show comparatively little variation between a wide variety of tissues, so that most of the investigation of the molecular aspects of this enzyme have been carried out with PDH from bovine heart and kidney, whereas its hormonal regulation has been extensively studied in white adipose tissue (for reviews see Randle, 1981; Denton et al., 1981).

The PDH complex is organized around a core of dihydrolipoyl transacetylase subunits (E2) to which pyruvate decarboxylase (E1) and dihydrolipoyl dehydrogenase (E3) subunits are noncovalently bound. E1 is a tetramer with a subunit composition of $\alpha_2\beta_2$ and E3 is apparently a homodimer. The composition of the complete bovine heart PDH complex is 30 E1 : 60 E2 : 6 E3 and is represented in Fig. 3. More recently, a further subunit of mammalian PDH has been discovered called *Component X* (De Marcucci and Lindsay, 1985). It was previously thought to be a proteolytic product of one of the other components of the PDH complex but has now been identified as an immunologically distinct polypeptide tightly bound to the E2 core. The function of Component X is unknown, but it is readily acetylated and is thus suspected of some role in the processing of acetyl units by the PDH complex. The activity of PDH is inhibited by its end products, acetyl-CoA and NADH, and these

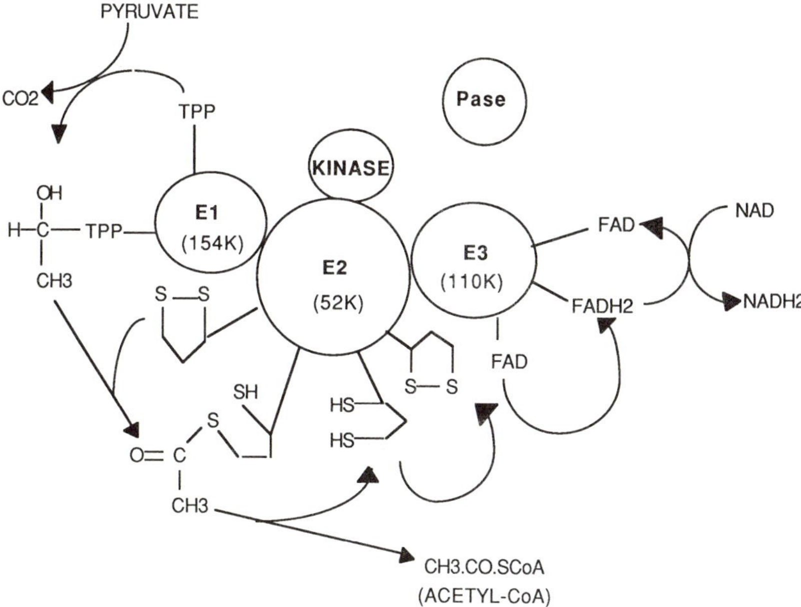

Figure 3. Schematic representation of the pyruvate dehydrogenase complex.

inhibitions are antagonized by CoA and NAD, respectively. Thus, activity is regulated by the concentration ratios of acetyl-CoA : CoA and of NADH : NAD. This is a potential mechanism of regulation in the lactating mammary gland in starvation where an increased utilization of ketone bodies is likely to increase the mitochondrial acetyl-CoA : CoA ratio (see Section 3). However, end-product inhibition is known to be quantitatively much less important than regulation by reversible phosphorylation.

The PDH complex is phosphorylated and inactivated by a specific intrinsic kinase bound to the dihydrolipoyl transacetylase moiety [E2] and is dephosphorylated and activated by a specific phosphatase that is more loosely associated with the complex (Fig. 3). The phosphorylation is confined to the α subunit of the pyruvate decarboxylase [E1] (Barrera et al., 1972; Sugden and Randle, 1978). Amino acid sequencing of tryptic phosphopeptides of the α subunit from bovine heart or kidney PDH reveals multisite phosphorylation at three separate serine residues (Yeaman et al., 1978; Sugden et al., 1979).

Peptide A

Site 1 Site 2
TYR-HIS-GLY-HIS-SER(P)-MET-SER-ASP-PRO-GLY-VAL-SER(P)-
TYR-ARG

Peptide B

Site 3
TYR-GLY-MET-GLY-THR-SER(P)-VAL-GLU-ARG

The relative rates of phosphorylation of these three sites are 1>>2>3, and it is phosphorylation at site 1 that inactivates the complex (Kerbey et al., 1979). It has been reported that phosphorylation of sites 2 and 3 inhibits the rate of reactivation of the complex by the phosphatase (Sugden et al., 1978). However, Teague et al. (1979) observed no decrease in the rate of reactivation in response to phosphorylation of sites 2 and 3 and have reported that phosphorylation of site 2, in addition to site 1, inactivates PDH. PDH kinase activity is modulated by a number of key metabolites: ADP, CoA, NAD, and pyruvate are inhibitors; acetyl-CoA and NADH are activators. Therefore, in mitochondria, the phosphorylation state of PDH can be regulated by ATP : ADP, NADH : NAD, and acetyl-CoA : CoA ratios and by pyruvate concentration (see Randle, 1981). A second mechanism, slower in onset, activates PDH kinase in heart and skeletal muscle. It involves a stable nondialysable factor that is independent of metabolites and renders the kinase insensitive to pyruvate inhibition (Hutson and Randle, 1978). This factor is a mitochondrial protein formed by cytoplasmic protein synthesis and can be separated from PDH by high-speed centrifugation. Its synthesis is increased in response to starvation and diabetes in these tissues (Kerbey and Randle, 1981, 1982).

The relative rates of dephosphorylation of the three sites are 2>3>1 (Teague et al., 1979). The PDH phosphatase requires Mg^{2+} (K_m = 0.7 mM) and Ca^{2+} (K_m = 1–30 μM), both of which are potential regulators in vivo (Kerbey et al., 1979). Ca^{2+} appears to lower the K_m of the phosphatase for phosphorylated PDH. It increases the binding of the phosphatase to transacetylase (E2), thereby facilitating access to the α subunit of E1 (Pettit et al., 1972). In starvation and diabetes, the activity of PDH phosphatase in bovine heart does not change. However, its effectiveness in reactivating PDH may be decreased by the phosphorylation of sites 2 and 3 in response to the increased kinase activity brought about by the mitochondrial protein factor (Sale and Randle, 1982a,b).

4.2. Regulation of Pyruvate Dehydrogenase in Mammary Gland

Rat mammary gland PDH exhibits many of the regulatory properties associated with reversible phosphorylation that have been demonstrated in other tissues. It is inactivated in extracts by incubation with MgATP, the rate of which is slowed by the presence of pyruvate, and it can be reactivated by the addition of Mg^{2+} and Ca^{2+} to the extract (Coore and Field, 1974). Measurement of the ratio of initial PDH activity to total PDH activity (i.e., activity following treatment with exogenous pig heart PDH phosphatase in vitro) is usually taken to represent the activation state of the enzyme, which varies according to the extent of its phosphorylation. Coore and co-workers showed that, in parallel with increased lipogenesis and increased concentration of the enzyme, the proportion of mammary gland PDH in its dephosphorylated active form is increased threefold during lactation (Coore and Field, 1974). The short-term changes in PDH activity in lactating mammary gland according to nutritional status are also achieved via changes in its phosphorylation state. In response to 24- or 48-h starvation, mammary gland PDH is phosphorylated and inactivated. The proportion of enzyme in its active form decreases by 71 and 77%, respectively (Kankel and Reinauer, 1976; Baxter and Coore, 1978). PDH is also inactivated (85%) by short-term insulin deficiency induced by 3-h streptozotocin treatment (Baxter et al., 1979). These inactivations are remarkably similar in extent to those reported for PDH in white adipose tissue of 48-h-starved or alloxan-diabetic nonlactating rats (Stansbie et al., 1976). The phosphorylation and inactivation of PDH in mammary gland in response to starvation correlates with an increase in PDH kinase activity (Baxter and Coore, 1978) and a decrease in the activity of PDH phosphatase (Baxter and Coore, 1979a). An important feature of the increased PDH kinase activity in mammary gland after 24-h starvation is the apparent loss of sensitivity of the kinase to inhibition by pyruvate (Baxter and Coore, 1979b; Baxter et al., 1979).

These observations provide evidence that, following starvation or diabetes, the mechanism that activates PDH kinase in heart and skeletal muscle via the synthesis of a mitochondrial protein activator (Section 4.1) may also be operable in the lactating rat mammary gland under these conditions. This mechanism for inhibiting PDH activity is not readily reversed by inhibition of the kinase (Kerbey et al., 1976) or activation of PDH phosphatase (Illingworth and Mullings, 1976). Consequently, the apparent resistance of PDH in white adipose tissue from starved or alloxan-diabetic rats, to reactivation by insulin in vitro, has been attributed to this mechanism (Stansbie et al., 1976). Similar resistance is seen in mammary acini from 24-h-starved lactating rats. High concentrations of insulin can neither restore rates of lipogenesis nor reactivate PDH activity, as estimated by the accumulation of pyruvate and lactate in these cells (Munday and Williamson, 1981). However, incubation with dichloroacetate, which is a more potent inhibitor of PDH kinase than pyruvate (Whitehouse et al., 1974), substantially reactivates both PDH and lipogenesis in these starved cells (Munday and Williamson, 1981).

There is no direct evidence, but it is assumed that the phosphorylation of mammary gland PDH occurs on the α subunit of E1. Steady-state labeling with ^{32}P shows this to be true in adipocytes, where under control conditions all three serine residues in the two tryptic phosphopeptides are labeled (Hughes et al., 1980). Incubation of these adipocytes with insulin causes equivalent dephosphorylation of each of the three serine residues and activates the PDH complex (Hughes et al., 1980). Insulin administered with glucose to starved or streptozotocin-treated lactating rats completely reactivates PDH in the mammary gland within 1 h (Baxter and Coore, 1978; Baxter et al., 1979). This insulin effect is somewhat at variance with the absence of an insulin effect on PDH in acini in vitro described above (Munday and Williamson, 1981). It may indicate that factors important in the action of insulin in vivo are lost in the preparation of isolated acini. The reactivation of PDH by insulin in the lactating mammary gland is associated with a decrease in PDH kinase activity (Baxter and Coore, 1978), accompanied by restoration of the kinase's sensitivity to pyruvate (Baxter et al., 1979), and a reactivation of PDH phosphatase (Baxter and Coore, 1979a). In white adipose tissue, insulin dephosphorylates the α subunit of E1 and activates PDH via the stimulation of PDH phosphatase (Sica and Cuatrecasas, 1973; Mukherjee and Jungas, 1975; Denton and Hughes, 1978). Despite the sensitivity of PDH phosphatase to Ca^{2+}, the activation by insulin appears to occur without an increase in mitochondrial Ca^{2+} concentration (Marshall et al., 1984). It has been demonstrated that α-adrenergic agonists, like insulin, stimulate PDH and lipogenesis in white adipocytes. However, these effects are Ca^{2+} dependent, because the depletion of intracellular Ca^{2+} by incubation with EGTA abolishes the effects of α-agonists, but not of insulin, on PDH activity (Cheng and Larner, 1985). The effects of adrenaline and noradrenaline on PDH in adipocytes have been variously reported as stimulatory (Taylor et al., 1973; Weiss et al., 1974), inhibitory (Coore et al., 1971), and biphasic (Sica and Cuatrecasas, 1973; Smith and Saggerson, 1978). These effects appear to depend very much on the concentration of the hormone and probably reflect the fact that these hormones have α- as well as β-adrenergic receptor activities. Whereas the α effect on PDH is due to mobilization of intracellular Ca^{2+} (Cheng and Larner, 1985), adrenaline and glucagon have been reported to inhibit the uptake of $^{45}Ca^{2+}$ into the mitochondrial fraction of isolated adipocytes (Severson et al., 1976). The mechanisms by which increases in cAMP could control mitochondrial Ca^{2+} transport remain to be elucidated.

There is clearly much evidence to suggest that the regulation, by reversible phosphorylation, of the PDH complex via its specific kinase and phosphatase activities is broadly similar in all mammalian tissues including the lactating mammary gland of the rat. In this tissue, PDH is inactivated–activated by phosphorylation–dephosphorylation, in parallel with changes in lipogenic rate, emphasizing the importance of this regulatory step. Changes in phosphorylation state are achieved via reciprocal changes in the activities of PDH kinase and PDH phosphatase. At present, only insulin has been identified as exerting short-term hormonal control over this regulatory mechanism in the lactating mammary gland. However, the reported effects of α- and β-adrenergic agonists on PDH in white adipose tissue suggest that there might yet be other unidentified hormonal signals controlling the PDH system in rat mammary gland.

5. ATP-Citrate Lyase

There is an 8- to 10-fold induction of ATP-citrate lyase activity in the mammary gland of the rat in response to lactation (Gumaa et al., 1973; Martyn and Hansen, 1981). However, at peak lactation, the activity of this enzyme is at least 10-fold greater than the activities of either PDH or acetyl-CoA carboxylase in this tissue (Gumaa et al., 1973), casting doubt on its regulatory significance. ATP–citrate lyase has been purified from the rat mammary gland and shown to exist as a tetramer of subunit M_r 116,000 daltons (Guy et al., 1981). The mammary enzyme contains approximately 0.5 mol of phosphate/mol subunit but can be phosphorylated further (0.6–0.8 mol phosphate/mol subunit) in vitro by cAMP-dependent protein kinase (Guy et al., 1980, 1981), by Ca^{2+}- and phospholipid-dependent protein kinase, and Ca^{2+}- and calmodulin-dependent multiprotein kinase (Hardie et al., 1986). These phosphorylations all occur on a single serine residue in a tryptic peptide with the sequence THR-ALA-SER(P)-PHE-SER-GLU-SER-ARG (Hardie et al.,

1986). These properties of mammary ATP–citrate lyase together with its amino acid composition, and sequence around its phosphorylation site, suggest that it is identical to the enzyme from rat liver (Singh et al., 1976; Pierce et al., 1981).

The phosphorylation, by cAMP-dependent protein kinase, of ATP–citrate lyase from rat mammary gland (Guy et al., 1981) or rat liver (Ranganathan et al., 1982) was originally reported to have no effect on the activity of the enzyme. Houston and Nimmo (1985) have recently reported a twofold increase in the K_m for MgATP of rat liver ATP–citrate lyase following phosphorylation by cAMP-dependent protein kinase. However, this effect is unlikely to be physiologically significant since this increased K_m is still 10-fold lower than intracellular MgATP concentrations. In addition, the effect of the protein kinase was not shown to be reversible, so it remains possible that the inactivation is an artifact not connected with the phosphorylation. Further doubt about the physiological significance of ATP–citrate lyase phosphorylation arises from the results of treatment of isolated hepatocytes with insulin and glucagon. These hormones have opposing effects on lipogenesis (Geelen et al., 1978), but both increase the phosphorylation of ATP–citrate lyase at the same serine residue phosphorylated by cAMP-dependent kinase, and in neither case does the level of phosphorylation exceed 0.1–0.15 mol/mol subunit (Alexander et al., 1982; Pierce et al., 1982).

The lack of physiologically relevant control of ATP–citrate lyase by reversible phosphorylation and its high activity in the lactating mammary gland suggest that this enzyme is not involved in the regulation of mammary gland lipogenesis by phosphorylation–dephosphorylation mechanisms.

6. Acetyl-CoA Carboxylase

6.1. Structure and Regulation

Acetyl-CoA carboxylase (ACC) purified from the lactating rat mammary gland has a single subunit of M_r 240,000 daltons. This subunit contains a single molecule of biotin and is multifunctional, carrying its two active sites on the same polypeptide chain (Ahmad et al., 1978; Hardie and Guy, 1980; see Hardie, 1980). The protomeric form (~13S) of ACC is a homodimer (Gregolin et al., 1966a), which in the presence of high concentrations of citrate forms polymers (~50S) of up to 30 subunits in a linear array (Gregolin et al., 1966b; Ahmad et al., 1978). The polymerized form of the enzyme is more active than the protomer and there is some evidence for the occurrence of the protomer–polymer transition in vivo (Meredith and Lane, 1978; Ashcraft et al., 1980). However, it has recently been shown that activation of ACC by citrate is considerably more rapid than polymerization of the enzyme (Beaty and Lane, 1983). This suggests that the polymerization is a consequence, rather than a cause, of the enzyme activation.

ACC catalyzes the first step committed to the synthesis of fatty acids (Fig. 1), and considering the high energy requirement of this biosynthetic pathway, it would seem logical for ACC to be a regulatory enzyme. Regulation at this step would also determine what proportion of the flux from glucose to acetyl-CoA would enter fatty acid synthesis rather than the TCA cycle. Studies with purified ACC have shown that the enzyme can be regulated both by allosteric effectors and by reversible phosphorylation (see Hardie, 1980; Hardie et al., 1984). There are two allosteric effectors likely to be of physiological importance:

1. Citrate, acting as a classical feed-forward activator of the enzyme. Citrate activates ACC, purified from the mammary glands of lactating rats fed chow ad libitum, by approximately 50-fold within 1 min. The concentration of citrate required to half-maximally activate this enzyme ($A_{0.5}$ citrate) is approximately 2 mM (Table II). Therefore, changes in the intracellular citrate concentration in mammary gland (0.2–0.5 mM, Williamson et al., 1975; Robinson and Williamson, 1977b) are likely to affect ACC activity.
2. Fatty acyl-CoA, acting as a classical feedback inhibitor. Fatty acyl-CoA specifically inhibits ACC purified from rat liver at concentrations below the critical micelle concentration. The K_i values for saturated fatty acyl-CoA with chain lengths of 16–20 vary from 1 to 10 nM (Nikawa et al., 1979).

It is increasingly evident that the allosteric regulation of ACC interacts strongly with regulation by reversible phosphorylation to effect overall control of enzyme activity. ACC in lactating rat mammary gland was identified as a phosphoprotein by Ahmad et al. (1978) and Hardie and Guy (1980), in confirmation of previous observations in lactating rabbit mammary gland (Hardie and Cohen, 1978). The enzyme purified from mammary glands of rats fed chow ad libitum contains approximately 3 mol of alkali-labile phosphate per subunit (Hardie and Guy, 1980; Table II). However, the purified enzyme can be further phosphorylated and inactivated in vitro by incubation with MgATP and the catalytic subunit of cAMP-dependent protein kinase (Hardie and Guy 1980; Munday and Hardie, 1984) or certain cyclic nucleotide-independent protein kinases (see Section 6.3). These effects are reversed by treatment with purified protein phosphatases. The phosphorylation and inactivation of ACC by cAMP-dependent protein kinase have been shown to be of considerable physiological significance in liver and adipose tissue. It is an integral part of the mechanism by which hormones that raise intracellular cAMP concentrations, that is, glucagon in liver and glucagon or adrenaline in white adipose tissue, bring about the phosphorylation and inactivation of ACC and inhibit rates of lipogenesis (for reviews see Hardie et al., 1984; Munday et al., 1986). The inhibition of ACC in response to phosphorylation by cAMP-dependent protein kinase is achieved largely through an increase in the $A_{0.5}$ of the allosteric activator, citrate (see Section 6.3), exemplifying the interaction between phosphorylation and allosteric regulation. Given the importance of the reversible phosphorylation of ACC in the control of fatty acid synthesis in the major lipogenic tissues of nonlactating rats, our laboratory has examined its importance in the rat mammary gland at peak lactation.

6.2. Role of Phosphorylation in the Physiological Regulation of Mammary Gland ACC

6.2.1. Measurement of ACC Activity in Crude Extracts of Lactating Mammary Gland

In parallel with increased rates of fatty acid synthesis, there is a 30- to 40-fold increase in the amount of immunotitratable ACC in the rat mammary gland from parturition to peak lactation (Mackall and Lane, 1977). The ratio of *initial* ACC activity (measured in crude tissue extracts without preincubation) to *total* ACC activity (measured after preincubation with Mg^{2+} and citrate) is also higher in the mammary glands of lactating rats compared with 20-day pregnant (McNeillie and Zammit, 1982) or virgin control animals (Munday and Williamson, 1982).

Numerous studies have used the ratio of initial to total enzyme activity as an index of the state of activation of ACC. Figure 4 shows the activation of ACC following preincubation with Mg^{2+} and citrate, in mammary extracts from chow-fed, 24-h-starved, and high-fat-fed lactating rats. This activation is clearly blocked if homogenization and incubation are carried out in the presence of the protein phosphatase inhibitor NaF, indicating that it occurs via a dephosphorylation of the enzyme by endogenous phosphatases in the extract. Evidence for the existence of such phosphatases in mammary gland extracts has been reported (McNeillie et al., 1981). Therefore, the ratio of initial to total ACC activity is a measure of the degree of phosphorylation of the enzyme.

A role for ACC in the short-term control of mammary gland

lipogenesis was inferred from the results of Munday and Williamson (1981). Activation of PDH by the addition of dichloroacetate to acini from starved and refed rats increased lipogenesis by 250 and 100%, respectively. However, in the presence of dichloroacetate, only 70% of the increased flux through PDH was converted into lipid in acini from starved rats, whereas all the increase passed to lipid in acini from refed rats. The further addition of insulin was required to obtain maximal rates of lipogenesis in acini from starved rats (Munday and Williamson, 1981). This further stimulation of lipogenesis by insulin was accompanied by an increase (50%) in the initial activity of ACC in crude extracts of these acini (Munday, 1983). Thus, in certain circumstances, ACC may regulate the overall lipogenic flux in the mammary gland of the lactating rat.

The initial to total ACC activity measured in crude extracts of lactating rat mammary glands decreases by 30–40% in response to 24-h starvation or streptozotocin-induced insulin deficiency (McNeillie and Zammit, 1982; Munday and Williamson, 1982). In 24-h-starved rats, the activation state of ACC is totally restored to chow-fed control levels after 2.5-h refeeding chow or 1 h after administration of insulin with glucose (McNeillie and Zammit, 1982; Munday and Williamson, 1982). These changes in the ratio of initial : total ACC activity occur in parallel with changes in the lipogenic rate (Table I) and are likely to be the result of changes in the phosphorylation state of the enzyme. Figure 4 shows that the initial activities of ACC (t = 0 min), measured at a saturating citrate concentration (20 mM), in crude extracts of mammary glands from chow-fed, 24-h-starved and high-fat-fed lactating rats are 4.11 ± 0.17 (n = 6), 0.68 ± 0.21 (n = 3), and 2.11 ± 0.40 (n = 6) μmol/min/g wet wt tissue, respectively. The difference in activity between ACC from high-fat-fed and chow-fed rats is abolished by incubation with Mg^{2+} and citrate in the absence of fluoride (Fig. 4B) and may thus be attributed to an increased phosphorylation and inactivation of ACC in response to the high-fat diet. The residual difference in activity of ACC from chow-fed and 24-h-starved rats after activation by Mg^{2+} and citrate is likely to represent a decrease in concentration of the enzyme following 24-h starvation (Fig. 4A). However, the extent of ACC activation is much greater in extracts from 24-h-starved rats (200%) than from chow-fed rats (70%). Thus, the 80% inhibition of ACC activity in response to 24-h starvation remains unchanged throughout incubation in the presence of fluoride but decreases to 60% in its absence (Fig. 4A). The decrease in ACC activity produced by 24-h starvation may therefore be accounted for both by a decrease in enzyme concentration and by an increased phosphorylation and inactivation of the enzyme.

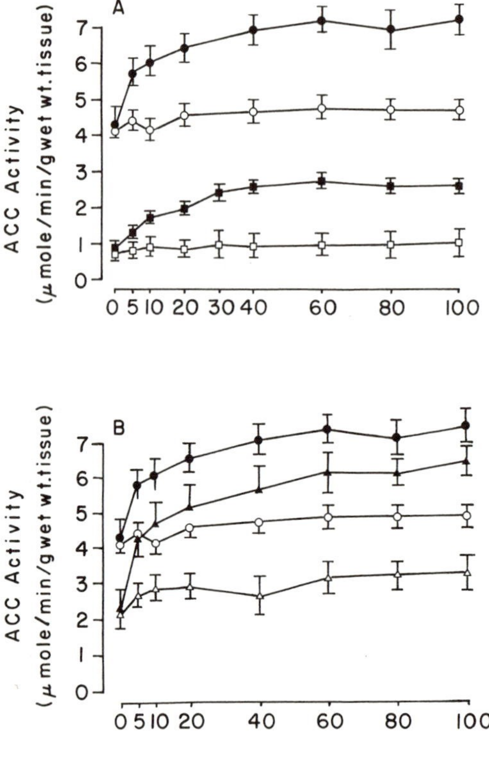

Figure 4. Activation of acetyl-CoA carboxylase in crude extracts of lactating rat mammary gland by incubation with Mg^{2+} and citrate. For experimental details, see Munday and Hardie (1986). Crude extracts from chow-fed control rats (●, ○), 24-h-starved rats (■, □), or high-fat biscuit-fed rats (▲, △) were prepared and incubated at 37°C in the presence of (○, □, △) or absence (●, ■, ▲) of 50 m*M* NaF. Incubations were carried out in the presence of 20 m*M* $MgCl_2$, 20 m*M* sodium citrate, and bovine serum albumin (10 mg/ml). Samples (10 μl) were removed at the time points shown and ACC activity was assayed at 37°C for 1 min in the presence of 20 m*M* $MgCl_2$, 20 m*M* sodium citrate, and bovine serum albumin (10 mg/ml). Each point represents the mean of six experiments for chow-fed controls, three experiments for 24-h-starved rats, and six experiments for high-fat-fed rats. Vertical lines represent SEM.

6.2.2. Studies on ACC Purified from Lactating Mammary Gland

6.2.2a. Effects of Starvation and Refeeding. To confirm that these changes in ACC activity are due to phosphorylation–dephosphorylation of the enzyme, ACC has been purified from the mammary glands of lactating rats in various physiological states. The purification uses avidin–Sepharose affinity chromatography in the presence of EDTA to inhibit protein kinase activity, NaF to inhibit phosphatase activity, and a range of protease inhibitors to maintain the integrity of the ACC (Munday and Hardie, 1986). Table II shows that, as predicted from measurements in crude extracts, 24-h starvation produces a large and significant decrease in the V_{max} (73%) and a similar increase in the $A_{0.5}$ citrate (75%) of ACC purified from the lactating rat mammary gland. These changes are accompanied by an increase in the alkali-labile phosphate

Table II. Kinetic Parameters and Alkali-Labile Phosphate Content of Acetyl-CoA Carboxylase Purified from Lactating-Rat Mammary Gland under Different Physiological Conditions[a]

Treatment	Number of observations	V_{max} (μmol/min/mg)	$A_{0.5}$ (mM)	Phosphate content (mol/mol subunit)
(a) Sacrificed 10.00 h				
Chow-fed control	(26)	2.55 ± 0.24	2.10 ± 0.13	3.31 ± 0.21
24-h starved	(19)	0.70 ± 0.09***	3.67 ± 0.54**	4.46 ± 0.42*
24-h starved/2.5-h refed chow	(8)	2.12 ± 0.23	2.40 ± 0.22	3.72 ± 0.17
24-h starved/2.5-h streptozotocin/2.5-h refed chow	(10)	0.78 ± 0.10***	4.13 ± 0.35***	4.05 ± 0.27*
Chow-fed/2.5-h streptozotocin	(7)	2.56 ± 0.21	2.54 ± 0.36	3.44 ± 0.20
High-fat biscuit-fed	(9)	0.99 ± 0.19**	2.85 ± 0.38*	4.33 ± 0.43*
(b) Sacrificed 14.30 h				
Chow-fed control	(6)	1.92 ± 0.26	3.04 ± 0.41	3.64 ± 0.41
6-h starved	(8)	1.96 ± 0.13	2.94 ± 0.42	3.84 ± 0.29

[a]For experimental details see Munday and Hardie (1986). Animals were sacrificed by stunning and cervical dislocation at the individual times shown. Results are means ± SEM for the number of observations shown. Values significantly different from their respective controls (by Student's t-test) are indicated: $^{*}p < 0.05$; $^{**}p < 0.005$; $^{***}p < 0.0005$. $A_{0.5}$ is for citrate.

content of approximately 1 mol/mol of ACC subunit. Strong evidence that this inactivation is caused by the increased phosphorylation is its reversal by dephosphorylation. ACC purified from chow-fed or 24-h-starved lactating rats and incubated with the catalytic subunit of protein phosphatase-2A purified from rabbit skeletal muscle undergoes a time-dependent activation until, after 90 min, the activity of ACC from either source is indistinguishable (Munday and Hardie, 1986). At the end of the incubation, ACC from chow-fed rats had been dephosphorylated by approximately 1 mol phosphate/mol ACC subunit, whereas the phosphate content of ACC from 24-h-starved rats had decreased by 2 mol/mol subunit. As a result of this dephosphorylation, there was no significant difference between the kinetic parameters of either enzyme, the V_{max} of each enzyme increasing to approximately 4 μmol/min/mg and the $A_{0.5}$ citrate decreasing to approximately 1 m*M* (Munday and Hardie, 1986). Thus, the effects of 24-h starvation on the phosphate content and activity of purified mammary ACC can be completely reversed in vitro by dephosphorylation with protein phosphatase-2A.

Despite the dramatic decline in the rate of mammary gland lipogenesis during the first 6 h of starvation (Table I), 6-h starvation does not significantly alter either the kinetic parameters or the phosphate content of purified mammary ACC compared with chow-fed animals killed at the same point in the diurnal cycle (Table II). This agrees with the lack of effect of 6-h starvation on the ratio of initial : total ACC activity measured in crude mammary gland extracts (Williamson et al., 1983). Similarly, while short-term insulin deficiency, induced by streptozotocin treatment, inhibits mammary gland lipogenesis (Table I) and decreases ACC activity measured in crude extracts (McNeillie and Zammit, 1982; Munday and Williamson, 1982), it has no effect on the V_{max}, $A_{0.5}$ citrate or the phosphate content of the purified enzyme (Table II). It therefore appears that phosphorylation of ACC in the lactating mammary gland does not occur rapidly in response to starvation or insulin deficiency. One must assume that the rapid decline in mammary gland lipogenesis in response to starvation or insulin deficiency (Table I) is due to a decreased substrate supply to the tissue or to the inhibition of one or more of the other regulatory steps already discussed in this chapter (Sections 2, 3, 4). Inhibition of earlier steps in the pathway would decrease flux through ACC either by reducing the supply of its substrate or by decreasing the concentration of its allosteric activator, citrate. These noncovalent effects on ACC may be measurable in crude tissue extracts but would be lost on purification of the enzyme. This may explain the apparent discrepancy, in the effect of streptozotocin treatment, between measurements of ACC activity made in crude extracts and with the purified enzyme. Clearly, ACC does become phosphorylated after a period of prolonged starvation and this has profound inhibitory effects on its kinetic parameters. This inhibition is likely to play a significant part in the further dramatic inhibition of lipogenesis (from 85 to 98%) that occurs in the lactating rat mammary gland between 6 and 24 h after food withdrawal (Table I). The reason for the slow onset of ACC phosphorylation during starvation is not clear. It certainly lags behind the fall in arterial plasma insulin concentration (Jones et al., 1984a) and it is possible that changes in protein synthesis are required, for example, induction of a protein kinase or repression of a protein phosphatase.

Whatever the underlying mechanism for the phosphorylation and inactivation of ACC during prolonged starvation, it is clear that this must be rapidly reversed when food is available again. Refeeding 24-h-starved lactating rats with chow for 2.5 h returns the V_{max} and the $A_{0.5}$ citrate of the purified enzyme to chow-fed control levels (Table II). This is associated with a decrease in the alkali-labile phosphate content of 0.75 mol/mol ACC subunit. In the course of refeeding starved lactating rats, the arterial plasma insulin concentration is restored to normal (Robinson et al., 1978). It is this increase in plasma insulin that is responsible for the reversal of the effects of starvation, since administration of streptozotocin immediately before refeeding prevents both the reactivation of lipogenesis (Table I) and the dephosphorylation and reactivation of ACC (Table II). Neither the kinetic parameters nor the phosphate content of purified mammary ACC differ significantly between 24-h-starved and 24-h-starved/2.5-h-streptozotocin-treated/2.5-h-refed lactating rats (Table II). It would therefore appear that in the mammary gland of 24-h-starved lactating rats, in response to refeeding, insulin brings about an activation of ACC by causing a dephosphorylation of the enzyme.

If the total activity of ACC in extracts, following preincubation with Mg^{2+} and citrate, is a reliable measure of total enzyme protein, then the results of Fig. 4A suggest that there is a 60% decrease in the concentration of ACC after 24-h starvation. Refeeding 24-h-starved rats for only 2.5 h completely restores mammary gland lipogenesis without increasing total enzyme protein as judged by the same criterion (Munday and Williamson, 1982). Thus, during the fed to starved to refed transition, regulation of ACC by phosphorylation–dephosphorylation or substrate supply is probably more important in the control of mammary gland lipogenesis than changes in enzyme concentration.

6.2.2b. Effects of a High-Fat Diet. In response to high-fat feeding, the mammary gland reduces the rate of fatty acid synthesis by 50% to compensate for the increased influx of dietary fatty acids (Table I). This is likely to involve the specific inhibition of the pathway that is committed to the synthesis of fatty acids rather than a complete inhibition of glucose utilization. ACC catalyzes the first step in this pathway and the work of Munday and Williamson (1987), with isolated acini, infers that in contrast to the effects of 24-h starvation, the inhibition of lipogenesis by high-fat-feeding is mediated solely through the inhibition of this enzyme. The activity of ACC in crude tissue extracts has been shown to be inhibited by 50–60% in the mammary glands of rats fed a high-fat biscuit diet (Fig. 4B; M.R. Munday, unpublished data). This inhibition appears to be the result of an increased phosphorylation of the enzyme. Purification of ACC, by avidin–Sepharose affinity chromatography, revealed a significant decrease in V_{max} (64%) accompanied by a smaller increase in the $A_{0.5}$ citrate (36%) of the enzyme in the mammary glands of lactating rats fed a high-fat biscuit diet compared with chow-fed controls. This correlated with an increase in total alkali-labile phosphate content of 1 mol/mol ACC subunit (Table II).

While the signal for the inhibition of lipogenesis by high-fat feeding may not be a decrease in circulating insulin (Section 1.3), the inhibition is readily reversed by insulin in isolated acini in vitro. This has therefore proved a more useful model than the 24-h-starved rat for studying the effects of insulin on ACC. Throughout the preparation and subsequent incubation of isolated mammary acini from high-fat-fed lactating rats, the inhibition of lipogenesis and the inhibition of ACC activity measured in crude extracts is maintained (Table III; Fig. 5). It is notable that the extent of these inhibitions is smaller than that measured in the intact tissue. Incubation of these acini with insulin totally restores rates of lipogenesis to the values measured in chow-fed controls (Table III). This occurs with a concomitant increase in the ACC activity in crude acinar extracts such that it is no longer significantly different from the activity

Table III. Fatty Acid Synthesis in Isolated Mammary Acini[a]

		Fatty acid synthesis	
		Control	Insulin
Acini from chow-fed rat	(4)	0.54 ± 0.06	0.52 ± 0.03
Acini from high-fat-fed rat	(7)	0.33 ± 0.03**	0.58 ± 0.09

[a]Mammary acini were isolated from chow-fed and high-fat biscuit-fed lactating rats and incubated at 37°C for 60 min in the presence and absence of 50 mU insulin/ml, as described by Robinson and Williamson (1977a). Rates of fatty acid synthesis were determined from ^3H_2O incorporation into fatty acids (Robinson and Williamson, 1977b) and are expressed as μmol ^3H_2O incorporated/min/100 mg dry defatted acini. Results are means ± SEM for the number of observations in parentheses. Values significantly different (by Student's *t*-test) from chow-fed controls are shown: $^*P < 0.05$; $^{**}P < 0.005$.

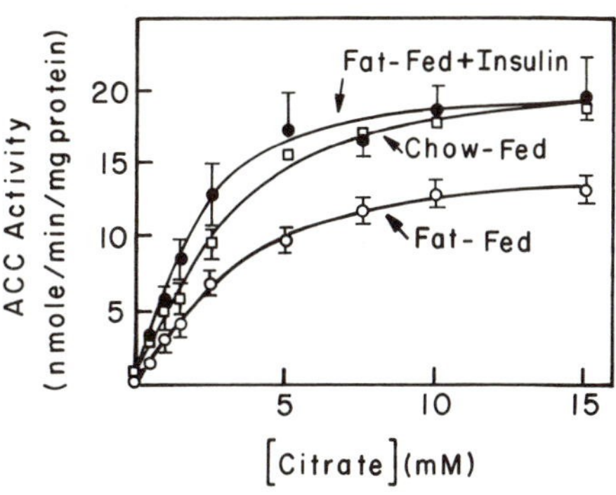

Figure 5. Acetyl-CoA carboxylase activity in crude extracts of acini from mammary glands of high-fat-fed lactating rats. Mammary acini were prepared from chow-fed (□) and high-fat biscuit-fed (○, ●) lactating rats and incubated at 37°C in the presence (●) and absence (□, ○) of 50 mU insulin/ml, as described by Robinson and Williamson (1977a). Crude extracts of these acini were prepared, and acetyl-CoA carboxylase activity was assayed, as described by Munday and Williamson (1987). Each point represents the mean of four experiments with SEM represented by vertical bars.

in extracts from chow-fed control cells (Fig. 5). Insulin has no effect on lipogenesis (Table III) or ACC activity (not shown) in acini from chow-fed lactating rats. The increase in ACC activity in acini from high-fat-fed rats incubated with insulin is observed at all citrate concentrations (Fig. 5) and, when analyzed, represents an increase (34%) in the V_{max} of the enzyme. There is no significant difference between the $A_{0.5}$ citrate values for ACC in extracts from any of the acini incubations shown in Fig. 5.

ACC purified from control and insulin-treated acini from high-fat-fed lactating rats exhibits a significant increase in V_{max} in response to insulin (Table IV). This increase (36%) is very similar to that observed in crude extracts, and while the $A_{0.5}$ citrate is unaltered, the phosphate

Table IV. Properties of Acetyl-CoA Carboxylase Purified from Mammary Acini from High-Fat-Fed Lactating Rats[a]

	Control	Insulin
V_{max} (μmol/min/mg)	1.35 ± 0.18	1.83 ± 0.13*
$A_{0.5}$ citrate (m*M*)	2.53 ± 0.36	2.74 ± 0.32
Phosphate content (mol/mol subunit)	5.3 ± 0.1	4.7 ± 0.2*

[a]Mammary acini were isolated from high-fat biscuit-fed lactating rats, as described by Robinson and Williamson (1977a). The acini were incubated at 37°C for 60 min in the presence of ^{32}P to achieve steady-state labeling and then for a further 60 min in the presence and absence of 50 mU insulin/ml. Acetyl-CoA carboxylase was purified and its kinetic parameters measured as described by Munday and Hardie (1986). The phosphate content was determined from the ^{32}P labeling of the enzyme as described for hepatocytes (Holland et al., 1984). Results are means ± SEM for five separate acini preparations. Values significantly different from controls (by Student's *t*-test) are shown: $^{*}p < 0.05$.

content of the enzyme decreases by 0.6 mol/mol ACC subunit in insulin-treated cells (Table IV). Thus, in acini from high-fat-fed lactating rats, insulin promotes a dephosphorylation and activation of ACC. This is identical to the apparent role of insulin in the mammary gland in vivo during the starved–refed transition (Section 6.2.2a). From this evidence it can be concluded that, in the lactating mammary gland, the activation of ACC by insulin is an important component of its stimulation of fatty acid synthesis and that this occurs via a dephosphorylation of the enzyme.

These observations are in marked contrast to the increased phosphorylation of ACC that occurs in response to insulin in isolated adipocytes (Brownsey and Denton, 1982; Witters et al., 1983) and hepatocytes (Holland and Hardie, 1985). However, it seems unlikely that increased phosphorylation is the direct cause of the activation of ACC observed in crude extracts of such cells. Unlike the effects of insulin on the mammary gland, the stimulation by insulin of ACC activity in crude extracts of adipocytes or hepatocytes is lost during the purification of the enzyme on avidin–Sepharose (Witters et al., 1983; Holland and Hardie, 1985). Furthermore, the addition of purified protein phosphatase-2A to crude extracts of control and insulin-treated adipocytes removes more than 80% of the phosphate from ACC, but the activation of ACC by insulin in these extracts remains (Haystead and Hardie, 1986). An insulin-stimulated dephosphorylation of ACC has not been observed in hepatocytes or adipocytes, and the presently favored mechanism of activation is via a low-molecular-weight effector of the enzyme (Saltiel et al., 1983; Haystead and Hardie, 1986). The reason for the different actions of insulin on ACC in mammary gland and adipose tissue is a matter for speculation, although a role for a low-molecular-weight effector in the dephosphorylation of ACC in the lactating mammary gland cannot be ruled out.

The catalytic subunit of protein phosphatase-2A dephosphorylates and activates purified ACC in vitro. However, it remains to be ascertained whether this protein phosphatase is responsible for the effect of insulin in the mammary gland in vivo. Mammary gland ACC phosphorylated by cAMP-dependent protein kinase is a substrate for protein phosphatases-1, -2A, and -2C in rat liver cytosol fractions (Ingebritsen et al., 1983). Protein phosphatase-1 has been shown to be present in lactating rabbit mammary gland (Burchell et al., 1978), but although protein phosphatase activity has been detected in extracts of lactating rat mammary gland (McNeillie et al., 1981), no attempts to identify and characterize the protein phosphatases in this tissue have been reported.

6.3. ACC Kinases in the Lactating Mammary Gland

Having considered the role of insulin in the activation of ACC in the lactating rat mammary gland, it is pertinent to consider the signals and mechanisms responsible for the inactivation of ACC in response to prolonged starvation and high-fat feeding. ACC is phosphorylated and inhibited in isolated hepatocytes in response to glucagon (Holland et al., 1984) and in isolated adipocytes in response to adrenaline and glucagon (Brownsey and Hardie, 1980; Witters et al., 1983; Holland et al., 1985). In each case, the increased phosphorylation occurs on a proteolytic peptide of ACC that is identical to the peptide containing the major site phosphorylated in vitro by cAMP-dependent protein kinase (Witters et al., 1983; Holland et al., 1984, 1985). Phosphorylation at this site by cAMP-dependent protein kinase causes inactivation of ACC, which can be reversed by dephosphorylation (Hardie and Guy, 1980; Munday and Hardie, 1984). Therefore, adrenaline and glucagon, which can raise cAMP concentrations in these cells, activate cAMP-dependent protein kinase, leading to direct phosphorylation and inactivation of ACC (Hardie et al., 1984; Munday et al., 1986). Since adrenaline, glucagon, and cAMP have apparently little effect on rates of lipogenesis or ACC activity in the lactating mammary gland (Section 1.3), it would seem unlikely that cAMP-dependent protein kinase is responsible for the in-

Table V. Protein Kinases that Phosphorylate Purified Mammary Gland Acetyl-CoA Carboxylase in Vitro[a]

	Phosphate incorporation (mol/mol subunit)	Effect on kinetic parameters of acetyl-CoA carboxylase	
		V_{max}	$A_{0.5}$ citrate
cAMP-dependent protein kinase	1.3	43% ↓	107% ↑
Acetyl-CoA carboxylase kinase-2	0.7	40% ↓	86% ↑
Casein kinase-1	0.7	None	None
Casein kinase-2	0.4	None	None
Ca^{2+}–calmodulin-dependent multifunctional protein kinase	1.2	None	None
Ca^{2+}–phospholipid-dependent protein kinase	0.9	28% ↓	None

[a]The data were taken from Munday and Hardie (1984) and Hardie et al. (1986). cAMP-dependent protein kinase and Ca^{2+}–calmodulin-dependent protein kinase were purified from rabbit muscle, Ca^{2+}–phospholipid-dependent protein kinase from rat brain and the remaining protein kinases were purified from lactating rat mammary gland.

creased phosphorylation of ACC in the mammary glands of 24-h-starved or high-fat-fed lactating rats. We must therefore consider the role of cyclic nucleotide-independent ACC kinases in the rat mammary gland.

Table V lists the protein kinases that are known to phosphorylate mammary gland ACC in vitro. Of these protein kinases, cAMP-dependent kinase, ACC kinase-2, casein kinase-1, and casein kinase-2 have been partially purified and characterized from the lactating rat mammary gland (Munday and Hardie, 1984). A Ca^{2+}- and calmodulin-dependent protein kinase has also been identified and characterized in isolated mammary acini from the lactating rat (Brooks and Landt, 1985). Protein kinase C activity has not yet been demonstrated in this tissue. Phosphorylation of ACC by casein kinase-1, casein kinase-2, or the calmodulin-dependent multiprotein kinase has no effect on the activity of the enzyme (Munday and Hardie, 1984; Hardie et al., 1986; Table V). The phosphorylation of ACC by casein kinase-2 and calmodulin-dependent multiprotein kinase occur on the same distinct phosphopeptide generated by tryptic digestion of ACC (Fig. 6). This tryptic peptide, termed T4 in this laboratory, has the following amino acid sequence:

```
                                    *                *
PHE-ILE-ILE-GLY-SER-VAL-SER-GLU-ASP-ASN-SER-GLU-ASP-
                   GLU-ILE-SER-ASN-LEU
```

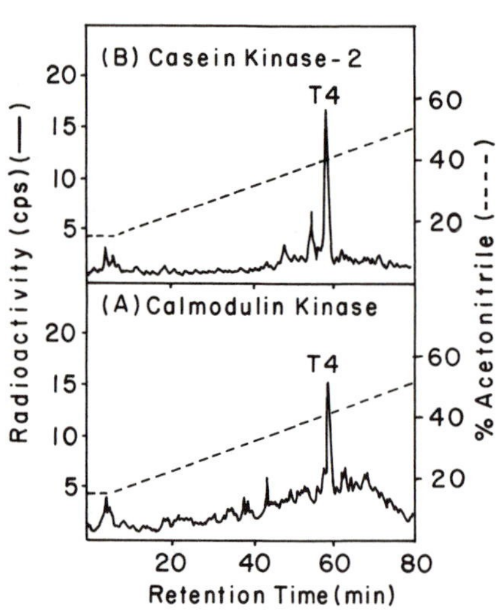

Figure 6. Analysis of tryptic phosphopeptides derived from ACC phosphorylated by Ca^{2+}–calmodulin-dependent multiprotein kinase (A) or casein kinase-2 (B). Acetyl-CoA carboxylase was phosphorylated using [γ-^{32}P]ATP and the kinase indicated in incubations described by Hardie et al. (1986). Trichloroacetic acid precipitates were digested with trypsin and analyzed by reversed-phase HPLC in 0.1% trifluoroacetic acid using the indicated gradient from water to acetonitrile. Radioactivity in the eluate was measured continuously by Cerenkov counting using a Reeve analytical monitor.

The asterisks denote the serine residues phosphorylated by the calmodulin-dependent multiprotein kinase. Although the serine residues phosphorylated by casein kinase-2 have yet to be identified, this peptide contains two classic recognition sites for casein kinase-2, that is, a cluster of acidic residues immediately C-terminal to the phosphorylated serine residue (Meggio et al., 1984). This peptide is of particular interest because it comigrates, both on reversed-phase HPLC and thin-layer isoelectric focusing, with the tryptic peptide of ACC whose phosphorylation is increased by insulin treatment of hepatocytes (Holland and Hardie, 1985) and adipocytes (Witters et al., 1983; T.A.J. Haystead and D.G. Hardie, unpublished data). Work in this laboratory has confirmed that the sequence of the *insulin-stimulated* peptide from adipocytes is identical to that shown above and the identity of the serine residue(s) phosphorylated in response to insulin is presently under investigation. It is an interesting possibility that the increased phosphorylation of ACC in response to insulin may be ascribed to either casein kinase-2 or calmodulin-dependent multiprotein kinase. It is important to note, however, that phosphorylation of this peptide by either kinase or in response to insulin treatment of adipocytes and hepatocytes does not result in increased activity of the purified ACC. The role of the phosphorylation of this peptide, and whether it is of physiological relevance to ACC in the lactating mammary gland, is still to be investigated.

Phosphorylation of purified ACC both by cAMP-dependent protein kinase and by the cAMP-independent ACC kinase-2 leads to inactivation of the enzyme (Munday and Hardie, 1984; Table V). These phosphorylations occur on a tryptic peptide that is distinct from T4 and has been termed T1 in this laboratory (Fig. 7). T1 has the following amino acid sequence:

```
          *
SER-SER-MET-SER-GLY-LEU-HIS-LEU-VAL-LYS
```

The asterisk denotes the serine residue phosphorylated by cAMP-dependent protein kinase. As this is a tryptic peptide, ARG or LYS must be the amino acid directly N-terminal to this peptide and thus this is a classic recognition site for cAMP-dependent protein kinase, that is, basic amino acid-X-serine (Cohen, 1985). That this serine is the residue phosphorylated by ACC kinase-2 has yet to be confirmed. The above peptide corresponds to peptide T1, which is labeled in isolated hepatocytes (Holland and Hardie, 1985) and to the peptide of isoelectric point about 7 (the p*I* 7 peptide), which is labeled in intact adipocytes and shows in-

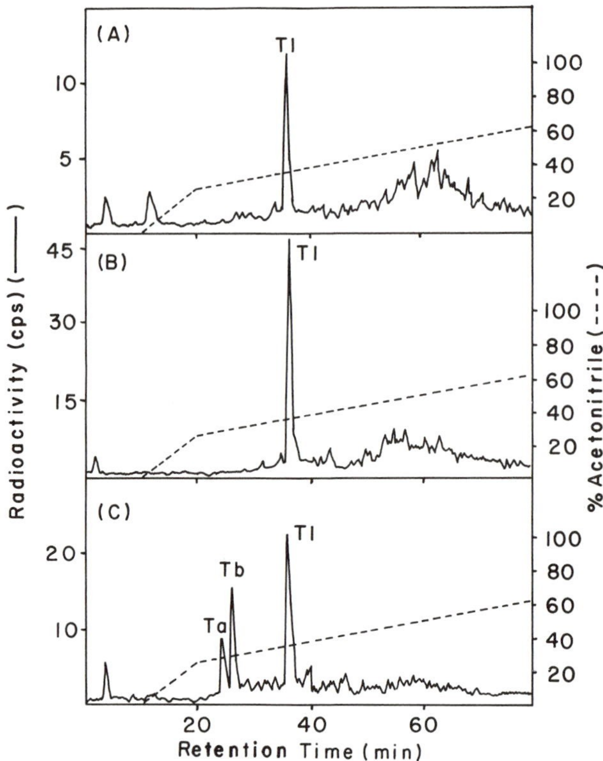

Figure 7. Analysis of tryptic phosphopeptides derived from ACC phosphorylated by cAMP-dependent protein kinase (A), ACC kinase-2 (B), or Ca^{2+}–phospholipid-dependent protein kinase (C). Acetyl-CoA carboxylase was phosphorylated using [γ-^{32}P]ATP and the kinase indicated in incubations described by Munday and Hardie (1984) and Hardie et al. (1986). Trichloroacetic acid precipitates were digested with trypsin and analyzed by reversed-phase HPLC in 0.1% trifluoroacetic acid using the indicated gradient from water to acetonitrile. Radioactivity in the eluate was measured continuously by Cerenkov counting using a Reeve analytical monitor.

creased phosphorylation in response to adrenaline (Brownsey and Hardie, 1980).

Protein kinase C phosphorylates three tryptic peptides, Ta, Tb, and T1 (Fig. 7). By comparison with the effects of cAMP-dependent protein kinase, it is the phosphorylation of T1 that is likely to explain the small degree of inactivation of ACC by this kinase (Hardie et al., 1986; Table V). Phorbol esters are known activators of protein kinase C (Castagna et al., 1982) and treatment of adipocytes with the active phorbol ester tetradecanoyl phorbol acetate (TPA) stimulates lipogenesis (van de

Werve et al., 1985) but not ACC activity (Haystead and Hardie, 1987) in these cells. TPA does increase the level of phosphorylation of ACC in adipocytes, but this occurs on peptide T4 (identical to the insulin-stimulated peptide) and not on peptides Ta, Tb, or T1 (Haystead and Hardie, 1987). Thus, the relevance of the phosphorylation of ACC by protein kinase C to the control of lipogenesis in mammary gland or other tissues is unclear and requires further investigation.

If ACC phosphorylated by cAMP-dependent protein kinase (Fig. 8) or ACC kinase-2 (not illustrated) is digested with trypsin plus chymotrypsin, two phosphopeptides (TC1 and TC2) are recovered after reversed-phase HPLC analysis. The sequence of TC1, -LYS/ARG-SER-SER-MET-SER-GLY-LEU-, shows that it is derived from the same site as tryptic peptide T1 (Fig. 7). TC2 is derived from a distinct site that is apparently not recovered in good yield after digestion with trypsin alone. This peptide has the amino acid sequence -LYS/ARG-ARG-MET-SER(P)-PHE-, which contains the classic recognition site for cAMP-dependent protein kinase (Cohen, 1985).

ACC kinase-2 is distinct from the catalytic subunit of cAMP-dependent protein kinase as judged by their apparent molecular weights (~76,000 and ~40,000, respectively), their substrate specificities (e.g., the ratio of initial rates of phosphorylation of phosphorylase kinase : ACC are

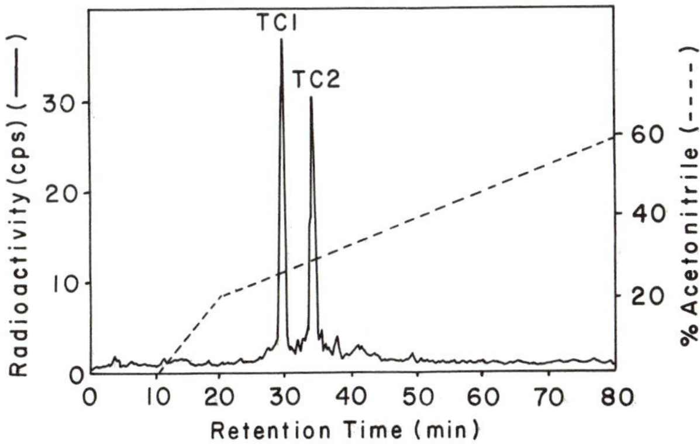

Figure 8. Analysis of phosphopeptides derived from combined tryptic and chymotryptic digestion of ACC phosphorylated by cAMP-dependent protein kinase. Acetyl-CoA carboxylase was phosphorylated using [γ-^{32}P]ATP and cAMP-dependent protein kinase in an incubation described by Hardie et al. (1986). Trichloroacetic acid precipitates were digested with trypsin and chymotrypsin simultaneously and were analyzed by reverse-phase HPLC in 0.1% trifluoroacetic acid using the indicated gradient from water to acetonitrile. Radioactivity in the eluate was measured continuously by Cerenkov counting using a Reeve analytical monitor.

1 : 10 and 10 : 1, respectively), and the insensitivity of ACC kinase-2 to the specific protein inhibitor of cAMP-dependent protein kinase (Munday and Hardie, 1984). However, they phosphorylate sites on the same proteolytic peptides and inactivate ACC in vitro in a very similar, reversible, manner (Munday and Hardie, 1984; Table V). Therefore, in the lactating rat mammary gland, ACC kinase-2 is a candidate for a cyclic nucleotide-independent kinase that could function in the regulation of ACC and lipogenesis in the same way as cAMP-dependent protein kinase functions in liver and adipose tissue.

The question remains as to whether ACC kinase-2 could be responsible for the phosphorylation and inactivation of ACC in the mammary glands of 24-h-starved and high-fat fed lactating rats. Table V shows that the phosphorylation of ACC by either ACC kinase-2 or cAMP-dependent protein kinase produces a much larger effect on the $A_{0.5}$ citrate of the enzyme than on V_{max}. This is in contrast to the changes in the kinetic parameters of the enzyme in mammary gland in vivo. After 24-h starvation, V_{max} is decreased (73%) to the same extent that $A_{0.5}$ citrate is increased (75%), and in the high-fat-fed rat, V_{max} is decreased (64%) to a greater extent than the increase in the $A_{0.5}$ citrate (36%). Recently, in this laboratory, a cAMP-independent ACC kinase, which we have termed ACC kinase-3, has been partially purified from rat liver. Phosphorylation of mammary gland ACC by ACC kinase-3 to stoichiometries similar to those shown in Table V produces an inhibition of enzyme activity in excess of 70% measured at saturating citrate concentrations, and greater than 90% measured at physiological (0.5 m*M*) citrate concentrations (D. Carling and D.G. Hardie, unpublished data). As shown in Fig. 8 and described above for cAMP-dependent protein kinase and ACC kinase-2, the phosphate incorporated by ACC kinase-3 is also recovered almost entirely in peptides TC1 and TC2 (unpublished results). However, although all three protein kinases phosphorylate the same serine residue in TC2, ACC kinase-3 exclusively phosphorylates serine-4, rather than serine-2, in TC1:

```
                    *
SER-SER-MET-SER-GLY-LEU
```

This subtle difference in the exact site of phosphorylation may explain the much larger decrease in V_{max} after phosphorylation by ACC kinase-3 compared with cAMP-dependent protein kinase or ACC kinase-2.

Preliminary experiments have identified ACC kinase-3 in the mammary gland of the lactating rat. Given the effects of this kinase on the

V_{max} of ACC, it is an attractive possibility that this is the kinase responsible for the inactivation of ACC in response to 24-h starvation or high-fat feeding. At present, we have no conclusive evidence on the signals or mechanisms regulating ACC kinase-2 or ACC kinase-3. We have observed that the activity of ACC kinase-3 is stimulated twofold by nanomolar concentrations of fatty acyl-CoA, which is very interesting given that ACC is phosphorylated and inactivated in lactating mammary gland in response to high-fat diets. It is also possible, as discussed in the previous section, that the phosphorylation state of ACC in the lactating mammary gland is regulated by insulin through the activity of phosphatases working against a background of kinase activity. These questions will be resolved by identification of the serine residues whose phosphorylation state is modulated in vivo in response to physiological manipulations. Such studies will enable the identification of the protein kinases and phosphatases that are physiologically important in the regulation of ACC, and measurement of changes in the activities of these interconverting enzymes in response to hormones or metabolites should reveal the signals responsible for the regulation of ACC in the lactating rat mammary gland.

7. Summary and Conclusions

It should be clear from our review that fatty acid biosynthesis in the mammary gland of the lactating rat is stringently regulated in response to changes in the quantity and fat content of the diet and also by at least one hormone—insulin. Regulation is effected at several sites within the pathway from extracellular glucose to fatty acid, particularly the steps catalyzed by the glucose transporter, 6-phospho-fructo-1-kinase pyruvate dehydrogenase, and acetyl-CoA carboxylase. The quantitative distribution of control between these regulatory sites in the pathway warrants further investigation, as it appears to be asynchronous.

On transition from the fed to the starved state, the inactivation of pyruvate dehydrogenase and acetyl-CoA carboxylase in the lactating rat mammary gland appears to be slower than the inhibition of lipogenesis (Williamson et al., 1983; Munday and Hardie, 1986). Refeeding starved rats with chow produces an immediate increase in plasma insulin concentration, rising to a peak within the first 15 min, and this increase is very closely accompanied by reactivation of glucose uptake by the gland (Page and Kuhn, 1986). There is a distinct lag between this rise in plasma insulin/increased glucose uptake and the reactivation of lipogenesis, which occurs some 30 min later (Mercer and Williamson, 1986), or the reactivation of lactose synthesis, which occurs later still (Bussman et al., 1984). A major proportion of the increased glucose uptake during the first 30 min of refeeding appears, from measurements of arteriovenous differences across the mammary gland, to be released back into the circulation as lactate (D.H. Williamson, personal communication). These results clearly suggest that, in response to insulin on refeeding, the glycolytic segment of the pathway is activated faster than pyruvate dehydrogenase and probably acetyl-CoA carboxylase.

It seems likely that the primary control point is glucose transport, based on the close parallels between overall rates of glucose utilization and the rates of uptake of the nonmetabolizable analogs 2-deoxyglucose and 3-*O*-methylglucose. This is particularly apparent in their similar and immediate response to refeeding (Bussman et al., 1984; Page and Kuhn, 1986). When glucose transport is reactivated by insulin, the activation of phosphofructokinase-1, pyruvate dehydrogenase, and acetyl-CoA carboxylase probably then occurs in ordered sequence, although still fairly rapidly (at least within 2.5 h). The implication of these observations is that the lactating rat mammary gland is cautious in committing a valuable substrate like glucose to irreversible pathways such as fatty acid synthesis. This makes good physiological sense under the conditions of starvation. For this reason, regulation of acetyl-CoA carboxylase is likely to be important because this enzyme lays beyond the branch point at mitochondrial citrate and consequently may determine the distribution of flux between fatty acid synthesis proper and the Krebs cycle. In at least two situations, that is, effects of fat-feeding in vivo and effects of insulin in dichloroacetate-treated acini from starved rats, changes in acetyl-CoA carboxylase activity are closely mirrored by changes in overall fatty acid synthesis, while there is no evidence for regulation at the other steps.

Of the four steps that may be the major sites of acute regulation of fatty acid synthesis in lactating rat mammary gland, we have discussed evidence that for at least two, pyruvate dehydrogenase and acetyl-CoA carboxylase, protein phosphorylation is the most important mechanism by which regulation is achieved. For the other two steps, glucose transport and 6-phosphofructo-1-kinase, the situation is less clear in the case of the mammary gland. However, in the other lipogenic tissues, liver and adipose tissue, there is evidence for a role of protein phosphorylation in both cases. In the case of glucose transport, this may be via a direct phosphorylation of the transport protein, whereas for hepatic phosphofructokinase-1 it is an indirect effect via phosphorylation of 6-phosphofructo-2-kinase. The relevance of these observations to lactating rat mammary gland remains an intriguing subject for future study.

Note added in proof. We have now purified ACC kinase-3 several thousandfold from both rat liver (D. Carling and D.G. Hardie) and lactating rat mammary gland (K.A. Ottey and M.R. Munday). Phosphorylation of purified mammary ACC by the kinase from either tissue results in a substantial 85–90% decrease in its V_{max}. ACC kinase-3 activity is stimulated by adenosine 5′ monophosphate and is itself regulated by reversible phosphorylation. ACC kinase-3 is phosphorylated and activated by a separate kinase activity that is as yet uncharacterized, and preliminary experiments in rat liver have demonstrated that it is this ACC kinase-3 kinase that is activated by nanomolar concentrations of long chain fatty acyl-CoA. We also have good evidence that ACC kinase-3 from rat liver phosphorylates and inactivates hydroxy methyl glutaryl-CoA reductase, an important regulatory enzyme in cholesterol biosynthesis in this tissue. This infers a potential coordinate regulation of the fatty acid and cholesterol biosynthetic pathways in rat liver that may also occur in lactating rat mammary gland.

References

Agius, L., and Williamson, D.H., 1980, Rapid inhibition of lipogenesis *in vivo* in lactating rat mammary gland by medium- or long-chain triacylglycerols and partial reversal by insulin, *Biochem. J.* **192:**361–364.

Agius, L., Robinson, A.M., Girard, J.R., and Williamson, D.H., 1979, Alterations in the rate of lipogenesis *in vivo* in maternal liver and adipose tissue on premature weaning of lactating rats. A possible regulatory role of prolactin, *Biochem. J.* **180:**689–692.

Agius, L., Rolls, B.J., Rowe, E.A., and Williamson, D.H., 1980, Impaired lipogenesis in mammary glands of lactating rats fed on a cafeteria diet. Reversal of inhibition of glucose metabolism *in vitro* by insulin, *Biochem. J.* **186:**1005–1008.

Agius, L., Rolls, B.J., Rowe, E.A., and Williamson, D.H., 1981, Increased lipogenesis in brown adipose tissue of lactating rats fed a cafeteria diet. The possible involvement of insulin in brown adipose tissue hypertrophy, *FEBS Lett.* **123:**45–48.

Ahmad, F., Ahmad, P.M., Pieretti, L., and Watters, G.T., 1978, Purification and subunit structure of rat mammary gland acetyl coenzyme A carboxylase, *J. Biol. Chem.* **253:**1733–1737.

Alexander, M.C., Palmer, J.L., Pointer, R.H., Kowaloff, E.M., Koumjian, L.L., and Avruch, J., 1982, Insulin-stimulated phosphorylation of ATP–citrate lyase in isolated hepatocytes. Stoichiometry and relation to the phosphoenzyme intermediate, *J. Biol. Chem.* **257:**2049–2055.

Ashcraft, B.A., Fillers, W.S., Augustine, S.L., and Clarke, S.D., 1980, Polymer–protomer transition of acetyl-CoA carboxylase occurs *in vivo* and varies with nutritional conditions, *J. Biol. Chem.* **255:**10033–10035.

Bar, H.P., 1973, Epinephrine- and prostaglandin-sensitive adenyl cyclase in mammary gland, *Biochim. Biophys. Acta* **321:**397–406.

Barrera, C.R., Namihara, G., Hamilton, L., Munk, P., Eley, M.H., Linn, T.C., and Reed, L.J., 1972, α-Ketoacid dehydrogenase complexes. XVI. Studies on the subunit structure of the pyruvate dehydrogenase complexes from bovine kidney and heart, *Arch. Biochem. Biophys.* **148:**343–358.

Baxter, M.A., and Coore, H.G., 1978, The mode of regulation of pyruvate dehydrogenase of lactating rat mammary gland. Effects of starvation and insulin, *Biochem. J.* **174:**553–561.

Baxter, M.A., and Coore, H.G., 1979a, Reduction of mitochondrial pyruvate dehydrogenase phosphatase activity in lactating rat mammary gland following starvation or insulin deprivation, *Biochem. Biophys. Res. Comm.* **87:**433–440.

Baxter, M.A., and Coore, H.G., 1979b, Starvation of lactating rats leads to alterations in the behaviour of pyruvate dehydrogenase kinase which persist in the semi-purified pyruvate dehydrogenase complex of the mammary gland but are partly reversible *in vitro, FEBS Lett.* **98:**195–198.

Baxter, M.A., Goheer, M.A., and Coore, H.G., 1979, Absent pyruvate inhibition of pyruvate dehydrogenase kinase in lactating rat mammary gland following various treatments. Removal of circulating insulin and prolactin and exposure to protein synthesis inhibitors, *FEBS Lett.* **97:**27–31.

Beaty, N.B., and Lane, M.D., 1983, Kinetics of activation of acetyl-CoA carboxylase by citrate. Relationship to the rate of polymerisation of the enzyme, *J. Biol. Chem.* **258:**13043–13050.

Brosnan, M.E., Ilic, V., and Williamson, D.H., 1982, Regulation of the activity of ornithine decarboxylase and *S*-adenosylmethionine decarboxylase in mammary gland and liver of lactating rats, *Biochem. J.* **202:**693–698.

Brooks, C.L., and Landt, M., 1985, Calmodulin-dependent protein kinase in acini from lactating rat mammary tissue: Subcellular locale, characterisation and solubilization, *Arch. Biochem. Biophys.* **240:**663–673.

Brownsey, R.W., and Hardie, D.G., 1980, Regulation of acetyl-CoA carboxylase: Identity of sites phosphorylated in intact cells treated with adrenaline and *in vitro* by cyclic AMP-dependent protein kinase, *FEBS Lett.* **120:**67–70.

Brownsey, R.W., and Denton, R.M., 1982, Evidence that insulin activates fat-cell acetyl-CoA carboxylase by increased phosphorylation at a specific site, *Biochem. J.* **202:**77–86.

Burchell, A., Foulkes, J.G., Cohen, P.T.W., Condon, G.D., and Cohen, P., 1978, Evidence for the involvement of protein phosphatase-1 in the regulation of metabolic processes other than glycogen metabolism, *FEBS Lett.* **92:**68–72.

Burnol, A.-F., Leturque, A., Ferre, P., and Girard, J., 1983, Effect of lactation on insulin sensitivity of glucose metabolism in rat adipocytes, *Am. J. Physiol.* **245:**E351–E358.

Bussman, L.E., Ward, S., and Kuhn, N.J., 1984, Lactose and fatty acid synthesis in lactating rat mammary gland—effects of starvation, re-feeding, and administration of insulin, adrenaline, streptozotocin and 2-bromo-α-ergocryptine, *Biochem. J.* **219:**173–180.

Castagna, M., Taka, Y., Kaibuchi, K., Sano, K., Kikkawa, U., and Nishizuka, Y., 1982 Direct activation of calcium-activated, phospholipid-dependent protein kinase by tumor-promoting phorbol esters, *J. Biol. Chem.* **257:**7847–7851.

Cheng, K., and Larner, J., 1985, Unidirectional actions of insulin and calcium-dependent hormones on adipocyte pyruvate dehydrogenase, *J. Biol. Chem.* **260:**5279–5285.

Clegg, R.A., and Mullaney, I., 1985, Acute change in the cyclic AMP content of rat mammary acini *in vitro.* Influence of physiological and pharmacological agents, *Biochem. J.* **230:**239–246.

Clegg, R.A., Mullaney, I., Robson, N.A., and Zammit, V.A., 1986, Modulation of intracellular cyclic AMP content and rate of lipogenesis in mammary acini *in vitro, Biochem. J.* **240:** 13–18.

Clegg, R.A., West, D.W., and Aitchison, R.E.D., 1987, Protein phosphorylation in rat mammary acini and in cytosol preparations *in vitro:* Phosphorylation of acetyl-CoA carboxylase is unaffected by cyclic AMP, *Biochem. J.* **241:**447–454.

Cohen, P., 1985, The role of protein phosphorylation in the hormonal control of enzyme activity, *Eur. J. Biochem.* **151:**439–448.

Coniglio, J.G., and Bridges, R., 1966, The effect of dietary fat on fatty acid synthesis in cell-free preparations of lactating mammary gland, *Lipids* **1:**76–80.

Coore, H.G., Denton, R.M., Martin, B.R., and Randle, P.J., 1971, Regulation of adipose tissue pyruvate dehydrogenase by insulin and other hormones, *Biochem. J.* **125:**115–127.

Coore, H.G., and Field, B., 1974, Properties of pyruvate dehydrogenase of rat mammary tissue and its changes during pregnancy, lactation and weaning, *Biochem. J.* **142:**87–95.

Cushman, S.W., and Wardzala, L.J., 1980, Potential mechanism of insulin action on glucose transport in the isolated rat adipose cell. Apparent translocation of intracellular transport systems to the plasma membrane, *J. Biol. Chem.* **255:**4758–4762.

Czech, M.P., 1976, Regulation of the D-glucose transport system in isolated fat cells, *Mol. Cell. Biochem.* **11:**51–63.

Czech, M.P., 1977, Molecular basis of insulin action, *Ann. Rev. Biochem.* **46:**359–384.

Czech, M.P., 1985, *Molecular Basis of Insulin Action,* Plenum Press, New York.

De Marcucci, O., and Lindsay, J.G., 1985, Component X. An immunologically distinct polypeptide associated with mammalian pyruvate dehydrogenase multi-enzyme complex, *Eur. J. Biochem.* **149:**641–648.

Denton, R.M., and Hughes, W.A., 1978, Pyruvate dehydrogenase and the hormonal regulation of fat synthesis in mammalian tissues, *Int. J. Biochem.* **9:**545–552.

Denton, R.M., Brownsey, R.W., and Belsham, G.J., 1981, A partial view of the mechanism of insulin action, *Diabetologia* **21:**347–362.

El-Maghrabi, M.R., Claus, T.H., Pilkis, J., and Pilkis, S.J., 1981, Regulation of 6-phosphofructo-2-kinase activity by cyclic AMP-dependent phosphorylation, *Proc. Natl. Acad. Sci. USA* **79:**315–319.

El-Maghrabi, M.R., Claus, T.H., Pilkis, J., Fox, E., and Pilkis, S.J., 1982, Regulation of rat liver fructose 2,6-bisphosphatase, *J. Biol. Chem.* **257:**7603–7607.

Field, B., and Coore, H.G., 1976, Control of rat mammary-gland pyruvate dehydrogenase by insulin and prolactin, *Biochem. J.* **156:**333–337.

Flint, D.J., 1982, Regulation of insulin receptors by prolactin in lactating rat mammary gland, *J. Endocrinol.* **93:**279–285.

Foe, L.G., and Kemp, R.G., 1982, Properties of phospho and dephospho forms of muscle phosphofructokinase, *J. Biol. Chem.* **257:**6368–6372.

Forn, J., and Greengard, P., 1976, Regulation by lipolytic and antilipolytic compounds of the phosphorylation of specific proteins in isolated intact fat cells, *Arch. Biochem. Biophys.* **176:**721–723.

Garton, G.A., 1963, The composition and biosynthesis of milk lipids, *J. Lipid Res.* **4:**237–254.

Geelen, M.J.H., Beynen, A.C., Christiansen, R.Z., Lepreau-Jose, M.J., and Gibson, D.M., 1978, Short-term effects of insulin and glucagon on lipid synthesis in isolated rat hepatocytes. Covariance of acetyl-CoA carboxylase activity and the rate of ^3H_2O incorporation into fatty acids, *FEBS Lett.* **95:**326–330.

Gibbons, G.F., Pullinger, C.R., Munday, M.R., and Williamson, D.H., 1983, Regulation of cholesterol synthesis in the liver and mammary gland of the lactating rat, *Biochem. J.* **212:**843–848.

Green, A., 1983, Glucagon inhibition of insulin-stimulated 2-deoxyglucose uptake by rat adipocytes in the presence of adenosine deaminase, *Biochem. J.* **212:**189–195.

Gregolin, C., Ryder, E., Warner, R.C., Kleinschmidt, A.K., and Lane, M.D., 1966a, Liver acetyl-CoA carboxylase: The dissociation–reassociation process and its relation to catalytic activity, *Proc. Natl. Acad. Sci. USA* **56:**1751–1758.

Gregolin, C., Ryder, E., Kleinschmidt, A.K., Warner, R.C., and Lane, M.D., 1966b, Molecular characteristics of liver acetyl-CoA carboxylase, *Proc. Natl. Acad. Sci. USA* **56:**148–155.

Grigor, M.R., and Warren, S.M., 1980, Dietary regulation of mammary lipogenesis in lactating rats, *Biochem. J.* **188:**61–65.

Gumaa, K.A., Greenbaum, A.L., and McLean, P., 1973, Adaptive changes in satellite systems related to lipogenesis in rat and sheep mammary gland and in adipose tissue, *Eur. J. Biochem.* **34:**188–198.

Gumaa, K.A., Greenbaum, A.L., and McLean, P., 1971, in: *Lactation* (I.R. Falconer, ed.), Butterworths, London, pp. 197–238.

Guy, P.S., Cohen, P., and Hardie, D.G., 1980, Rat mammary gland ATP-citrate lyase is phosphorylated by cyclic AMP-dependent protein kinase, *FEBS Lett.* **109:**205–208.

Guy, P.S., Cohen, P., and Hardie, D.G., 1981, Purification and physicochemical properties of ATP-citrate (pro-3S) lyase from lactating rat mammary gland and studies of its reversible phosphorylation, *Eur. J. Biochem.* **114:**399–405.

Hamosh, M., Clary, T.R., Chernick, S.S., and Scow, R.O., 1970, Lipoprotein lipase activity of adipose and mammary tissue and plasma triglyceride in pregnant and lactating rats, *Biochem Biophys. Acta.* **210:**473–482.

Hardie, D.G., 1980, The regulation of fatty acid synthesis by reversible phosphorylation of acetyl-CoA carboxylase, *Mol. Aspects Cell Reg.* **1:**33–62.

Hardie, D.G., and Cohen, P., 1978, The regulation of fatty acid biosynthesis. Simple procedure for the purification of acetyl-CoA carboxylase from lactating rabbit mammary gland, and its phosphorylation by endogenous cyclic AMP-dependent and -independent protein kinase activities, *FEBS Lett.* **91:**1–7.

Hardie, D.G., and Guy, P.S., 1980, Reversible phosphorylation and inactivation of acetyl-CoA carboxylase from lactating rat mammary gland by cyclic AMP-dependent protein kinase, *Eur. J. Biochem.* **110:**167–177.

Hardie, D.G., Holland, R., and Munday, M.R., 1984, Regulation of fatty acid synthesis by insulin, glucagon and catecholamines, *Horm. Cell Regulation* **8:**117–138.

Hardie, D.G., Carling, D., Ferrari, S., Guy, P.S., and Aitken, A., 1986, Characterisation of the phosphorylation of rat mammary ATP–citrate lyase and acetyl-CoA carboxylase by Ca^{2+} and calmodulin-dependent multiprotein kinase and Ca^{2+} and phospholipid-dependent protein kinase, *Biochem. J.* **157:**553–561.

Hawkins, R.A., and Williamson, D.H., 1972, Measurements of substrate uptake by mammary gland of the rat, *Biochem. J.* **129:**1171–1173.

Haystead, T.A.J., and Hardie, D.G., 1986, Evidence that activation of acetyl-CoA carboxylase by insulin in adipocytes is mediated by a low-M_r effector and not by increased phosphorylation, *Biochem. J.* **240:** 99–106.

Haystead, T.A.J., and Hardie, D.G., 1987, Insulin and phorbol ester stimulate phosphorylation of acetyl-CoA carboxylase at similar sites in isolated adipocytes. Lack of correspondence with sites phosphorylated on the purified enzyme by protein kinase C, *Eur. J. Biochem.* (in press).

Hers, H.G., and Van Schaftingen, E., 1982, Fructose 2,6-bisphosphate 2 years after its discovery, *Biochem. J.* **206:**1–12.

Hers, H.-G., Hue, L., and Van Schaftingen, E., 1982, Fructose 2,6-bisphosphate, *Trends Biochem. Sci.* **7:**329–331.

Holland, R., and Hardie, D.G., 1985, Both insulin and epidermal growth factor stimulate fatty acid synthesis and increase phosphorylation of acetyl-CoA carboxylase and ATP–citrate lyase in isolated hepatocytes, *FEBS Lett.* **181:**308–312.

Holland, R., Witters, L.A., and Hardie, D.G., 1984, Glucagon inhibits fatty acid synthesis in isolated hepatocytes via phosphorylation of acetyl-CoA carboxylase by cyclic AMP-dependent protein kinase, *Eur. J. Biochem.* **140:**325–333.

Holland, R., Hardie, D.G., Clegg, R.A., and Zammit, V.A., 1985, Evidence that glucagon-mediated inhibition of acetyl-CoA carboxylase in isolated adipocytes involves increased phosphorylation of the enzyme by cAMP-dependent protein kinase, *Biochem. J.* **226:**139–145.

Houston, B., and Nimmo, H.G., 1985, Effects of phosphorylation on the kinetic properties of rat liver ATP–citrate lyase, *Biochim. Biophys. Acta* **844:**233–239.

Hughes, W.A., Brownsey, R.W., and Denton, R.M., 1980, Studies on the incorporation of [^{32}P]-phosphate into pyruvate dehydrogenase in intact rat fat-cells, *Biochem. J.* **192:**469–481.

Hutson, N.J., and Randle, P.J., 1978, Enhanced activity of pyruvate dehydrogenase kinase in rat heart mitochondria in alloxan-diabetes or starvation, *FEBS Lett.* **92:**73–76.

Illingworth, J.A., and Mullings, R., 1976, Pyruvate dehydrogenase activation after an increase in cardiac output, *Biochem. Soc. Trans.* **4:**291–292.

Ingebritsen, T.S., Blair, J., Guy, P., Witters, L., and Hardie, D.G., 1983, The protein phosphatases involved in cellular regulation. 3. Fatty acid synthesis, cholesterol synthesis and glycolysis/gluconeogenesis, *Eur. J. Biochem.* **132:**275–281.

Ip, C., Tepperman, H.M., Holohan, P., and Tepperman, J., 1976, Insulin binding and insulin response of adipocytes from rats adapted to fat feeding, *J. Lipid. Res.* **17:**588–599.

Jones, R.G., Ilic, V. and Williamson, D.H., 1984a, Regulation of lactating-rat mammary-gland lipogenesis by insulin and glucagon *in vivo.* The role and site of action of insulin in the transition to the starved state, *Biochem. J.* **223:**345–351.

Jones, R.G., Ilic, V., and Williamson, D.H., 1984b, Physiological significance of altered insulin metabolism in the conscious rat during lactation, *Biochem. J.* **220:**455–460.

Joost, H.G., Weber, T.M., Cushman, S.W., and Simpson, I.A., 1986, Insulin-stimulated glucose transport in rat adipose cells. Modulation of transporter intrinsic activity by isoproterenol and adenosine, *J. Biol. Chem.* **261:**10033–10036.

Jung, C.Y., 1975, in: *The Red Blood Cell,* 2nd ed. (D.M. Surgenor, ed.), Academic Press, New York, pp. 705–759.

Kahn, C.R., 1985, The molecular mechanism of insulin action, *Ann. Rev. Med.* **36:**429–451.

Kankel, K.-F., and Reinauer, H., 1976, Activity of the pyruvate dehydrogenase complex in the mammary gland of normal and diabetic rats, *Diabetologia* **12:**149–154.

Karnieli, E., Zarnowski, M.J., Hissin, P.J., Simpson, I.A., Salans, L.B., and Cushman, S.W., 1981, Insulin-stimulated translocation of glucose transport systems in the isolated rat adipose cell. Time course, reversal, insulin concentration dependency, and relationship to glucose transport activity, *J. Biol. Chem.* **256:**4772–4777.

Kerbey, A.L., and Randle, P.J., 1981, Thermolabile factor accelerates pyruvate dehydrogenase kinase reaction in heart mitochondria of starved or alloxan-diabetic rats, *FEBS Lett.* **127:**188–192.

Kerbey, A.L., and Randle, P.J., 1982, Pyruvate dehydrogenase kinase/activator in rat heart mitochondria. Assay, effects of starvation, and effect of protein-synthesis inhibitors in starvation, *Biochim. J.* **206:**103–111.

Kerbey, A.L., Randle, P.J., Cooper, R.H., Whitehouse, S., Pask, H.T., and Denton, R.M., 1976, Regulation of pyruvate dehydrogenase in rat heart. Mechanism of regulation of proportions of dephosphorylated and phosphorylated enzyme by oxidation of fatty acids and ketone bodies and of effects of diabetes: role of coenzyme A, acetyl coenzyme A and reduced and oxidised nicotinamide-adenine dinucleotide, *Biochem. J.* **154:**327–348.

Kerbey, A.L., Radcliffe, P.M., Randle, P.J., and Sugden, P.H., 1979, Regulation of kinase reactions in pig heart pyruvate dehydrogenase complex, *Biochem. J.* **181:**427–443.

Kuhn, N.J., and White, A., 1975, Milk glucose as an index of the intracellular glucose concentration of rat mammary gland, *Biochem. J.* **152:**153–155.

Kuroda, M., Simpson, I.A., Honnor, R.C., Londos, C., and Cushman, S.W., 1985, cAMP-independent modulation of rat adipocyte glucose transporter intrinsic activity by the adenylate cyclase regulatory system, *Fed. Proc.* **44:**480.

Lavandero, S., Donoso, E., and Sapag-Hagar, M., 1985, β-Adrenergic receptors in rat mammary gland, *Biochem. Pharmacol.* **34:**2034–2035.

Lavau, M., Fried, S.K., Susini, C., and Freychet, P., 1979, Mechanism of insulin resistance in adipocytes of rats fed a high-fat diet, *J. Lipid Res.* **20:**8–16.

Libertini, L.J., and Smith, S., 1978, Purification and properties of a thioesterase from lactating rat mammary gland which modifies the product specificity of fatty acid synthase, *J. Biol. Chem.* **253:**1393–1401.

Libertini, L.J., and Smith, S., 1979, Synthesis of long-chain acyl-enzyme thioesters by modified fatty acid synthetases and their hydrolysis by a mammary gland thioesterase, *Arch. Biochem. Biophys.* **192:** 47–60.

Livingstone, J.N., and Lockwood, D.H., 1974, Direct measurements of sugar uptake in small and large adipocytes from young and adult rats, *Biochem. Biophys. Res. Commun.* **61:**989–996.

Louis, S.L., and Baldwin, R.L., 1975a, Changes in the cyclic AMP system of rat mammary gland during the lactation cycle, *J. Dairy Sci.* **58:**861.

Louis, S.L., and Baldwin, R.L., 1975b, Effect of adrenalectomy and insulin insufficiency upon the cyclic AMP system of the rat mammary gland, *J. Dairy Sci.* **58:**502.

Mackall, J.C., and Lane, M.D., 1977, Changes in mammary gland acetyl-coenzyme A carboxylase associated with lactogenic differentiation, *Biochem. J.* **162:**635–642.

Marshall, S.E., McCormack, J.G., and Denton, R.M., 1984, Role of Ca^{2+} ions in the regulation of intramitochondrial metabolism in rat epididymal adipose tissue. Evidence against a role for Ca^{2+} in the activation of pyruvate dehydrogenase by insulin, *Biochem. J.* **218:**249–260.

Martin, R.J., and Baldwin, R.L., 1971, Effects of insulin and anti-insulin serum treatments on levels of metabolites in rat mammary glands, *Endocrinology* **88:**868–871.

Martyn, P., and Hansen, I.A., 1980, Initiation of fatty acid synthesis in rat mammary glands, *Biochem. J.* **190:**171–175.

Martyn, P., and Hansen, I.A., 1981, Initiation of lipogenic enzyme activities in rat mammary glands, *Biochem. J.* **198:**187–192.

McNeillie, E.M., and Zammit, V.A., 1982, Regulation of acetyl-CoA carboxylase in rat mammary gland. Effects of starvation and of insulin and prolactin deficiency on the fraction of the enzyme in the active form *in vivo*, *Biochem. J.* **204:**273–280.

McNeillie, E.M., Clegg, R.A., and Zammit, V.A., 1981, Regulation of acetyl-CoA carboxylase in rat mammary gland. Effects of incubation with Ca^{2+}, Mg^{2+} and ATP on enzyme activity in tissue extracts, *Biochem. J.* **200:**639–644.

Meggio, F., Marchiori, F., Borin, G., Chessa, G., and Pinna, L.A., 1984, Synthetic peptides including acidic clusters as substrates and inhibitors of rat liver casein kinase TS (Type-2), *J. Biol. Chem.* **259:**14576–14579.

Mercer, S.W., and Williamson, D.H., 1986, Time course of changes in plasma glucose and insulin concentrations and mammary gland lipogenesis during refeeding of starved conscious lactating rats, *Biochem. J.* **239:**489–492.

Meredith, M.J., and Lane, M.D., 1978, Evidence for polymeric filament to protomer transition in the intact avian liver cell, *J. Biol. Chem.* **253:**3381–3383.

Miller, A.L., Geroch, M.E., and Levy, H.R., 1970, Rat mammary-gland acetyl-coenzyme A carboxylase. Interaction with milk fatty acids, *Biochem. J.* **118:**645–657.

Miller, A.L., and Levy, H.R., 1969, Rat mammary acetyl coenzyme A carboxylase. Isolation and Characterisation, *J. Biol. Chem.* **244:**2334–2342.

Mukherjee, C., and Jungas, R.L., 1975, Activation of pyruvate dehydrogenase in adipose tissue by insulin. Evidence for an effect of insulin on pyruvate dehydrogenase phosphate phosphatase, *Biochem. J.* **148:**229–235.

Mullaney, I., and Clegg, R.A., 1984, Cyclic AMP phosphodiesterase and cyclic GMP phosphodiesterase activities of rat mammary tissue, *Biochem. J.* **219:**801–809.

Munday, M.R., 1983, The hormonal regulation of lipid metabolism in the lactating rat, D.Phil. Thesis, Oxon., U.K.

Munday, M.R., and Hardie, D.G., 1984, Isolation of three cyclic AMP-independent acetyl-CoA carboxylase kinases from lactating rat mammary gland and characterisation of their effects on enzyme activity, *Eur. J. Biochem.* **141:**617–627.

Munday, M.R., and Hardie, D.G., 1986, The role of acetyl-CoA carboxylase phosphorylation in the control of mammary gland fatty acid synthesis during the starvation and refeeding of lactating rats, *Biochem. J.* **237:**85–91.

Munday, M.R., Haystead, T.A.J., Holland, R., Carling, D., and Hardie, D.G., 1986, The role of phosphorylation/dephosphorylation of acetyl-CoA carboxylase in the regulation of mammalian fatty acid biosynthesis, *Biochem. Soc. Trans.* **14:**559–562.

Munday, M.R., and Williamson, D.H., 1981, Role of pyruvate dehydrogenase and insulin in the regulation of lipogenesis in the lactating mammary gland of the rat during the starved–refed transition, *Biochem. J.* **196:**831–837.

Munday, M.R., and Williamson, D.H., 1982, Effects of starvation, insulin or prolactin deficiency on the activity of acetyl-CoA carboxylase in mammary gland and liver of lactating rats, *FEBS Lett.* **138:**285–288.

Munday, M.R., and Williamson, D.H., 1983, Diurnal variations in food intake and in lipogenesis in mammary gland and liver of lactating rats, *Biochem. J.* **214:**183–187.

Munday, M.R., and Williamson, D.H., 1987, Insulin activation of lipogenesis in isolated mammary acini from lactating rats fed a high-fat diet: Evidence that acetyl-CoA carboxylase is a site of action, *Biochem. J.* **242:**905–911.

Murray, K.J., El-Maghrabi, M.R., Kountz, P.D., Lukas, T.J., Soderling, T.R., and Pilkis, S.J., 1984, Amino acid sequence of the phosphorylation site of rat liver 6-phosphofructo-2-kinase/fructose-2,6-bisphosphatase, *J. Biol. Chem.* **259:**7673–7681.

Newsholme, E.A., and Start, C., 1981, *Regulation in Metabolism,* Wiley, New York.

Nikawa, J., Tanabe, T., Ogiwara, H., Shiba, T., and Numa, S., 1979, Inhibitory effects of long-chain acyl coenzyme A analogues on rat liver acetyl coenzyme A carboxylase, *FEBS Lett.* **102:**223–226.

Ottaway, S., and Robinson, D.S., 1968, The significance of changes in tissue clearing factor lipase activity in relation to the lipaemia of pregnancy, *Biochem. J.* **106:**677–682.

Page, T., and Kuhn, N.J., 1986, Arteriovenous glucose differences across the mammary gland of the fed, starved, and re-fed lactating rat, *Biochem. J.* **239:**269–274.

Pettit, F.H., Roche, T.E., and Reed, L.J., 1972, Function of calcium ions in pyruvate dehydrogenase phosphatase activity, *Biochem. Biophys. Res. Commun.* **49:**563–571.

Pierce, M.W., Palmer, J.L., Keutmann, H.T., and Avruch, J., 1981, ATP–citrate lyase. Structure of a tryptic peptide containing the phosphorylation site directed by glucagon and the cAMP-dependent protein kinase, *J. Biol. Chem.* **256:**8867–8870.

Pierce, M.W., Palmer, J.L., Keutmann, H.T., Hall, T.A., and Avruch, J., 1982, The insulin-directed phosphorylation site on ATP–citrate lyase is identical with the site phosphorylated by the cAMP-dependent protein kinase *in vitro*, *J. Biol. Chem.* **257:**10681–10686.

Pilch, P.F., Thompson, P.A., and Czech, M.P., 1980, Co-ordinate modulation of D-glucose transport activity and bilayer fluidity in plasma membranes derived from control and insulin-treated adipocytes, *Proc. Natl. Acad. Sci. USA* **77:**915–918.

Pilkis, S.J., Chrisman, T., El-Maghrabi, M.R., Colosia, A., Fox, E., Pilkis, J., and Claus, T.H., 1983, The action of insulin on hepatic fructose 2,6-biphosphate metabolism, *J.Biol. Chem.* **258:**1495–1503.

Pilkis, S.J., El-Maghrabi, M.R., McGrane, M., Pilkis, J., Fox, E., and Claus, T.H., 1982, Fructose 2,6-bisphosphate: A mediator of hormone action at the fructose 6-phosphate–fructose 1,6-bisphosphate substrate cycle, *Mol. Cell Endocrinol.* **25:**245–266.

Pilkis, S.J., Regen, D.M., Stewart, B.H., Chrisman, T., Pilkis, J., Kountz, P., Pate, T., McGrane, M., El-Maghrabi, M.R., and Claus, T., 1984, Rat liver 6-phosphofructo-2-kinase/fructose 2,6-bisphosphatase: A unique bifunctional enzyme regulated by cyclic AMP-dependent phosphorylation, *Mol. Aspects Cell Regul.* **3:**95–122.

Plucinski, T.M., and Baldwin, R.L., 1982, Effects of hormones on mammary adenosine 3′,5′-monophosphate levels and metabolism in normal and adrenalectomised lactating rats, *Endocrinology* **111:**2062–2065.

Randle, P.J., 1981, Phosphorylation–dephosphorylation cycles and the regulation of fuel selection in mammals, *Curr. Top. Cell Regul.* **18:**107–129.

Randle, P.J., Newsholme, E.A., and Garland, P.B., 1964, Regulation of glucose uptake by muscle. 8. Effects of fatty acids, ketone bodies and pyruvate, and of alloxan-diabetes and starvation, on the uptake and metabolic fate of glucose in rat heart and diaphragm muscles, *Biochem. J.* **93:**652–665.

Ranganathan, N.S., Linn, T.C., and Srere, P., 1982, Phosphorylation of dephospho-ATP–citrate lyase by the catalytic subunit of cAMP-dependent protein kinase, *J. Biol. Chem.* **257:**698–702.

Rao, G.A., and Abraham, S., 1975, Stimulatory effect of glucose upon triglyceride synthesis from acetate, decanoate, and palmitate by mammary gland slices from lactating mice, *Lipids* **10:**409–412.

Rider, M.H., Foret, D., and Hue, L., 1985, Comparison of purified bovine heart and rat liver 6-phosphofructo-2-kinase. Evidence for distinct isoenzymes, *Biochem. J.* **231:**193–196.

Robinson, A.M., and Williamson, D.H., 1977a, Comparison of glucose metabolism in the lactating mammary gland of the rat *in vivo* and *in vitro*. Effects of starvation, prolactin or insulin deficiency, *Biochem. J.* **164:**153–159.

Robinson, A.M., and Williamson, D.H., 1977b, Effects of acetoacetate administration on glucose metabolism in mammary gland of fed lactating rats, *Biochem. J.* **164:**749–752.

Robinson, A.M., and Williamson, D.H., 1977c, Control of glucose metabolism in isolated acini of the lactating mammary gland of the rat. The ability of glycerol to mimic some of the effects of insulin, *Biochem. J.* **168:**465–474.

Robinson, A.M., and Williamson, D.H., 1978a, Control of glucose metabolism in isolated acini of the lactating mammary gland of the rat. Effects of oleate on glucose utilisation and lipogenesis, *Biochem. J.* **170:**609–613.

Robinson, A.M., and Williamson, D.H., 1978b, Control of lactating rat mammary gland metabolism by insulin, *Biochem. Soc. Trans.* **6:**1316–1318.

Robinson, A.M., Girard, J.R., and Williamson, D.H., 1978, Evidence for a role of insulin in the regulation of lipogenesis in lactating rat mammary gland. Measurements of lipogenesis *in vivo* and plasma hormone concentrations in response to starvation and refeeding, *Biochem. J.* **176:**343–346.

Robson, N.A., Clegg, R.A., and Zammit, V.A., 1984, Regulation of peripheral lipogenesis by glucagon. Inability of the hormone to inhibit lipogenesis in rat mammary acini *in vitro* in the presence or absence of agents which alter its effects on adipocytes, *Biochem. J.* **217**:743–749.

Sakakibara, R., and Uyeda, K., 1983, Differences in the allosteric properties of pure low and high phosphate forms of phosphofructokinase from rat liver, *J. Biol. Chem.* **258**:8656–8662.

Sale, E.M., and Denton, R.M., 1985a, Adipose-tissue phosphofructokinase. Rapid purification and regulation by phosphorylation *in vitro, Biochem. J.* **232**:897–904.

Sale, E.M., and Denton, R.M., 1985b, β-Adrenergic agents increase the phosphorylation of phosphofructokinase in isolated rat epididymal white adipose tissue, *Biochem. J.* **232**:905–910.

Sale, G.J., and Randle, P.J., 1982a, Role of individual phosphorylation sites in inactivation of pyruvate dehydrogenase complex in rat heart mitochondria, *Biochem. J.* **203**:99–108.

Sale, G.J., and Randle, P.J., 1982b, Occupancy of phosphorylation sites in pyruvate dehydrogenase phosphate complex in rat heart *in vivo.* Relation to proportion of inactive complex and rate of reactivation by phosphatase, *Biochem. J.* **206**:221–229.

Saltiel, A.R., Doble, A., Jacobs, S., and Cuatrecasas, P., 1983, Putative mediators of insulin action regulate hepatic acetyl-CoA carboxylase activity, *Biochem. Biophys. Res. Commun.* **110**:789–795.

Sampson, D.A. and Jansen, G.R., 1985, The effect of dietary protein quality and feeding level on milk secretion and mammary protein synthesis in the rat, *J. Pediatr. Gastroenterol. Nutr.* **4**:274–283.

Sapag-Hagar, M., and Greenbaum, A.L., 1973, Changes of the activities of adenyl cyclase and cAMP-phosphodiesterase and of the level of 3′5′ cyclic adenosine monophosphate in rat mammary gland during pregnancy and lactation, *Biochem. Biophys. Res. Commun.* **53**:982–987.

Sapag-Hagar, M., and Greenbaum, A.L., 1974, Adenosine 3′ : 5′-monophosphate and hormone interrelationships in the mammary gland of the rat during pregnancy and lactation, *Eur. J. Biochem.* **47**:303–312.

Severson, D.L., Denton, R.M., Bridges, B.J., and Randle, P.J., 1976, Exchangeable and total calcium pools in mitochondria of rat epididymal fat pads and isolated fat cells. Role in the regulation of pyruvate dehydrogenase activity, *Biochem. J.* **154**:209–223.

Sica, V., and Cuatrecasas, P., 1973, Effects of insulin, epinephrine, and cyclic adenosine monophosphate on pyruvate dehydrogenase of adipose tissue, *Biochemistry* **12**:2282–2291.

Simpson, I.A., and Cushman, S.W., 1986, Hormonal regulation of mammalian glucose transport, *Ann. Rev. Biochem.* **55**:1059–1089.

Singh, M., Richards, E.G., Mukherjee, A., and Srere, P.A., 1976, Structure of ATP citrate lyase from rat liver. Physicochemical studies and proteolytic modification, *J. Biol. Chem.* **251**:5242–5250.

Smith, S.J., and Saggerson, E.D., 1978, Regulation of pyruvate dehydrogenase activity in rat epididymal fat-pads and isolated adipocytes by adrenaline, *Biochem. J.* **174**:119–130.

Smith, V., Kuroda, M., and Simpson, I.A., 1984, Counter-regulation of insulin-stimulated glucose transport by catecholamines in the isolated rat adipose cell, *J. Biol. Chem.* **259**:8758–8763.

Sochor, M., Greenbaum, A.L., and McLean, P., 1984, Fructose 2,6-bisphosphate, sugar phosphates and adenine nucleotides in the regulation of glucose metabolism in the lactating rat mammary gland, *FEBS Lett.* **169:**12–16.

Stansbie, D., Denton, R.M., Bridges, B.J., Pask, H.T., and Randle, P.J., 1976, Regulation of pyruvate dehydrogenase and pyruvate dehydrogenase phosphate phosphatase activity in rat epididymal fat-pads. Effects of starvation, alloxan-diabetes and high-fat diet, *Biochem. J.* **154:**225–236.

Sugden, P.H., and Randle, P.J., 1978, Regulation of pig heart pyruvate dehydrogenase by phosphorylation. Studies on the subunit and phosphorylation stoichiometries, *Biochem. J.* **173:**659–668.

Sugden, P.H., Hutson, N.J., Kerbey, A.L., and Randle, P.J., 1978, Phosphorylation of additional sites on pyruvate dehydrogenase inhibits its re-activation by pyruvate dehydrogenase phosphate phosphatase, *Biochem. J.* **169:**433–435.

Sugden, P.H., Kerbey, A.L., Randle, P.J., Waller, C.A., and Reid, B.M., 1979, Amino acid sequences around the sites of phosphorylation in the pig heart pyruvate dehydrogenase complex, *Biochem. J.* **181:**419–426.

Sun, J.V., Tepperman, H.M., and Tepperman, J., 1977, A comparison of insulin binding by liver plasma membranes of rats fed a high glucose diet or a high fat diet, *J. Lipid Res.* **18:**533–539.

Taylor, S.I., Mukherjee, C., and Jungas, R.L., 1973, Studies on the mechanism of activation of adipose tissue pyruvate dehydrogenase by insulin, *J. Biol. Chem.* **248:**73–81.

Taylor, W.M., and Halperin, M.L., 1979, Stimulation of glucose transport in rat adipocytes by insulin, adenosine, nicotinic acid and hydrogen peroxide. Role of adenosine 3′ : 5′-cyclic monophosphate, *Biochem. J.* **178:**381–389.

Teague, W.M., Pettit, F.H., Yeaman, S.J., and Reed, L.J., 1979, Function of phosphorylation sites on pyruvate dehydrogenase, *Biochem. Biophys. Res. Commun.* **87:**244–252.

Threadgold, L.C., Coore, H.G., and Kuhn, N.J., 1982, Monosaccharide transport into lactating-rat mammary acini, *Biochem. J.* **204:**493–501.

Threadgold, L.C., and Kuhn, N.J., 1984, Monosaccharide transport in the mammary gland of the intact lactating rat, *Biochem. J.* **218:**213–219.

Van de Werve, G., Proietto, J., and Jeanrenaud, B., 1985, Tumour-promoting phorbol esters increase basal and inhibit insulin-stimulated lipogenesis in rat adipocytes without decreasing insulin binding, *Biochem. J.* **225:**523–527.

Van Schaftingen, E., Davies, D.R., and Hers, H.-G., 1981, Inactivation of phosphofructokinase 2 by cyclic AMP-dependent protein kinase, *Biochem. Biophys. Res. Commun.* **103:**362–368.

Van Schaftingen, E., Davies, D.R., and Hers, H.-G., 1982, Fructose-2,6-bisphosphatase from rat liver, *Eur. J. Biochem.* **124:**143–149.

Van Schaftingen, E., and Hers, H.-G., 1986, Purification and properties of phosphofructokinase 2/fructose 2,6-bisphosphatase from chicken liver and from pigeon muscle, *Eur. J. Biochem.* **159:**359–365.

Vinten, J., Gliemann, J., and Osterlink, K., 1976, Exchange of 3-*O*-methyl glucose in isolated fat cells. Concentration dependence and effect of insulin, *J. Biol. Chem.* **251:**794–800.

Ward, S., and Kuhn, N.J., 1985, Role of fructose 2,6-bisphosphate in mammary gland of fed, starved and re-fed lactating rats, *Biochem. J.* **232:**931–934.

Weiss, L., Loffler, G., and Wieland, O.H., 1974, Regulation by insulin of adipose tissue pyruvate dehydrogenase. A mechanism controlling fatty acid synthesis from carbohydrates, *Hoppe-Seyler's Z. Physiol. Chem.* **355:**363–377.

Whitehouse, S., Cooper, R.H., and Randle, P.J., 1974, Mechanism of activation of pyruvate dehydrogenase by dichloroacetate and other halogenated carboxylic acids, *Biochem. J.* **141:**761–774.

Wilde, C.J., and Kuhn, N.J., 1979, Lactose synthesis in the rat, and the effects of litter size and malnutrition, *Biochem. J.* **182:**287–294.

Wilde, C.J., and Kuhn, N.J., 1981, Lactose synthesis and the utilisation of glucose by rat mammary acini, *Int. J. Biochem.* **13:**311–316.

Williamson, D.H., 1980, Integration of metabolism in tissues of the lactating rat, *FEBS Lett.* **117:**K93–K105.

Williamson, D.H., McKeown, S.R., and Ilic, V., 1975, Metabolic interactions of glucose, acetoacetate and insulin in mammary-gland slices of lactating rats, *Biochem. J.* **150:**145–152.

Williamson, D.H., Munday, M.R., Jones, R.G., Roberts, A.F.C., and Ramsey, A.J., 1983, Short-term dietary regulation of lipogenesis in the lactating mammary gland of the rat, *Adv. Enzyme Regul.* **21:**135–145.

Williamson, D.H., Munday, M.R., and Jones, R.G., 1984, Biochemical basis of dietary influences on the synthesis of the macronutrients of rat milk, *Fed. Proc.* **43:**2443–2447.

Williamson, D.H., Ilic, V., and Jones, R.G., 1985, Evidence that the stimulation of lipogenesis in the mammary glands of starved lactating rats re-fed with a chow diet is dependent on continued hepatic gluconeogenesis during the absorptive period, *Biochem. J.* **228:**727–733.

Witters, L.A., Tipper, J.P., and Bacon, G.W., 1983, Stimulation of site-specific phosphorylation of acetyl coenzyme A carboxylase by insulin and epinephrine, *J. Biol. Chem.* **258:**5643–5648.

Witters, L.A., Vater, C.A., and Lienhard, G.E., 1985, Phosphorylation of the glucose transporter *in vitro* and *in vivo* by protein kinase C, *Nature* **315:**777–778.

Yamanishi, K., Nishino, H., and Iwashima, A., 1983, Ca^{2+}-dependent stimulation of hexose transport by A23187, 12-*O*-tetradecanoylphorbol-13-acetate and epidermal growth factor in mouse fibroblasts, *Biochem. Biophys. Res. Commun.* **117:**637–642.

Yeaman, S.J., Hutcheson, E.T., Roche, T.E., Pettit, F.H., Brown, J.R., Reed, L.J., Watson, D.C., and Dixon, G.H., 1978, Sites of phosphorylation on pyruvate dehydrogenase from bovine kidney and heart, *Biochemistry* **17:**2364–2370.

Zammit, V.A., 1979, Effects of citrate on phosphofructokinase from lactating rat mammary gland acini, *FEBS Lett.* **108:**193–196.

Index